# Florence Nightingale on Health in India

Gérard Vallée, editor
Lynn McDonald, general editor

Volume 9
of the Collected Works of
Florence Nightingale

Wilfrid Laurier University Press
www.wlupress.wlu.ca

We acknowledge the financial support of the Government of Canada through the Book Publishing Industry Development Program for our publishing activities.

**Library and Archives Canada Cataloguing in Publication**

Nightingale, Florence, 1820–1910.
Florence Nightingale on health in India / Gérard Vallée and Lynn McDonald, editors.

(Collected works of Florence Nightingale ; v. 9)
Includes bibliographical references and index.
ISBN-13: 978-0-88920-468-3
ISBN-10: 0-88920-468-3

1. Medical care — India — History — 19th century. 2. Public health — India — History — 19th century. 3. Great Britain — Armed forces — India — Medical care — History — 19th century. 4. Royal Commission on the Sanitary State of the Army in India — History. 5. Nightingale, Florence, 1820–1910. I. Vallée, Gérard, 1933– II. McDonald, Lynn, 1940– III. Title. IV. Series.

RA529.N44 2006 362.1′095409034 C2006-905313-8



Cover design by Leslie Macredie. Front cover image: Santal village near Santiniketan, Bengal, 1968. Photograph: Carolyn Kinsley. Front flap: Bronze bust of Nightingale by Sir John Steel. Photograph courtesy of the Victoria Memorial Hall, Calcutta. Back cover image: Water wheel near Udaipur, Rajasthan, 2005. Photograph: Ann Rempel.

∞

Printed in Canada



Wilfrid Laurier University Press
Waterloo, Ontario, Canada N2L 3C5
E-mail: press@wlu.ca
Web: www.wlupress.wlu.ca

*Collected Works of Florence Nightingale* website:
www.sociology.uoguelph.ca/fnightingale

# CONTENTS

# ACKNOWLEDGMENTS

Acknowledgments are due to a large number of individuals and organizations for assistance on this volume, and even more for assistance at earlier stages in the *Collected Works* project. First of all acknowledgments are due to the Henry Bonham Carter Will Trust for permission to publish Nightingale original manuscripts, and indeed for treating Nightingale material generally as being in the public domain. To the owners of Nightingale manuscripts thanks are due for their important role in conservation, for permitting scholarly access and for permitting copies to be made for this *Collected Works*.

Archivists and librarians around the world provided skilled assistance, often beyond the call of duty. Many people worked on the preparation of the texts, many as volunteers. Thanks are due to transcribers: Gwyneth Watkins, Kelly Thomas, Leo Uotila and Victoria Rea; volunteer verifiers of texts: Cherry Ambrose, Linda Elliot, Joyce Donaldson, Jean Harding, Mary Parfitt and Marcia Macrae; to volunteers who assisted with proofreading: Sandra Hunter and Cherry Ambrose; for research assistance on the history of India: Dr Nancy Cassels; for advice on British India: Dr Richard Rempel; and for reading a section of the manuscript: Dr Charles Roland.

Sue Goldie's Calendar of Letters was used in the search for sources, in the electronic version made available through the Florence Nightingale Museum by Hugh Small and Alex Attewell.

At the Press thanks are due to Dr Brian Henderson, director; Carroll Klein, managing editor; Doreen Armbruster, typesetter; Leslie Macreadie and Penelope Grows, marketing; Steve Izma, production; and Jacqueline Larson, peer review. Thanks are due to the anonymous peer reviewers for helpful comments. The copy editing was done by Kristen Pederson Chu. Acknowledgments for photographs and other illustrations are given where they appear.

Thanks to the Library of Parliament (of Canada) for assistance with British Parliamentary Papers.

In spite of the assistance of so many people undoubtedly errors remain, which are the responsibility of the editors. We would be grateful for notification of any errors, and for information on missing identifications. Corrections will be made in the electronic text and any later print publication.

We note that this volume goes to press at the 150th anniversary of the launching of Nightingale's career as a social reformer. That is, she returned to England from the Crimean War in August 1856, and began her work for social and health care reform in September 1856, at Balmoral Castle, the guest of Queen Victoria, lobbying the war minister for a royal commission on sanitary reform.

Gérard Vallée and
Lynn McDonald
*August 2006*

# Dramatis Personae

Parthenope Nightingale, Lady Verney (**1819-90**), sister
(Sir) Harry Verney (**1801-94**), brother-in-law
Samuel Smith (**1794-1880**), "Uncle Sam"
Hilary Bonham Carter (**1821-65**), cousin
Henry Bonham Carter (**1827-1921**), cousin, secretary of the Nightingale Fund
Captain (Sir) Douglas Galton (**1822-99**), husband of cousin
Mary Clarke Mohl (**1793-1883**), "Mme Mohl," friend
Julius Mohl (**1800-76**), Orientalist, friend

(Sir) Edwin Chadwick (**1800-90**), sanitary expert
Lord Cranborne (**1830-1903**), marquess of Salisbury, secretary of state for India
Dr James M. Cuningham (**1829-1905**), sanitary commissioner
Dr William Farr (**1807-83**), medical statistician
(Sir) Bartle Frere (**1815-84**), governor of Bombay
Lord de Grey (marquess of Ripon) (**1827-1909**), viceroy, friend
Dr Thomas Gillham Hewlett (**1832-89**), sanitary commissioner for Bombay
(Sir) John Lawrence (**1811-79**), later Lord, viceroy, friend
(Sir) Louis Mallet (**1823-90**), permanent under secretary of state for India **1874-83**
(Sir) James Ranald Martin (**1793-1874**), Army Sanitary Commission
(Sir) John McNeill (**1795-1883**), surgeon, friend and ally
(Sir) Robert Rawlinson (**1810-98**), civil engineer
Lord Stanley (15th earl of Derby) (**1826-93**), chair of second royal commission
(Sir) John Strachey (**1823-1907**), Bengal Sanitary Commission
Dr John Sutherland (**1808-91**), surgeon and sanitarian, close collaborator
(Sir) Charles Edward Trevelyan (**1807-86**), governor of Madras, friend
Dr James Pattison Walker (**1823-1906**), Bengal Sanitary Commission
(Sir) Charles Wood (Lord Halifax) (**1800-85**), secretary of state for India

# List of Illustrations

# FLORENCE NIGHTINGALE: A PRÉCIS OF HER LIFE

Florence Nightingale was born in Florence, Italy, 1820, the second daughter of wealthy English parents taking an extended European wedding trip. She was raised in England at country homes, Lea Hurst, in Derbyshire, and Embley, in Hampshire. She was educated largely by her father, who had studied classics at Trinity College, Cambridge. At age sixteen Nightingale experienced a "call to service," but her family would not permit her to act on it by becoming a nurse, then a lower-class occupation and thoroughly unthinkable for a "lady." Lengthy trips to Rome and Egypt were allowed (1847-48 and 1849-50 respectively). She had earlier (1837-39) been taken on a long trip with her family, mainly to Italy and France. These European trips not only improved her language skills (she was fluent in modern French, German and Italian as well as competent in ancient Latin and Greek) but exposed her to republican politics and Italian independence (she was in Rome and France during the revolts of 1848).

Nightingale was finally permitted to spend three months at the (Protestant) Deaconess Institution in Kaiserswerth, near Düsseldorf, Germany, in 1851 and several weeks with Roman Catholic nursing orders in Paris in 1853. Her father gave her an annuity in 1853 to permit her to become the superintendent of the Establishment for Gentlewomen during Illness, Upper Harley Street, London. She left there in 1854 to lead the first team of British women nurses sent to war. The British Army was poorly prepared for that war and the death rate from preventible disease was seven times that from wounds. The Barrack Hospital at Scutari where she was stationed was structurally unfit to be a hospital, had defective drains and had to be re-engineered by a team of visiting experts before the death rate could be brought down.

Nightingale's work as a social and public health reformer effectively began on her return from the Crimean War in 1856. Recognized as a national heroine, she chose to work behind the scenes for structural changes to prevent that war's high death rates from ever recurring. She began by lobbying to get a royal commission established to investigate the causes of the medical disaster and recommend changes. She herself briefed witnesses, analyzed data and strongly influenced the thrust of the report, despite falling ill even before it was finished. It is thought that Nightingale suffered from the chronic form of brucellosis, after nearly dying from the disease during the war. She spent most of the rest of her life as an invalid, seeing people on a one-to-one basis and continuing to exert influence through her research and writing. The illness was certainly painful and incapacitating, but Nightingale learned how to work around it, focusing her hours of working time on the most important projects, those that had the best prospect of saving lives.

Nightingale was baptized in the Church of England and remained in it for the rest of her life, although often despairing of its paltry role for women, the minimal demands it made of its adherents generally and its social conservatism. Her experience of religious conversion in 1836 and call to service in 1837 (the latter specifically dated 7 February, and frequently referred to) were both shaped by reading the work of an American Congregational minister, Jacob Abbott, notably *The Corner-stone.* Her faith was nourished by broad reading, from the medieval mystics, liberal theologians and the German historical school to sermons, devotional books, tracts and religious novels. The family had been largely Unitarian in earlier generations, but a grandmother was evangelical Church of England. There is a strong Wesleyan element in Nightingale's faith, from dissenting chapels in Derbyshire, and Lutheran influences from Kaiserswerth.

God for Nightingale was a perfect Creator who made and runs the world by *laws,* which human beings can ascertain by rigorous, preferably statistical, study. With the knowledge thus gained we can then intervene for good, thus becoming God's "co-workers." Ongoing research is required, for human interventions, however well intentioned, may have negative, unintended consequences. This approach appears in all the work Nightingale did, whether in health care or social reform more broadly.

To guide her in doing the research necessary to discover "God's laws," Nightingale developed an effective methodological approach. Her sources were statistician L.A.J. Quetelet on the conduct of research and J.S. Mill on the philosophical grounding. *Society and Politics* shows what Nightingale learned from these two persons and how she further developed their ideas. The successful use of this methodology is evident in *Public Health Care,* as it is here and in later volumes.

Nightingale's ardent and consistent liberal politics are another theme informing her social reform work. Her family (and the Verney family, into which her sister married) were strong Liberal supporters. Her brother-in-law was a Liberal MP, as were cousins and family friends. She herself gave money to the Liberal Party and even wrote campaign letters for a small number of Liberal candidates. At a time of considerable political flux Nightingale's politics were consistent: she was a thorough "small l" liberal in her ideas, a supporter of freedom of inquiry and expression and an advocate of religious toleration. The Liberal Party seemed to be the best political manifestation of these goals. Again, as with the Church of England, the Liberal Party often failed to live up to its principles—she desperately wanted Liberal governments to be liberal on India as well as Ireland.

For most of her long working life Nightingale was confined to her room, describing herself variously as "a prisoner to my room" or even "a prisoner to my bed." Some days she could not see anybody but usually she had interviews, sometimes several and sometimes lengthy ones, with nursing leaders, medical experts, politicians and Indian officials. Many people who requested interviews with her over their various concerns were turned down. Time with family and friends took second place, fitted around this "business," God's business, "my Father's business," in her understanding. People who did not get interviews, however, normally got letters in reply, often long and careful explanations, and offers of assistance.

Nightingale's own network of colleagues and advisors was impressive and she continued to add to it as newer, younger experts, MPs and officials came into office. She always worked collectively, seeking advice and getting her own questionnaires, draft articles and reports vetted by knowledgeable people. When she herself could not aid someone's cause, she suggested someone who could.

Nightingale continued to produce papers and reports of various kinds well into her seventies. She did not do any serious writing in her eighties, when blindness and failing mental faculties gradually stopped her. There are brief messages only from 1902 on. She was given honours in her last years (the Order of Merit in 1907) and enjoyed the company of younger relatives and several close nursing friends. She died at ninety and was buried in the churchyard of St Margaret's, Wellow, the family's parish church. Consistent with her wishes, the family declined an offer of burial at Westminster Abbey.

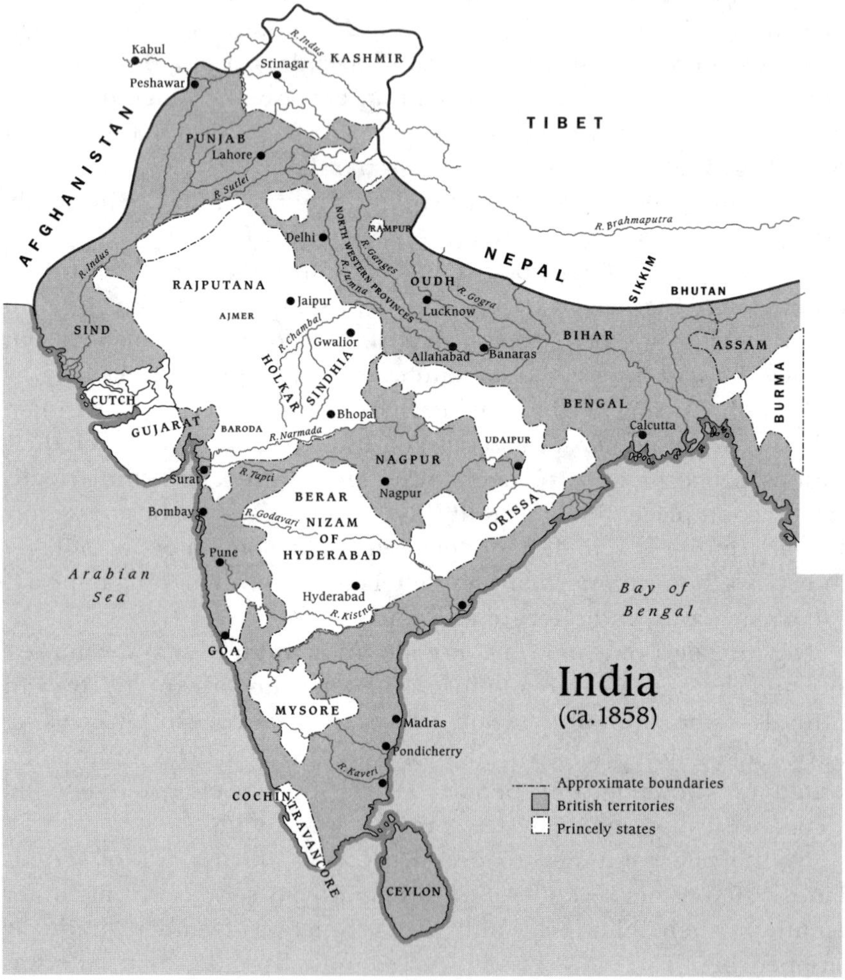


Produced by Wilfrid Laurier University Press.

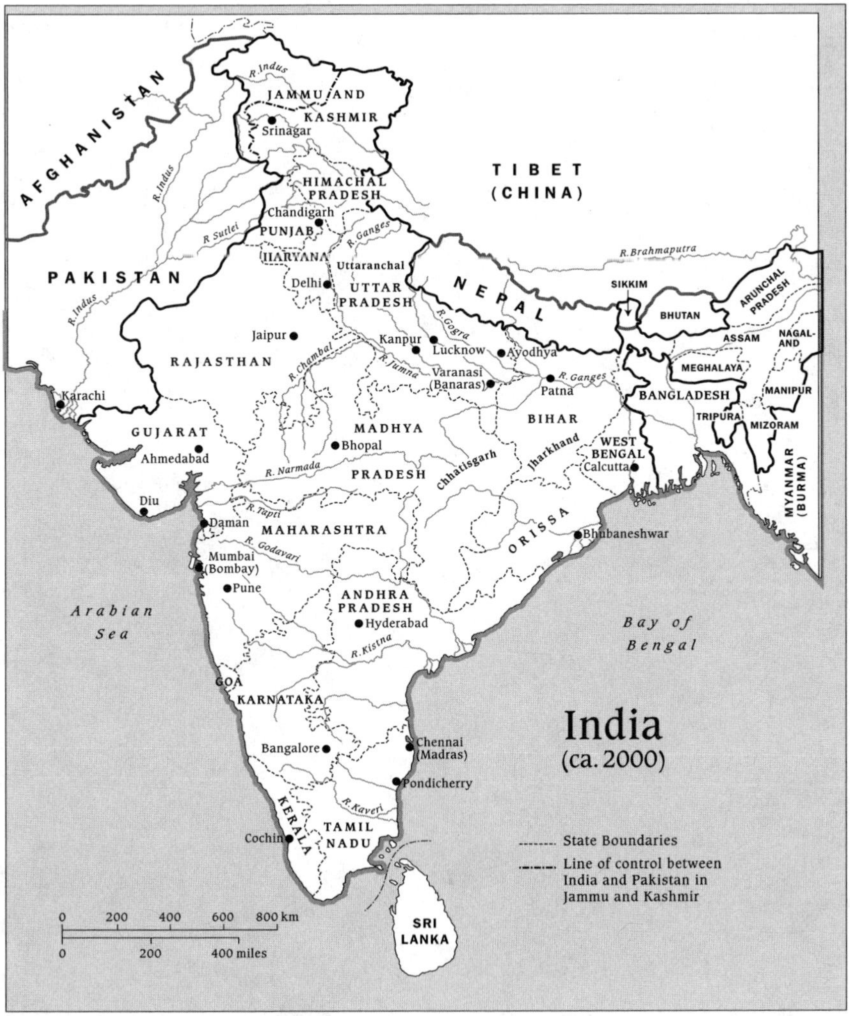


Produced by Wilfrid Laurier University Press.

# Nightingale's Work on India

Florence Nightingale devoted some forty years of her life to bringing about a number of reforms to improve public health and the condition of life of the people of India. Initially her focus was on British soldiers serving there, but increasingly she worked at promoting the health and well-being of Indian nationals. Nightingale turned to Indian concerns soon after her return from the Crimean War in August 1856 as the Mutiny of 1857-58 broke out. Her interest quickly shifted to basic, long-term measures in order to deal with the underlying problems. Preventible mortality from poor sanitary conditions and famine became major preoccupations in her work from the early 1860s to the end of her life.

Nightingale's India work can be seen as a major response to her "call to service" of 1837, a mission she interpreted as being to save lives. Where better could a social reformer save lives than in India, Britain's greatest possession? The chance of making a difference, of actually saving lives, was probably greatest there. China, of course, then had, as it still does, a larger population, but India was the place where a British person could more readily have an impact. The fact that direct British administration of India began in 1858 made it an even better opportunity and further justified Nightingale's involvement.

The purpose of this general introduction is to present background information necessary to understand the place and meaning of the material, published and unpublished, found in volumes 9 and 10 of the *Collected Works*. Here we briefly give the context of Nightingale's India work: historical, political, social and scientific, both in India and in England.

## The British Presence in India

It is not possible, nor would it be desirable here, to give a detailed description of the complex period of British rule in India. Excellent recent studies of the penetration and conquest of India can be consulted and we refer the reader to them.[1] The following remarks should suffice to map out the context of Nightingale's involvement.

Because of the tremendous market opportunities that India's riches offered to European powers eager to expand their reach over all continents, it was to be expected that India would become a major object of colonial ambitions. This was generally done under the cover of bringing and spreading "civilization" to more or less hapless populations. The imperial assumption was that India itself did not know the blessings of civilization enjoyed in Europe. It could be helped out of its unfortunate stagnation, in that period of decline of the Mughal Empire, by a dynamic injection of Western techniques and practices. Moreover, imperial ambition was coupled, after 1800, with churches' efforts to spread "true religion" to peoples considered prisoners of superstition, and to remodel them according to European notions. Merchants and missionaries typically shared a feeling of superiority when meeting non-European populations.

Early in the seventeenth century the British presence in India was essentially limited to the activities of the East India Company, itself in competition with Portugese, Dutch and French merchants for the conquest of the Indian market. The Company, through its Court of Directors, primarily fostered its own commercial interests, at least initially. But it was gradually given "rights" that made it into a state unto itself. Local Mughal princes were more and more inclined to seek the protection of the Company, and to that end granted it land and rights. Thus Robert Clive,[2] governor of Bengal in the mid-eighteenth century, became a man of formidable power by exploiting Indian fears and divisions, installing puppet rulers and looting the country. His victory at Plassey (1757) sealed the position of the Company and put the British on the road to territorial power in India. Now much

1 For example, Christopher Alan Bayly, *Indian Society and the Making of the British Empire*; Sarvepalli Gopal, *British Policy in India 1858-1905*; Lawrence James, *Raj: The Making and Unmaking of British India*; Thomas R. Metcalf, *Ideologies of the Raj*; and Sara Suleri, *The Rhetoric of English India.*

2 Robert Clive (1725-74), governor of Bengal 1755-60 and 1764-67.

more than a mere commercial body, the Company was able to direct military operations and to supervise the administration of provinces (it became *diwan* or finance manager for Bengal, Bihar and Orissa in 1765, with the licence to trade without charge). It acquired a monopoly over the collection, sale and importation of goods with power to levy taxes. As governor general of Bengal (and also of Bombay and Madras) from 1773 to 1785, Warren Hastings increased British penetration to such an extent that Parliament unsuccessfully tried to have him impeached for his scandalous exploitation of the colony. Even so, he ranked among the governors most attuned to Indian culture.

The British Parliament passed the India Act in 1784 to temper the Company's vast ambitions. Through this legislation power eventually passed from the Company's Court of Directors to the Crown's Board of Control, which included members of the British Cabinet. Lord Cornwallis's Permanent Settlement of 1793 aimed at limiting the rights of zemindars or landlords who collected taxes from the peasants, while insisting on their duties to improve the life of peasants and the productivity of the land. In reality, however, it had but few practical consequences; zemindars remained favoured by the colonial establishment and their behaviour selfishly condoned by British officials. Until 1856, governors general and high officials were seen as "high-principled aristocrats from Britain's political elite . . . on loan to India"; they saw themselves "not as India's conquerors but as its emancipators."[3] But few of those gentlemen were lofty altruists. At the beginning of the nineteenth century the governor general, Richard Wellesley, himself felt no inhibition at all in declaring that "officials should be allowed 'the means of acquiring a competent fortune' with which they could return home" (152). Indeed, many of these aristocrats viewed their stay in India merely as a springboard for a brilliant career. It then comes as no surprise that they were more interested in their own status and riches than in the well-being of Indians. Greed, social arrogance (toward those they sometimes called "niggers"), racial contempt and blindness toward Indian culture (especially its philosophy and religion): these attitudes planted the seeds of future discontent and rebellion.

3 Lawrence James, *Raj* 151.

## The Mutiny of 1857-58 and Its Aftermath

The rebellion came in the form of the Mutiny of 1857-58. Numerous grievances brought about this pivotal event in the history of the British in India: resentment of princes, Indian frustration at being kept away from the consultative process, the unpopular annexation of Oudh, demobilization of the army and overtaxing of the peasants, as well as the fear of Christianity being forced upon Hindus and Muslims, especially among the Bengali sepoys (soldiers). Rebellion in the army led to a violent confrontation between the occupying force and various groups of Indians, in the course of which atrocities were perpetrated on both sides. Both sides had grown ill-disposed toward each other; as Colonel Chardin Johnson said: "We despise niggers, they hate us."[4] Not exactly a proto-war of national independence, the Mutiny is understood today rather as an exercise in settling scores; Indians rebelled against British arrogance and encroachments, wishing to take their piece of the profits flowing into British pockets and to return to the Mughal situation antedating the British conquest. The London press saw it differently, broadcasting pointed disinformation: it reported unilaterally on the slaughter of Europeans and remained largely silent on the racial ferocity with which the British punished the rebels. C.A. Bayly comments:

> The most dramatic and immediate consequences of the revolt were felt, of course, by the sepoy army itself and its rural allies. No quarter was given by the British, enraged at the atrocities committed against their women and children. Tens of thousands of soldiers and village guerrillas were hanged, shot or blown from guns. . . . The Indian sepoy was at no time to outnumber European troops in the subcontinent by more than two to one and Europeans were placed in charge of artillery in well-fortified and segregated army cantonments.[5]

It cannot be denied that the conquerors did suffer, although it became clear that health conditions killed more British than the war itself: trauma and infection, ill-adapted clothing, heat, flies, fever and thirst.

The Mutiny was a decisive incentive for Nightingale, whose interest in India was already manifest in 1856, to study and reform the Indian Army. In fact, the sepoys had voiced grievances that were shared by

4 Lawrence James, *Raj* 267.

5 Christopher Alan Bayly, *Indian Society* 194-95.

the population at large. Thus the uprising they started soon became a national battle that uncovered the need for essential changes in the ways things were done in India. Once the Mutiny had been brought under control, important adjustments had to be made in the administration of India.

The events surrounding the Mutiny, as Nightingale said in 1857, "have led to a universal conviction that this vast empire must henceforth be held by British troops," and by healthy British troops. The British Army was exposed to health hazards peculiar to the Indian climate. "The British race," she continued, "has carried with it into those regions of the sun its habits, its customs and its vices, without considering that under a low temperature man may do with impunity what under a higher one is death." Special care had to be taken of the soldiers' lives under these new conditions. "The observance of sanitary laws should be as much part of the future *régime* of India as the holding of military positions or as civil government itself. It would be a noble beginning of the new order of things to use hygiene as the handmaid of civilization" (see p 46 below). Thus in 1857 Nightingale was able to anticipate and grasp the work to be done in India, and she committed herself to see to it that it be done. A letter to Sir John McNeill shows her looking at the Mutiny as instigating a "beginning of things," as had the French Revolution: "so this affair in India must end in the entire doing away of the caste system or in the overthrow of the British power there" (see p 49 below).

## British India 1858-1900

The Mutiny marked the end of the "Company raj" and the beginning of the "British raj," leaving "a deep and abiding mark both on the fabric of Indian society and on the nature of British rule."[6] When the India Act was adopted by Parliament in 1858, the Company's rule was terminated and the crown took over with two instances of executive power: the secretary of state for India (with his Council of India) and the viceroy (governor general in Calcutta seconded by a kind of Cabinet that eventually included Indians). Greater sensitivity was thereafter shown to the interests and feelings of Indians.

After 1858 measures to reform the army, which the Mutiny had demonstrated to be essential, were introduced. In the three presiden-

6 Thomas R. Metcalf, *The Aftermath of Revolt* vii.

cies (Bengal, Bombay and Madras) the army was reorganized as a well-co-ordinated machine with fewer Indian and more British soldiers; by 1866 Indian soldiers had declined from 256,000 to 122,000, while British soldiers had increased from 45,000 to 61,000.[7] Concerns about the army as both an effective and humane organization moved to the forefront. It is in these circumstances that the fate of all soldiers, British and Indian, became Nightingale's "business."

British India, as Nightingale knew it, was a huge country with a baffling mixture of races, religions, languages, occupations and climates. It had, however, frontiers different from those of present-day India, as the map shows. We get an idea of the size of the country she was interested in by looking at the following sample: Without the "princely states" but including Mysore, the total population in 1872 was given as 238,830,958 (Nightingale used only approximate figures at different times). The *Memorandum on the Census of the British India 1871-72,* the first general census to be carried out, detailed the populations of some states as follows:

| | |
|---|---|
| Bengal | 62,680,633 |
| Madras presidency | 33,308,225 |
| Bombay presidency | 25,647,818 |
| Hyderabad | 10,666,080 |
| N.W. Provinces | 31,688,217 |
| Oudh | 11,220,232 |
| Punjab | 22,910,946 |
| Rajputana | 9,981,588 |
| Central Provinces | 9,251,229 |
| British Burma | 2,747,148 |
| Mysore | 5,055,412 |

Calcutta, the capital of British India, situated on the banks of the Hugli River, had a population of 892,429 in 1872. It comes as no surprise that we often read, in the documents of the period, worries about how to "hold" such a massive country with a few thousand officials and soldiers.

At the time of the 1872 census, one quarter of British India was Muslim. That huge population was dispersed in cities, towns and villages. Cities had experienced the beginnings of "modernization" (some "civil lines" had gas lights, tarmac roads, industries) and were

7 Robin James Moore, *Sir Charles Wood's Indian Policy 1853-1866* 215.

places of a nascent middle class. Technological innovations such as canals for irrigation and transport, railways, telegraph, postal service and steam transport were introduced into India within years of their appearing in Europe, marking the beginnings of a sound infrastructure. But towns and villages were often poor and delivered to the hands of ravenous local landlords. The "second royal commission" doubtless overshot the evidence when its report described India as a vast reservoir of filth and dirt, and some of the material collected below espoused the same exaggeration. Not everything was ugly in India, and Nightingale found much to praise in its village life and social institutions. But the need for basic improvements in living was glaring.

## Nightingale's Interest in India

Nightingale's involvement with Indian matters began in the first years of her public career. Once initiated, it remained one of her major concerns and fields of action. There is no period of her active life when her energies and initiatives were not deployed on behalf of India, its soldiers and its people. The last years of her life saw her still practically interested in India, so that it can be said that her interest in India and her "India work" never abated.

Nightingale's concerns for India go back to 1856, to the months following her return from the Crimean War, and intensified during the "Royal Commission on the Sanitary State of the Army in India" (1859-63) and its sequels, of which more will be said soon. In 1879 she could in fact say: "My interest in India can never abate."[8] In 1889 she wrote a retrospect of her continuous Indian work, and as late as 1898 she was welcoming the Aga Khan to discuss the Indian situation. Her interest in India, it will be shown in these volumes, covered a vast range of issues, from sanitation and public health to education, social reform, political development, philosophical and religious questions. She kept abreast of events and personalities, and volunteered concrete suggestions for the improvement of life in India. When her life story is considered as a whole and with the benefit of hindsight, Nightingale's commitment to India can be seen as a major realization

8 Letter to Priyaranjan K. Sen 13 October 1879, in Priyaranjan Sen, ed., *Florence Nightingale's Indian Letters: A Glimpse into the Agitation for Tenancy Reform, Bengal 1878-82* 20.

of the "call to service" she had heard in her early years and eagerly tried to interpret. "'Lord, here I am, send me' has always been religion to me. I must be willing to go now as I was to go to the East," she wrote to Sidney Herbert.[9] She believed that the India work was an instance of being God's co-worker. "How to create a Public Health Department for India, how to bring a higher civilization into India. What a work, what a noble task for a government—no 'inglorious period of our dominion' [quoting Edmund Burke] that, but a most glorious one! That would be creating India anew. For God places His own power, His own life-giving laws in the hands of man. He permits man to create mankind by those laws, even as He permits man to destroy mankind by neglect of those laws" (see p 193 below).

Was Nightingale's keen interest in India matched by an adequate knowledge of the real situation of the country? Here we must largely rely on inferences. She was reading seriously on India by December 1857 (see p 50 below) and beginning to work through such issues as mortality and climate. She never went to India, and thus the kind of knowledge gathered through immediate contact with the land cannot be expected. She worked from her home, often as "a prisoner to my bed" (see p 562 below). However, her authorized biographer[10] expresses respect for the quality of her information based on reading, personal contact, the work of the royal commission on India and an abundant exchange of letters and notes. She kept reading reports and minutes of Indian committees and was in correspondence with the most knowledgeable persons involved in the country's administration. Questions of public health, sanitation and, of course, nursing were familiar to her.

Nightingale's desire to see India with her own eyes could not be realized, and she lamented the fact. She would have loved to go to India herself (see p 47 below), as she declared to Lady Canning, wife of Lord "Clemency" Canning, the first viceroy.[11] Lady Canning wrote

---

9 Letter 26 November 1857, ADD MSS 43394 f190, quotation from Isa 6:8.

10 E.T. Cook, *The Life of Florence Nightingale* 2:25, 27, 273-75.

11 Earl Charles John Canning (1812-62), governor general of India during the Mutiny and first viceroy of India 1856-62, favoured reconciliation, hence "Clemency Canning," but brought in land revenue settlement in Oudh unduly favourable to landlords. He resigned in 1862.

to her own mother: "Miss Nightingale has written to me; she is out of health and at Malvern, but says she would come at twenty-four hours' notice if I think there is anything for her to do in her 'line of business.' "[12] Cook adds that Nightingale had already twice made the offer to go to India at the time of the Mutiny: "She thought of herself as a soldier in the ranks; and absorbed intently though she was in her work for the army at home, she would have considered active service in the field a superior call" (1:371). In 1857 Nightingale asked her friend John McNeill for guidance: "We may have to reconquer India. I should like much to go out; we shall have dreadful sickness there, but I have no one to advise me. I want to see you about this" (see p 49 below). She repeated her wish to go out to India to Sidney Herbert (see p 507 below). In the following years she often expressed her desire to go to India, as she wrote to various correspondents: "I asked him [Dr Walker] whether I should ever be able to go to India. He said, had you not better first be able to walk?"[13] "While others try to run away from India, I would desire more than anything else which I do desire ... to go to India. I have studied the country so much, I seem to know so well what I want to do there, that it appears to me as if I would be going home, not going to a strange country. But alas for me, it is quite impossible. I shall never leave London, except for the grave" (see p 507 below). "I wish I could go out to India. . . . " (see p 121 below) "Oh that I could come to Calcutta and organize at least the hospital accommodation for the poor wretches in the streets. There is nothing I should like as much. But it is nonsense to wish for what is an impossibility" (see p 212 below). As late as 1888 she still claimed: "I wish I were going too."[14] That wish was, of course, not to be fulfilled.

Nightingale knew the social conditions of India very well, certainly better than she knew its intellectual traditions. Her knowledge of India and her desire to see it were combined with a real sense of respect for the country and its population. She never expressed anything that would approach the lofty, indeed bizarre and arrogant view found in James Mill's *History of British India*, that "whatever is worth seeing or hearing in India can be expressed in writing. As soon as everything of importance is expressed in writing, a man who is duly

12 Letter of 14 November 1857, in Cook, *The Life of Florence Nightingale* 1:371.
13 Letter to W.E. Nightingale 4 April 1861, in *Life and Family* (1:246).
14 Letter to Henry Bonham Carter 19 October 1888, Add Mss 47721 f141.

qualified may obtain more knowledge of India in one year in his closet in England than he could during the longest life by the use of his eyes and ears in India."[15]

Nightingale's dealings with Indian matters unveil precious information on various topics, deepening our received history of the British raj and uncovering aspects of the raj that are less known. Given the time period to which her activities belonged, it can be expected that the "benefits" of empire would occupy the fore. For instance, Nightingale unquestionably believed that Britain was bringing "civilization" to the subcontinent, and she had virtually no doubt as to the rightness of the "ideologies of the raj"[16] and the legitimacy of British rule in India. At least in the early stages of her India work she did not escape a form of colonial paternalism, sharing the imperialists' view of their role as benefactors and educators of Indians. In the words of T.R. Metcalf, she could "represent an aggressive English imperialism in the guise of a mother's curative care for the 'sick child' that was India" (109). Civilization and science were thought to benefit Indians and in that sense Nightingale was fundamentally optimistic, sharing the Enlightenment view that science could help solve most practical problems. In particular she rejected the common opinion that "disease and death must be the penalty for subduing the earth" (see p 59 below). Yet, over against a strong stream of British opinion, she came to believe that the function of colonialists was to prepare Indians for self-government, and agreed with the efforts of such people as Thomas Munro, Mountstuart Elphinstone and Lord Ripon in that regard.

Early on, Nightingale was critical of the practice of empire, increasingly so over the years. She found great shortcomings in British agrarian, judicial, educational and administrative policies. She resented the administrators' resistance to change and slow pace of action when the necessity of introducing measures had become evident. She could be caustic when denouncing the complacency of officials, the self-interest, the merciless exploitation and even brutality of some agents of London in the name of civilization. She was tacitly aware that commercial attachés, planters and traders were in the process of destroying local industries and impoverishing populations, and that colonial agents denied those populations markets for their produce and flooded them with their own surpluses.

15 James Mill, *History of British India*, 5th ed., Preface of the Author.
16 See Thomas R. Metcalf, *Ideologies of the Raj*.

She was often frustrated by the discontinuity created by numerous changes in the home government: she repeatedly had to adjust to a new minister and staff, and to confusing political arrangements. In particular, she regularly complained about the removal of the incumbent secretaries of state for war and for India "every four months," mainly due to recurrent changes of government, and about seeing a "minister taken away just as he is carrying measures you have been hatching for years."[17] That play at musical chairs irritated her. However, there was an important exception to that state of affairs in the case of viceroys/governors general: they remained in office to the end of their appointed term in spite of any change in government. The new government naturally appointed a member or sympathizer of its own party at the next occasion. Lord Ripon's decision in 1884 to leave office early to ensure that a sympathetic successor was appointed, i.e., a Liberal, was high-minded and effective: Lord Dufferin, another Liberal, became the next governor general. Secretaries of state, of course, as members of Cabinet, were out as soon as a new party came into power.

### Nightingale's Health Care Background

Nightingale's early agenda for India was shaped by her experiences in hospital work in London, nursing during the Crimean War and, thereafter, her part in reforming the army. Those three topics are the material of other volumes in this series, but they must be addressed briefly here in order to highlight the abilities she brought to her India work.

Informal work in the care of the sick and hands-on training periods in Germany and France preceded Nightingale's appointment as superintendent of the Harley Street "Establishment for Gentlewomen during Illness" in 1853. Her management of the institution received praise and caused other hospitals to seek her services in the training of nurses. But history was to take her elsewhere.

In October 1854 the *Times* reported on the nursing deficiencies manifested in the course of the Crimean War (1854-56). Nightingale immediately volunteered to lead a group of nurses to Scutari at the very same time that Sidney Herbert, then secretary at war, fortuitously asked her to do precisely that. Thus she spent twenty-one months of active service in the East, in the course of which she had to deal with

17 *Women* (8:905).

all sorts of problems: care of the wounded and convalescents, hospital organization, diet of the sick, shortcomings of the army structures—all aspects that kept her busy in the field and upon her return to England.

Back in London she met with Sidney Herbert and decided to devote her energies and efforts to the reform of the army, with special attention to the health of the soldiers. The Crimean War had exposed blatant deficiencies in the operations of the British Army that had to be attended to. Nightingale had personally witnessed disturbing problems in her own domain, notably in an inadequate treatment of the sick and wounded, a shaky chain of command and the deplorable state of barracks and hospitals. In the aftermath of the war frenetic calls for reform were voiced; they were accentuated by the inaction of departments and ministers. But Sidney Herbert was determined to tackle the reforms and his daily co-operation with Nightingale on these initiatives was to be remembered with affection until her own death. Thanks to this commission's work and her previous activities, she accumulated an extremely rich experience that prepared her well for her India work.

## Nightingale's "First Royal Commission"

Herbert's and Nightingale's collaborative reform work on behalf of the British Army effectively commenced in 1856. With patient energy they pressed for a thorough inquiry into the army's health conditions. Nightingale used her reputation acquired in the course of the war to push for changes. Herbert used his own contacts among politicians. Their joint efforts resulted in the summoning of the "Royal Commission appointed to Inquire into Regulations affecting the Sanitary Condition of the Army, the Organization of Military Hospitals, and the Treatment of the Sick and Wounded" (1857-58), which is typically called Nightingale's "first royal commission." The commission was concerned with the home army in the aftermath of the Crimean debacle. Nightingale gave written evidence to the commission, investigated barracks and hospitals, wrote substantial essays on the health of the army, female nursing and hospitals, and took considerable part in the writing of the report of the commission.

By that time the general mode of operation of a royal commission had become customary. Appointed by the crown for the purpose of investigating particular matters and recommending measures to improve a given situation, it originated from the relevant offices of the executive government. The objects of inquiry were carefully defined in the warrant constituting the commission. The choice of members to sit on the commission was crucial. The commission held its sittings in any part of the United Kingdom, but normally in London; it took evidence from experienced experts and, as in the case of the royal commission on India, could receive information from abroad. At the conclusion of the inquiry all of the information was sifted and a report, including recommendations, was presented to the crown and Parliament through the concerned departments, which were to see to its implementation. The royal commission constituted a main engine of governmental and administrative reforms.

Sidney Herbert chaired the "first royal commission" on the reform of the army, working with Nightingale. The two succeeded in "packing" it with their own preferred members. The commission was appointed in April 1857. It is of interest to give here the composition of the commission, since some of the names will reappear in the texts edited below.

Sidney Herbert, chair;
Augustus Stafford (MP);
General Henry Storks (general);
Dr Andrew Smith (army doctor);
Dr Thomas Alexander (army doctor);
Sir Thomas Phillips (examining lawyer);
Sir James Ranald Martin (civil doctor);
Sir James Clark (the queen's physician);
Dr John Sutherland (sanitarian);
Dr Graham Balfour (army doctor), secretary.

The "inner cabinet" was made up of Herbert, Sutherland and Nightingale. Nightingale of course was not a member of the commission and did all her work behind the scenes.

The report of the first commission was written by Herbert in August 1857 with Nightingale's help. Issued in January-February 1858, it called for sweeping reforms in the conduct of the army's life and for the formation of four subcommissions for the implementation of the report's recommendations. The four subcommissions were appointed in the same year. Foremost among them was the Barrack and Hospital Improvement Commission (called the Army Sanitary Commission from 1865 on); the three others dealt with the establishment of the Army Medical School, the organization of the Army Medical Department and army medical statistics. Sidney Herbert chaired all four subcommissions. All were involved in the India work. A brief appendix on India appeared at the end of the massive report. Nightingale and some members of the commission urged the use of the press to make sure that the attention of the public and the politicians would be focused on the necessary reforms. This focus was relatively easy to secure when special emphasis was put on the most shocking fact uncovered in the course of the inquiry: that the rate of mortality in the army in time of peace was double that of the civil population. Obviously not everything was fine with the army and some changes were urgent.

In 1857 Nightingale wrote an extensive background document, *Notes on Matters Affecting the Health, Efficiency and Hospital Administration of the British Army Founded Chiefly on the Experience of the Late War* (567 pages in normal pagination, plus numerous additions with Roman numerals). A postscript dealt with "sanitary matters in India." The document was supplemented by her *Subsidiary Notes as to the Introduction of Female Nursing into Military Hospitals in Peace and in War* (133 pages), both of which she circulated the following year. The research required by the commission and by these writings brought her into contact with most of the personalities important to the field and to her future work.

Throughout this work Nightingale insisted on extending the investigation to the army in India, both British and Indian (sepoys). Having already collected statistics on the mortality of soldiers in India and information on their living conditions, she was determined to investigate the appalling situation of the soldiers in India whose lives were sacrificed, as she believed, to sanitary neglect, more than to combat.

## The Royal Commission on the Sanitary State of the Army in India

Nightingale's concerns for the well-being of the India Army were not abstract or Platonic. They took form and reality in what can be referred to as her "second royal commission," the "Royal Commission on the Sanitary State of the Army in India," which occupied the years 1856-63, more specifically 1859-63. Early expressions of her concern for India are found in her 1857 writings. Then, in a letter to Edwin Chadwick of October 1858, she declared: "I hope we shall hear that something is being done by the government about Indian sanitary matters soon" (see p 70 below). The commission was appointed in May 1859 by Lord Stanley, secretary of state for India, who was first approached with a proposal for an aide-mémoire on India by Edwin Chadwick (see p 69 below). It operated jointly with the War Office. Nightingale's intense lobbying among politicians, the press and the public led again to the strategic placing of sympathetic members on the commission, most of whom were to be important in her future work:

Sidney Herbert, chair, succeeded by Lord Stanley;
Dr John Sutherland (army sanitarian);
Dr James Ranald Martin (sanitarian, inspector general of hospitals);
Dr William Farr (statistician of the General Register Office);
Dr Thomas Alexander (sanitarian);
Sir Robert Vivian (member of the Council of India);
Sir Proby T. Cautley (member of the Council of India);
Colonel Edward H. Greathed ("Queen's officer of acknowledged Indian experience").

William E. Baker was secretary, but in fact Sutherland and Nightingale did the work of secretary, Baker being Sutherland's clerk and being sometimes called "assistant secretary."

As in the case of the first royal commission, there was an "inner cabinet" made up of Sutherland, Farr and Nightingale. Questionnaires, mainly drafted by Nightingale, went out to all stations in India (some 150, perhaps 200: Nightingale's statements vary here), and their replies ("Stational Returns") were received in London to be analyzed by Nightingale and Dr Sutherland. Oral evidence was taken in London and some witnesses were briefed by Nightingale prior to their giving evidence. The bulky report (2028 pages) produced by the commission and completed in May 1863 was mostly written by her, as she told her mother: "I have now written the biggest part of their report, but I have not begun my own evidence, nor the digest of the reports from our Indian stations, 150 in number. . . . "[18] The recommendations for reform contained in the report were also her own work.

She also prepared the terrain for the reception of the report. In 1861-62 she had submitted her *Observations on the Evidence Contained in the Stational Reports Submitted to the Royal Commission on the Sanitary State of the Army in India* (92 pages), which embodied the gist of the report and were aimed to make its findings available to the public; this text

18 *Life and Family* (1:152).

was widely circulated in India and at home (to the queen, to influential friends, to John Lawrence,[19] Charles Trevelyan,[20] etc.), and is reproduced below.

It is important to underline Nightingale's role in and impact on the work of the commission. Once the idea of a royal commission had been accepted and the commission appointed, she engaged on a course of daily prompting of its members and spurring of the War and India Offices. Her diligence was not always rewarded, but she succeeded in devising appropriate machinery for the inquiry and in providing the propelling energy to the work of the commission.

In spite of all her efforts the actual presentation of the report to the House of Commons was botched and Nightingale was understandably furious. Due to an incomprehensible blunder, a poorly abridged version of the report prepared by the clerical staff was presented to the House. It left out Nightingale's *Observations* and gave only a short summary of the stational returns, thus omitting the rationale for the changes sought. She protested and had the "mistake" corrected by having a copy of the full report deposited in Hansard's office. In the process she had her *Observations* privately printed and circulated; it became known as her "little red book," as opposed to the Blue Book of the official report. The incident added a bitter note to her dealings with officials. However, Nightingale could greet the completion of the report as "the dawn of a new day for India—not only for our army there, but for the poor natives" (see p 129 below).

Once the report had been completed, Nightingale's ingenuity was devoted to getting it known to a large public through the press. She wanted not just reviews but good reviews. To that end she solicited friends and competent persons to write about the report in respected journals. A great deal of correspondence was devoted to selecting the right persons for the right journals and persuading them to write the reviews. Throughout this activity she emerged as a consummate strategist in planning the dissemination and reception of the commission's report.

Knowing too well that "reports are not self-executive," the commission recommended an effective machinery for the implementation of

---

19 On Sir John Lawrence see the biographical sketch below in Appendix A.

20 Sir Charles Edward Trevelyan (1807-86), a staunch Liberal, administrator in India 1826-38, assistant secretary to the Treasury in London 1840-59, governor of Madras 1859-60. See the biographical sketch in Appendix A below.

recommendations. There was to be: a sanitary commission in each presidency (Bengal, Bombay, Madras, i.e., the areas formerly governed by the local presidents of the East India Company); a sanitary commission or committee at the War Office: the Barrack and Hospital Improvement Commission, which had been appointed in 1857 and became in 1865 the Army Sanitary Commission or Committee; an India Office Sanitary Commission or Committee. Nightingale proceeded to press for implementation of the recommendations, notably with Lord de Grey (of the War Office) and Sir Charles Wood (of the India Office) and their successors. She agitated to have John Lawrence made viceroy (he became viceroy in November 1863 and took up his post in January 1864). Before embarking for India he paid a visit to Nightingale, on 4 December 1863, when the two established an effective working relationship. She assiduously saw all people who could help the cause, wrote to them and pressed them to action.

The papers, letters and notes published here abundantly show Nightingale's relentless efforts and actions to secure first the advancement of sanitary conditions in India and then the evolution of social-political institutions in India that conditioned sanitary progress.

## Medicine and Nursing in the Mid-Nineteenth Century—India and the West

Any study of Nightingale's contributions to hygiene and health care must take into account the state of medicine and nursing in the second half of the nineteenth century, both in the West and in India, and refrain from precipitate judgments based on today's medical knowledge. More precise information on the state of health care will be given at the appropriate places in these volumes. In general it can be said that, by 1860, Western (imperial in our case) medicine was successfully emerging from its dark ages (with its bloodlettings,[21] purges and mercurials) into a scientific phase. Progress in related scientific disciplines (chemistry, physics, zoology, botany, pharmacology, climatology, and above all in anatomy, based on the dissection of bodies) helped medicine to decisive developments in clinical observation, experimentation, theory and technique. The encounter with tropical,

21 Nightingale herself was bled while in Greece in 1850; see *European Travels* (7:419).

epidemic and endemic diseases stimulated research and opened the door to new vistas. Medical discoveries were not always met with speedy acceptance, as was shown by Nightingale's stubborn adherence to the environmental or "miasma" theory over germ, but gradually the test of practice was allowed to validate promising avenues of diagnostics and therapeutics.

In fact one may be puzzled by Nightingale's reluctance to accept germ theory, a mere "theory" with no evidence for it at the beginning of her career, but one for which substantial evidence appeared in the 1870s and 1880s. Interestingly, it was Robert Koch's identification of the cholera bacillus in Calcutta water during an epidemic in 1883 that gradually led to her "conversion." Her colleague Dr Sutherland was the intermediary, purchasing a microscope in 1884 in order to see the bacilli for himself. By 1891 she was recommending public lectures in Indian villages to show "the noxious living organisms in foul air and water."[22] Nightingale, though, continued to prefer "miasma" or environmental theory for its stress on what we would understand to be the breeding grounds for disease germs. Germ theory was "dangerous," she believed, when germs were considered the "origin, not the product, of the disease, of which uncleanliness, bad drainage, bad water supply, etc., are the origin" (see p 864 below). Obviously the strenuous measures she recommended to remove dirt and ensure a clean water supply and safe sewerage and drainage prevented germs from breeding.

The state of nursing in England at the beginning of Nightingale's career was deplorable, particularly when compared with France and Germany. It was considered a "profession" of ill repute and certainly not suitable for "gentlewomen," as evidenced by Nightingale's difficulties with her own family at the thought of her entering it. That state of affairs began to change in the 1850s, with Nightingale playing an important role in its evolution. Other volumes of this series elaborate on these developments in nursing.

As for India, health care still consisted chiefly of indigenous forms of healing and treatment as found in Ayurveda (Hindu), Unani (Islamic) and folk medicines. Nightingale compared the sanitary state of India with that of Europe in the Middle Ages (see p 125 below). As Europe had to "toil its way up to safety" from pestilence, so would

22 Letter to the Poona Sarvajanik Sabha December 1891, in *Social Change in India.*

India, but now it would have "the advantage of European experience." Timidly, health care in India began to interact with Western medical systems, then mainly confined to British enclaves. One impact of the royal commission on India was to clear the way for a system of state medicine and public health for India. However, plague was still current in India in the 1860s (see p 434 below) and "the moment of transition from enclavism to public health came only in the 1890s with the establishment of a new 'tropical medicine,' based on the germ theory of disease, and a corresponding intensification in state medicine in India . . . epitomized by the measures taken during the Indian plague epidemic of the 1890s and 1900s."[23] Much time was needed to overcome the view of Western and indigenous medicines as rival systems, to regard them rather as widely complementary, as will appear shortly.

Nightingale remarked on the health conditions of Indian nationals: "Everywhere the people are suffering from epidemic diseases, fevers, dysenteries, cholera: constant epidemics we may call them, and constant high death rates" (see p 190 below). Care of the sick among Hindus and Muslims was almost exclusively the domain of the family, with the help of traditional healers and cures. Nightingale worked hard to try to introduce nursing and female nursing to India, as will be shown below. She claimed that the royal commission report aimed at "nothing less than to bring the appliances of a higher civilization to the natives of India" (see p 190 below). There was not a town in India that did not need "water supply, draining, paving, cleansing, healthy plans for arranging and constructing buildings. . . . These things the people cannot do for themselves. But the India government can do them" (see p 192 below).

On the other hand, Nightingale emphasized how backward the administrative structure for sanitary improvements was. In England the legislation had been in place for years, so that "not a local administrative body but has its sanitary powers," but in India "no such progress has been made and no such powers exist" (see p 248 below).

In the end the conquest of cholera, smallpox and plague was to be the result of prolonged collaborative efforts based in numerous countries (see p 861 below), while the treatment of diseases increasingly required willingness to overcome prejudices. It also required convic-

---

23 David Arnold, *Colonizing the Body: State Medicine and Epidemic Disease in Nineteenth-Century India* 13.

tion of the practical utility of sanitary measures to justify expenditures on public health. To Lord de Grey Nightingale pointed out that a "single epidemic costs the country more than all the works" of sanitation, further noting that "none but Sir John Lawrence" was "enlightened enough" to see that (see p 524 below). It is in this light that the impact of the royal commission on India must be seen; it was "the first of several similar bodies appointed over the next eighty years to investigate and report on such matters as plague research, irrigation, industrial development and agriculture."[24]

Reading the material collected below, one gets the impression that, in matters of public health in India, the initiative came unilaterally from British agents, both in the medical field and in nursing. Did the colonial "sanitarians" encounter nothing in India to which they could associate themselves in the task of constructing a public health system? Were they confronted with an empty field they had to cultivate from ground zero?

Recent historians of India have given renewed attention to the question of the Western encounter with indigenous medicine, and often came up with fresh findings showing that indeed there was an Indian partner to British efforts. There was wider interaction between the two partners than the material of the present two volumes would indicate. Already in the seventeenth century they well knew of each other and were willing to borrow from each other in therapeutic practice: the use of plants, drugs and metals. "A respectful dialogue between Europeans and Indians was made possible by their shared commitment to a humoural conception of the human body."[25] At that time both disliked vivisection and lacked a precise knowledge of causation. In an atmosphere of perceived equality some Europeans early thought "that they could learn something from India,"[26] and some Indian practitioners were open to European methods.

The Indo-Islamic world had a long tradition of medical knowledge that could, and did, compete with the European system. Points of contact between the two systems have now been identified: British doctors serving at the court of the nawab of Arcot or some raja; colonial

24 David Arnold, *Science, Technology and Medicine in Colonial India* 85.

25 Mark Harrison, "Medicine and Orientalism," in Biswamoy Pati and Mark Harrison, eds., *Health, Medicine and Empire: Perspectives on Colonial India* 80.

26 M.N. Pearson, "The Thin End of the Wedge: Medical Relativities as a Paradigm of Early Modern Indian-European Relations" 158.

health officers consulting local doctors and healers; Western scientists making inventories of plants, herbs and metals linked with healing; the translation of Indian medical texts, etc. Borrowings and mutual reception have been documented.[27] There was a tendency to consider Indian medical knowledge "to be part of mankind's treasury" (273) that could be used for the profit of European medicine. Nightingale was made aware by Dr Murdoch[28] that "Hindu medical literature is enormous"; Dr Murdoch even considered "that medicine is the only Hindu science."[29] Conversely, some Indian practitioners thought that their own methods could be invigorated, purified and brought to a level of universal validity with the help of Western science. Company doctors and their successors mediated the reception and assimilation of European medicine by Indian practitioners. While the Indian Medical Service in the 1860s (between 650 and 820 surgeons) was staffed almost exclusively by Europeans, Indian subordinates performed some duties and soon native medical institutions in presidencies began to teach European medical science.[30]

The attitude of mutual respect began to decline when anatomy made decisive inroads in the West due to the practice of dissection allowing surgery to become more reliable and the discovery of the circulation of blood. Thus, after the seventeenth century, "the beginning of scientific medicine based on observation"[31] emerged in the West, and although traditional practices, such as bleedings, persisted until the middle of the nineteenth century, Western medical science gained definite ascendancy in India.

A feeling of scientific superiority on the part of Europeans was standard in Nightingale's lifetime. The British used Western science in India to "reinforce" their domination[32] and to secure intellectual

---

27 See Christopher Alan Bayly, *Empire and Information: Intelligence Gathering and Social Communication in India 1780-1870* 247-83.

28 John Murdoch (1819-1904), Christian evangelist and author of a number of publications on sanitation. He helped found the Christian Literature Society for India and was secretary of the Christian Vernacular Education Society in India.

29 Letter to John Sutherland 18 August 1886, ADD Mss 45758 f225.

30 See David Arnold, *Science, Technology and Medicine in Colonial India* 57-91.

31 M.N. Pearson, "The Thin End of the Wedge" 163.

32 Christopher Alan Bayly, *Empire and Information* 255.

hegemony. While some agents, astronomers and physicians tried to promote co-operation, combining the better parts of Indian knowledge with Western science, Western ideas tended to dislodge traditional beliefs, at least among the elite. European doctors, without totally disparaging Indian practice, were more and more critical of the Indian "continued adherence to Aristotelian humoural notions which had only recently been abandoned in Europe" (281). In the end, however, elite and wealthy Indians "used both Western-trained and Indian physicians, trusting the former for surgery, the latter for internal remedies" (281).

Complete hegemony over the "native mind" was in fact never achieved. "British medicine in India, before the beginning of the twentieth century, was too poorly funded and too riven with internal contradictions" (282) for it to triumph definitely over indigenous systems. Some of that complex state of affairs is reflected in the texts below.

The health situation of Indian populations was gravely jeopardized by the recurrence of famines. Famine left people defenceless against infectious diseases and thereby led to elevated mortality. Colonial powers were slow in realizing such connections, but gradually famine control found its place on the public health agenda. Nightingale was an active participant in that evolution, as her writings in the 1870s witness.

## Major Collaborators in the India Work

Nightingale enjoyed the collaboration of well-placed, qualified and dedicated officials in her India work. Among them were public figures at home and in India whom she knew thanks to family connections or whom she took the initiative to meet, sanitary experts whom she was eager to encourage and consult and friends whose influence she was able to put to use. Only the most important co-workers are mentioned here.

First of all there was Sidney Herbert (1810-61),[33] with whom she had already worked on the first royal commission. He chaired the second one until he had to resign on account of illness in December 1860. He remained the model against whom other officials were judged. Nightingale particularly appreciated his diligence, skill at negotiating with difficult ministers and determination to carry objectives through the necessary stages of implementation. They saw eye-to-

33 See the biographical sketches in *European Travels* for both Sidney and Elizabeth Herbert (7:771-75).

eye on major issues and had an especially good working relationship. That he was a man of exceptional character was widely recognized by his political colleagues.

Superlatives abound in descriptions of his work. To John McNeill Nightingale declared her belief that "the sanitary salvation of India depends upon Mr Herbert" (see p 93 below). And to Harriet Martineau: "He never wanted anything but a reason to go himself straight to any minister and get it done" (see p 230 below). After Herbert's death she memorialized him on every occasion; she was inclined to idealize his qualities and the years of collaboration with him.

As secretary at war Sidney Herbert was responsible for sending her to the Crimea at the head of a contingent of nurses. Shortly after her return to England in 1856, her collaboration with Herbert began, to become almost daily in these last five years of his life: writing of the *Notes on the Army*, the first royal commission on the health of the army at home, implementation of reforms of the army, agitating for and launching of the Royal Commission on the Sanitary State of the Army in India. Her devotion to Herbert and to what he stood for was total and passionate. In turn he greatly appreciated her help, advice and insights. He was committed to the reform of the army as much as she was. Their unity of mind and purpose functioned as a mutual incentive to offer a remarkable instance of productive collaboration.

The day of his death was experienced by Nightingale as a catastrophe and she commemorated it with nostalgia all her life long. With the passing of time she might have lionized him a little, but he clearly remained the great inspiration of her life work, her "dear master," whose work she felt called upon to bring to completion, although since her return from the Crimea she lived in the constant fear of her own death. For her part, Elizabeth Herbert (1822-1911) was more than an admiring observer of her husband's activity. She took an active role as advisor and collaborator. She not only knew what was going on but could in her own way substitute for her husband when his health began to decline, corresponded with other actors and did her share in hospital administration. In 1865 she converted to Roman Catholicism, to Nightingale's chagrin it must be said.

On Herbert's resignation Lord Stanley (1826-93)[34] assumed the chair of the royal commission. Clearly Nightingale preferred Sidney

34 On Lord Stanley see the biographical sketch below in Appendix A.

Herbert as chair, politely arguing to Stanley, when the commission was first set up, that "I know no man, except yourself, who could preside over such a commission but Mr Herbert" (see p 54 below). Lord Stanley was certainly capable, informed and diligent in his India work, entirely open to discussing the most confidential matters with Nightingale. Being a member of the House of Commons he could raise questions in the House and call for information. Nightingale several times asked for his assistance in that respect. For example, she asked him to be in the House on the evening when it was to debate Dr Sutherland's salary in the Estimates: "*Could you defend us? tonight?* There is no time to prime any MP who did not know the subject. And if there were, he would be of no use. No one but you would have any weight" (see p 528 below).

For many years Nightingale's relationship with Lord Stanley was steady; after rather cool beginnings it became more and more wholehearted. Nightingale often had to press him to action, but he regularly responded and became an agent of the measures she wished to see carried out. A closer relationship was inevitable when Lord Stanley took over the chair of the royal commission on India; it grew even closer at the time of the implementation of the report of that commission. At times impatient with him, she learned to appreciate his personality and did not hesitate to communicate to him all the information she received privately from India. Sometimes she also confided in him.

Yet Nightingale felt that Lord Stanley was not quite as apt as Sidney Herbert would have been at achieving implementation of the recommendations of the commission. She had to prod, cajole and remind, but in the end Lord Stanley acted. That is why favourable comments about him are mixed with negatives. Sometimes she thanks him for his kindness: "Your offer to act for us is too good to be wasted" (see p 285 below), but then complains: "Lord Stanley does nothing for us" (see p 219 below). Altogether, however, Nightingale found in Lord Stanley a faithful and devoted collaborator.

At the time the royal commission was at work the governors general were Lord Canning, whose wife Nightingale knew from the management committee of her Harley Street institution, and Lord Elgin, a person Nightingale did not know personally, although she had known his mother in Paris. Lord and Lady Elgin were approached by Nightingale indirectly via a mutual friend, Harriet Martineau (see p 231 below).

Direct involvement with governors general began with the appointment of Sir John Lawrence in 1863, on Lord Elgin's death. John

Lawrence was an experienced Indian official, having served both in India and at the India Office. He was fully open to working with Nightingale, and both were conscious of the need to act quickly. To an Indian official late in 1864 she said, "I feel so strongly, with regard to India, that what is to be done must be done now, or not at all. I mean, during Sir John Lawrence's time—in sanitary matters. We had a Sidney Herbert at the War Office—with his life, all progress passed away. So may it *not* be with Sir John Lawrence's. But I fear it will" (see p 504 below).

For Nightingale Lawrence's action was heroic—her admiration for him was almost as great as that for Sidney Herbert. Of him she said: "His is the greatest government under God's. And he is the only man to fill it" (see p 264 below). His major failing was his inability to delegate, his "caesarism" (see p 621 below) as she called it. She had more understanding for his lack of knowledge of sanitary matters, for his career had been military. There were differences of opinion, and sometimes Lawrence did things against the advice of Nightingale and her team, a matter to be dealt with delicately, for he was overall the most supportive person they had to work with. He had "not the least idea how the governors of the minor presidencies thwart and insult the sanitary principle. If he had, I think it would in some degree modify his view" (see p 545 below). Lawrence was thus faulted on a particular position he had taken, but he remained with Nightingale and her group on the principles. It was his virtue of thinking "every man like himself" that misled him. Altogether Nightingale was inclined to find Christlike features in John Lawrence, willing to be "crucified every day" (see p 493 below). Because of the central place Lawrence occupied in Nightingale's career, sections below will deal with his activity prior to his departure for India as viceroy in 1864, his part in carrying out the commission's recommendations, his establishment of the Bengal Sanitary Commission (see p 278 below) and his further correspondence with Nightingale.

Nightingale's collaboration with Lord Ripon,[35] both in England and in India, is documented in *Social Change in India*. Their agreement on policies toward India was unique and corresponded to Nightingale's final views of the British role in a colony about to come of age. We will see that Lord Ripon eventually surpassed Lawrence in Nightingale's estimation.

---

35 On Lord Ripon see the biographical sketch in *Social Change in India*.

Nightingale's team in London included doctors and public health experts or "sanitarians." Dr John Sutherland,[36] who was employed by the War Office, was her closest collaborator; he was not only a constant source for necessary medical and "sanitary" expertise, but even drafted material for her and acted as intermediary with other officials. He was the only paid member of the Army Sanitary Commission. Douglas Galton, a Royal Engineer, was a much-liked and respected relation by marriage. He vetted material for her and was a frequent consultant on all engineering and building matters. William Farr,[37] both a doctor and a leading statistician, was her statistics expert. From his position as head of the Statistics Branch at the General Register Office he could obtain the latest data. He also vetted questionnaires and papers for her. Robert Rawlinson, England's leading water expert, was a reliable and much-used source on all matters concerning water supply, drainage and sewers. These four were constant co-workers.

Nightingale knew Sir Charles Trevelyan, governor of Madras, prior to his taking up the post, through a Crimean War connection. There were family connections as well through his Macaulay relations; indeed Nightingale wrote him with condolences on the death of Lord Macaulay. There is correspondence between her and Trevelyan from 1858 to 1881, often warm and chatty, and often including messages for Lady Trevelyan.[38] When he went out to India as governor in 1859 she evidently considered him to be a major ally. Her questionnaires were only just then going out to the Indian stations. She optimistically told him that she was "sure that the answers to the copies sent to your presidency will be both the best filled up

36 On Dr John Sutherland see the biographical sketch in *Public Health Care* (6:674-76).

37 Dr William Farr (1807-83), superintendent of statistics at the General Register Office, closely associated with Nightingale's work and member of the second royal commission. See the biographical sketch in *Society and Politics* (5:831-32).

38 After Lady Trevelyan died, Nightingale wrote to Harry Verney: "I found almost accidentally such an interesting letter of *Lady Trevelyan's* to me from India. *Do you think that Sir C. Trevelyan would like to see it?* He has so forgotten me, of late years, that I felt it would be an intrusion to write to him on her death what I felt for her. And I did not. Save that she was rather worldly, I did feel much for her. . . . For a few years my communications with them were incessant. I don't know anyone who seemed to enter into my work more than *Sir C. Trevelyan.* Now that is all over." Letter 14 March 1873, Wellcome (Claydon copy) Ms 9006/30.

and the soonest sent back to us." She also intimated her hope that he should have "already set on foot the improvements which are intended to be suggested by these queries." She hoped that "no farther authority" would be needed in his presidency (see p 95 below).

Among other important collaborators in Nightingale's work was Sir Bartle Frere,[39] governor of Bombay 1862-67, then a regular visitor in London. She also had important contacts with Lady Dufferin, whose work is reported in *Social Change in India.* She had an especially good relationship to the governors general Ripon (whose work at the War Office she had appreciated already in 1859), Dufferin and Lansdowne. On all these and other collaborators much material will be presented below and in *Social Change in India.* An immense network of experts and friends developed over the years to support Nightingale's India work.

## Nightingale's Working Style

Her education and family milieu doubtless helped to shape Nightingale's work habits and method of dealing with persons and issues. Her method[40] or *modus operandi* was not particularly original, but she practised it with an impressive intensity and success, as the work she did for the second royal commission clearly illustrates. She was extremely good at data collecting. Faced with a problem, she would first hunt for the facts. Where to find them? She would read reports, official records, Blue Books, minutes and memoranda. She displayed an amazing capacity at digesting reports and analyzing them. When she could not rely on personal observations, as was largely the case in her India work, she knew how to research a question. Points to be clarified would be discussed with experts, and consultants were drawn into the enterprise. Letters addressed to governors general, British officials at home and in India, retired British administrators, ordinary citizens at home and in India brought her complementary information, with the result that she often knew as much as the experts and officials themselves, sometimes even more.

Armed with the factual evidence, she would go to work and write down her view of the problem and her proposal. This was done methodically, paying great attention to the organization of reports, memoranda, articles or lengthy letters. When proposing the introduc-

39 On Sir Bartle Frere see the biographical sketch below in Appendix A.

40 On Nightingale's method see Jharna Gourlay, *Florence Nightingale and the Health of the Raj* 18-21.

tion of a new measure (e.g., reform of army hospitals, the introduction of female nursing in the army, water supply in a given town), she regularly insisted that the beginning should be modest and only upon initial success be expanded to a larger area.

Her writing ability was remarkable. Writing was second nature to her, as is manifest in the flowing style of her abundant correspondence and in the forceful drafting of articles, memoranda and reports.

When her written text called for a specific public action, after completing it she began agitating: securing publicity, calling upon persons in place to help in its circulation and reception, lobbying officials, going to the press or "leaking information to the press," e.g., confiding to journalist Harriet Martineau. In that respect Nightingale was a consummate publicist and could mobilize public opinion "as she did in the case of Indian famines and land tenancy in Bengal."[41] Her lobbying activity naturally irritated some people, or she continued to be, as Lord Panmure (secretary of state for war) had called her, "that turbulent fellow" (see p 273 below).

After action was decided upon, she would follow it up and keep the actors on their toes. Being concerned with results as she was, she thought it essential to be in direct contact with the secretary of state for India at home and the governor general in India: personal contacts with most of them helped the cause and gave her the occasion to "inform" them and influence policies.

## Sources and Scope of the India Material

The vast amount of often pioneering work produced by Nightingale in relation to India is still little known. As this *Collected Works* goes to print there has been only one full-length book on the subject, Jharna Gourlay's *Florence Nightingale and the Health of the Raj*. Barbara Dossey gives one chapter to India in her excellent book on Nightingale as a "visionary."[42] Yet there is no lack of primary material. Of the daunting amount of articles, letters and reports Nightingale wrote, often with lengthy and sometimes several drafts, only a small amount has heretofore been published. Hence the present two volumes.

Nightingale's writings on Indian matters fall into two groups. First, there are the writings which were published and therefore come to us

41 Jharna Gourlay, *Florence Nightingale* 20.

42 Barbara M. Dossey, "The Birth of Indian Nationalism," in *Florence Nightingale: Mystic, Visionary and Healer*, discussed in *Social Change in India.*

as a finished and final product that has to be respected; changes made to her texts here merely relate to punctuation and to minor orthographic variations. These writings are made up of more or less extensive essays, reports, conference papers, articles for journals and newspapers, official letters and published correspondence. Titles are clearly indicated in the Source, with quotation marks for articles and italics for books.

Second, there is the huge archival material spread over the world and consisting of unpublished letters and drafts of letters, drafts of reports and essays, memoranda, notes from conversations, personal notes and diaries.

The contents of the two India volumes are grouped according to themes or subject areas. Each theme contains material published by Nightingale (reports, articles, pamphlets) and archival pieces (letters and notes). Letters and notes pertaining to the preparation of a publication and its sequels are, as much as could be done, placed before and after the publication. While not all letters and notes could thus be assigned a location because of occasional lack of contextual information, all efforts were made to indicate their likely place in Nightingale's mental landscape.

While all the printed and published writings are included in full, the archival material is selective (it covers some 20,000 manuscript pages). They were chosen so as to present a representative, yet substantial, sample of her production. The amount of writing Nightingale produced throughout her life cannot fail to amaze the reader who looks at the archival material. The huge literary output found there was achieved in spite of her ill health and busy schedule, both conditions that are repeatedly mentioned in her letters as an obbligato motif. For example: "I am an incurable invalid, entirely a prisoner to my bed (except during a periodical migration) and overwhelmed with business. . . . "[43] " . . . under the pressure of overwork and illness. . . . "[44] "Work and illness prevent me from seeing you. . . . "[45]

The present two volumes roughly reflect two great stages in Nightingale's India work. Volume 9, *Florence Nightingale on Health in India,* mainly deals with concerns central to her first twenty years of

43 From a letter to Mrs Chalmers 2 October 1866, *Life and Family* (1:807).

44 From a letter to John C. Barnard 12 February 1879, Columbia University, Presbyterian Hospital School of Nursing C.134.

45 From a letter to Kate Marsden 27 January 1893, *Theology* (3:508).

work: sanitation and sanitary improvements in the health of soldiers and civilians. Gradually she came to realize that social and political structures would have to be modified substantially in order to achieve these improvements. Such structural changes were then seen as a prerequisite of efficient sanitary measures and moved to the centre of her concerns; hence volume 10 is titled *Florence Nightingale on Social Change in India.* The two volumes differ in emphasis, but they show considerable overlapping of concerns. "Health" must always be understood in the broader sense. Famine caused deaths from starvation and disease, hence agriculture, irrigation, land tenure, taxation and efficiency in government departments became issues of public health. It remains that Nightingale evolved from being concerned with sanitation as such to being preoccupied with social change as a condition for "civilizing" India.

Much care was taken to provide in the Appendixes information useful to understand Nightingale's work and its context (the War and India Offices, and other administrative structures) and to facilitate reading (a glossary, the spelling of place names). Particularities in the spelling of place names are explained in the "Key to Editing."

Finally, it would be wrong to look at the present volumes as constituting a biographical essay in the style of a sustained narrative of Nightingale's forty years of work on India. Even the narrative parts encountered below are disjointed and serve only the purpose of highlighting themes and topics of her work relating to India. This is the goal the material collected here is intended to serve. The decision to arrange the material thematically carries with it the risk of doing some violence to chronology. A certain crisscrossing of dates could not be avoided in the effort to retrace developments in the perception of various problems which, in life, obviously ran parallel. In other words, each section of the two volumes deals with one major problem, but within each section chronological order is followed, leading necessarily again and again to the covering of the same years.

The inconvenience of steering clear of a biographical sketch can fortunately be remedied now. Readers interested in a more sequential account of Nightingale's involvement with India can find an excellent narrative in Jharna Gourlay's *Florence Nightingale and the Health of the Raj,* 2003; her work also contains a judicious assessment of Nightingale's contribution to military and civil health in India. Of course E.T. Cook's *The Life of Florence Nightingale* remains indispensable for the general context and various aspects of Nightingale's life and work. *A*

*Bio-Bibliography of Florence Nightingale* by W.J. Bishop and Sue Goldie served as a useful secondary source. Sue Goldie's *Calendar of Letters* was consulted in the search for letters.

## An Overview of Nightingale's India Work

The following bio-bibliography of Nightingale's India work[46] provides an overview of her work on India and the general context of the various items found in these two volumes of the *Collected Works.* It summarizes the main activities and writings of her four decades of Indian work.

1857-58 Worked for the Royal Commission on the Sanitary Condition of the Army with Sidney Herbert. Wrote *Notes on Matters Affecting the Health, Efficiency and Hospital Administration of the British Army* (1857) with an appendix on India. Urged friends and colleagues to publicize the royal commission's report.

1859-63 Worked for the Royal Commission on the Sanitary State of the Army in India. Wrote a questionnaire to collect data on stations, sorted the evidence gathered, chose members for the working committee, prepared the *Report* and wrote *Observations* (dated 1862). Collaborated with Sidney Herbert and Lord Stanley on the planning and work of the commission, Dr Sutherland and Dr Farr on the report and its publication, and with Chadwick and Martineau on publicizing the report.

1863 Worked for the appointment of the sanitary commissions in India. Established rapport with Sir John Lawrence, exchanged ideas with him about barrack improvement and the choice of personnel for Indian sanitary commissions. Defended the royal commission's report in the face of criticism. Wrote *How People May Live and Not Die in India* (1863) for the Social Science Conference in Edinburgh.

1864-68 Corresponded and collaborated with Lawrence in India about army sanitary organization; wrote *Suggestions in Regard to Sanitary Works for Improving Indian Stations* (1864); liaised with the India Office and the War Office for prompt action; wrote a Memorandum to answer Dr Leith's criticism on behalf of the Barrack and Hospital Improvement Commission and *Suggestions on a System of Nursing for Hospitals in India* (1865) in collaboration with Sir John McNeill; con-

46 Adapted from Cook, *The Life of Florence Nightingale* 2:437-58, 488-97, and Jharna Gourlay, *Florence Nightingale* 275-77.

sulted with Mary Carpenter, Dr Hathaway, Dr Pattison Walker and Lord Napier on the progress of public health in India; started to make unofficial contacts with Indians (1867); wrote *Memorandum on Measures Adopted for Sanitary Improvements in India Up to the End of 1867* (1868); lobbied Lord de Grey and Sir Stafford Northcote for military and civil sanitary reforms in India.

1869-70 Collaborated with Sir Bartle Frere, former governor of Bombay and now president of the India Office Sanitary Committee. Wrote a Memorandum on Indian sanitary measures for Lord Mayo, and the introduction to the *Report on Measures Adopted for Sanitary Improvements in India 1868-69* (1869). Accepted honorary membership in the Bengal Social Science Association; wrote an Address to the members on Indian sanitation, which was included in the *Report on Measures Adopted for Sanitary Improvements in India 1869-70* (1870) as well as her "Sanitary Progress in India."

1871-73 Wrote *Observations on Sanitary Progress in India* (1872); worked with the India Office Sanitary Committee. Became involved with famine, irrigation and the poverty of people in India; wrote *Life or Death in India, with an Appendix on Life or Death by Irrigation* (1873) for the Social Science Conference in Norwich; finished the proof copy of *The Zemindar, the Sun and the Watering Pot as Affecting Life or Death in India* (1873-74); liaised with Lord Northbrook and Lord Cranborne about military and civil sanitation in India. Started to focus more on the poverty of the people than on sanitation.

1874-76 Alliance with Sir Arthur Cotton to fight for irrigation in India. Lobbied Lord Salisbury (Cranborne) for irrigation canals; became involved in the railways vs canals dispute; published "Irrigation and Means of Transit in India" (*Illustrated London News,* 1874).

1877-79 Focused on famine, the *ryots* and irrigation; tried to build up public opinion in Britain about India's plight; published "Irrigation and Water Transit in India" (*Illustrated London News,* June 1877), "The Indian Famine" (*Daily Telegraph,* August 1877), "The United Empire and the Indian Peasant (*Journal of the National Indian Association,* 1878), "The People of India" (*The Nineteenth Century,* 1878), "A Water Arrival in India By a Commissioner" (*Good Words,* 1878). Became involved with land tenancy issues in Bengal and rural education; corresponded with P.K. Sen; published three articles, all titled "A Missionary Health Officer in India" (*Good Words,* 1879), "Co-operation in India" (*Journal of the National Indian Association,* 1879), three articles, all titled "Irrigation and Water Transit in India" (*Illustrated London*

*News,* 1879), three articles, all titled "Can we Educate Education in India to Educate Men?" (*Journal of the National Indian Association,* 1879); spurred Gladstone to promote agricultural banks in India.

1880-84 Continued to agitate for tenancy reform in Bengal; wrote "The Dumb Shall Speak and the Deaf Shall Hear, or the Ryot, the Zemindar and the Government" (*Journal of the East India Association,* 1883), "Our Indian Stewardship" (*The Nineteenth Century,* 1883), "The Bengal Tenancy Bill" (*The Contemporary Review,* 1883). Worked for Native Army Hospital Corps and village sanitation with Lord Ripon; supported Ripon's reforms; wrote Gladstone and the queen on behalf of Ripon. Established rapport with Lord Dufferin.

1885-89 In contact with William Wedderburn, A.O. Hume, Dadabhai Naoroji; supported the Indian National Congress. Received Indian delegates from abroad, helped them to publicize their cause. Corresponded with Lord Dufferin on sanitation. Focused on female health education in villages. Worked with Lady Dufferin to get sanitary "primers" written, established contact with John Murdoch, Dr Mary Scharlieb, Manmohun Ghose and others toward the adoption of suitable books. Worked for an amended Bombay Village Sanitation Bill; established contact with the Poona Sarvajanik Sabha and the Bombay Presidency Association, to which she wrote letters. Helped Lord Roberts to select nurses for army hospitals in India. Corresponded with Catherine Grace Loch, the first lady superintendent of the army hospitals in India; did background work on the Rukhmabai child-marriage case.

1889-92 Established contact with Lord Lansdowne through Benjamin Jowett; criticized the idea of sanitary boards in India. Wrote a Memorandum for Lord Cross on village sanitation in India. Worked on the amended draft of the Bombay Village Sanitation Bill with the Poona Sarvajanik Sabha and the Bombay Presidency Association, to which she wrote more letters; acted in favour of an Indian committee in the International Hygiene Congress; invited Indian delegates to take part; offered them hospitality at Claydon; organized a Memorandum to be sent to the secretary of state regarding village sanitation. Publicity in the journal *India.* Wrote an introduction to a biography of Malabari (1892).

1893-96 Published "Health Lectures for Indian Villages" (1893) and "Health Missioners for Rural India" (1896) in *India.* Collaborated with Wedderburn and Malabari. Advocated rural health education using women health workers; wrote "Village Sanitation in India" for the International Hygiene Congress in Budapest.

1897-98 Continued to receive Indian sanitary papers from the India Office for her comments; met the Conservative MP M. Bhownaggree, leading Indian politicians Dinsha Wacha, G.K. Gokhale, and the Aga Khan; continued correspondence with nurses in India and some Indian acquaintances; briefed Vaughan Nash on famine.

1902 on Did not do any serious writing due to blindness and failing mental faculties; only brief messages.

1906 India Office asked to stop sending her sanitary papers.

## Events Mentioned in Volumes 9 and 10

Important historical events referred to or implied in the two volumes.

| | |
|---|---|
| 1839-42 | First Afghan War |
| 1845-51 | Great Famine in Ireland |
| 1845-49 | Sikh Wars; annexation of the Punjab |
| 1846 | Repeal of the Corn Laws |
| 1850 | Irish Tenant League established |
| 1851 | First Sanitary Conference, Paris |
| 1854-56 | The Crimean War |
| 1856-61 | Cholera epidemics in India |
| 1857-58 | The Indian Mutiny |
| 1857-58 | Royal Commission on the Sanitary Conditions of the Army |
| 1858 | Rule of the East India Company terminated and beginning of crown rule (raj); Queen's Proclamation |
| 1859 | Second Sanitary Conference, Paris |
| 1859-63 | Royal Commission on the Sanitary State of the Army in India |
| 1860 | International Statistical Congress, London |
| 1861-67 | Famines in India |
| 1861-65 | The American Civil War |
| 1862 | Cholera Commission Report |
| 1863 | International Statistical Congress, Berlin<br>Social Science Congress, Edinburgh |
| 1864 | Poor Law Reform |
| 1866 | Third Sanitary Conference, Constantinople |
| 1867-77 | Cholera epidemics in India |
| 1869 | Inauguration of the Suez Canal |

| | |
|---|---|
| 1869-70 | Cholera Inquiry |
| 1870, 1881 | Ireland's Land Acts adopted |
| 1870-71 | Franco-Prussian War |
| 1870 | Home Rule League formed in Ireland |
| 1873 | Social Science Congress, Norwich |
| 1874 | Fourth Sanitary Conference, Vienna |
| 1876 | Queen Victoria proclaimed empress of India |
| 1876-79 | Famines in India (the "Great Famine") |
| 1878-80 | Second Afghan War |
| 1878 | Vernacular Press Act in India |
| 1879 | Anglo-Zulu War |
| 1880 | Famine Commission Report |
| 1881 | Fifth Sanitary Conference, Washington |
| 1882 | Repeal of Vernacular Press Act |
| | Ripon's Resolution on Local Self-Government |
| 1883 | First Conference of the Indian Association of Bengal |
| 1883-85 | Ilbert Bill controversy |
| 1884 | First Cholera Conference, Berlin |
| 1885 | Bengal Tenancy Act |
| | Foundation of the Indian National Congress |
| | Second Cholera Conference, Berlin |
| | Sixth Sanitary Conference, Rome |
| 1892 | Limited Indian representation on legislative councils in India |
| | Dadabhai Naoroji elected to British Parliament |
| 1894 | Eighth International Congress of Hygiene and Demography, Budapest |
| 1896-97 | Famines in India; plague in Bombay |
| 1899-1902 | Boer War |
| | Famines in India |

# Key to Editing

All the manuscript material in the *Collected Works* has been carefully transcribed and verified (for a description of the process of obtaining and processing this information see "Research Methods and Sources," Appendix E in *Life and Family*. Illegible words and passages are so indicated, with [illeg], or [?] inserted to indicate our best reading of the word or words in question. Dates for material cited or reproduced are given wherever possible, in square brackets if they are estimates only (by an archivist, previous scholar or the editor). Any controversy about date is indicated. The type of material, whether a note, actual letter, draft or copy is given as precisely as possible. Designations letter/draft/copy signify that the source was Nightingale's own files, given to the British Library or to St Thomas' Hospital and then the Florence Nightingale Museum, and are probably drafts or copies kept by her. The designation of "letter" is used only when there is good reason to believe that it was actually sent and received (a postmarked envelope, for example, or the archive being other than Nightingale's own files). In some cases both the original letter and Nightingale's draft or copy are extant, and these show that the copies she kept are reliable. We do not use the convention of ALS (autograph letter signed), but our "letter" is close to it, bearing in mind that Nightingale often used initials rather than her signature. The electronic I-text (that is, the transcriptions as "input," before editing) gives full information on supporting material (envelopes, postmarks), and whether the piece was in pen, pencil, dictated or typed.

The practice was naturally to use the best source possible, the original letter where available. Where a draft or copy was also available this is noted. Sometimes the original was no longer available and a typed copy in an archive or a published copy had to be used.

All sources indicated as "ADD MSS" (Additional Manuscripts) are British Library, the largest source of Nightingale material. The Wellcome Library for the History and Understanding of Medicine Library is abbreviated "Wellcome." Most of those materials are copies of correspondence at Claydon House, indicated as (Claydon copy). If not so indicated they are originals. Where only short excerpts from a letter are used (because the rest is on another subject) these are indicated as "from a letter" and the address and ellipses at the beginning and end are omitted. Postscripts that merely repeat points or move on to a completely different subject are omitted without ellipses.

To avoid use of "ibid." and "op. cit.," and to reduce the number of footnotes generally, citations are given at the end of a sequence if the same source is cited more than once. Subsequent citations are noted in the text with the new page or folio number given in parentheses. The term "folio" (abbreviated as f or ff in the plural) is used for reference to manuscript pages, p and pp for printed pages, where needed, or page numbers are given after the date or volume number without p or pp. References to material that appears in earlier volumes of the *Collected Works* are identified by our title, volume number and page number rather than the archival source.

To make the text as accessible as possible spelling, punctuation and capitalization have been modernized and standardized, and most abbreviations replaced with full words. British spellings have been maintained and standardized (labour, honour). We have kept her old-fashioned "farther," but change "shew" to "show," "civilise" to "civilize," "inclose" to "enclose," "staid" to "stayed" and her occasional abbreviation "ye" to "the." We change "story" to "storey" when it refers to a floor. We use modern spellings of words with "ae," such as gynecology, pyemia, septicemia and hemorrhage. Nightingale's terms for a student nurse, "probationer," and a maternity hospital, "lying-in," remain as they are.

We have followed the trend to lesser use of capitals, even to kings, queens and viceroys (but Viceroy-in-Council for his Cabinet). Nightingale was fond of dialect and we trust that the meaning will be clear enough, as with other old-fashioned words she used and which we did not edit. The electronic text gives a full glossary of edited words.

Roman numerals are replaced with Arabic (except for royalty, popes and the citation of classical texts). We have left Nightingale's use of masculine generics as they are, hence "man," "men," "he," etc., referring to human beings generally. Some, but not all, excessive "and," "but" and "the" have been excised. Nightingale's "Esq." titles for men have been omitted. Any words the editor has added to make sense (usually in the case of rough notes or faint writing) appear in square brackets.

Italics are used to indicate underlining and small capitals for double (or more) underlining. All indications of emphasis in texts are Nightingale's (or that of her correspondent or source), *never* the editor's. Foreign words are not italicized, unless Nightingale did. Any use of (sic) also is Nightingale's, never the editor's. When taking excerpts from written material Nightingale indicated ellipses with x x and we have kept these. Ellipses for editorial purposes are indicated with . . . for skipped material within a sentence, . . . . if to the end of the sentence or more than a sentence has been dropped. Passages that break off abruptly (or in which folios are missing) are so indicated.

Editorial notes appear in footnotes or, if very brief, in square brackets in the text. Articles (the, a, an) and the appropriate form of the verb to be have been supplied where necessary to make sense. Persons who changed their names (usually through marriage or the acquisition of a title, sometimes for purposes of inheritance) are referred to by the more commonly used name, cross-referenced in the index to the other if another name is also used. Dates to identify people are given at the first appropriate moment, not where there is only passing mention of the person or the name appears on a list or in a footnote; italicized entries in the index indicate entries with identifying information. Of course, for many people, notably servants and acquaintances, identifying information is not available.

The bibliography provides full information on most books cited. Newspaper sources, government reports and periodical references are given in footnotes only. References to classical and other works available in many editions (now often on the Internet) are by book, chapter, canto, scene, line, etc., as appropriate, and are not repeated in the bibliography.

We refer to Nightingale and indeed all adult women by their surnames, the normal practice for references to men. We note with some dismay the frequent practice in the secondary literature of using first names, even nicknames, for women, reserving surnames, initials and honorifics for men only. We use correspondents' names in the source headings but normally refer to them by the name Nightingale used: hence Dr Sutherland, Mme Mohl.

In Nightingale's day British officials serving in India were usually called "Indians," Indian nationals "natives." So they appear in her, and other, texts. In editorial introductions we follow modern usage, to make clear who are British officials and who real Indians, Indian nationals. A bazaar refers to a market area. Ryots are peasants, who may also riot.

Nightingale used various spellings for Muslim: Muhammadan, Muhammedan, Mussulman, Mahometan, Mahomedan. "Muhammadan" is generally used in the present volumes. Further, the form "zemindar" is preferred to "zamindar," following Nightingale's usage.

Editing the "Indian" material called for a series of important decisions as to the spelling of place names. Given the many "archaic" ways of spelling Indian names of provinces and states, cities, towns and villages encountered in Nightingale's writings, the way they were to be reproduced here had to be determined. When possible, spellings have been modernized and made to follow the present-day usage every time there was no risk of misunderstanding or confusion; when the identity of a place could not be ascertained with a fair degree of confidence, Nightingale's spelling usage was retained, in particular in her printed texts. Editorial notes follow modern usage with some major exceptions, as indicated below. Bombay (now Mumbai) and Madras (now Chennai) were left in the old form, and the old spelling Calcutta (now Kolkatta) kept as these spellings appear in so many proper names, notably of the presidencies and their sanitary commissions. Thus:

| Banaras is kept instead of the "new" | Varanasi |
|---|---|
| Baroda | Vadodara |
| Berhampore | Brahmapur |
| Bombay | Mumbai |
| Calcutta | Kolkatta |
| Cochin | Kochi |
| Ganges | Ganga |
| Madras | Chennai |
| Oudh | Awadh |
| Quilon | Kollam |
| Simla | Shimla |
| Trichinopoly | Tiruchchirappalli |

Appendix D in volume 10 gives a complete list of the other place names in their actual spelling as encountered in the two volumes.

# Introduction to Volume 9

The material of the present volume documents Nightingale's efforts to improve the sanitary conditions of soldiers and civilians in India, and identifies the issues she was confronted with in her work. It is presented thematically. It begins with the planning for and the formation of the Royal Commission on the Sanitary State of the Army in India; next comes the work of the commission, its report and actions toward implementation of its recommendations; there are then sections on irrigation and the prevention of famine, sanitation and the prevention of epidemics, and nursing. In each case there are actual published papers, correspondence and notes toward their preparation, dissemination and follow-up action. There is some overlap, of course, as new issues emerge and old ones require further work. Efforts were made to avoid duplication as much as possible, but some remains. Sometimes the same issue had to be explained many times (to different people), with some nuance in the explanation. Sometimes also Nightingale simply did not succeed in getting the requisite action and had to return to the problem time and again.

First, the correspondence shows Nightingale anxiously working toward getting the right members on the royal commission. A large number of candidates was proposed and evaluated, then chosen or rejected. In each case a lively exchange of information took place and judgments on persons were expressed, always with a view to securing the most competent candidate. In general Nightingale succeeded in having her preferences accepted.

Once the commission was appointed and its work launched, a frustrating situation emerged: there was reluctance on the part of the India Office to open its books: "The office throws all kinds of obstacles in the way" (see p 97 below). It was difficult to get to the relevant data concerning the sanitary conditions of the army, which were buried in reports that the India Office wanted to keep confidential to avoid the risk of showing how deplorable the situation was. That is why, on many occasions, the information had to be obtained by a personal contact willing to leak it. Nightingale makes her frustration abundantly clear in her letters. But in the end the commission got the necessary data from the India Office and, additionally, plenty of data from India thanks to the questionnaires sent there and the corresponding returns. The result was a thorough survey of the health condition of the army and, indirectly, of that of the Indian population at large. Detailed recommendations for remedy were made, including precise points for administrative changes.

In the implementation stage of the commission's recommendations, Nightingale could count on an impressive network of well-placed and qualified collaborators: public figures at home and in India, sanitary experts, whom she was eager to encourage and consult, and friends whose influence she was able to put to use. Of all those collaborators many were congenial and willing to act; others had to be prompted. But all had to be kept on their toes, so Nightingale felt, and reminded of their duties. Typical of her attitude was her relationship with John Lawrence, whom she admired so much, with whom she was basically in agreement, but with whom also she recognized important differences, as the correspondence shows. Her differences with Lord Cranborne (later Lord Salisbury)[1] in his various functions are also revealing; she was angered by his reluctance to undertake irrigation works due to financial constraints, yet she remained civil in her criticism though firm in her proposals.

An important shift is evident in this volume as Nightingale's interest in the health of the army gradually widened to include the civilian population and even the establishment of a public health system in India. Her early position appears first in the remark that the army cannot enjoy good health if the surrounding area is unhealthy. Attention to the sanitary state of the "native lines" or "native lanes" then led step by step to a concern with the entire civilian population. In time the health of Indian nationals became the end, not a mere means to an end. Added to her insistence on sanitation in general were concerns to prevent famines by promoting irrigation and increasing food production, and her efforts to battle epidemics by spreading information on hygiene and basic health precautions. In fact the main obstacles to public health were seen in famines and epi-

1 See Jharna Gourlay, *Florence Nightingale* 130-32.

demics, interrelated curses which jacked each other up in a kind of macabre dance. The enterprise of overcoming those obstacles was obviously aimed at the entire Indian population and not only soldiers. The material below reflects this important development of Nightingale's interest in India and the scope of her intervention.

A further development manifest here was Nightingale's concern with social and political change in India. Such concern appears significantly in this volume. It will become dominant in *Social Change in India.* While some overlap in material between the two volumes was inevitable, the vantage points are different, as will become evident.

The present volume shows Nightingale at work, studying reports and statistics, producing memoranda, notes and letters, and trying to move every office and every person in charge toward implementing the recommendations of the royal commission and improving public health in India. She kept complaining about illness and overwork, but she delivered.

Evaluation of the long-term success or failure of this work is a subject mainly for future scholarship. A few final words toward it are found at the end of this volume, and an Epilogue with somewhat more assessment closes out *Social Change in India.*

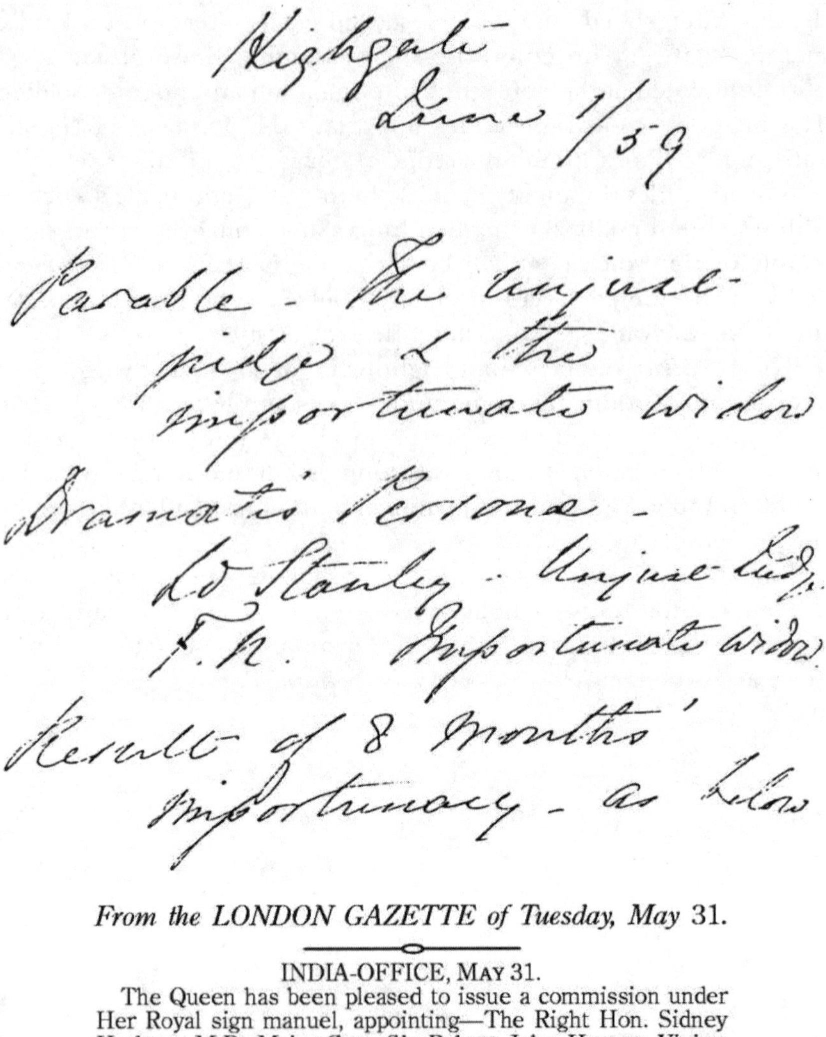

Highgate
June 1/59

Parable – The unjust judge & the importunate widow

Dramatis Personae –
Ld Stanley – Unjust Judge
F.N. Importunate widow

Result of 8 months' importunacy – as below

*From the LONDON GAZETTE of Tuesday, May* 31.

INDIA-OFFICE, MAY 31.

The Queen has been pleased to issue a commission under Her Royal sign manuel, appointing—The Right Hon. Sidney Herbert, M.P., Major-Gen. Sir Robert John Hussey Vivian, K.C.B., Col. Sir Proby Thomas Cautley, K.C.B., Thomas Alexander, Esq., C.B., Col. Edward Harris Greathed, C.B., William Farr, Esq., M.D., James Ranald Martin, Esq., John Sutherland, Esq., M.D., to be Her Majesty's Commissioners to inquire into, and report upon, the measures which it may be expedient to take for maintaining and improving the health of all ranks of Her Majesty's army serving in India.

Announcement of Royal Commission on India. Courtesy of Sir Edmund Verney and the Claydon House Trust.

# THE ROYAL COMMISSION ON INDIA

Nightingale's "India work" properly began at the time of the Royal Commission on the Sanitary State of the Army in India (1859-63), but already in 1857 she was hoping to extend the inquiry into the conditions of the Home Army to the army's situation in India. As soon as the work of the first royal commission on the health of the army (1857-58) was completed, she started active lobbying to have the second commission launched, and agitated to have the "right" members placed on it. It seems that Edwin Chadwick was the first person to have had the idea of an inquiry on India, which he communicated to Lord Stanley as a proposed "aide-mémoire." Nightingale picked up the idea and confidently expressed in detail to Lord Stanley how she would structure such an inquiry and turn it into a royal commission (see p 54 below). The abundant correspondence with Lord Stanley after he became president of the commission is rich with her often-unsolicited advice. Even before the commission submitted its report, she warned Lord Stanley that "when the commission is closed, its real work will begin" (see p 121 below). In the meantime, especially with the help of Sutherland and Farr, Nightingale rushed to work, drafting and sending questionnaires to all military stations in India and analyzing the numerous returns. Along with the oral evidence taken in London, those data were organized into a massive report, to the writing of which she was the main contributor. At the same time, she produced her *Observations* distilling the report and, with Dr Sutherland, the *Abstract of the Same Report* (or *Abstract of the Evidence*) summarizing the stational returns. Published writings as well as an extensive correspondence witness to this, her first active involvement on behalf of India.

The first item below is a short postscript Nightingale added to her monumental *Notes on Matters Affecting . . .* , at the end of its 800-plus pages. It reveals the understanding she brought to the subject at the beginning of her work, notably the assumption of the desirability of

British rule in India. It shows her disdain for complacency and a high-minded ambition: "It would be a noble beginning of a new order of things to use hygiene as the handmaid of civilization" (see p 47 below). It also shows that already in 1857 Nightingale had concerns for soldiers in India that soon developed into the idea of a royal commission. Writing to Sidney Herbert on Christmas Day 1857, she suggested that the report of the first commission be circulated "also in India" (Add Mss 43394 f211).

Source: From a flyleaf or postscript added to Nightingale's *Notes on Matters Affecting the Health, Efficiency and Hospital Administration of the British Army Founded Chiefly on the Experience of the Late War* (London: Harrison & Sons 1858) 565-67

1857

The subjects discussed in the preceding pages have been dealt with, as required by Lord Panmure's[1] instructions, with special reference to the experience obtained during the Crimean War. While the sheets were passing through the press, those lamentable occurrences [the Mutiny] took place in India which have led to a universal conviction that this vast empire must henceforth be held by British troops. If we were to be led by past experience of the presumed effect of Indian climates on European constitutions, our country might almost despair of being able to supply men enough for the military occupation of so vast a region. The art of preserving health has hitherto made but small progress in our Eastern possessions. The British race has carried with it into those regions of the sun its habits, its customs and its vices, without considering that there are penalties exacted by nature in her tropical dominions from those who neglect or transgress her laws far more severe than in the more temperate climates of our own country. Under a low temperature man may do with impunity what under a higher one is death. Our vast Eastern Empire consists of many zones, of many regions, of many climates. Its plains, rivers, deltas, table lands, its sub-alpine districts and regions of eternal snow present, perhaps, all the climates of the earth. On the mere question of climate, it is surely within human possibility so to select and arrange military stations and service that at all ordinary times our troops may have the opportunity of recruiting their health and strength, to a considerable degree at least, without interfering materially with military service.

1 The 2nd Baron Panmure (1801-74), secretary at war.

Might it not be possible, even in the great majority of instances, so to arrange the stations and so to connect them by railroads and telegraphs that the troops would hardly be required to occupy unhealthy districts? Even with regard to such districts the question arises to what extent the unhealthiness is inevitable, and to what extent it would be remediable. There have been and there are eminent men in the Indian service who entertain no doubt as to the practicability of introducing sanitary reform into almost every barrack and cantonment in the East. Considerable progress has indeed been made in this very matter within the last half century and there can be little doubt but that, aided by the clearer light of modern discovery and especially by the complete experience of the Crimean War, a great deal may be done to diminish the disease and mortality in a large army of occupation by which we must hereafter hold our Indian Empire.

The subject is one which, it cannot be doubted, will receive the immediate attention of her majesty's government.

As an illustration of the necessity of government interference in the matter, it may be stated, on the very first authority, that, after a campaign, perhaps one of the most arduous and successful on record, and when the smallness of the British force and the season of the year required every sanitary precaution to be taken for the preservation of the force, a certain earnest, energetic officer appointed a sanitary inspector to attend to the cleansing of a captured city and to the burial of some thousand dead bodies of men, horses, asses, bullocks, camels and elephants, which were poisoning the air. The Bombay government, to which the appointment was referred, "would not sanction it," "*because there was no precedent for it.*"

In future, it ought to be the duty of the Indian government to require no "precedents" for such procedure. The observance of sanitary laws should be as much part of the future régime of India as the holding of military positions or as civil government itself. It would be a noble beginning of the new order of things to use hygiene as the handmaid of civilization.

Source: From a letter to Lady Canning, West Yorkshire Archive Service 177/2/3

16 September 1857

I need not say that, should you think it possible for me to be of the smallest use, I would come out, at twenty-four hours' notice, to serve in any capacity, in my "line of business" that you would direct.

**Editor:** Nightingale's correspondence on India in 1857 moves quickly from concerns raised by the Mutiny to what practically might be done. The appointment of a royal commission, its terms of reference and the choice of its members will soon dominate. She succeeded in getting her vision of the basic principles of the royal commission's mode of operation accepted. It had to be based in England, with power to institute inquiries in India. It had to have a small number of men with great experience, or better not to exist at all. From the correspondence it is evident that she had to persuade Lord Stanley of this strategy; he had proposed a committee of three, to review "existing opinions," in England. A letter she wrote him argued that to collect evidence "*merely* in England" would not do. Research in India might be required to refute the conventional wisdom that India was "essentially unhealthy." The merely "medical" subject matter he thought adequate had to be broadened to matters "engineering, military, sanitary and medical," the "sanitary" of course implying a broad public health, preventive, approach (see p 61 below). One of the people he had proposed for the committee of three was John Simon, then medical officer for the Privy Council and a leading public expert, to be sure, but one with whom Nightingale disagreed on several key issues. He had notably published a report decrying preventive sanitary measures. He was not appointed.

Nightingale exchanged much correspondence with both Stanley and Herbert. Finally, late in December 1858, she asked Stanley (most apologetically) to come to see her, for "a few minutes' conversation" (see p 73 below). Their differences were evidently resolved, for, as Nightingale reported to Sidney Herbert, he agreed to ask him to be chair of the commission and to select his "own tools" (see p 73 below).

Source: From two letters to Sir John McNeill,[2] Florence Nightingale Museum (LMA) H1/ST/NC3/57/SU90 and 93, copy Add Mss 45768 ff60 and 66

15 July 1857

I don't think that you are at all more "nervous" about the Indian affairs [Mutiny] than the best informed here. I speak like a parrot. But my impression is from all I hear that this "row" is but the begin-

2 Sir John McNeill (1795-1883), assistant surgeon on the East India Company's Bombay establishment, one of Nightingale's strongest allies in her India work. He went to the Crimea for inspection with Colonel Alexander Tulloch; their report was unpopular at the War Office.

ning of things. As the revolution of 1793 in France was but the beginning of what ended in the total overthrow of the feudal system, so this affair in India must end in the entire doing away of the caste system or in the overthrow of the British power there. We may have to reconquer India. I should like much to go out; we shall have dreadful sickness there, but I have no one to advise me. I want to see you about this.

10 October 1857

I will not say a word about India. You know so much more about it than anybody here. We have seen terrible things in the last three years, but nothing to my mind so terrible as Panmure's [secretary of state for war] unmanly and stupid indifference on this occasion! I have been three years "serving" the War Department. When I began there was incapacity but not indifference. Now there is incapacity and indifference. What are the murders committed by these miserable Hindus compared to the murders committed by an educated Englishman?

Panmure's coming up to town last Thursday week was the consequence of reiterated remonstrances. I have heard men in office say that he deserved to be impeached and he is going away again after the next Indian mail! That India will have to be occupied by British troops for several years, I suppose there is no question. And so far from the all-absorbing interest of this Indian subject diminishing the necessity of immediately carrying out the reforms suggested by our [first] commission, I am sure you will agree that they are now the more vitally important to the very existence of our army.

Source: From an undated letter to Sidney Herbert, Wiltshire County Record Office, Pembroke Collection 2057/F4/67

Great Malvern
[1857]

The Indian news is terrible [the Mutiny], or rather the goings on of this War Department with regard to it. We have seen terrible things for the last three years, but nothing, I think, like Panmure's unmanly and brutal indifference. What are the murders committed by these miserable Bengalis compared to the murders committed by the insouciance of an educated and cultivated Englishman?

However, you have begun at the root of the matter, the physical and moral efficiency of the army. And, by carrying your reforms, all the rest will follow and the Indian matter indirectly, too. . . .

I wrote to Lord Stanley a letter (in my usual temperate terms and with the moderation which is my characteristic) about the affair at Dum Dum, where 1800 women and children, having been packed into a space for 300, 500 of them died of dysentery and all within five miles of Calcutta. And the government officer, instead of dispersing them immediately, drives back to Calcutta and makes a minute. Really I can remember nothing in the Crimea (for a want of all organization) to compare with this. And then people say, "It's all the climate. What can you expect? Women and children WILL die in India."

I wrote to Lord Stanley, pointing out how urgent such facts make a commission of inquiry. He answers: "I can only say at this moment that the Dum Dum affair shall be fully inquired into." (I hope *not* by *old Indians.*) I had seen it, but thank you nonetheless for reminding me." If it has "reminded" him to do it the old way, it will be no good. I hope "at this moment" means that *another* "moment" is coming.

Martin[3] and Tulloch[4] were not examined yesterday before the reorganization commission, as intended, but General Franks and Major Holland were. Martin and Tulloch are to be examined on Monday, and I have written a sentence for Martin (which he has inserted into some written evidence of his to be given in) as to the necessity of a sanitary commission.

The Dum Dum inquiry, if fairly gone into, must bear so heavily on somebody (possibly Linton who is at Calcutta) that I should *hope* it would initiate a real and searching sanitary commission.

Source: Letter, Wiltshire County Record Office, Pembroke Collection 2057/F4/66

30 Old Burlington St.
Christmas Eve [24 December 1857]

Dear Mr Herbert

I have gone through Ewart's[5] "Colonization in India" four reports (which are only evidence) and marked all the passages which refer to sanitary business. If you would like to have the marked copy rather than the trouble of doing the same thing, I will send it you.

---

3 Dr James Ranald Martin (1793-1874). See the biographical sketch below in Appendix A.

4 Sir Alexander Tulloch (1803-64), major general in India; his tables showing the death rates at stations in India were so shocking that investigation into the conditions of the army was made imperative.

5 Joseph Ewart (1831-1906), member of the Bengal Medical Service. He authored *A Digest of the Vital Statistics of the European and Native Armies in India*, 1859, and *The Sanitary Condition and Discipline of Indian Jails*, 1861.

The impression it leaves upon my mind is, through much evidence often contradictory, generally clumsy, flimsy and always vague, that the thing can be done, i.e., the sanitary reform can be worked, that practical insight in the details is utterly wanting, but that there is a prima facie case which is entirely irresistible, that men may live in India as well as in England, if people will set about it, but that nobody has set about it.

An immense number of other subjects is treated in the report, supply, revenue, etc. The impression it leaves is that the only persons who understand any of the subjects are the civil administrative people, and that all the rest are idle bunglers.

I have besides (through Mr Arthur Mills[6]) certain India House returns of mortality, very good, or rather very bad. And Balfour[7] is going (as a Christmas present) to make me up some returns of diseases. One curious fact I have got at, that at Dugshai, Sabathu, Mussoorie stations, as healthy as any English climate, the troops suffer intensely from diarrhea. Why? Because in the plains the skin does the whole eliminating function. And then they are sent up to these hill stations, without a rag more clothing. Why, if they did *not* have diarrhea, every man of them would die. Oh how poor nature is abused and blamed, who is only doing her very best to save us from our own folly, which ought to be the thing blamed.

There are very good, useful, popular sanitary materials even in Ewart's report. But I am more and more convinced that no real good will ever be done except by a report calculated to carry weight with it and compel observance by regulation.

Please don't suppose that I am staying in town on account of the business. Williams [Nightingale's physician] is very recalcitrant (and was when you spoke to me) about my going to Malvern at all. I have not made up my mind, but if I stay here it will only be on account of my own health.

yours sincerely

F. Nightingale

Martin's evidence (in said report) is all good, and sound on general principles. But, like the man, there is not a single practical suggestion.

---

6 Arthur Mills (1816-98), MP and cousin of Selina Bracebridge.

7 Dr T. Graham Balfour (1813-91), secretary of the first royal commission, head of the Army Statistical Department.

Source: From an undated note, Wiltshire County Record Office, Pembroke Collection 2057/F4/65

[1857]

Note on the Monthly Return of Sickness and Mortality. Two important deductions are drawn from this return by Sir A. Tulloch, that (1) acclimatization has "no perceptible advantage in India, even when troops are serving under the most disadvantageous circumstances"; (2) that it would be advantageous to send Sikh troops to China. The second of these is an important suggestion, especially at the present time, but the first requires to be seriously examined.

1. No satisfactory conclusion can be drawn from three months' statistics. But, as Sir A. Tulloch has used this period, we must do so, too, and show that his conclusion is not borne out by the facts.

2. He acknowledges that the Bengal returns are for the three healthiest months in the year, and yet the mortality was at the rate of 39 per 100 per annum, Madras 54 per 100 per annum, Bombay 58 per 1000 per annum, the returns for the two last Presidencies being for the more unhealthy seasons. This fact alone destroys his argument.

Source: Letter to Lord Stanley (secretary of state for India), Liverpool Record Office, Derby Collection 920/7/146/1

30 Old Burlington St.
21 July 1858

Dear Lord Stanley

Pray excuse me, in the first place, for this note. It has occurred to me (although probably it has occurred to you, if feasible, long ago) that, as the new government for India will soon be initiated [i.e., the crown's taking over of the administration of India from the East India Company], the sanitary state of stations and cantonments, to be henceforth occupied by British troops is one of the very first subjects for attention. I suppose it is not questioned that our Indian Empire must now be held by British troops. And a great point to be considered will be where these troops can best be placed for the twofold purpose of preserving their health and retaining possession of the country; without attention to the first, the drain upon us may prevent us from accomplishing the second. Perhaps an inquiry into the whole subject of the sanitary state of the Indian Army, the positions it has hitherto occupied and the more healthy positions where it may be possible to place it, without risking its military efficiency, might be entrusted to competent people, who should also point out the special precautions required as to barrack, hospitals, encampments and the selection of "*sanatoria*" to which invalids might be sent for recovery within a reasonable distance of their corps. There would be many kindred subjects of inquiry. I will not weary you with excuses, but remain, as shortly as I can, which is the best excuse,

yours faithfully
Florence Nightingale

Source: From two letters to Lord Stanley, Liverpool Record Office, Derby Collection 920/7/146/2 and 3. Copy of (1) and (2) in the second letter was also sent to Sidney Herbert, Wiltshire County Record Office, Pembroke Collection 2057/F4/67

24 July 1858

I ought to apologize for writing again, but that I take a much more hopeful view of the Indian sanitary case than you do. I know that you have been in India and understand it much better than I do. On the other hand, the greatest sanitary remedies are those discovered within the last five or eight years. The difficulties are, as you say, very great. But what is really wanted, in the first instance, is intelligent inquiry.

Formerly the loss in India was much greater than it is now. It has been reduced by various sanitary measures and there is no reason to doubt that it can be much further reduced. Formerly the West Indian stations were far more unhealthy than any in India. The losses were considered inevitable, until, after careful inquiry, it appeared that the chief causes were quite removable and they were removed accordingly. I believe there is no reason to fear but that India may be held quite safely by Englishmen. All the accounts I have received from these stations show that they are in what we should consider, even in England, a detestable sanitary state; I mean what would produce a dreadful sanitary destruction even here; and that they may be greatly improved. The difficulties you mention about the stations are precisely those which modern science has coped with and has overcome, and may cope with and overcome again, in order to render the military tenure of the country compatible with the safety of the army. When you have time to consider this subject more fully, I need not say that any help you thought we could give would be most eagerly given.

Much information already exists in this country. Should you be willing to grant us permission and afford us facilities for obtaining it, I think the first thing we could do would be to reduce it into a tangible shape for you.

Great Malvern
4 August 1858

Pray forgive me, once for all, the impertinence necessary for writing such a letter in answer to your note of 27 July. And take for granted the "I think"s and "in my opinion"s and "I humbly suggest"s, which, I perhaps feel in more sincerity than if I were to write them, ought to begin every sentence of mine to you. I entirely see the difficulty but I see no impossibility in an efficient sanitary inquiry for India.

1. It must be conducted in England, because in India there are not the men for it.

2. There are very few men in England who can do it. The Netley inquiry, of which you may have heard, shows this. It is alarming, not because we have lost a good army model hospital by it, though that is a great loss, but because it shows what an amount of error in opinion and information is always at the command of government. What should be now obtained from India are facts, not opinions. The opinions should be deduced at home by competent people.

3. I can see no way of doing this but by a course something similar to that adopted by the Royal Commission on the Sanitary State of the Army. Had the India bill passed before that commission sat, would it not have had to include an Indian inquiry? If so, this is only an extension and a continuation of that commission.

4. There is a great deal of documentary evidence at the India House. There are a great many Indians who might be examined at home by a commission. Lastly, the most important information would be obtained by forms of returns and printed questions to be constructed and sent out to India by, and returned to, the commission, filled up. This is always a much safer plan than that of sending for opinions, instead of facts, provided there is someone capable of *reading* these sanitary statistics and showing what they indicate. Therefore I think that:

1. this inquiry must be instituted in England,
2. by a commission of a few men of great experience, or it will fail,
3. the course taken by the royal sanitary commission gives good hints for it,
4. it must have power to institute inquiries in India and to issue circulars of printed questions to be filled up in India.

Sanitary matters are such a speciality and so new, and the subject is so enormous and of such immense importance, when applied to India, that I know no man, except yourself, who could preside over such a commission but Mr Herbert. I have not the least idea whether he would, and venture to mention him only with the proviso that I know nothing at all about it. Should you have time to preside over such a commission, I conclude that it is always best and shortest for the minister to do his work himself. I venture to enclose a kind of sketch of

1. what a commission would have to do,
2. what papers will be wanted for the very outset.

Should you think well to ask me to suggest names of commissioners or plan a proceeding for your consideration, I need not say I should be too glad. I could fancy something like the following commission working well:

| | |
|---|---|
| Chairman: | Lord Stanley or Mr Herbert |
| Sanitary members: | Dr Sutherland and Mr Martin |
| Medical: | Mr Alexander, director general |
| Engineering and Topographical: | Indians |
| Military: | Indians |
| Statistical: | Dr Farr |

(1)

1. Although the subject of inquiry is in India, the inquiry itself would be best conducted in England and extended to India, if necessary.

2. The best means of conducting such an inquiry would be by constituting a special commission, composed of persons conversant with the various matters connected with the inquiry, viz., sanitary, medical, engineering and topographical, military, statistical.

3. The commission should have ample powers of obtaining information and documents. It should have access to all documents in the India House relating to topography, diseases and mortality among the troops, supplies, etc., of every district in India where military stations have been or are likely to be placed. Likewise, to all documents relating to hospitals.

4. It should examine retired or acting medical, engineering and military officers, conversant with the stations in each of the presidencies. It should inquire into the sanitary condition of existing stations, with a view of recommending improvements. It should recommend improvements in existing stations, barracks and hospitals and in the diet, drink, dress, duties and exercises of soldiers.

5. It should point out the best positions for sanatoria and the method of using them so as to be most conducive to the health and efficiency of the troops.

6. It should inquire into the whole question of hill stations and recommend the best positions available for troops in a military and sanitary point of view.

7. It should further indicate the special provisions necessary for field hospital and field sanitary service, suitable to the different presidencies.

8. Also, any specialties in the organization of general and field hospitals, to make them more suitable for Indian service.

9. Also, the organization of medical boards for regulating the medical and sanitary service in the presidencies.

10. The commission to have power to extend its inquiries to India and to appoint persons for the purpose, subject to the approval of the minister.

(2) *Wanted*

1. The best India House map of India;
2. The trigonometrical survey, as far as completed;
3. List of all military stations, to be marked also on the maps;
4. Copies of all periodical reports of medical boards in presidencies which have been published;
5. Copies of all published army (Indian) statistical tables; same [of] queen's troops;
6. Lists of all places where there are permanent barracks and hospitals;
7. Access to catalogue of documents at India House and to all documents there, bearing on the inquiry;

Note. Upon the above data might be constructed forms of returns or printed questions to be sent out to India and returned, filled up for the commission to work upon.

Source: From a letter to Douglas Galton, Add Mss 45759 ff7-8

Great Malvern
31 July 1858

Private. I ought to tell you (PRIVATELY) the chief reason why I want him [Dr Sutherland] here, which is about Indian sanitary matters, referred to me by Lord Stanley. . . .

I feel quite raised in the scale of creation by being the cousin of a colonel in the Royal Engineers [Douglas Galton[8]].

8 Captain Douglas Galton (1822-99), permanent under secretary at the War Office, from which he retired in 1869 to work on the Army Sanitary Commission. He married Nightingale's cousin Marianne Nicholson in 1851. He was knighted in 1887.

Source: From a letter to Sidney Herbert, Wiltshire County Record Office, Pembroke Collection 2057/F4/67

Great Malvern
4 August 1858

As to what you say about the Indian sanitary inquiry, I entirely agree as to its difficulty, but not as to its impossibility.

1. I think it must be conducted in England, because in India there are not the men (to do it).

2. I think there are only a few men in England who can do it so as to be of any use because much of the information which will have to be obtained from India will be erroneous, or rather it will consist of opinions, not facts, and will have to be sifted by those who can sift. . . .

3. Again, I think this inquiry must be carried on, if undertaken at all, in something like the way your royal sanitary commission was, although I acknowledge the greater difficulty. Because you had, on that, some people whose conclusions were all ready-made in their heads, founded on experience of their own, which nothing could alter and nothing could take away from.

Still, had the India Bill [transferring the administration of India from the East India Company to the crown] passed before your royal sanitary commission sat you would have necessarily had to include the Indian inquiry in it and it is only an extension and continuation of that commission.

4. There are, I assure you, in England people from India who have *both* "livers" and "heads." And there is an immense deal of accumulated documentary evidence at the India House which, if sifted by those who are capable, would give a great deal of information not open to the objection which would attach to the information received at home from an inquiry instituted in India, which would transmit home opinions, not facts.

At the same time, this commission, if commission there be, must have power to institute inquiries of its own in India. And the most valuable part of this information would probably be derived from forms of returns which it would itself construct and send out, to be returned to it filled up. But these must be read by people who are capable of reading them.

I have just seen an instance of the reverse. I have just seen [W.H.] Burrell's [member of the Netley inquiry] notes on the South Eastern barracks enclosing returns filled up, Galton's notes, who has not seen the returns, and Sutherland's. Burrell has written his, as if he had not seen the returns. And nevertheless the readings from these will make the most important part of the South Eastern inspections report.

To sum up, I think:

1. that the inquiry as to Indian sanitary things must be instituted in England and by a commission;

2. that this must consist of a few men of great experience in this way, or it had better not sit at all;

3. that it must follow much the course of the former royal sanitary commission;

4. that it must have power to institute inquiries and to issue circulars of printed questions to be filled up in India.

I assure you that I have not been so good as to offer your services to Lord Stanley, which I am afraid you will think I have. But I enclose copies of suggestions I have made to him this day. (I had a second letter from him saying "only show me how we are to set to work," and offering and asking for "information.")

My belief is that, if he has a commission with any other chairman, he will bring together a great mass of blunders instead of information, as the commission for the Indian Army is, as you say, a blunder. You call Hawes[9] an "inconvenient little dolt." But that commission will prove an inconvenient large dolt. Believe me, I do not even wish, much less hope, that you will undertake this. I only think Lord Stanley had better let it alone, if you don't.

Source: From an incomplete letter to Lord Stanley, Liverpool Record Office, Derby Collection 920/7/146/4

Great Malvern
10 August 1858

Thank you very much for your note of 5 August and for your promise of consideration. From you to whom the subject is not new, from you who have already given so much attention to it, the promise of consideration is equivalent to the greatest benefits accruing from it for India.

The history of all our wars and of all our possessions has clearly shown how much it may cost the mother country, *un*necessarily, in valuable life, to keep possession of even a few square miles, unless we

9 Sir Benjamin Hawes (1797-1862), permanent under secretary of war 1857-62. He typified Nightingale's difficult collaborators among officials at the War and India Offices.

master the conditions on which the soil of a country can be held by foreigners. Over and over again our troops have been actually destroyed without an effort to save them, and it has never (hitherto) been, until public attention has been called to the subject, that very ordinary and very well-known precautions adapted to the climate have been put in force, when our mortality has immediately diminished. In India, the same problems are presented in another way. They must be carefully examined and studied by themselves. In this way will be found what are those natural laws which must be obeyed before the white man can hold this vast empire with the least risk to himself. These laws will vary of course (within limits in such an extent of country), of such different degrees of elevation and occupying such very different zones. Your commission will have to determine what these laws are. The subject, as a government inquiry, is a special one, probably, except to yourself, almost a new one. But there is no doubt that, by bringing European experience to bear upon it, many of the problems affecting the health of this white man in our Eastern Empire, will be speedily solved and the military occupation of the country rendered much more easy in time to come.

I need not say that, whatever experience we have is at your disposal a month hence, or any time you may choose to call for it, if you think it will be of any good. I have hesitated even to write thus much, in your present press of business. You have doubtless heard of a discovery which seems likely to afford a test you were inquiring after. Angus Smith[10] has clearly proved the possibility of testing the quantity of organic matter in any given air. He has not yet determined the scale. But he has shown that the scale is *determinable.* He finds that blood, when shaken together [breaks off]

Source: From two memoranda and a letter to Lord Stanley, Liverpool Record Office, Derby Collection 920/7/146/5-7

12 August 1858

PRIVATE. The remarks which you have been so good as to send (enclosed) contain the substance of the objections generally raised against India. They are founded on the assumption that there is something deadly, inherent in all tropical climates. And that, somehow or other, disease and death are to be the penalty of "subduing the

---

10 Robert Angus Smith (1817-84), chemist, water expert.

earth."[11] The discovery of the reasons for local unhealthiness is often difficult. And when people unaccustomed to such inquiries come in contact with these problems, they are apt to overlook such reasons and take refuge in fatalism. Ague prevailed in temperate climates, until draining was discovered, and the fevers mentioned (in the enclosed) as growing in gardens will grow there, until man has learnt how to use water in tropical climates. This, in fact, is the main problem to be solved by your committee.

The very last report[12] which proceeded from the defunct board of health but a few days ago lays the blame of the excess of infantile mortality (which, since the first board was broken up, it has taken no pains to present) on infection and contagion. It adduces a scheme of statistics to prove that sanitary measures are not of much use, a scheme which everyone conversant with statistical inquiries knows to be simply nonsense. If this be done in the green tree, what will be done in the dry?[13]

So far from blaming the "old Indians," let science and experience be brought to bear on the Indian question; there is no doubt it can be solved. The enclosed is the case against us. Let us give the case for.

15 August 1858

Private. In re Mr Simon.[14] There are few things more painful to have to do than to discredit a professional man. And one would only do it for the sake of numbers. Mr Simon's work has always been what may fairly be called "scampish," in the language of the trades: his writings must always be considered as the result of a "prospecting" expedition, as they call it in the gold countries. The last report of the board of health, to which I have alluded, and the report on Netley Hospital are indications of this. "All sanitary precautions are to be undervalued" because they have become unpopular; "epidemics to be declared inevitable" and "quarantine to be substituted for sanitary

11 An allusion to Gen 1:28.

12 *Papers Relating to the Sanitary State of the People of England,* June 1858, included an introduction by John Simon to a major paper by E.H. Greenhow, "The Results of an Inquiry into the Different Proportions of Death Produced by Certain Diseases in Different Districts in England," which Nightingale felt disparaged preventive sanitary measures.

13 An allusion to Luke 23:31.

14 John Simon (1816-1904), later Sir, medical officer of the Board of Health, later of the Privy Council.

improvement"—quarantine, which it was well nigh hoped, had become an extinct superstition. This last report of the board of health has all the error of what Dr Farr's forthcoming report will have all the truth.

Great Malvern
15 August 1858

*Private.* [I] I will lose no time in answering your note. From the experience of similar committees, it may be gathered:

1. that to collect evidence *merely* in England will not fulfill the object. Sir G. Clerk's[15] memorandum is an example of this. For although it states facts, it grounds opinions, now considered untenable, upon them. Present knowledge leads us to believe that the very unhealthiness of which he complains might be prevented. Similar statements would be repeated before the committee without end. And the practical result would be "voted to be this," viz., that India is *essentially* an unhealthy country, a result upheld by every "old Indian" till *now.* Hence

2. the committee might have to make personally, or to direct to be made by practised persons, inquiries on the spot, in order to test the truth of such allegations. Considering the supreme importance of the subject, it would be necessary to give the committee or commission as wide a scope as possible.

II. As to the constitution:

1. It would not answer the object to exclude every element from the inquiry except the medical. The subjects of inquiry, engineering, military, sanitary and medical, must be exhausted before it can draw up its report. Persons acquainted with only one of these departments would never be able to draw up either report, regulations or instructions, involving necessarily the duties of engineers, military and sanitary officers. Whether committee or commission, it should consist of (1) Indian military officers of high rank, (2) Indian military engineer (Colonel [Henry] Goodwyn, Bengal Army???) and topographer (Colonel [Andrew Scott] Waugh? I suppose one might as soon ask for Sir C[olin] Campbell), (3) Indian medical officer conversant with san-

15 Sir George Clerk (1800-89), permanent under secretary of state for India 1858-60, the highest-ranking civil servant. Nightingale had a rather bleak opinion of the staff at the India House. But she knew how important senior bureaucrats were, as they could help as well as hinder her cause.

itary subjects (Mr Martin), (4) civil sanitarian conversant with army arrangements, barracks, camps, etc. (Dr Sutherland), (5) civil engineer conversant with sanitary practice (Mr Rawlinson, C.E., by far our best water engineer), (6) statistician (Dr Farr): the statistics could not be "*read*" without him.

2. AND MOST IMPORTANT: I cannot conceive any practical result coming out of a committee without a chairman who, from his position as well as from his knowledge, can keep them in order. There will otherwise be no consistency in the whole inquiry and there will be infinite difference of opinion. Committees never do anything very well or very ill. They come to a compromise. Who is to reconcile jarring opinions? The chairman must be conversant with such subjects, in order to direct the inquiry in a proper channel, and must be selected with special reference to his experience and to his capacity *for good principle.* (I only know of two such.)

3. The inquiry cannot be a hurried one. And those who undertake it would have to devote themselves to it for such time and in such manner as may be (and will be) found to be indispensable for success.

III. The result of forming a committee of the three persons you have named and of making the inquiry in the manner proposed would be this, viz., to arrive at nothing more than an abstract of existing opinions, valuable in itself, but it could be nothing more than an *aide-mémoire.* (One of the persons named—Mr Simon—has no practical opinion at all and no experience of *army* or *topographical* questions. Of him more anon.)

To sum up: the object of the inquiry is, undoubtedly, to obtain the practical results you mention. But, to do so, there must be competent engineering assistance and evidence, because the result of the inquiry ought not to be *only* to point out positions for cantonments, but also the precautions to take in order to make sites more healthy. Such precautions being for the most part engineering works, it is necessary that such works should be recommended by capable engineers and the proposed "manual" stamped with engineering authority. Such a manual would be useful. But proper regulations to be always followed would be far more useful. The committee or commission should draft these for consideration. And such regulations will involve military, engineering and medical points. The committee must, therefore, contain all these elements. Also, it must speak "as one having authority."[16] Its

16 An allusion to Matt 7:29.

report must command attention with the country. A report from the three men *alone* mentioned by you would not. If you were to be minister for India for the next quarter of a century, this would, comparatively, not signify, but, with an India Council to be composed probably generally of "old Indians," what would the report of such a commission do as to influencing them without you? It would simply carry no weight. . . .

If you think a royal commission unadvisable, at all events it will be as much more "distingué" (as Lord Castlereagh[17] was without orders) to be without one. The only points to be secured are:

1. that the men are specially suited for all departments of the work,
2. that the committee have power enough,
3. that the chairman be *au fait* of the subject,
4. that there be power to extend the inquiry to India, if necessary.

If you see fit, I would write down a few heads for the instructions.

F.N.

P.S. Out of the following list of names of Indian engineering officers, now in England, I believe a really good man might be chosen to serve on the committee: Colonel Henry Goodwyn, Colonel G.T. Greene (Bengal Army), Captain J. Ouchterlony (Madras Army), Lieutenant Colonel C.N. Grant (Bombay Army).

Source: From an incomplete letter to Sidney Herbert, Wiltshire County Record Office, Pembroke Collection 2057/F4/67

19 August 1858

At the risk of annoying you, I think I had better tell you how Lord Stanley is going on. He wrote to me [14 August 1858] thus:

"How would this do? Drs Martin, Sutherland, Simon, to conduct the inquiry here, without royal commissions or any such pompous delays, without compulsory powers, but with all that we could give them in collecting evidence from Indian witnesses; special instructions to them not to produce a last Blue Book, but to embody in their report whatever facts they thought worth preserving; the subjects of inquiry to be health of troops, in first instance, and next, the sanitary conditions under which European life is possible in India; their report to be in size, style and subject such that it might serve as a manual to

17 Viscount Robert Stewart Castlereagh (1769-1822), 2nd marquess of Londonderry, foreign secretary and plenipotentiary at peace congress of Vienna in 1814.

engineers planning cantonments, to officers in charge of troops and to intruding settlers in India. Tell me if you approve and I will speak to the chairs and get the thing in train at once."

He enclosed a long letter to himself from Sir G. Clerk, approving of a "commission of inquiry," but giving all the arguments of the "*old Indians*" to prove that India *must* be unhealthy, as it was from the beginning, is now and ever shall be, world without end.[18] Lord Stanley concludes, "I have heard the same thing propounded by others. Possibly you may know whether it is a vulgar prejudice or a scientific truth."

Fortunately for you I have no copy of my answer. But unfortunately for you I think it expedient to recapitulate my arguments, viz.,

1. That from experience it may be found that (1) it will not do merely to collect evidence in England. Sir G. Clerk's letter confirms this, for, although it states facts, it grounds opinions on them now known to be untenable. Present knowledge tells us the very unhealthiness of which he complains might have been prevented. Before such a commission as that named by Lord Stanley similar statements would be repeated without end, and the practical result would be that every "old Indian" will uphold that India is *essentially* unhealthy. Hence (2) the committee would have to make personally, or to direct to be made on the spot by practical persons, inquiries to test the truth of such allegations.

Considering the supreme importance of the subject, it would be necessary to give the committee or commission as wide [a] scope as possible.

2. As to the constitution, it would not do to exclude every element except the medical. The subjects of inquiry, engineering, military, sanitary and medical, must be exhausted before the report is drawn up. People acquainted with only one of these subjects would never be able to draw up either. . . .

MOST IMPORTANT. There must be a chairman over all to *direct* the inquiry, to give consistency to it and to prevent differences of opinion. He must not only have experience in this special subject, but be of such a position as will carry weight with public opinion.

3. The inquiry must not be hurried and the men who undertake it will have to work at it long and hard. To conduct the inquiry by the three men named (alone) and in the manner named by Lord Stanley would be to arrive at nothing more than an abstract of existing opin-

---

18 An allusion to a liturgical formula based on Matt 24:21 and Eph 3:21.

ions, an aide-mémoire or manual—very useful. But regulations which must be followed would be much more useful. Also, Lord Stanley might be out of office before the report or manual was ready. And then, what influence would it have with a council of "old Indians"? There MUST be a chairman to carry weight with the country.

Also, if Lord Stanley wants an abstract of existing opinion, one of the persons he names, Mr Simon, has no opinions at all and has had no practical experience of army topography whatever. The object of the inquiry should be, certainly, to obtain the practical results Lord Stanley mentions. In order to do so, however, there must be competent engineering assistance and evidence, because the result should not be *only* to point out positions for cantonments, but precautions to be taken in making sites more healthy. Such precautions being for the most part engineering works, they must be recommended by capable engineers; a manual for engineers must be stamped with engineering authority.

But the committee or commission must also draft regulations for consideration and such regulations involving military, engineering and medical points; it must contain all these elements.

Sir G. Clerk's letter contained the substance of the objections generally raised against India, founded on the *assumption* that there is something deadly inherent in all tropical climates and that, somehow or other, disease and death must be the penalty of subduing the earth. The discovery of the reasons for local unhealthiness is often difficult. And when people unaccustomed to such inquiries come in contact with these problems, they are very apt to take refuge in fatalism. We used to have ague here till draining was discovered. Sir G. Clerk mentions fevers as growing in gardens in India. And so they will, till man has learnt how to use water in tropical climates.

The very last report which proceeded from the defunct Board of Health (by Mr Simon) only a few days ago lays the blame of the excess of infantile mortality—which, since the first board was broken up, it has taken no means to prevent—on infection and contagion, two exploded superstitions. And it puts forward a scheme of statistics (simply trash) to prove that sanitary precautions have been greatly overvalued, that epidemics are inevitable and that quarantine is to be substituted for sanitary improvements.

Mr Simon's publications must be considered in the light of a "prospecting" expedition, as they call it in the gold countries. His work may fairly be called "scampish," in the language of the trades.

So far from blaming the "old Indians," they are a green tree compared with the dry one of our old Board of Health. But the Indian question will not be solved by them and we must do it for them.

If Lord Stanley does not like a royal commission, it will be more "distingué" (as Lord Castlereagh was without any orders) to have none. And it does not matter much, provided the inquiry be conducted by men specially suited for all departments of the work, by a chairman who can give unity and precision to it, and with power to extend it to India, if found necessary. . . .

Mrs Herbert will say that I give you the best possible argument for not coming back to England [he was in Salzburg, Austria], which I acknowledge.

Source: From a letter to Lord Stanley, Liverpool Record Office, Derby Collection 920/7/146/8

Great Malvern
31 August 1858

Do you think that you would be so good as to let me see a copy of your instructions under which the royal commission on the reorganization of the Indian Army is acting? if not illegitimate the asking.

Source: From a copy of a letter to A.H. Clough,[19] British Library RP 3451

31 August 1858

I do not really mind about Mr Herbert's coming back, in connection with the "thing." *That* does not signify. But I am afraid there will be a great deal that will very much signify, in connection with his coming back and with an *Indian* sanitary commission, which I am agitating about, as I dare say you know.

Source: From two letters to Lord Stanley, Liverpool Record Office, Derby Collection 920/7/146/9 and 10

5 September 1858

I have no doubt that the amount of amateur advice you receive is to you the "intolerable deal of sack" to the "ha'porth of bread"[20] which

---

19 Arthur Hugh Clough (1819-61), married to Nightingale's cousin, Blanche Smith. See the biographical sketch in *Life and Family* (1:841-42).

20 Shakespeare, *King Henry IV*, Act 2, scene 4. See the breakfast scene in chapter 5 of Charles Dickens, *Nicholas Nickleby*.

last you don't get. Nevertheless I remembered what you said, that you wished to turn your attention to the sanitary subject, after you were crowned king of the Indian Council. And seeing that event had taken place, I came to town. Since I wrote to you, I have received farther information and made more inquiries. The farther I go, the deeper in importance to the interests of the empire does the subject appear.

I also wrote to Mr Herbert who is (or was) in Austria; he fully sees the immense importance of the question and its connection with the general army sanitary question (which came before his own commission), as well as with the spécialités of the Indian Army. And he will give every aid, I know, in any proceedings you may wish to take in the matter, if you wished it.

12 September 1858

Thank you for your note, received from Malvern. I expected that the "organization" commission would not touch the sanitary question. And I am glad it does not, as the subject is *special* and will require very careful and full investigation by persons competent. The experience of the royal sanitary commission is important and will afford much assistance. The report gives the results simply, but it does not show the immense care required in dealing with the question. There was hardly anything to begin with. The thing, in fact, from the statistical inquiry with which we began, up to the final recommendations (with the important practical proceedings now flowing from them), had all to be worked quietly and with the utmost care. And the result was that we laid the basis of a military sanitary system for the first time in Europe, and which promises to bear fruit.

The same course will have to be taken with the Indian inquiry. Those who touch it must devote themselves to it. And I have no doubt, if you fairly launch it and select the proper working men, similar results will follow. What we found of most use was practical sanitary experience. Mere figures and scientific talk did very little for us. I am sure that the men who did the practical work of the royal sanitary commission will be willing in the public interest to do the Indian work also. I did not expect that, with the immense interests now in your hand, you could attend immediately to the sanitary question, however important. And I should apologize for having written to you, had you not named the period of the meeting of the Council for the time you would wish to attend to this.

Source: From two letters to Sidney Herbert, Wiltshire County Record Office, Pembroke Collection 2057/F4/67

15 September 1858

About the Indian matter, I think it is "as well as can be expected." Since you were so very good as to say that YOU would undertake the matter, the chief fear has been that Lord Stanley would say his "organization" commission could do it. He is however convinced:

1. That it has neither men nor "instructions" to touch it at all. "The best means of securing the efficiency" of troops raised for India service is the only sentence in their instructions which can be construed to mean sanitary reform at all. And Lord Stanley says it does *not.* I am glad of it.

2. He is convinced that the subject *ought to* be dealt with and "separately" and "fully" and "urgently." These are all his own words. He says he cannot do anything *directly*. But I do not think he will do anything without consulting you. And that is the main matter. And as he will do no mischief, which is satisfactory, I hope in a few weeks he will be able to do good. He has not committed himself to anything either way.

I am going to Malvern tonight, because I know, if I were to stay, I could not keep my hands off tormenting you. But I hope you will be so very good as to let me know when you come to town. I suppose you may perhaps be "looking up" the creatures in a fortnight's time? Please don't deceive me. Because it is nothing to me to come up.

8 October 1858

One of Alexander's[21] best men, Muir,[22] has been appointed sanitary officer at Bombay. He reports to his chief that the sanitary abominations there are quite enough to account for our mortality. The same at Calcutta.

I had a note from Lord Stanley this morning. But not a word about the commission. The wretch is at Knowsley. How dare he be at Knowsley?[23] Is he persuading his Papa?

---

21 Dr Thomas Alexander (1812-60), director general of the Army Medical Department.

22 Sir William Muir (1819-1905), head of the intelligence department at Agra during the Mutiny, foreign secretary under Sir John Lawrence. He was lieutenant governor of the North West Provinces 1868-74 and a lecturer at Cambridge.

23 The earls of Derby owned the Knowsley estate in Lancashire; Lord Stanley's father was the 14th earl of Derby, prime minister. Nightingale later had to write to Lord Stanley regarding the system of cultivation and settlement he recommended, which she considered to be unsafe (see p 71 below).

## Relations with Edwin Chadwick

**Editor:** Among Nightingale's collaborators in London was Edwin Chadwick (1800-90), later Sir, Britain's leading sanitarian and a skillful publicist.[24] Although by then he held no public office, his friendship was important for his strategic contacts. For a while Chadwick had been insisting that something be done for India, and trying to influence Lord Stanley in that direction. He wrote to Nightingale on 18 August 1858:

> On Friday I had an interview with Lord Stanley on the Indian Army question to give him explanations preparatory to making an application to him in writing, which I may hereafter get called for. I proposed the preparation of a sanitary aide-memoire officially for India, prepared in the way in which I once explained to you. I proposed to act for the purpose, if he thought fit, with Dr Sutherland. The answer I got was that nothing would be done on the subject until the new Indian Council was appointed. I told him that I should probably open the subject at the Liverpool meeting, to which he said there would not be the slightest objection. I intimated my resolve not to let the subject drop though the government might not do so. He stated that his attention had been called to my article in the *North British* which he had as yet only read cursorily.[25]

To Nightingale's request for further assistance on India Chadwick wrote: "I have thought it my duty to avail myself of desperate chances to get into the House for the sake of the cause, but I have been jockeyed at all points in electoral matters. . . . By political differences, at present, I am shut out from any aid . . . , but I wish you to be assured that I shall be watchful to contend against odds. I will endeavour to get another interview with Lord Stanley on the Indian Army [sanitary] question."[26]

Then on 10 May 1859 Chadwick sent Nightingale an important letter:

> I was about to send a reminder to Lord Stanley of my suggestion to him eight months ago of a commission for the sanitary improvement of the Indian Army, when I received your note of information [of 9 May]. I have heard nothing, though he promised me immediate attention at the time. It might be well to urge on Mr Sidney Herbert particular attention as to his colleagues on the commission, as

---

24 See the biographical sketch in *Society and Politics* (5:828-29).

25 ADD Mss 45770 ff34-37; Chadwick's article is "Our Army in India," 29 (August-November 1858):211-43.

26 Letter 4 May 1859, ADD Mss 45770 ff96-97.

> the choice, which should be given to him, involves the extent of his labour if not his entire success.
>
> The Indian Army sanitary commission may be made the means of sharpening up and advancing all sanitary doctrines and doing more than make good the deficiencies of the first sanitary commission as respects the army at home; the definitions as to what is preventible may be made more clear and sharp; the subject may be got beyond mere medical generalia, where medical sanitary professors mostly stay; it may be advanced to more clear perceptions of the means, the sanitary and special engineering works; and it may be got beyond these, where the sanitary engineers stay, to the administrative machinery, the financial and the official, organization, returns, reports, checks, etc., and the whole, medical, structural and official, combined to an executive result. I shall be most happy to give Mr S. Herbert any assistance in my power to these ends, but it makes one of my disamusements that, as the sanitary cause or sanitary science advances, it becomes more and more difficult to act otherwise than directly. I would gladly have crammed members of Parliament or anyone, and the cram sufficed for the first generalia but, when we advance to executive particulars, the cram fails; you cannot foresee objections and there are few who can be crammed to sustain *themselves* upon them or to cross-examine witnesses urging [?] them. It is the increased trouble required for indirect, as we get on, that I find so discouraging after being used to more direct action, from the time required being greater, every day remaining to me being equal to two formerly, and strength and certainty of result diminishing. I shall however do whatsoever I may.[27]

Obviously Nightingale used several points in this letter to define the parameters of the second commission. It should also be pointed out that Chadwick was also, for Nightingale, the conduit to John Stuart Mill.

Source: From a letter to Edwin Chadwick, Add Mss 45770 ff50-51

7 October 1858

So little is known and so much has to be done as to sanitary affairs in India that I think you must treat it [in his article] from your own point of view. I know no one who can do it so well. You see no one has come up to yours in the *North British*. . . . I hope we shall hear that something is being done by the government about Indian sanitary matters soon.

---

27 Add Mss 45770 ff100-03.

Source: From a letter to Edwin Chadwick, ADD Mss ff60-61

11 October 1858

From the information which I have received, I should say that it would be unsafe to recommend the system of cultivation and settlement to which you allude. For you might be met by a statement that clearing and cultivation are uniformly attended by pestilence. One of the great points with regard to Indian inquiry is to ascertain how to cultivate (not only with safety but) with increase of salubrity. The statement almost amounts to a proverb in India, wherever you make a garden, you make a graveyard. The West India experience is too limited to establish a rule.

Source: From two letters to Lord Stanley, Liverpool Record Office, Derby Collection 920/7/146/11 and 12

9 October 1858

I am glad you received the volumes which I sent to you. You will see that they are strictly "confidential." I thought you would like to see them. And indeed I felt bound to send them, as they have so direct a bearing on the subject of our correspondence about the sanitary state of the Indian Army.

You will find at page VIII, Preface to section X, p 234, the statistics of the present state of that army, and I am persuaded that four fifths, if not five sixths, of that dire loss may be saved to the country. The Indian inquiry, which one would be glad to see begun, is a necessary pendant to that regarding the army at home. Its hospital questions are identical. Indeed the whole hospital question as regards India must be gone into. They require reorganization as much as our own home and war hospitals. The barrack arrangements also require to be considered. I constantly receive evidence to show that remov*able* defects *are* destroying and have destroyed (in times past) the lives of multitudes who might have lived to serve their country. And there is no doubt that many lives are annually sacrificed by the state of the hospitals. The subject is of far too great importance to the interest of the empire and of humanity to be left in abeyance.

16 October 1858

*Private.* A more painful case in point could hardly have occurred than the one I feel bound to enclose to you, although you may have seen it. It illustrates all that has been said, all our administrative defects. It is as bad on a small scale as anything which happened in the Crimea on a large one.

Observe: commanding officers, medical officers, government officers, all doing the same thing. All ought to have been brought to a court martial. What was Shah Sorja [Siraj] and his Black Hole[28] to this? and all within five miles of Calcutta. Observe the want of any military organization of the most ordinary sanitary knowledge. And then the man drives back to Calcutta and makes a minute. Meanwhile the women are dead. Yet I know the people existing now who will say, "the ordinary and inevitable effect of the Indian climate! what could you expect? women and children *will* die in India"!

I understand that Sir A. Tulloch and Mr Martin are to be examined on the 23rd before your organization commission, Sir A. Tulloch on sanitary points. After what you told me, that there was not a man on that commission fit to touch these points, it is perhaps an excess of caution to tell you that Sir A. Tulloch is quite unfit to be examined upon them. His figures are unimpeachable. He and Sir J. McNeill were the saving of the Crimean Army as to supply. But as to sanitary things, Tulloch has never turned his attention to them and will only mislead. The subject is a special one and demands a special inquiry, as you say. With many apologies for again troubling you.

Source: From a letter to Lady Canning, West Yorkshire Archive Service 177/2/3

5 November 1858

There is sufficient evidence to show that a great amount of disease in India springs from intoxication among the troops, especially on landing, and that the evil is greatly increased by poisonous liquors sold in the native bazaars. There is evidence also of great saving of health and life having been effected by supplying the men with wholesome liquors *under suitable regulations.* Could not something more be done in providing proper canteens under proper regulations at all the stations and in putting down all other traffic in liquor near the men's quarters?

To me, who have seen Scutari in the year of its drunkenness and Scutari in the year of its sobriety, the soldier appears the most hopeful member of mankind for this experiment. I have described the process of cure at Scutari at page 452 of my report.[29] Of course the same pro-

---

28 A reference to the infamous "Black Hole of Calcutta," the name given to a tiny airless cell in which members of the British contingent at Fort William were imprisoned during a siege of the garrison by Shah Siraj-ud-Daula in 1756. John Zephaniah Holwell, a survivor of the siege, became famous for his account of the incident, published in 1758.

29 *Notes Affecting the Health, Efficiency and Hospital Administration. . . .*

cess will not do for India, I am well aware. Games under cover and amusements must be necessary for the men everywhere.

2. The terrible catastrophe at Dum Dum and the evidence as to the enormous rate of mortality among soldiers' wives and children prove the necessity of providing proper "married quarters" at every station. Space and fresh air are wanted as well as needful conveniences. It is terrible to think of these poor women and children suffering when so much of it can be prevented. Could not something more be done in India to remedy this defect?

Source: From a letter to Lord Stanley, Liverpool Record Office, Derby Collection 920/7/146/13

23 December 1858

Might I ask a very few minutes' conversation with you, as I am going out of town for some time in a few days. I am quite aware of the presumption of this proposition. Please refuse it, if it is very inconvenient.

Source: From a letter to Sidney Herbert, Wiltshire County Record Office, Pembroke Collection 2057/F4/67

27 December 1858

On Friday I took my courage by the forelock and wrote to Lord Stanley to ask him to come and see me. The reason of my doing this wild act was that I thought, if it failed, it would only pass for a foolish woman's love of being busy, and if it succeeded it would succeed. I took care to let Lord Stanley know when he came that you were not particeps [involved].

He came today. There are so many things that both he and I could say which it would not be fair upon him to ask him to write and which it would not be fair upon you to ask me to write. Bref [in short], he *says* he will write to you *directly* to ask you to be chairman and to select your own tools. I confine my eloquence or my stupidity to these three points. I confine my reasons to merely showing him an Indian map which I have now completed with the mortality of Queen's and East India Company troops, written under each station, and to telling him the practical results which you have given to your first royal *sanitary* commission, also recapitulating to him what you had said in your letters from [Bad] Gastein [Salzburg], the substance of which he had seen before. . . .

Lord Stanley says that he was only waiting for the end of organization commission, but says that he will not now wait for that. "At all events," he added, "the work of that commission will be finished by the meeting of Parliament." . . .

Lord Stanley said that he must speak to Lord Derby [his father, the prime minister] first. So he has not done it yet. I am afraid I am a bad ambassador. I am too anxious. But if Lord Stanley will just write to you and put the matter into your hands, I shall be satisfied and leave you to fight your own battles. And I promise, as the old Prussian general said in his prayers, only give me this once, and I never will pray to you again.

Source: From a letter to Sidney Herbert, Wiltshire County Record Office, Pembroke Collection 2057/F4/68

Great Malvern
1 January 1859

I think, with you, that you must use Lord Stanley's proposal, when it comes, as a lever to get the regulations and the council. But there will be much preliminary work to do in preparing the ground for your Indian inquiry. I should, if I were you, accept first, when Lord Stanley writes, and then put in the lever. If Lord S. understands that you must and will have the army matters settled before you move, he will then give General Peel[30] a little shove. But as the regulations and council will go on moving through the War Office, till they have a corporal of sappers and miners, a hospital sergeant and a purveyor's clerk sitting upon you, with an apothecary's boy in the chair, I bet you a penny that the Indian inquiry is all done, which will take at least three years (interim reports and interim action having been set agoing in the meantime) *before the other.* General Peel can't manage his subordinates and Lord Stanley can.

2. With regard to the commissioners, Lord Stanley asked whether the former commission, *minus* Andrew Smith,[31] would do. I left it to you to answer that question, my impression being that, except Alexander and Sutherland, you found them heavy in hand. What would you think of having those two again (Alexander for his own instruction)?

3. Martin, who is necessary for his Indian knowledge.

4. Farr, without whom the statistics would be with difficulty done, as he has clerks; Tulloch and Balfour have not an idea of doing figures, except with their *own* pens.

---

30 Jonathan Peel (1799-1879), general, brother of Sir Robert Peel, secretary of state for war.

31 Dr Andrew Smith (1797-1872), later Sir, director general of the Army Medical Department during the Crimean War, and for Nightingale a major cause of the lack of planning and disastrous results.

Does it not seem to you essential to have one Indian military engineer and one Indian military officer? If desirable to have members of the Indian Council, Sir Proby Cautley[32] might do for the first and Sir Richard [member of the Council of India 1858-74] for the second. But Lord Stanley volunteered to say that there was not one member on the Council who knew anything about sanitary things or how to spell the word, and specially instanced Sir P. Cautley as prominent in ignorance. In this, Lord S. differs from Mr Martin, who gives them rather a good character. I did not press, for I did not feel sure of what you might think about having a member of the Council on.

Colonel Goodwyn, Bengal Engineers, now at home, bears a very high character. Lieutenant Colonel Waugh, Bengal Engineers, surveyor general of India, now in India, is I suppose the first topographer in Europe (that is Irish). Would you think it well to make inquiries about these men? (It might be as impossible to let Colonel Waugh, as Lord Canning, come home. That I don't know.) With regard to Balfour as secretary, it might be difficult to find a better man. To have a man who knows more of India would have advantages and also disadvantages. He would be prejudiced. Balfour is not a little in that line too, however. His great value lay in having materials in his possession of so much value, of which he did not know the value before. (There would not be this for India.)

I think it would be worthwhile to see what they have got at the India House that would do as a secretary, though very likely to return to Balfour. I should like to know whether you decide for or against a man of the Indian Council to be on the commission.

N.B. Lord Stanley told me that Lord Canning insisted upon large masses of troops as necessary at Allahabad and objected to having them at Dugshai, Mussoorie, etc., our hill stations. Now it so happens that Allahabad stands highest but one of all our stations in mortality—115 per 1000. To decide what can be done to make unhealthy stations healthy will be the aim of your commission. It does not require Tulloch to tell us that troops will be healthy if removed to healthy stations. But, if it be necessary for our holding of India to have numbers at a place with a loss of 11½ percent, can you conceive our holding India at such a price? . . .

Do you know John Stuart Mill? a most intelligent but very odd man, now at liberty. He did the foreign relations at the India House, Sir

32 Sir Proby Thomas Cautley (1802-71), irrigation expert and paleontologist, best known for the construction of the Ganges Canal.

George Clerk the others. Perhaps this would prevent his being useful as a commissioner in the way you want. What the *Times* said of him was quite unfair.

## Relationship with John Stuart Mill (1806-73)

**Editor:** Nightingale read Mill's writings early in her life and learned much from his philosophy, although she had problems with his views on free will, necessity, law and God. They never met, but collaborated on matters of Poor Law reform, nursing, women's rights and suffrage. See the biographical sketch of Mill in *Society and Politics* (5:829-31) and material in *Public Health Care* (6:418-19, 423-27). The India question remained a marginal one in Mill's relationship with Nightingale. Mill had been an employee of the East India Company until its demise in 1858. For that reason Nightingale thought he could be of help in her India work. In 1859 she entertained the idea of proposing him as a member of the second royal commission, but wondered whether "it would be infra his dig to ask him to be secretary" in the first item below. The idea was altogether rejected because he was seen as too much identified with the "old" regime and the Company (see p 88 below). In 1862 she confided to Chadwick, always the intermediary between Mill and herself, that Mill "had been excessively kind to me" (see p 120 below), doubtless for having consented to read her *Suggestions for Thought.* Again via Chadwick she sent him the proof of her *Observations* for information and comment. It is not clear that he received the paper. Mill's election to Parliament in 1865 led Nightingale to hope for his help "in India sanitary matters" (see p 532 below), and to ask Chadwick whether she should write to Mill and solicit his support (see p 530 below), a query she repeated a year later (see p 557 below). She eventually did write to Mill on 11 August 1867 (*Society and Politics* 5:394-97), asking him "for his influence on" the India Public Health Service. Mill did not react to the invitation, which left Nightingale disappointed, saying in 1868 that "Mr Mill has never helped me about India" (see p 614 below). Mill died in 1873 and Nightingale wrote to Mme Mohl: "When Mill left the India Office he might most materially have helped all my sanitary commissions, irrigation and civilizing schemes for India. He did nothing."[33]

33 Cook, *The Life of Florence Nightingale* 2:316.

Source: From a dictated letter to A.H. Clough, Balliol College Archives lot 305/4

Great Malvern
2 January [1859]

Do you think John Stuart Mill would do for the Indian sanitary commission as a commissioner? I suppose it would be infra his dig to ask him to be secretary. I make this inquiry quite privately and am not authorized.

Source: From a dictated letter signed by Nightingale to Sir John McNeill, Florence Nightingale Museum (LMA) H1/ST/NC3/59/SU108

Great Malvern
13 January 1859

I am sorry that Sir Charles Trevelyan is going to Madras. I think they might have found many a man to make as good or better a governor, I doubt whether they will find many or perhaps any to make as good a Treasury secretary. But I think he may be of great use to us in sanitarizing the condition of the troops at Madras.

Lady Trevelyan does not go. She remains in London for the sake of the children.

Source: From a dictated letter to Sir Charles Trevelyan, signed by Nightingale, Newcastle University Library 35/7

Great Malvern
14 January [1859]

Thank you very very much for your kind note and for your permission to send you any suggestions about the sanitary state of the troops in India. You will do us essential good there. I cannot write to you at present, but I engage to do so as ardently as you like. The opportunity is too good to be lost. We shall avail ourselves of it in due time—more ardently perhaps than you will like. You are going to Madras but all India is what you are going for, no doubt. A Madras governor general could easily have been found or made, without such a sacrifice, I mean to the country in losing such an officer at home, and to you in leaving home.

Source: From a letter to Lord Stanley, Liverpool Record Office, Derby Collection 920/7/146/14

22 March 1859

I have just been put in possession of the general tenor of the report of your commission on the organization of the Indian Army. I find, as you yourself were good enough to write to me once would be the case, that it enters little into that which most interests us all, viz., the best way of preserving the soldier's health and employing his energies in a country and climate like that of India. The number of European troops which you have proposed (in that report) to place permanently in India is, I believe, 80,000 and the period of service twelve years. Yet nothing has been as yet considered as to how the waste of life (70 per 1000) on such a service is to be prevented or diminished. The problem before the country is how to keep up an army of 80,000 men under such conditions. And not one consideration seems to have presented itself on this subject, except that possibly the mother country will be able to supply this great annual loss *inevitably* following (at present) from *evitable* disease.

Men may flock to our colours when there is to be fighting, but will they come when there is to be dying, especially from disease which they will very soon learn can be prevented or diminished? I believe they will not. And now seems to be the time to institute inquiry, to be followed by active measures, having for their object how to hold India with 80,000 British troops, every man of whom, who does not die in the interim, will be exposed for twelve years to the climate and—what is far worse—to the sanitary neglects *abounding* in every station in India. This is a question which will very soon be raised by the country unless taken up by ministers.

Source: From a letter to Sidney Herbert, Wiltshire County Record Office, Pembroke Collection 2057/F4/68

12 April 1859

I am afraid you will think me overbusy. But you cannot think how that Indian business has lain at my heart. After you were gone, I wrote to Lord Stanley (quite tame, believe me, but I repeated what he had said last December, without preamble). And this is his answer, the oddest thing of all, I think: Don't destroy it, please. J'y tiens—et pour cause [I care for it—and for good reason].

Source: From a letter to Lord Stanley, Liverpool Record Office, Derby Collection 920/7/146/16

14 April 1859

In relation to your wish that Mr Herbert should act as chairman to your proposed Indian sanitary inquiry, he says this morning, "I am ready to begin. I have no contest and could run up to town twice a week without difficulty. If a contest should arise, I can but adjourn for a few days. There must too, I should think, be some preliminary work in getting at documents, maps, etc."

Source: From five letters to Sidney Herbert, Wiltshire County Record Office, Pembroke Collection 2057/F4/68

18 April 1859

I have heard nothing from Lord Stanley, whom however I gratified (not with the sight but) with the substance of your note. I was rather in hopes that he would have written to you. I did not expect to hear from him because, I think, he is angry (notwithstanding his mansuetude), which doesn't signify, as if he will but do this one thing. I am very sure never to want anything from him again—Lord Stanley is a kind of Robinson Crusoe of humanity. He has no fellow creatures. He never communicated with anybody, nor anybody with him on any subject that I ever heard of. He is a species *in himself* and will be described as such by any future Cuvier.[34] Genus – Homo; Species Lord Stanley.

20 April 1859

Enclosed I send:

1. the list of commissioners,
2. heads for the instructions, to which I hope you will add a great deal . . . ,
3. a list of a few of the "documents which we want, if they can be obtained from the India House,"
4. a list of good witnesses, which you *don't* want now. Only perhaps Lord Stanley will say there are none to be had. . . .

It occurred to me, what should you think of Colonel Sir W. Russell, MP, for the "queen's man"? Probably you know him. But if not, he is a man of about poor Stafford's calibre, with zeal and generosity, without sense or judgment, but without Stafford's tendency to gross exaggeration. He has enthusiasm, a quality something scarce on your commission. He would follow you and not be obstinate. He has Indian experience now. And I suppose it is rather a good thing to have a MP, is it not? He is a cavalry officer, which is a bad thing. I knew him in the Crimea. For an army man, he is wonderfully "go ahead" and would astonish the old Indians out of their ruts.

34 Georges Cuvier (1769-1832), French naturalist, founder of comparative anatomy and vertebrate paleontology.

[continued] 28 April 1859

Brigadier Greathed,[35] the man of the wonderful march from Delhi to Agra (?), is come home. He is a first-rate soldier and a good Indian name. Would he do? It is sometimes better to begin on a "table rase," like this Russell or Greathed. They have no prejudices.

28 April 1859

For a "queen's officer" on the Indian sanitary commission it is much easier to say whom *not* to have than whom to have. But

1. Sir E. Lugard,[36] to educate? able and honest, *not* independent (but what army man is?), with Indian experience.

2. Sir J. Burgoyne,[37] a faithful friend of the sanitary cause, his rank would help, not a wise man, no Indian experience.

3. Colonel Kennedy,[38] assistant quartermaster general at Aldershot, very highly thought of by all good army men, has Indian experience. It is true the man ought to be an engineer, but no queen's engineer has been in India till the war [the Mutiny]. And *all* these men know just this of India to recommend and no more: "If you want to make the soldier healthy in India, take him *out* of it."

Therefore you will have to educate your man anyhow, and I had rather educate Sir E. Lugard.

29 April 1859

If your mind has inclined to have Sir E. Lugard, I conceive it will be the best. After making every inquiry, I don't see anyone who will do as well. He has been twenty-four years in India, an adjutant general there, has great local knowledge, is *un*energetic, honest and fair. In what little official intercourse Galton has had with him about your barrack matters, he has been sensible. That he is a Horse Guards "organ" there is no doubt. But the commission will always be called "one-sided" by its enemies, if there is no such "organ." . . .

---

35 William Wilberforce H. Greathed (1826-78), Royal Engineer, later Major General, C.B. He served in India and China, was the directing engineer for the siege of Lucknow and was an expert on irrigation.

36 Edward Lugard (1810-98), later Sir, spent his career in the army in India and Persia and served as under secretary for war 1861-71.

37 John Fox Burgoyne (1782-1871), made general upon his return from the Crimean War.

38 John Clark-Kennedy (1817-67), with whom Nightingale worked for many years on military hospitals.

I have ascertained that no *royal* engineer or artillery officer ever went to India before the war and that none has as yet returned.

West Hill Lodge<br>Highgate Rise<br>30 April 1859

I told Sutherland you wish that he and Martin should immediately draw up the paper of questions to send out to the Indian stations. He will have to look at any documents, which the E.I. [East India] House has to show, first. And as there was not time for you then to get them the authority before he started for Ireland, he put it off till he came back.

Do not you think that it will be advisable for a good deal of this preliminary work to be done before the commission meets for business? because whereas, in the Crimean case, *we* had all the experience on our side, in the Indian case, *they* will have all the experience on theirs.

It will not take long to do a good deal. If you would get us access to all the information at once by asking Lord Stanley to put Dr Sutherland and Mr Martin (and, if you thought well, Dr Farr) into communication with the India House? The two first would then prepare the forms of questions as soon as they had abstracted the documents necessary. Farr, I suspect, would find no statistics but what we have already.

Dr Sutherland and Mr Martin might be asked by you at once to examine all records, etc., and to abstract the information already available for you as chairman, to draw up forms for local inquiries: questions for getting local information from all the stations in India, perhaps to cause these forms to be accompanied by skeleton maps and plans.

Dr Farr might be asked in the same way to do the same thing as to the present state of Indian statistics. . . .

Mr Martin *ditto* as to the present sanitary state of Indian stations and position of Indian medical service in regard to it (a short abstract for you). It would not do to be (from want of experience) in the power of the India Council men.

The commission work will include (according to its instructions)

| | |
|---|---|
| *topography* | *barracks* |
| climate | camps |
| productions | stations |
| diseases | hospitals |
| localities | sanatoria |

waters strategic points
statistics

1. Selection of healthy sites;
2. inquiry into causes of sickness and mortality in unhealthy stations . . . ;
3. sanitary improvements required in existing stations;
4. organization of an Indian sanitary department.

Source: From three letters to Sidney Herbert, Wiltshire County Record Office, Pembroke Collection 2057/F4/68 (all written from West Hill Lodge, Highgate Rise)

6 May 1859

I am *very* glad, on the whole, that you have Sir E. Lugard. I wish Lord Stanley would give the word to Open Sesame to his treasures. . . .

Do you know Sir Robert Napier,[39] Bengal Engineers who made the roads in the Punjab for Sir J. Lawrence? He is now on his way home, is a good sanitarian and will give capital information as a witness.

7 May 1859

Dr Sutherland is here and he meets Dr Farr here tomorrow for the purpose of talking over together some of the preliminary work of the Indian commission. On Monday he calls upon Mr Martin for the same purpose. But the work which could be done between this and Thursday . . . would be very much facilitated by having the permission for the India House. You know, of course, that the barrack commission are planning a ten days' inspection in Scotland from next Thursday. And you, I believe, mean to meet them yourself at Edinburgh on the 17th. Much of the Indian preliminary work cannot therefore begin effectually (if this plan is carried out) till Monday fortnight. . . . We have been going over the heads of questions to be sent out to the stations in India.

9 May 1859

It occurs to me, do you know Colonel Alison, late military secretary to Lord Clyde?[40] If we cannot have the bird, at least the stake the bird sat

39 Robert Cornelius Napier (1810-90), later Lord Napier of Magdala, commander-in-chief in India 1870-76. He met Nightingale in December 1869.

40 Archibald Alison (1826-1907), later, Sir, decorated for his service in the Crimean War. He lost an arm at the siege of Lucknow. He served as military secretary to Lord Clyde (Sir Colin Campbell) when the latter was commander-in-chief in India, and later rose to the rank of general.

upon may taste of it. Colonel Alison has the credit of being a highly educated man and very good officer. I don't know what more we shall get than good sense and local knowledge in any *queen's* officer, because H.M. has no sanitary engineers in India at all, poor thing! Colonel Alison was to be at home from Italy about this time.

I will send you every word I can gather about Greathed or anybody else tomorrow.

Source: From a letter to Edwin Chadwick, Add Mss 45770 f99

West Hill Lodge
Highgate Rise
9 May 1859

I think your article in the *North British* and at the Social Science Meeting, together with your interview with Lord Stanley, has already borne fruits. Lord S. has asked Mr Herbert to be chairman to another sanitary commission to do in India what the first has done at home.

Source: Letter, Add Mss 45759 ff26-27

West Hill Lodge
Highgate Rise
9 May 1859

*Private*

My dear Captain Galton

Sir E. Lugard refuses (on account of pressure of work) to serve on the Indian sanitary commission. In his default, I had proposed (to Mr Herbert) Brigadier [Edward H.] Greathed, he of the wonderful march from Delhi [to] Agra (?), of whom I know nothing but that he is a first-rate soldier and that he is returned home. Mr Herbert inclines now to him. Could you get Greathed's measure for us in things such as we want? or could you mention any fresh name which would be for this commission? "A queen's officer of acknowledged Indian experience" is the only stipulation made. Advise me, pray. Or tell me anyone through whom I could get information.

yours ever most truly
F. Nightingale

Source: From a letter to Sir John McNeill, Florence Nightingale Museum (LMA) H1/ST/NC1/59/SU115, typed copy Add Mss 45768 ff98-99

West Hill Lodge
Highgate Rise
9 May 1859

Sir E. Lugard has declined to serve on the Indian sanitary commission on account of the present pressure of business at the War Office. And we are again at our wits' ends for a "queen's officer of acknowledged Indian experience." And again it is left to us to choose.

I mentioned Brigadier Greathed, now in England, the man of the wonderful march from Delhi. And Mr Herbert seems inclined to have him, merely because I cannot name anyone else. But I know nothing of him but his reputation. Nor do I know anyone through whom to get his measure. In this dilemma, could you help us again? both by saying what you think of Greathed and by mentioning any other queen's officer now at home, whom you think well of for this purpose.

Would you look at the enclosed list of heads for inquiries to be sent out to the stations in India and tell us your opinion as to the different queries therein? Would you also kindly give an opinion as to the general direction which the inquiry should take?

Source: From a letter to Uncle Samuel Smith, Add Mss 45792 ff83-84

10 May 1859

*Private.* Her Majesty has stipulated for a "queen's officer of acknowledged experience in India" to be seventh on the Indian sanitary commission! No one who has not made the inquiries which I have can possibly imagine the difficulty which this stipulation has put us into. There does not appear to be any "queen's officer" of any ability at all who is now at home. Tulloch is out of the question; Sir E. Lugard declines on the score of the pressure of business. Brigadier Greathed and Colonel Alison, late military secretary to Lord Clyde, I am now hesitating between.

Now, if I could get Sir John Lawrence's opinion to recommend one of these two or any other man, I should be a happy woman. He must know all the (Indian) queen's officers. (And, he will say, what a pack they are!) Could you either directly, or indirectly through Sir R. Vivian, get Sir J. Lawrence's opinion? In the latter case, Sir R. Vivian must be taken into the confidence which I shall not mind if only he will consider it as "confidential." . . .

The worst of it is I have not a day to lose. For I must give an answer. I have already consulted Galton, Martin, Sir J. McNeill and one of Clough's friends through Clough.

Source: From five letters to Sidney Herbert, Wiltshire County Record Office, Pembroke Collection 2057/F4/68 (all written from West Hill Lodge, Highgate Rise)

11 May 1859

I have a promise of Sir John Lawrence's answer on Friday (about a queen's officer for the commission), if you thought it worth waiting for. Unfortunately he was from home when I wrote to his friend. Do you think that, now at the eleventh hour, you could have him too on the commission and fence the queen's officer by him, as they have forced a queen's officer upon you? I feel that all these men whom we have got (or have lost) are such children, rogues or asses by the side of him—and he is the founder of anything that is sanitary in India. But you will be a better judge of this than I. I don't see how Lord Stanley or the queen could refuse. Sir J. Lawrence might.

I ought to remind you perhaps about Alison of the extremely bad reputation as to want of judgment that hangs about his family in Scotland.

11 May 1859

The substance of the information, various as it is, may thus be summed up. There are no superior queen's officers in India, therefore superior Indian queen's officers cannot be had. Except in the late war and those are not come back. I am just where I was, after having got all this information: (1) Colonel Alison, (2) Brigadier Greathed, though nothing favourable or unfavourable is to be known as to our matters about this officer. He can give information about strategic points and positions and is a most efficient man. (3) Sir W. Colebrooke:[41] this man appears to have far more general ability and experience than anyone else mentioned. But he is old and his experience is *not* recent. He is however a genuine sanitarian and a very remarkable man and admirable reformer. He is an officer of the R.A., served as such in Java and India, was A.D.C. to Lord Hastings in the Maratha War 1816-17 when cholera first appeared, Q.M.G. with Sir W.K. Grant, many years in India, always in tropical climates, governor of New Brunswick, recently of Barbados. He is a man of a much higher class of mind and character than anyone we have had recommended. . . .

41 Sir William MacBean George Colebrooke (1787-1870), served with the Royal Artillery throughout the East and then on a royal commission that recommended social, economic and political reforms in Ceylon. He became a general in 1865.

Now I am come to an end. Martin strongly praises Colonel Alison (No. 1). Sir J. McNeill has often told me of Sir Colebrooke's high character and abilities (No. 3). The Senior U.S. [United Services] Club would be sufficient address. Everybody speaks well of Greathed. But then they say nothing that would not do for a man like General [Charles Ash] Windham just as well. . . . The worst of it is that Sir W. Colebrooke is the only man who has been the least tried in our line of business. The others may be geniuses or altogether wanting.

I have asked Sir John Lawrence to recommend (through a common friend) but have not yet his answer. What would you think of asking Sir E. Lugard to send you (not one but) several names for you to choose amongst?

[Captain R.M.] Laffan has at last resigned on account of ill health. They will not do anything in the way of change in that office till your committee has reported, perhaps not for a twelvemonth. It would be well worthwhile to get Galton in for a twelvemonth. The office is very troublesome against the barrack commission. Galton might not accept it, even if offered to him, because of the Board of Trade. This is what I hear from the Whitehall people. Of course many things may happen between this and then.

The only *definite* and *positive* information I have obtained from the united researches of Drs Sutherland, Farr and Martin (relative to beginning the Indian sanitary inquiry) is that there is a clerk who has been 150 years (sic) in the India House, who will know all about the documents there when we have got the entrée.

13 May 1859

I wish that Sir John Lawrence would answer, which he was to do today, but he has not yet. Through Sir R. Vivian who, whatever his prejudices, is as honest and anti-jobbing as Lawrence himself, I have tried to get opinions on the *general* merits of the queen's officers (who have been named) from some of the old Indian officers at the India House. One and all agree that Greathed is fit for nothing. I tell this for what it is worth. I know not. I have heard Lord W. Paulet and other officers of high standing in the Crimea, without as much judgment as your little Mary, say the same thing of Storks and others who certainly had some (i.e., judgment). The man most highly spoken of by Sir Robert Vivian and company is Colonel David Russell, CB, Inspecting Field Officer, Recruiting Dept., Horse Guards, long in India in command of a regiment and a very good (queen's) officer. (It may be that his name will turn up on [Major General Richard] Airey's[42] or somebody else's recommendation.)

---

42 Sir Richard Airey (1803-81), later Lord, quartermaster general.

13 May 1859

At the last moment Sir J. Lawrence's answer has come. He evidently thinks that you might as well "ask him to dance, having tied up his legs" (in fact, he says so) as choose a queen's officer. He would choose, he says, if he must, Colonel Campbell of the 52nd, or Colonel Orlando Felix, who has been eighteen years in India. He does not know Colonel David Russell, he says. He does not like Greathed or Alison. He does not *highly* extol even his Colonel Campbell (he knows him by character only) but calls him "the only officer he would name." He puts Colonel Felix second to Campbell.

I am afraid this kind of information will only obfuscate you. But if Airey or Lugard have sent you lists, it may help to have Sir J. Lawrence's imprimatur. . . . Lawrence is of course very careful not to commit himself in any general condemnation of the queen's service. He only speaks "of these matters" "for this purpose," etc.

14 May 1859

This is the last vero ultimo [the truly last one]. Ross Mangles,[43] a poor judge you will say, says Greathed is a man of great ability. But do you know old Martin says that, when he was presidency surgeon and Mangles secretary at Calcutta, he (Mangles) was the only person who ever gave him help in improving that sink of all unsanitary abomination, viz., our capital of India. Greathed is about fifty, a nephew of Glyn, the banker. Probably you have decided long since. I only report my last.

Source: From a letter to Harriet Martineau,[44] ADD MSS 45788 ff54-55

19 May 1859

I must tell you a secret, because I think it will please you. For eight long months I have been "importunate widow"-ing my "unjust judge,"[45] viz., Lord Stanley, to give us a royal sanitary commission to do exactly the same thing for the armies in India which the last did for the army at home. We have just won it. The queen has signed the warrant [issued 31 May]. So it is safe. Mr Sidney Herbert is chairman, of course. Drs Sutherland, Martin, Farr and Alexander, whose names will be known to you, Sir R. Vivian and Sir P. Cautley of the India Council, are on it.

---

43 Ross Lowis Mangles (1833-1905), one of only five civilians to be awarded the Victoria Cross, which he won for his bravery during the Indian Mutiny.

44 Harriet Martineau (1802-76), author and journalist at *The Daily News*. See the biographical sketch in *Women* (8:1033-35).

45 An allusion to Luke 18:1-8.

Source: From a letter to Sidney Herbert, Wiltshire County Record Office, Pembroke Collection 2057/F4/68

West Hill Lodge
Highgate Rise, N.
19 May 1859

As Greathed is to be only ornamental, it is a good name to have. And Sir E. Lugard's letter is the letter of a man of thought and feeling, though not of a man of the world (I wish he would not appeal to Hawes). I shall not break my heart about Sir J. Lawrence, though he is a much better sanitarian than Lord Stanley. What he seems to have said is absurd enough. But whatever was done in India by him or his brother was good sanitary action. However, it does not do to have a man of that weight second on a commission who, if he were to go wrong, might go and write a report all to himself, which would be awkward. I had another reason for wishing Sir J. Lawrence to become intimate with you. But that you can do anyway, if you like. He says that things may ripen for another uproar in India, that there are seeds and that he cannot get ministers in England to attend to him.

Source: From a memorandum to Sidney Herbert, Wiltshire County Record Offic, Pembroke Collectione 2057/F4/68

| Chairman | Mr Herbert | [1859] |
|---|---|---|
| 1. Medical member | *Mr Alexander* | |
| 2. Statistical | *Mr Farr* | |
| 3. Sanitary Indian | *Mr Martin* | |
| 4. Sanitary, General | *Dr Sutherland* | |
| 5. Military, Indian (queen's) and Indian Councillor | *Sir R. Vivian* | |
| 6. Engineer, Indian Council | Sir Proby Cautley or *Colonel Waugh* . . . OR Colonel *Baker*. . . . | |

N.B. *John Stuart Mill* you thought of once. But I think you considered him too much identified with the "old" for a commissioner.

Engineers and Medical Officers who will give good evidence

*Bengal Army*

Engineers In India

Col. Boileau
Lt. Col. Waugh Surv. Genl
Major Ommanney
Capt. C.B. Young
Lieut. J.M. Innes
Lieut. R. de Bourbel

| | | |
|---|---|---|
| | At Home | Col. H. Goodwyn |
| | | " G.T. Greene |
| MEDICAL | In India | Surgeon Grant |
| | | Asst. Surgeon Norman Chevers |
| | | Surg. John McClelland |
| | | " H.M. McPherson |
| | | Asst. Surgeon Macnamara |
| | | " Marcus Hill |
| | At Home | Surgeon Dempster |
| | | " K. Mackinnon |
| | | Dr Julius Jeffreys |
| *Madras Army* | | |
| ENGINEERS | In India | Col. Cotton |
| | | Major Lawford |
| | | Capt. Collyer |
| | | Lt. Col. Atkinson |
| | At Home | Capt. Ouchterlony |
| | | " Harsley |
| | | " Hitchins |
| MEDICAL | In India | Duncan MacPherson, Director General |
| | | Surgeon E.G. Balfour |
| | | " Maclean |
| | | Asst. Surgeon Waring |
| | | " Francis Day |
| | At Home | Surgeon Key |
| | | " Geddes |
| | | " R. Wight |
| *Bombay Army* | | |
| ENGINEERS | In India | Col. Scott |
| | | Major Crawford |
| | | Capt. Marriott |
| | | " Ballard |
| | At Home | Lt. Col. C.N. Grant |
| | | " H.B. Turner |
| | | Major Wingate |
| | | " John Hill |
| MEDICAL | In India | Surgeon Gibson |
| | | " Collier |

| | |
|---|---|
| | " Morehead |
| | " Arnott |
| At Home | Major McLennan |
| | " Glen |
| | " Stovell |

Manner of Inquiry:

1. Examination of documents in possession of the India House regarding the health of troops and stations.
2. Parole evidence from persons on leave in England, acquainted with stations.
3. Obtaining all maps, plans, etc., which throw light on the subject.
4. Issuing printed lists of questions to all stations in India.

These documents will be wanted from the India House:

1. The best India House map of India.
2. Trigonometrical survey, as far as completed.
3. List of all military stations to be marked also on the maps.
4. Copies of all published periodical reports of medical boards in presidencies.
5. Copies of all published army Indian statistical tables.
   Same, queen's troops.
6. Lists of all places where are permanent barracks and hospitals.
7. Access to catalogue of documents at India House and to all documents there bearing on the inquiry.

To ask Lord Stanley for a general power of examining all documents respecting health of army in India House.

Should Sir John McNeill be on the commission?

Don't be limited to any time for finishing the inquiry.

## Work on the Commission

**Editor:** After all this preparatory work the Royal Commission on the Sanitary State of the Army in India was formally appointed and received royal assent, 31 May 1859, Nightingale was more than ready to tackle the work of evidence gathering, but officials were slow to act. She complained that "much absurd and ignorant commentary" is heard, and that the India Office "throws all kinds of obstacles in the way" (see p 97 below). The correspondence shows that she had to reproach almost everybody, but never had any criticism to direct at Sidney Herbert; her only regret was that the royal commission could not sit while the House was in session, as he was busy there. She immediately started to work on designing the "queries," or questionnaires, to go to the Indian stations. She consulted Dr Farr on 2 June and wrote John McNeill on 11 June with an early draft seeking his advice. She was also aware, as the work started, of Sidney Herbert's failing health, and sought to save him the "labour of detail" (see p 93 below), reserving him for the handling of meetings for which his particular gifts and diplomacy were needed. Even close collaborators needed Nightingale's prompting; for instance, Dr Farr apparently declared himself "satisfied" with the disease and mortality statistics, before the stational data had been gathered (see p 98 below). Incidentally, it took five months to get the questionnaires processed through the India Office.

Source: Unsigned note, Wellcome (Claydon copy) Ms 8998/2

Highgate
1 June 1859

Parable: The unjust judge and the importunate widow.
Dramatis Personae:
Lord Stanley—Unjust Judge
F.N.—Importunate Widow
Result of eight months' importunacy—as below.

[Clipping from the *London Gazette* of Tuesday, 31 May]
India Office, 31 May.
The queen has been pleased to issue a commission under her royal sign manuel, appointing: the Right Hon Sidney Herbert, MP; Major General Sir Robert John Hussey Vivian, K.C.B.; Colonel Sir Proby Thomas Cautley, K.C.B.; Thomas Alexander, Esq., C.B.; Colonel Edward Harris Greathed, C.B.; William Farr, Esq., M.D.; James Ranald Martin, Esq.; John Sutherland, Esq., M.D., to be her majesty's commissioners to inquire into, and report upon, the measures which it may be expedient to take for maintaining and improving the health of all ranks of her majesty's army serving in India.

Source: From a letter to Sidney Herbert, Staatsbibliothek zu Berlin Preussischer Kulturbesitz

Highgate
2 June 1859

The enclosed draft of queries *for the Indian stations* is the result of examining the chief manuscript medical documents at the India House as well as of general sanitary experience. It is rough—perhaps too long—and perhaps must be added to, after discussion and further examination of papers at the India House. The statistical part is left incomplete for Farr to deal with.

A separate set of military queries must perhaps be added. The enclosed is only a rough draft of the *health* questions.

If you chose to propose at the first meeting that Martin, Farr and Sutherland should form a committee to draw up queries on health and statistics, they could then be printed and circulated among the other commissioners before being decided upon.

Or if, which would save a deal of valuable time, as many of the commissioners have not a sanitary notion in their heads, you would act upon your own authority to draw up and send out the queries yourself?

After you have gone over these, would you be so good as to let us have them back and to tell Sutherland, if you see him tomorrow, what are your remarks upon them?

yours sincerely
F. Nightingale

Source: Letter to William Farr, Wellcome Ms 5474/7, typed copy Add Mss 43398 f122

Highgate
2 June 1859

My dear Sir

Your commission was gazetted on 31 May and Mr Herbert is in town. As it will be necessary to obtain the statistics of sickness, mortality and invaliding of the Indian Army from the medical boards there, would not some of the proposed forms for the Army Medical Department be better than any other, filled up for each station with the diseases annually for a period say of ten years? Or would it be necessary to provide others?

We must of course have the most minute statistics, both for soldiers and officers in the queen's, Company's and native troops. And these we should get by this method for ten years. I suppose the medical boards have the presidency medical book records. Would it be necessary to get the returns for each corps separately? Would it not be important to get the ages—age and time of service at death or invaliding?

yours sincerely
F. Nightingale

Source: From a typed copy of a letter to Sir John McNeill, ADD Mss 45768 ff104-05, Florence Nightingale Museum (LMA) H1/ST/NC3/SU120

Highgate
11 June 1859

Enclosed is the list of proposed queries for the Indian stations. Could you be so kind as to look it over and make any corrections and additions you think fit. Also noting in the margin the person to whom the query ought to be addressed. These queries are printed only for correction and are to be rearranged according to the respective officers to whom they are to be sent, and printed on larger sheets with spaces for the replies.

Tabular forms to be filled up are also to be added, as well as a set of purely military questions for military officers, and a circular letter.

Sutherland has been studying at the India House, and the result is incorporated in these questions. As well as Martin's information. Farr is drawing up the statistical forms.

You will see the result of this morning's division. My satisfaction is of a very limited nature. Mr Herbert told me that if he were secretary of state for war, he would turn over this Indian matter to Lord Stanley. Now *I* can say *that* of Lord Stanley which Mr Herbert cannot because, as I read somewhere, the inferior details, the superior ignores.

I am sure that Lord Stanley has neither the grasp of the subject nor the faculty that some men have of putting themselves into the right hand, as to detail, and seeing who knows and who does not. I believe the sanitary salvation of India depends upon Mr Herbert doing it. And I should say the same, and a great deal more, if I were dead and there were no question of my work. Do you think we could make any proposal to Mr Herbert by which, saving him all labour of detail (which we could do), we could keep his hand over us for the meetings which might even be deferred till Parliament ceases to sit, and for the final report? Or we might have only (say) an hour of his time per week at a weekly meeting for parole evidence. I am not afraid to say that Sutherland, Farr and I could do all the detail work for him; Sutherland and I did it for the last.

Source: From a letter to William Farr, British Library of Political and Economic Science, Farr Collection 1/75

Highgate
16 June 1859

My proprietor, although already installed at the War Office, as I dare say you know, found time of Tuesday to expedite Indian matters here during the afternoon. As he is extremely anxious to get off the printed queries to India as soon as possible (those which I sent to you on Saturday for your criticism) we have thought it would save you time and consideration for us to draw up the forms to give us the information we want, if sent to the Presidency Medical Boards to be filled up for ten years last past, also a copy to each officer to whom the printed queries are sent, to be filled up for the last year.

Would you now give these your consideration and tell us whether they do give us the information we want, which it is obvious the organization Blue Book does not. And would you kindly return them to me *here* as soon as possible, with your corrections, additions and notes. A circular letter is to be sent with them.

Source: From a letter to William Farr, Wellcome Ms 5474/9, typed copy Add Mss 43398 f134

3 August 1859

We have not yet mastered sufficiently the processes of arithmetic to ascertain how many copies will be wanted. But, as soon as we do, we will send to you for your approval.

We should like to know whether any progress has been made in ascertaining how much of the information can be obtained at home, and which, if any, of the forms can be filled up at the adjutant general's, army medical departments or elsewhere at home.

Source: From a letter to Sidney Herbert, Wiltshire County Record Office, Pembroke Collection 2057/F4/68

10 August 1859

We have made a list of stations in the three presidencies to which to send copies of the Indian questions. We submitted this list to Colonel Baker[46] at the India House. And we have just received it back as correct. (Colonel Baker was informed what was the object.) There are no fewer than 166!!! of which there is accommodation for *queen's* troops at 82, for *Company's European* troops at 97 and for *native* at 148. About six are occupied by queen's troops alone. Will you tell us how we should send out the 82 copies for queen's troops? We would rather they should go out through the *War Office* by your orders to the queen's commanders in the presidencies. Or must they go with the others through the *India House*?

46 William E. Baker, clerk of the second royal commission, chair of the India Office Sanitary Committee 1872-74.

Source: From a letter to William Farr, Wellcome Ms 5474/10, typed copy ADD Mss 43398 f135

Hampstead, N.W.
31 August 1859

Sir C. Wood,[47] Mr Herbert tells me today, "has got a surgeon," after much search, who is to do your forms at the India House. I send into town every day. And whatever you please to send to 30 Burlington St. for Dr Sutherland or me suffers no delay.

Source: From a letter to Sir Charles Trevelyan, Newcastle University Library 35/9

25 September 1859

I dare say you know that we have got a royal commission, with Mr Sidney Herbert at its head, to do for the sanitary state of the army in India what the first one did for the army at home. I hope that, in a few days, the copies will be sent out (to all the stations in India) of certain queries which have been framed, the answers to which are to be filled up on the spot. I am sure that the answers to the copies sent to your presidency will be both the best filled up and the soonest sent back to us. And I should not wonder if you had already set on foot the improvements which are intended to be suggested by these queries and if no farther authority will be needed in your presidency.

But I recommend to your favourable consideration the getting these queries answered and sent back to us *as soon as possible.* For we are much in need of information. Two things you might strike at once (and I dare say have done so): (1) abolishing spirit-drinking, (2) ordering a list to be made of healthy hill stations, to which it may be possible (and compatible with military reasons) to remove the troops from the plains. . . .

Your inspector general of hospitals, Dr MacPherson, appeared to me the only (superior) medical officer in the Crimea who really knew his business. . . .

Mr Herbert's accession to the War Office has been the means of working out a good many things for the army, which we had in hand. But things in an old country go very slow. It often strikes me: if the House of Commons knew how little it has to do with the actual administration of the country! It turns out one ministry and puts in another and thinks it has done great things. It has done nothing at all. For the

47 Sir Charles Wood (1800-85), later Lord Halifax, president of the Crown's Board of Control 1853-55, secretary of state for India 1859-66.

clerks and the under secretaries in the offices are the real people who govern, at least in the War Office and somewhat, though not so much, in the India House. And unless the chief is a man really master of the details of business and with strong convictions and a strong will of his own, it really makes little matter *which* chief is in the office.

My health is declining and I am almost now confined to my bed. But you cannot tell (or at least you can tell) the pleasure it is to me to hear of such as you doing such things for our poor men, whom I know so well and know how much there is of good in them to be worked out. Any papers like those you are so good as to promise to send me will be most interesting to me.

ever yours truly and gratefully
Florence Nightingale

Source: From a typed copy of a letter to an unnamed recipient, Add Mss 45797 ff63-64

Hampstead, N.W.
27 September 1859

You asked us to read [F.G.] Monat's [Mouat's] [medical officer, inspector of jails for Bengal] blue pamphlet, "The British Soldiers in India." It is very satisfactory. But it would never have been written without the first royal sanitary commission, and is another of the many signs how wide its influence has been. It merely gives, in new language, most of the principles enunciated in that report. . . .

The best point of the whole book is what is set forth in the Preface, viz., that the news of the probability that a future commission upon the "sanitary state of the army in India" might be presided over by Mr Herbert had given an impulse to the whole practical inquiry throughout India. Without his name and authority, indeed, there would be little chance of any practical good coming out of it to the poor men.

Source: From two letters to Sidney Herbert, Wiltshire County Record Office, Pembroke Collection 2057/F4/68 (both written from Hampstead, N.W.)

7 October 1859

*In re India House.* If you would write a short and tempestuous note to Sir C. Wood, after the manner of the duke of Wellington in Spain to Mr Filder,[48] and say that our supplies *must* come (whether there be any

48 The 1st duke of Wellington (1769-1852), defeater of Napoleon; William Filder, commissary general at Sebastopol. On 27 January 1855, the *Times* quoted H. Drummond, MP for West Surrey, as stating (in error) that Filder was the

or not) or he will be hung—our supplies *would* come. The thing is after this wise: if the India House puts its washing out, everything is well and punctually done. What washing it does at home is not done at all.

Mr Prinsep has sent back our last form, with much absurd and ignorant commentary of his own upon it, and has written a note to Dr Farr, which I have, as also the form, saying that the Indian commission must seek for its information in India. Now we *know* that this is not true. The information *is* in the India House. And the only question is how to get it out.

The office throws all kinds of obstacles in the way. And for the sake of saving a few clerks at a few pounds a week (for a limited time) the results of the returns made for years with great labour and at great cost are not to be given to the commission. Mr Hornidge (of the India House) is entirely on our side. The information IS in the India House—*in Colonel Baker's department.* Dr Farr has seen the rolls there himself. And it would be a mere waste of time and labour to send to India for them. Our forms ask merely for information, which the rolls supply. To say they do not, is merely a "put-off."

The India House has not answered your letter, which they have had in the Military Department for three months, so I am informed. The only course is for you to write again, I am afraid, and ask them to supply the information which the commission requires. Two or three "writers" (or more if necessary) must be employed to do the work, under the supervision of Mr Hornidge, with whom Dr Farr would consult. I should consider it an honour, if I might be allowed to pay (through you) these "writers." The India department will not do our work as establishment work, for they have as much as they can do of their ordinary routine work. But a note from you to Sir C. Wood will bring Mr Prinsep to his senses. Surely it is of some importance to get at the results of their past experience, and to put them in the way of profiting by future observations in India.

The whole "fencing" is a mere matter of work and of a few good clerks for a short time, to pay whom, if you would allow me to put £100 in your hands, I should be delighted. Sir C. Wood is as sharp as a

---

man Sir Thomas Picton had wanted to hang for poor fulfillment of his duties during the Peninsular War. The man thus threatened was in fact Deputy Commissary General Lutchens, also erroneously accused. On 6 February J. Walter Wilkinson wrote a letter to the editor to point out the fact that Filder had not been the object of the threat.

needle. But he does not know anything at all about *our* work. And the comments of Prinsep and company pass muster with him and dispose fatally of questions of the utmost importance by simply putting them on the shelf. Mr Prinsep was happily (for us) married this week and is now out of the way, which is happier still.

29 October 1859

The queries for the queen's troops in India have arrived (after a very difficult voyage through the Strand) at the War Office in Whitehall Gardens. Dr Sutherland will go there, make them up into packets and send them to the W.O. in Pall Mall as soon as you have given the necessary instructions for their being forwarded to India, filled up and returned to you. Shall we write you a circular something like the enclosed for the three officers commanding in the three presidencies?

Source: From a letter to William Farr, Wellcome Ms 5474/12, typed copy Add Mss 43398 f150

Hampstead, N.W.
31 October 1859

Sir C. Wood has informed me that he has seen you and that "you are satisfied." Does your "satisfaction" include the statistics of disease and mortality at each STATION throughout India? I ask this because our sanitary questions on the stations are either gone or on their way to going to India. The replies to them will be of little use unless we have the stational statistics.

Source: From three letters to Sidney Herbert, Wiltshire County Record Office, Pembroke Collection 2057/F4/68 (all written from Hampstead, N.W.)

5 November 1859

No orders have come from Pall Mall to Whitehall[49] yet anent the Indian queries, though Whitehall has sent to Pall Mall every day for the same. If the utmost dispatch is made, I believe there is reason to hope, with a continuance of the present favourable weather, that the queries may reach Pall Mall in two months from Whitehall. They have only been five months in passing through the India House, not much more than they would have required to go to India and back, a circumstance which inspires me with the most cheerful anticipations.

---

49 "Pall Mall" refers to the area of London known for its men's social clubs and as the centre of networking; at the time this letter was written it was the home of the War Office. "Whitehall" refers to the government administrative centre.

I have made out a list of some sixteen W. Indian stations, but do not send it, for fear of overpowering the W.O.'s administrative abilities, till the E. Indian ones are gone.

10 November 1859

I have a "melancholy satisfaction"[50] in congratulating you on the fact that there is an office in this government worse organized than that which you have undertaken to reform. And this is the great India House. The great house has a head (so they say), but no hands, and Sir C. Wood had much better have accepted our proposal than have done what he has done, which is nothing.

We asked for no work from the overworked magnates, which we knew we should not get, but the appointment of two good clerks, selected by Mr Hornidge (the head of the Statistics Department) and paid by us. The men should have been set to work the next day and the work would have been done by this time. As it is, nothing has been done and nothing ever will be done, as there is no organization of labour in that house such as Sir C. Wood might see any day in Yorkshire. The fault lies with Sir G. Clerk, not with Sir C. Wood. That worthy Scot has no capacity for business, as I believe Sir C. Wood knows full well. And the inaction presided over by that man is general.

What we want now is for Sir C. Wood to give prompt and peremptory orders, i.e., orders that shall be obeyed, for carrying out our work. Or let him say that they cannot (or will not) do it. And we are quite ready with a plan of operations of our own, independent of them, and clerks of our own. It is a cruel waste of time and we might have been half through the business of the commission by now. Mr Hornidge was to speak yesterday to Sir C. Wood's secretary about it. But I despair of anything being done.

2. (This is another matter—the materials for which Mr Prinsep also said did not exist at the India House, but they *do.*) The *forms* for the STATIONAL returns are now ready and will be sent to Mr Hornidge to be filled up. . . .

If Lord Stanley declined the commission because he knew of this state of things and it bothered him, I rather admire the man's *canniness.*

One mystery I will tell gratis, the queen's minister, responsible to the House of Commons, is not master at the East India House: Sir G. Clerk is the minister for India. Let the wise man profit by this notice.

---

50 From Edgar Allan Poe, "The Man That Was Used Up," 1839.

14 November 1859

The India House accepts with transport *your* clerks and your paying them.

Source: From a letter to Sir Charles Trevelyan (governor of Madras), Newcastle University Library 35/11

12 November 1859

By this same mail you will receive, I hope, a copy of "sanitary queries" through the War Office, such as we have sent to every commanding officer of Queen's and E.I. [East India Company] troops throughout all the stations of the East. These queries cover a great deal of ground and will require some trouble in replying to. As it has taken just five months to get them through the India House, I am not filled with the most cheerful anticipations as to the time it will take to get the answers back from India, perhaps some ten years after you have come home. My hope is that you will be able to have the replies sent from your presidency long before the other people have had time to read the questions.

The information which the replies to these queries will afford is of the greatest importance to the public service, as you will see. We have nothing like it from India or indeed from any foreign possession. And, if it can be fully and correctly given and with as little delay as possible, the results in action must be most valuable. But if the present ministers are "out" by the time this information arrives, the result will be much longer delayed.

*Of all the presidencies, Madras has hitherto been the most forward in sanitary knowledge.* And we trust, now that a fair opportunity is given of stating the truth fully and fearlessly, that commanding officers, engineers and medical officers will *vie* with one another in helping it. I had three reasons for sending you a copy (as a private man): (1) the hope that you will forward the filling up of the replies as much as possible; (2) that you will be able to act upon them as much as possible, without waiting for farther authority, in carrying out the reforms they will indicate—which, with your knowledge, is all that is necessary; (3) that you will send us a list of all places where healthy stations might be placed, with the names of unhealthy stations for which they might be substituted.

I have a "melancholy satisfaction" in recording that there is one government office worse organized than the War Office, and that is the great India House. The queen's minister and the man who is responsible to the House of Commons [C. Wood] is not master there.

The under secretary of state [G.R. Clerk] is minister for India. Mr Herbert may plant and Sir Charles Wood may water. But Sir George Clerk alone giveth the increase.[51] I hate an under secretary of state, don't you? They have all the faults of popes and cardinal archbishops—the faults of irresponsible power, stupidity, cunning, ferocity. I wonder whether it is contagious, I think they should be placed under quarantine. However that may be, the double government certainly does not seem to answer there. There is no getting any business done in that office. . . .

With regard to my "Notes on Hospitals," I am glad that it affords you any suggestions. It was intended primarily for *temperate* climates and, if used in *tropical* climates, the following details should be added, which are known, of course, much better to Major Horsley than they are to me, but which have not been known to some English officers. [ten items are given]

Source: From two letters to William Farr, Wellcome Ms 5474/13 and 14, typed copy Add Mss 43398 ff154 and 161

Oak Hill House, Frognal
Hampstead, N.W.
14 November 1859

The India House accepts *your* clerks with transport. Mr Hornidge will write to you as soon as ever Sir G. Clerk has sanctioned it in writing. He did so sanction it today in words.

6 December 1859

In consequence of your intemperate desire to have the Indian Medical Service regulations, we have applied at the Great House for copies. And the answer is that they have only one office copy and if we want any we must send to India.

Knowing their weakness, we had (in our "queries") previously sent to two hundred stations in India for copies of all "regulations," and we hope the result will satisfy your literary appetite.

Please let me, for my own satisfaction, deposit the enclosed slip of paper in your hands.

51 An allusion to 1 Cor 3:6.

Source: From a letter to Sidney Herbert, Wiltshire County Record Office, Pembroke Collection 2057/F4/68

Hampstead, N.W.
18 November 1859

Even the offer of 12/ a day (the price of the two clerks) has failed to move the Great House of India to any exertion. On Monday Dr Sutherland went there and made the above handsome proposal viva voce. It was accepted viva voce. And he was requested to write it down (the Indians could not believe in the magnificent sum of 12/) and address it to Sir G.R. Clerk, which he did. Farr went there himself yesterday to set his two clerks to work, who are ready and waiting, but was told that Sir G. Clerk had given no authority. These people must be ordered forthwith to supply the information in their own way, if not in ours.

Our two men were to be employed exclusively on the *military* returns (otherwise called master rolls). Other two clerks will be required exclusively for the *medical* returns. Let them supply all or two or none. We will supply none or two or all and pay for all, just as they like. But such stiff-necked Israelites[52] were never to be found in the wilderness as in the India House.

Source: From a letter to William Farr, Wellcome Ms 5474/15, typed copy ADD Mss 43398 f164

Oak Hill House, Frognal
Hampstead, N.W.
9 January 1860

I am exceedingly anxious, as you may suppose, to see your charming New Year's gift. But I would much rather have it shown to me by you. And I do not like to ask you to come up here, as I am coming to town *incessantly*, when I hope to see you. If, however, for the sake of not delaying, you would send them [the stational statistics] me by post, I would take care that they be returned to you within twenty-four hours. And Dr Sutherland should see them in that time. But do not you think that they had better be printed *immediately* for *immediate* circulation? And if so I would waive my pleasure of seeing them, especially those returns showing the deaths, admissions, diseases and loss of efficiency at each station.

Your four clerks have been sanctioned at the Treasury. Mr Herbert comes back to town this week. . . . I send this note by a servant that you may, if you think well, send back by the returns by him.

52 An allusion to Exod 32:9.

Source: From a letter to Sir Charles Trevelyan, Newcastle University Library 35/13

10 January 1860

I read the minutes and reports which you were so good as to send me with the greatest interest. The principles set forth are clear, decided and good. And it augurs well for the future of sanitary reform in the Indian Army that, while the royal commission is taking evidence in London, you at Madras are acting so energetically.

I sent you through the India House a copy of suggestions issued by our "Barrack and Hospital Improvement Commission" to the royal *engineers* here to enable them to carry out improvements on uniformly correct principles. Perhaps something in it may be useful and applicable in India.

Source: From a letter to William Farr, Wellcome Ms 5474/17, typed copy ADD Mss 43398 ff168-69

2 April 1860

He [S. Herbert] looked over all your Indian commission papers, was not at all staggered by the expense, is to write to Dr [E. George] Balfour to desire him to fill up the forms you send (for returns of Indian *queen*'s troops) and to desire him to call for extra assistance for doing so.

But as this is more Sutherland's business than mine, I shall leave him to tell you all about it and to return to your little portfolio.

Source: From a letter to Sidney Herbert, Wiltshire County Record Office, Pembroke Collection 2057/F4/68

26 May 1860

This is only to say that I had a message from Lord Stanley (we are not on "speaking terms"!) to the effect that he would be very glad to know if you had time to attend to the Indian Sanitary Commission, whether you had meetings now and how it was going on, and that he would be very glad to offer himself as chairman (!) if you found you had no time to do it yourself. I have not answered this. Perhaps it was only a complimentary message, in the same way as "the weather" and "your health." Don't trouble yourself to answer this. But I thought it my duty to tell you that that queer individual had laid himself open to an offer.

Source: From a letter to Lord Stanley, Liverpool Record Office, Derby Collection 920/15/2

28 May 1860

My sister told me that you had inquired after the "Indian Sanitary Commission." It has had but four or five sittings in all—*none* since the session began. Mr Herbert has not had time. Still time has not been lost. For pointed sets of queries and forms of return have been sent out to every presidency, to each station, to commanding medical and engineer officers, *in each.* The reduction of the answers and of the (filled-up) forms will take a considerable time, when all have been received. And, in *this* sanitary commission, the viva voce examinations are intended more as cross-examinations upon the written returns, in this case, the most important.

But when Mr Herbert will have time to do anything in this matter is quite uncertain. Pardon me if I have taken your inquiry "au pied de la lettre" [literally]. It may have been made merely in the course of conversation.

**Editor:** The topic of Herbert's illness, his leaving of the House of Commons and of the royal commission chair, and his keeping his Cabinet position as secretary of state for war, is treated at length in the correspondence with Elizabeth Herbert in *Women* (8:651-710). The following letter, though, is not in *Women.*

Source: From a letter to Elizabeth Herbert, Wiltshire County Record Office, Pembroke Collection 2057/F4/68

5 December 1860

Dearest, Lord Stanley volunteers to say that his University Commission work is done and, if asked by Mr Herbert to take the presidency of the Indian Sanitary Commission, concerning the progress of which he has been making inquiry, he would (I suppose) "think about it."

Lord Stanley is quite beyond my comprehension. And I would not even have conveyed this message (which is the "third time of asking" from Lord Stanley) to Mr Herbert, had it not been that the present necessity to relieve him from as much work as possible makes any loophole right to speak about at least.

Source: From two letters to William Farr, Wellcome Ms 5474/34 and 41, typed copy ADD Mss 43399 ff1 and 17

9 January 1861

Mr Herbert's failing health (he has disease of the kidneys) and retirement from the House of Commons, which has cost him a severer struggle and greater pang than anybody knows of, of course makes a great difference to us, although, at the earnest request of those who know him best, he retains office. Lord Stanley has been offered and accepted the Indian commission. We are making haste to do as much as we can before he comes on, but anxiety has made me more unfit than I was before. Mr Herbert (I cannot bear to call him by his new name [Lord Herbert of Lea], nor will I) is just as eager about things, however, as ever.

20 April 1861

*In re* Angus Smith's evidence. Ask Sutherland to tell you the evidence I should give about disinfectants in the Crimea and how A. Smith's scheme of laying down India in disinfectants, which he unfolded to me by letter, strikes me.

Source: From a letter to Sir Harry Verney,[53] Wellcome (Claydon copy) Ms 8999/23

9 June 1861

We meet constantly with this remark: "These queries apply only to Europeans. No reply." It is not the least necessary for natives to have any of the requisites for life, or for exercising any one of its functions in a healthy manner.

And when they have said "caste," *tout est dit* [all is said]. "Caste" justifies the absence of air, water, light, drainage, cleanliness, care in hospital, etc. "P.G." (Patrick Grant)[54] makes some very racy and stern remarks here and there on the *laisser-aller* [carelessness] of his officers, no one of whom will ever allow that everything has not been done to make the station "as healthy as possible."

3. The third point which comes out strongly is the necessity of bringing the Indian canteens under the same or similar regulations as English canteens, of putting down the sale of spirits in the bazaar by the strong hand of power, which *can* be done and *has* been done.

---

53 Harry Verney (1801-94), Nightingale's brother-in-law. See the biographical sketch in *Life and Family* (1:837-39). His son, Edmund Hope Verney (1838-1910) went to India and sent material back to Nightingale (1:840-41).

54 It should probably read John Peter Grant, lieutenant governor of Bengal 1859-62. Patrick Grant was commander-in-chief in India 1856-57.

4. The necessity of providing *workshops*, covered grounds for athletic exercises and every means to save the men from eating (!), drinking and sleeping away the hot and the rainy seasons.

5. The necessity of providing well-lighted and comfortable and attractive reading rooms and day rooms etc. And how soon this "pays"!

**Editor:** Sidney Herbert died on 2 August 1861. Nightingale always believed that that day had been the saddest day of her life, and every year thereafter remembered the anniversary. A few days later she wrote to Galton: "The very last words I ever heard my dear master say were about your position in the War Office. . . . His last articulate words were (but I think I told you this) 'poor Florence, our unfinished work.' He said this twice. And I who know him know what depth of despair there was in those words."[55] On 9 August she sent W.E. Gladstone[56] information on Sidney Herbert's career, requested for use in an eulogy.[57]

The adversities she encountered in her work were often a reminder that, had Sidney Herbert lived, they could have been overcome more easily. In her mind nobody was able to replace him, his friendship, his political ability and his efficiency in implementing reforms; she was quick to compare, disadvantageously, most of her collaborators with him. As for Sidney Herbert himself, the evidence shows that he highly appreciated her collaboration and sought her advice on many matters. In a letter below Nightingale alludes to her effort to enlist Farr to write an obituary on Sidney Herbert.

---

55 Letter 16 August 1861, ADD Mss 45759 f257.

56 W.E. Gladstone (1809-98), Liberal statesman, chancellor of the Exchequer 1859-66, elected prime minister on four separate occasions between 1868 and 1894. On Gladstone's relation to India and Nightingale's efforts to win him over to her causes, see *Society and Politics* (5:427-76) and *Social Change in India.*

57 *Society and Politics* (5:430-34).

Source: From five letters to William Farr, the first one from the Private Collection of Susan Teagle, then Wellcome Ms 5474/43, 44, 45 and 46, copy ADD Mss 43399 ff41-42, 46-47, 50-53, 54-55 and 56-57 (all written from Hampstead, N.W.)

10 September 1861

I felt very downhearted about the Indian commission since his resignation. Since your paper I feel that his friends will rally round his memory to carry out that most important part of the work as he would have wished. The barrack commission starts tomorrow for the Mediterranean inspection, one of his last official acts. Till the day fortnight of his death, do you know, he struggled on doing to the last what he could in the office. That I should have survived him seems to me most curious. He who could do so much with me, I who can do nothing without him. My last tie is severed with that noble army which I have served so faithfully seven years next October, in weariness oft, in watchings oft, in prisons, I can truly say with St Paul.[58] For last month makes four years that I have been imprisoned by sickness.

17 September 1861

Would you kindly, at your leisure, see Mr Baker, at 4 Old Palace Yard, and ask him what was understood with Lord Stanley about printing the remainder of the abstracts of replies from Indian stations. I understand that it is proposed to give only those already in type as "specimens" of the whole.

How can one station be a "specimen" of another station? There are no two stations alike. You might as well say that Mr Rawlinson[59] could sewer Winchester from reading a description of Croydon. Or that you could give thirty weekly returns as "specimens" of the weekly mortalities of the year and not give the remaining twenty-two weeks.

Lord Stanley expressly said that he could not take Dr Sutherland's evidence as complete, *because* all the replies from India were not come in. Now, if he thinks the commission or anybody will read the replies in the original manuscript, I think, through whose hands every one of them had passed, he is very much mistaken.

---

58 An allusion to 2 Cor 6:5 and 11:27.

59 Robert Rawlinson (1810-98), later Sir, civil engineer. He had served as sanitary commissioner during the Crimean War. Nightingale kept in contact with him throughout her India work. His membership on the new joint commission was deemed very important.

Certainly the most valuable information, not only in the report but in the India House, will be the printed abstracts of all these stational replies and your statistics. I would have written to Lord Stanley direct, but that perhaps is unnecessary. He does not know (and I should have to explain) that every one of these manuscript replies, with the abstracts, proofs and revises, has passed through my hands, and therefore I am speaking "en connaisance de cause" [with expert knowledge].

2. Would you also ask Mr Baker whether the maps and plans, which Dr Sutherland chose as specimens to be reduced and lithographed for the report, *must* absolutely stand over till the commission meets again, before it is authorized to be done.

I was in hopes that it would be finished and ready by *November*, when the commission meets again, when Dr Sutherland comes back from the Mediterranean and when he and I begin our digest for the report, for which these maps and plans are necessary. I think Dr Sutherland might have reduced their number. But he says not.

Could Mr Baker give an idea as to the "enormous" expense the Stationery Office says it would be? What kind of sum? I would gladly do something at my own expense, if I knew what. Again I would have written to Lord Stanley about this, without troubling you. But if he has positively said that "it must stand over till the commission meets again"; he will not alter that decision for me. . . . Poor Lady Herbert was exceedingly gratified by your paper at Manchester.

28 September 1861

I ought to have answered your two kind letters before. I think it would be very desirable, as you say, to examine some non-commissioned officers and men from India. But I do not know the Indian Army. Colonel Greathed would be a good person to name some.

But I think it is still more desirable to examine somebody who would give you evidence about *caste*, how far it is a religious and how far a social institution, how far it can be got over and how far you must bow to it in civilizing and sanitizing our native troops.

As I have had every one of the manuscript books of replies to do, nothing has struck me so much as this, viz., that *caste* is made an excuse for not feeding, not cooking for, not cleansing or washing, not housing, not teaching, not amusing and not nursing them. The books of replies differ widely as to the *right* of this. Some say that nothing *can* be done. Others show that a great deal *has* been done in some places. Others, still, that it requires only a vigorous effort on the part of our government to do it. I refer particularly to the absence of almost all sanitary civilization (or effort to introduce any) into the native parts of our stations or among our native "lines."

I would propose that you should examine before the commission Mr Ballantyne, librarian to India House, Cannon Row, Mr John Muir, late Bengal Civil Service, Edinburgh, Lieutenant General Briggs, 2 Tenterden St. and perhaps General Ludlow.[60] Mr Ballantyne was thirteen years at Banaras, as I dare say you know. All these men would know, if any do, exactly the value to put upon how far caste is to be an obstacle in the way of sanitary civilization.

It is really horrible, the state of the native (troops), hospitals without any one sanitary appliance, except medicine, which they are far better without. And I, for one, should vote for destroying every hospital I have read about. The sick would be much better out of them. But then to be sure we have neglected the native *lines* just as much. So we must put back the sick into the hospitals.

I understand you that Lord Stanley is going to have a meeting this next month. I shall be glad if it expedites our matter of maps and printing abstracts. But I hope you will not let him consider it a final meeting. Dr Sutherland will not be back and he must be examined again. He wishes it himself. I told him his evidence was very tame, and he thought so too. There is a great deal more to be said.

You say his evidence has not yet been sent to you. The proof (corrected) of it was sent back to press more than a month ago. I too have not yet seen Tulloch's evidence and shall be glad to see it. We are very much obliged to you for what you have done in forwarding a part of the maps and plans, which saves much time. Would Mr Baker send me up here, or to Mrs Sutherland's,[61] 41 Finchley New Road, those which he says "are done."

I don't know what the "*proof*" is which he says "is done" now, because he has no abstracts in hand "to do." The *fourth* volume of printed abstracts is ready. But I have already received my two copies of it, some time ago. We have only one manuscript book now not abstracted. But I begin in time to make an "uproar" as to having the *power* to print abstracts of the remaining books, as they come in from India.

---

60 Major General John Ludlow (1801-82).

61 Sarah Elizabeth Sutherland (c1808-95), member of the Ladies' Sanitary Association, close assistant to her husband, a friend of Nightingale; see correspondence in *Women* (8:601-08) and biographical sketch (8:1037-38).

I should like to see Dr Mouat's report, as you kindly offer it. I know Dr Mouat and his works, which are very good, not like his brother's which are "of the devil."[62]

Have you seen Ganguly's India?[63] Ganguly is a converted Brahmin and his book touches on caste. I mean to get it. And, if it is worth reading, I will send it you, if you wish it. . . . Remember too that YOU are to be examined before the commission and are our sheet anchor.

2 October 1861

*India.* I will answer any "written questions" about the Indian hospitals, etc., provided they are "written" by you and provided you are pretty sure that the sense of the commission will not be: what does this woman know about India? She has never been there.

2. I agree with you that we have "scarcely any evidence as to the native army." Mouat would do. Martin ought to name someone else. Dr Sutherland could tell something from the "replies." But experienced witnesses tell more, *if there are any.* General *Ludlow* might do.

(N.B. The "replies" about the native troops are sometimes disgraceful, disgraceful both to commanding and to medical and engineering officers. We look upon the native troops, do you know? much as Virginians look upon slaves.)

But I do not give up my point as to having witnesses about "caste." I was told by an experienced and *learned* Indian that we had made the great mistake of encouraging "caste," whereas, in all India, the native idea is that military service does away with caste.

I wish someone would question Ballantyne before he appears as witness. If he shares all the superstitions about caste and will confirm them, he had better not appear at all. My poor master would have done this directly. But Lord Stanley (although "a deal better than nothing," as the nigger woman said of men in general) has not this *nous* [mind] or this talent.

3. As to the British Army hospitals in India, they have all the faults we affection so much, which, ceteris paribus [everything else being equal], must work more harm under that climate than under ours.

4. Dr Sutherland will be back in England at the end of this month.

---

62 An allusion to 1 John 3:8.

63 Perhaps Brajakishore Basu Ganguly, the father of Kadambini Ganguly (1861-1923), known as Kadambini Bose (or Basu), the first female graduate and female medical practitioner of Bengal. Her father was an enthusiastic supporter of women's education.

5. I have not yet received the evidence with Mr Baker's analysis.
ever yours sincerely
Florence Nightingale

My poor master has been dead two months today, too long a time for him not to be forgotten, and too long a time for the commander-in-chief not to have proved himself a "snob" and Sir G. Lewis[64] a "muff." The dogs have trampled on his dead body. Alas! seven years this month I have "fought the good fight"[65] with the War Office *and lost it*!

5 October 1861

*India.* I sent you yesterday (by post) Ganguly's India. I don't think however there is much of practical in it to guide us. Please return it to me at your leisure.

It is not what is inevitable in the "horrible results of caste," as you say, which I want to impress upon you, but the excuse for laziness which all those who are lazy (among the European authorities over the native troops) find in "caste." And it is this which I want some practical witnesses to settle, or to overthrow, before the commission. (General Ludlow and General Briggs *might* be better practically than Ballantyne or Muir to give evidence on this.)

I have received a copy of the "complete oral evidence," to use Mr Baker's expression, with his Index and thank him for it. But what alarms me is that he should think it "complete."

Independently of your and Dr Sutherland's evidence, there is much, much more still INcomplete especially as to native troops, and not only that, but as to engineering, for water supply, etc., in which our stations are *wholly* deficient. It does seem curious that we should still be drinking out of skins carried by "*bheesties*" [water carriers] there, when we think of the old Roman waterworks and when we think of their magnificent underground arrangements too, that we should be allowing native bazaars of half a quarter of a million inhabitants to grow up as at Secunderabad and Bangalore without one single such arrangement, poisoning us round our own stations.

I trust you will let me know *when* you expect your next meeting to take place, as also that you will not let Lord Stanley think that it is anything like the last.

---

64 Sir George Cornewall Lewis (1806-63), Sidney Herbert's successor as secretary for war 1861-63.

65 An allusion to 1 Tim 6:12.

I am going to write to Martin to the same effect that you may have an assistant and because Baker says, it was Martin who desired him to send me the oral evidence. But Martin is so absorbed by his one idea of "hill stations" that he will not be vigorous on our side.

I am going on with the abstracts of the Indian replies, of which some very important ones as Bombay have arrived since I wrote. For I hope that people will forget that "no more are to be printed." At least I mean to ignore it.

Source: From a letter to Sir James Ranald Martin, in Joseph Fayrer, *Inspector General Sir James Ranald Martin* 170-71

Hampstead, N.W.
7 October 1861

I have to thank you first for a volume of the "*completed oral evidence*" of the Indian sanitary commission (as Mr Baker calls it), and which I find I owe to your suggestion. I understand you are to have a meeting on the 11th (of the commission). So I write to hope that you do not consider the oral evidence "complete" and that you will not let Lord Stanley think so.

1. We have hardly any evidence about the native troops and I hope that you will name some witnesses on this subject.

In all the books of replies which have yet arrived from India, I have been struck with this, viz., that we make "caste" an excuse for doing next to nothing for the native troops in the way of cleansing, or bathing, or hutting, or feeding, or cooking for, or teaching, or amusing them, or nursing them in hospital. Some of the returns say that it is quite impossible to do anything on account of "caste"; others show that a great deal has been done in some places; and others say that government, if roused, could do almost anything. (I allude especially to sanitary measures for the native lines and bazaars.)

Could you not call some practical witnesses, especially on this matter of "caste," to say how much of this is inevitable, how much only an excuse for our laziness or want of judgment? x x

We are entirely without engineering evidence as to what can be done in the way of water supply, in the way of sanitary arrangements, etc., while the replies show that our state in India is far behind that of 2000 years ago in these respects. In fact, we are drinking dirty water carried by bheesties as Abraham did, to this moment.

3. I hope you will insist on Dr Farr being examined on the statistics, and on Dr Sutherland being further examined on these "replies," of which he has by no means given all the juice in his former examina-

tion. (Dr Sutherland does not return from the Mediterranean till the end of the month, where he is inspecting our stations—one of the last official acts of my dear master.)

4. I hope that you will carry with Lord Stanley the printing of the abstracts of all the remaining Indian "replies," not yet come in, which are not many. How can one station serve as a "specimen" for another? We must have all. Also the lithographing of all the plans and maps which were sent to be done (by Dr Sutherland) some months ago, as illustrations of the digest which is to be made of all the books of "replies."

If your meeting on the 11th carries this (viz., the maps and abstracts) it will be a very opportune meeting. But I rather hope both that you will have several more meetings and that you will not have them till November. For there are many things to bring before you which must stand over till Dr Sutherland returns. . . .

P.S. We must hang together now my dear master is gone. He was a leader we shall not find again. And I appeal to *you*, and shall appeal to you, to carry some very important points before the commission, as you *have* always permitted me to do so.

Source: From four letters to William Farr, Wellcome Ms 5474/48-51, copy ADD Mss 43399 ff60, 62, 63 and 64 (the first two written from Hampstead, N.W.)

21 October 1861

I think there can be no objection to the ending of your paper [on Sidney Herbert]. I like it very much. I like people to know that Sidney Herbert was not so raw a statesman (as his friends would have it appear) as to consider his work *finished*. Poor Lady Herbert would, I am sure, be glad to have a copy.

When is your next Indian commission meeting called for?

2 November 1861

If you could, without any trouble to yourself, lay your hand upon my letter to you giving the heads of an examination for non-commissioned officers and privates, on the Indian sanitary matter, it would help me in arranging the heads of my own evidence, to which I am sorry to say I have done little of late. I have been so ill and busy. Please, to direct it to *32 South St., W.*, where I shall be on Monday.

My dear master has been dead three months today. Poor Lady Herbert goes abroad this next week with the children and shuts up Wilton, the eldest boy going to school. It is as if the earth had opened and swallowed up even the name which filled my whole life these five years.

I do not go back to Burlington St., which is now to me deserted.

28 November 1861

Would you dine here at 6:00 o'clock with Sutherland? and would you sleep? I would ask Martin to stay [to] dinner too. But he and Sutherland agree so badly and nothing like business ever comes out of it.

I send you our poor Clough's books on Plutarch,[66] if you like to keep them all for your children, pray do. I shall like to think of them in your hands. I also return a portion of your Indian evidence.

20 December 1861

Dr Sutherland says he *must* see you about the maps and estimates for lithographing them (Indian) which are all here. Could you come in today or tomorrow and dine at 6:00 o'clock? Today would be more convenient to me.

## Producing the Report

**Editor:** Nightingale devoted much of 1862 to writing for the commission. First there was the massive report, which was substantially her own work, to be finalized amidst renewed difficulties at the War Office. In a letter to her mother in 1862 Nightingale described her work with the War Office and Lord Stanley as a "weary, hopeless struggle. . . . I have now written the biggest part of their report."[67] She had to intervene to see that Drs Farr and Sutherland were paid for the special work done for the commission (see p 118 below). Then there was the "Abstract from the same Reports," i.e., from the stational returns, done with Sutherland; a new "Abstract of the Evidence" was written by her. Finally she wrote her important summary of the report, *Observations*, prepared with utmost care; for visual presentation she asked her cousin, Hilary Bonham Carter, an artist, to produce woodcuts illustrating Indian activities. She also assembled the material for her paper, "How People May Live and Not Die in India," to be read in 1863. She sent a draft of her *Observations* to Dr Farr and to Sir John McNeill for criticism, also to John Lawrence.

Because Parliament prorogued on 7 August 1862, the presentation of the report to the House of Commons had to wait till February 1863. It was botched by Sir Charles Wood, who, "by mistake," submitted a mere summary of it, as already mentioned in the Introduction (see p 16 above).

---

66 A five-volume edition of Plutarch's *Lives*, based on John Dryden's translation and revised by A.H. Clough, appeared in 1859.

67 Letter 7 March, *Life and Family* (1:150-54).

Source: From a letter to Sir John McNeill, Florence Nightingale Museum (LMA) H1/ST/NC1/62/SU145, typed copy ADD Mss 45768 ff170-71

15 April 1862

I work on still for the War Office. But it is a guerilla warfare, of little profit although Lord de Grey is entirely on our side. I have written the greater part of the Indian sanitary report for Lord Stanley and am doing the digest of the stational reports. That for the Bombay presidency I have finished. Lord Stanley has asked me to write answers to written questions, under my own name. But these *I have scarcely begun.*

Source: From three letters to William Farr, Wellcome Ms 5474/52-54, copy ADD Mss 43399 ff67, 68 and 70-71

18 June 1862

Very many thanks for your police report. I read it with the greatest interest. And though I do not presume to say it is excellent, because everything you do is excellent, it will put the pensions and policemen on a much better footing.

We shall be glad to see you in India as soon as you can come out. I communicated both your note and police report to Dr Sutherland.

13 July 1862

Would you be so good as to look over my "evidence" and give me your suggestions, as you were godfather to it, in the first instance, I believe. It is entirely uncorrected and will want a good deal of correction. Also, I have done the digests of the two presidencies, Bengal and Bombay (stational reports), but not that of the Madras presidency. Therefore I shall still have illustrations from this last to insert into this said "evidence." . . .

Would you write on margin your criticisms and suggestions?

8 August 1862

You said, "write more, more." And I have written "more, more," and enclose you the result, begging for it to be returned to me with the former proof, and for you to make your remarks upon this one, in lieu of the former. (I have sent it to General-Register Office)

But this is not my object but my excuse in writing. I am miserably anxious about the report ("Indian sanitary"). There are so many (political) contingencies on the cards, not one favourable to us, that it would have been very important to have got the report presented this session—now to get it presented by next February to the House of Commons.

Lord Stanley wants to have a meeting *early next month* to consider the report. We have had his corrections upon our part of the report three months. If we could get your statistical introduction, our draft would be revised in two days and sent to press. By the beginning of next month the whole matter must be in the corrected proof. Any general statistical details may go in the appendix.

What is really wanted is the necessary statistical statement to precede the sanitary inquiry and conclusions in the report. In your hands indeed is placed the question whether India is to have sanitary reform or not. Pardon my importunity. If you *could* send me the statistical introduction as soon as possible, I shall be

your ever grateful
F.N.

Source: From a letter to Sir John McNeill, Florence Nightingale Museum (LMA) H1/ST/NC1/62/SU147, typed copy Add Mss 45768 ff174-75

Hampstead, N.W.
8 August 1862

I venture to send you by this post for your criticism my *Observations on the Stational Reports from India.* If you are so good as to look it through, will you note your remarks on the margin and return it to me? It is only a proof.

We have failed, owing to the dilatoriness of some of our members in getting our report, "Indian Sanitary," presented this session, as would have been most important. But next month Lord Stanley holds a meeting to consider the report. It now stands thus.

1. All the replies to the printed books of queries have come in from India, have been abstracted and are in print. My digests of these for the three presidencies are all written. Bombay is in type. Bengal and Madras not yet come back from press. Would you like to see these three digests?

2. Our part of the report (sanitary) is written and in type, and corrected by Lord Stanley, who pledges himself to carry it through the commission next month. This embraces the oral evidence, of course, rather more than or quite as much as the stational replies. My "observations," ordered by the commission (and which I now send), were limited to the stational replies.

I have little new, nothing good, to tell. Lord de Grey and Captain Galton miscalculated their powers or their intelligence when they promised to reorganize the War Office. The administrative work they do well.

Source: From a letter to William Farr, Wellcome (Claydon copy) Ms 5474/55, typed copy ADD Mss 43399 f74

12 August 1862

I do not understand from Lord Stanley's note that he wishes for a meeting until he is ready with the report. What he wants is the report. We thought to expedite matters by sending your part with the sanitary part to press, to get a proof of the whole so that you and Lord Stanley might see how the whole stood. That is all.

But if you prefer sending it direct to Lord Stanley, he will take means to have it put in connection with the part already in type. Then we shall have proofs of the whole. And a meeting will be held thereafter to discuss the report. But every day's delay counts for a year.

Source: Incomplete letter to Lord Stanley, Liverpool Record Office, Derby Collection 920/15/3

4 September 1862

Possibly you may remember, more possibly you have forgotten, that you, as chairman of the "Indian Sanitary Commission," desired me to do the enclosed. As you have been in India, I would rather submit it to you first for any corrections or suggestions that you will kindly make on the margin, before sending it in to the commission. It is only a proof. We have finished the abstracts of the stational reports of the three presidencies and illustrated them with woodcuts.

Source: From a letter to Hilary Bonham Carter, ADD Mss 45794 ff183-85

Hampstead, N.W.
4 September 1862

I have been waiting for five weeks to ask you to do the following for my Indian "evidence." And I think now I am doing you a benefit by calling for it loudly. I want it for woodcutting, the less picturesque, the fewer lines, the *less* laborious, therefore, the better:

1. An Indian bheestie (or water carrier) with his skin of water over his shoulder.

2. An Indian scavenger (or sweeper) carrying off the refuse on his head or in whatever way he does carry it. (These two I presume could be found in any Indian illustrated book.)

3. One of the vast Indian barrack rooms of more than 100 men, an interior view, with all the men lolling on their cots, being shut up during the hot hours—a *day* view. Ludlow Smith, or General Ludlow, or any Indian would supply you with the facts. And (I repeat) the more *barely* executed, the better. Only it must be *like*, being *for* Indians.

As all my other woodcuts are done, if I cannot have these in a few days to send to the woodcutters, it is of no use. And if you have no means of procuring the requisite Indian information, please tell me, and I will try elsewhere.

I do think this is a more useful thing to do, for you. So I make no apology.

Source: From two letters to Lord Stanley, Liverpool Record Office, Derby Collection 920/15/4 (both written from Hampstead, N.W.)

10 September 1862

With my late dear master, I had many discussions on this point,[68] becoming, as it is, unfortunately too important. But it is obvious that I can scarcely hope to press it on any man as I could on him. [folio missing]

It was then so improbable (perhaps the most improbable thing that could happen) that, of Sidney Herbert and me, *I* should be the survivor, that no record remains, as far as I am aware, of this [unknown] transaction, which was done verbally through me, in the spring of 1859 (immediately before Sidney Herbert, who was then to be chairman of this commission, took office).

This is my only excuse for bringing it before you, which would otherwise be a singular interference on my part. But a word in your note makes me think that you are unacquainted with it—although I know it was Sidney Herbert's intention to communicate it to you.

17 September 1862

1. About Dr Farr no rate of remuneration was mentioned. The understanding was, when Lord Herbert proposed through me that Dr Farr should act on the commission, that he should do the actuarial work and be paid a fee for it. (The same arrangement was made when Dr Farr served on Lord Herbert's subcommission for reforming our army statistical service and he was paid for it.)

Lord Herbert told me that he had communicated to you the arrangement by which Dr Sutherland was to act and be paid as secretary to the Indian Sanitary Commission, with Mr Baker as assistant. The work of both Dr Farr and Dr Sutherland is of course much more arduous than that performed by the unpaid commissioners.

Indeed I am aware that the expense of printing has already been great. And not to add my mite of cost, I have arranged with Mr Baker

68 The point concerned the proposed regulation of prostitution under the Contagious Diseases Acts. See *Women* (8:411-508).

for myself to pay for the woodcutting and printing of my paper. I may perhaps add that I have myself done the whole of Dr Sutherland's clerical work and a good deal of the other for him, as it would have been *absolutely* impossible for it to be accomplished without going to the Treasury for clerical assistance, of which we have had none. It is therefore the less impertinent of me, I hope, to measure the work which the Treasury *must* pay for.

2. I trust that a great deal may be done to prevent your report, when completed, from being "shelved." Lord Herbert set on foot four subcommissions, the moment his report was out, one for reforming barracks and hospitals, which is still at work, one for organizing the Army Medical School at Chatham, one for reorganizing the statistics, one for reforming the Army Medical Department and writing a code of regulations, the results of all of which, as you are aware, are now the active rules at the War Office. Three other commissions were subsequently formed. . . .

A great deal too was done in giving publicity to the report, in the *Times* and other papers, and in the reviews (as you are aware. For you were kind enough to offer to write an article, in the *Westminster* I believe, when you were yourself called to office). Also we reprinted the diagrams of army mortality, with their story attached, and these were sent to every commanding and medical officer in the army. I am not in the least inferring that these are instances for the Indian commission to follow. Probably your course of proceeding will have to be quite different. Probably a consultative board with an administrative head will have to be organized for each presidency.

But in the matter of publicity, the mere sending a copy of the abstracts of stational reports to each station will stir them up to do something. They will be read with avidity *there*, however much or however little we may read about India in England.

3. I am glad you have faith in Sir G. Lewis. For I have none. (And you probably see a different side of him from what I do.) He is the worst secretary of state I have ever seen. And I have served under five. His learning and his ignorance, his hurries and his delays, are alike against us. In one short year he has let down the War Office to the level from which Sidney Herbert was five years dragging it up. And this simply by letting the agencies work, against which Lord Herbert's official life was one continual struggle. He has not his equal for cramming a subject well for the House of Commons on Monday. But then he has not his equal for forgetting it all on Tuesday and acting quite

differently in the War Office, and on Saturday, if there *is* a "third course" open, for adopting that course with the Horse Guards.

*As far as he* is concerned, there is neither unity nor distinct responsibility (in each department), nor direct communication with him, nor promptitude of action, nor economy in administration in the War Office now. He is not head of his own office. He will, it is true, "not be appalled by the length of a report." But he will not see its *portée.* And well if he is not correcting his "astronomy" or his Latin "Hey diddle diddle," under the most important papers on the War Office table. Yet he is an honourable man.

You must excuse me for not answering your question about Dr Farr immediately. There are days and days when I am unable to write at all. And now you will think I have written too much.

Source: From a letter to Edwin Chadwick, ADD Mss 45771 ff5-6

Hampstead, N.W.
28 September 1862

As you are so good as to ask for a copy of my Indian paper for "John Mill" (who also has been excessively kind to me), I send you the only other proof I have, except the one I am engaged upon, for him. But you must be pleased to bear in mind that it is only a first proof, and that I can have no power to make it public till our report is out, which will be the beginning of next year. Then I will try and get you as many copies of my paper as you are so good as to make the use of which you mention. . . .

Where is "John Mill" now? and how is he?

Source: From a letter to Lord Stanley, Liverpool Record Office, Derby Collection 920/15/6

21 November 1862

My paper, which you have already seen, is done. But it occurred to me that it would be more conformable to discipline if I were to submit it to you in its state of "final revise" (in case you might have something to object), before I have it struck off and sent to your commission officially. . . .

The enclosed might interest you as enumerating the results which Lord Herbert gave to his first commission (sanitary). It was drawn up at the request of one of the present government. Please put it in the fire, when done with.

Source: From a letter to Sir Charles Trevelyan, Wellcome (Claydon copy) Ms 5482/48

22 November 1862

At least you will let me thank you for the precious five Hindustani books. I am afraid I am too old to learn Hindustani, though I should have thought nothing of it ten years ago. But they will remind me, if that were needed, of all the good you are doing in facilitating communication between our poor men and the people among whom they have to live. I wish I could go out to India.

We are forcing forwards the printing of the Indian sanitary papers, both because it is high time that the commission should finish its labours, and because I hope to put a good many into your hands by 4 December. But that (dreadful) General-Register Office has not finished our statistics yet. . . .

About the Ruam [?], it does not follow, as you say, that interceptory sewers are required to cleanse it. This is an engineering question which only a first-rate sanitary engineer could settle. In sanitary experience any influx of sewage into a river is bad (even here, and must be worse in India). And any delay of water in a riverbed requiring a periodic flushing is also bad. Sanitary engineering would prevent this.

Source: From a letter to Lord Stanley, Liverpool Record Office, Derby Collection 920/15/7

26 November 1862

I sent this morning my Indian paper to you "officially"(!) and I will send copies to the members of the commission. But, when the commission is closed, its real work will begin. (Is that Irish?) You will not rest the chance of sanitary reform in India on the recommendations of a report alone. (The very last Indian document I have seen, viz., a report from the "sanitary commission" of the Punjab, just arrived here, actually states that the best possible arrangement for India is one to which we know, in this country, are due severe outbreaks of cholera, one which killed poor Lord Raglan[69] in the Crimea, one which we consider to be one of the greatest sanitary defects in India.) This only confirms what all the reports have grievously impressed upon me, viz., that, although there is a certain outcry against bad sanitary conditions, nobody seems to know what they are, still less how to deal with them.

---

69 FitzRoy James Henry Somerset, later Lord Raglan (1788-1855), commander of the British Army in the Crimea. He died of dysentery following the disastrous assault on Sebastopol.

This was clearly seen when the report of the Royal Commission on the Sanitary State of the British Army (by Sidney Herbert) was under discussion. And it was determined, as you know, that practical work should succeed the declarations of principles. The result has been that the army at home is now healthier than the civil population, instead of its mortality being double.

(I venture to enclose you two diagrams which I had made to illustrate this—the first was published in the above report. I mean to publish these now with: "This is how he found the Army. This is how he left it." I will therefore beg you to return me these diagrams, as I have no other copies.)

May you live to see the Indian Army restored in the same way by your exertions. Would it not be possible to select a commission, consisting of experienced practical people, and let them guide the movement for a while, until it could go on itself? They could select agents in this country, and so enable the local presidential commissions to obtain men conversant with the details of works. And they could advise on all subjects connected with the welfare of the army as well as with the sanitary improvement of towns.

I think a good working commission might be got together without difficulty.

Source: From two incomplete letters to Sir Charles Trevelyan, Newcastle University Library 35/17 and 35/39

2 December 1862

I send you my abstract of the "Replies" from Indian stations together with my own paper [*Observations*] for your kind offer of study during the voyage.[70] You will see that it is all evils and no remedies at present.

I wish I could send you the conclusions. We are however still waiting for our statistics. But, with your kind permission, as soon as Lord Stanley arrives at any decision, I will send you out (by next mail, without waiting for publication) the papers, as they come out. If there is any particular way of sending them to you, you will kindly tell me.

From the papers I send, you will see at once that the condition of the country and people and, as a necessary consequence, of our army, are very much the same as the Middle Ages show as once the state of Europe. High death rate, occasionally ("now and then," as the reports naïvely put it) heightened by pestilence, is the result in India

70 He was posted to India as finance minister in 1862.

as once in Europe. This is one of the great problems of the future civilization of India. (I know you have other great problems towards its civilization to deal with and God bless you for undertaking it.) Europe had to toil its way up to safety by its own efforts. India may now have the advantage of European experience and science, if it is properly gone about.

[1862]

Unfortunately these stational returns, as you will see, tell us *nothing* of what ought to be done. Or where they do tell us anything, it is rather what should be avoided. (In the last sanitary report from the Punjab sanitary "commissioner," sent me by Sir John Lawrence, he positively states to be the best possible ideal for India that which has produced frightful choleras in Europe and which killed poor Lord Raglan in the Crimea.) In these things we must be guided by evidence and the evidence certainly is against the conclusion that sanitary improvement will be self-developing in India. What is wanted is to bring vigorous effort to bear on it from this country, the *administration* being, of course, left in *local* hands. Either way there is difficulty. There is a good illustration, as you yourself remarked, of "the way to do it" in Lord Herbert's subcommissions of practical working men who were appointed to give practical effect to his principles. I trust Lord Stanley will organize a working commission in England to draw up some general practical scheme for India and to guide it for a little time, until correct principles of improvement are in operation in each presidency.

Farewell and again God bless you. Since Sidney Herbert's death there has not been so great joy as that you should be going out to guide the financial matters of India. I would I were going to India too.

Source: From a letter to William Farr, Wellcome Ms 5474/59, typed copy ADD Mss 43399 f95

4 December 1862

Thank you very much for your Indian diagrams which are startling and painfully striking.

1. Would it not be well to add the *Home* Army comparison (executed just now by you and which is at this moment in Mr Hammick's hands) to both these valuable diagrams?

2. We have it on evidence that the mortality in the Indian Army might be reduced to 20 [from 69] per 1000. Ought there not to be a (square) diagram to show the effect of this?

3. Our improvement in statistical esthetics is not so conspicuous as our improvement in statistics. Our statistical art is somewhat in the same state as art before Cimabue [thirteenth-century Italian painter]. Could it not be improved?

4. I send the "abstract" of Indian stational reports.

Source: From a letter to Douglas Galton, Add Mss 45760 ff200-03

5 December 1862

I send back "Punjab" [Dr Hathaway's Punjab sanitary report]. He comes back to me (like the rats of Ehrenbreitstein[71]) again and again. And I can't prevent his getting upstairs. The India Office are so fond of him that every member sends me a copy.

All the reporting we can do, if we do it for 100 years, is no good, if this is the line prevalent and admired out there. What we give our lives to prevent, they advocate. What killed Lord Raglan in the Crimea, what has produced endless choleras in Europe, they approve. . . .

This report proves two things: (1) that it is impossible to exaggerate the sanitary defects of Indian stations; (2) that Indian medical officers (if this report fairly represents their intelligence on such subjects) are the best agents possible for increasing the high rate of mortality in the Indian Army.

Anything more hopeless than the infinite hiatus between the mischief described and the remedies recommended I have never seen. It is greater than that in the Crimea. I wish I *were* going out to India. Others dread it. There is *nothing* I should like so much, if it were only possible.

Source: From a letter to Harriet Martineau Add Mss 45788 f173

[November-December 1862]

I am working hard to get our Indian sanitary report through the press by February. I send you one paper which Lord Stanley (our chairman) insisted on being signed by my name. It is of course "confidential" till the report is laid on the table of the House of Commons. And I solicit your assistance, when the time comes, in pressing the reforms upon the public.

---

71 According to tradition, rats brought the plague to the fortress of Ehrenbreitstein on the Rhine and kept coming back.

Source: From a draft letter in Dr Sutherland's hand for Lord Stanley, ADD Mss 45781 ff74-75

[December 1862]

I send you the abstract of the sanitary state of Indian stations. You will be at no loss to discover that the condition of the country and people, and as a necessary consequence of our army, are very much the same as the historians of the Middle Ages describe as once the state of Europe. High death rate occasionally augmented by pestilence is the result in India as it used to be in Europe. This is the great problem of the future civilization in India. Europe had to toil its way up to safety by its own efforts. India may now have the advantage of European experience and science if it is properly gone about.

Unfortunately those returning, you will see, tell us nothing of what might be done. And anything they do tell us on this head is rather what should be avoided. In these things we should be guided by evidence and the evidence is certainly against the conclusion that sanitary improvement will be self-developing in India. What is wanted is to bring vigorous effort to bear on it from this country while the administration is left in local hands. I see no other way out of the difficulty.

We have a very good illustration of "the way to do it" in Lord Herbert's subcommissions, of practical working men who were appointed to give practical effect to the principles laid down in the report of his royal commission and this experience clearly points out the necessity of organizing a working commission in England to draw up some general practical scheme for India and to guide it for a little time until correct principles of improvement are in operation in each presidency.

Source: From a note to William Farr, Wellcome Ms 5474/60, typed copy ADD Mss 43399 f101

[1862 or 1863]

*Statistical.* The "defects of the existing organization" can be quite well "pointed out" in the *Report.* But it would have been most desirable, if possible, to call out *evidence* to prove that other classes, under the same climate, do not suffer as soldiers do.

No fact brought out by the first royal sanitary commission struck the public so much as this: that the soldier at home was nearly the most unhealthy of all trades. People who could understand nothing else understood this. The look of diagrams[72] again struck everybody. If something of the same kind could be done here—a comparison between soldiers and civilians in tropical climates—it would do more to convince such men as Sir Hope Grant[73] than all the rest put together.

The fallacy about the destructive effect of night duty being the cause of the soldier's mortality at home has disappeared in the minds of military men since the first commission. Could not the fallacy about climate being the *unavoidable* cause of the Indian mortality do the same before the commission? *Drainage.* It is most important to have Rawlinson or Austin upon *how* this is to be done.

Source: From a letter to Edwin Chadwick, ADD Mss 45771 f27

5 January 1863

I have sent (to the Athenaeum) a copy of my Indian paper (with woodcuts) for you, and one for Mr Mill. Please remember and remind him (though it seems impertinent to say so to two such distinguished officials) that it *must* be *strictly confidential* till the Indian Blue Book is laid on the table of the House of Commons.

Source: From a letter to Lord Stanley, Liverpool Record Office, Derby Collection 920/15/9

3 March 1863

I am afraid you will be surprised, though not so much surprised as I am, at my asking to see you. You will easily guess that it is on a point connected with your Indian sanitary report.

Could you find an hour soon which you could appoint to see me?

Source: Notes/draft letter for John Sutherland on meetings with Lord Stanley and Lord de Grey, ADD Mss 45751 f222

[ca. March 1863]

1. Lord Stanley is in earnest, however cautious.
2. He is going to Sir C. Wood today to try to persuade him to let the home commission work. He asked my leave since it will depend ultimately on Sir C. Wood. It was no use saying No!

---

72 It should be recalled that Nightingale the statistician pioneered the "pie chart," so common since, to graphically illustrate given data. She used it first at the time of the first royal commission.

73 Sir James Hope Grant (1808-75) became commander-in-chief of the Madras Army in 1862.

3. You are to go to Lord Stanley on Saturday at 11:00 with the draft [of the report?] proposed as we wish it (of course we have not done that already), to hear what Sir C. Wood has said.

4. Lord Stanley thinks it quite impossible to submit the money part to the commission,

5. neither to put it into direct communication with the presidency commissions.

6. He dwelt of course on the great jealousy of the India government against the India/home government and urged a Calcutta commission, which I answered and he gave up.

7. He said that the act was only for the three seats of presidency (in which I think he is wrong; he said afterwards he did not know).

8. Lord S. said that no India government would listen to a plan of sending their plans to be criticized by a W.O. commission. So I said, put it as if the commission were to be their own, Cautley and Martin upon it, and the W.O. commission added on to theirs, the detail can be arranged after.

9. Lord S. says that you must reckon *a year* as the average delay produced by reference home to England.

1. Lord de Grey entirely gives up his idea of a Calcutta commission and adopts ours. But

2. he strongly urges that it be put into the recommendations of report.

3. He will do nothing till the report comes out, unless he finds that the India balance, set apart for buildings, is to be expended at once, of which he will inform.

4. He says that the *practical* success of the commission will depend on whether we can make Lawrence, Cautley, Vivian defend its measures in the home commission.

5. He sees great difficulty in putting the home commission in direct communication with the presidency commissions.

6. He did not know that presidency commissions were recommended. He had read my paper, every word, and quoted it. I mean my letter to Lord S. Have you heard from Sir J[ohn Lawrence?]? . . .

Lord de Grey lays the *greatest* stress on a copy being sent privately to him *without delay*.

Source: From two letters to Lord Stanley, Liverpool Record Office, Derby Collection 920/15/10 and 12

16 April 1863

*Private.* Forgive me for addressing you again about your Indian sanitary report. Sir John Lawrence wrote to me a few days ago about these matters, among other things saying that there are now "barracks in India for full 25,000 men under consideration" and that "many are urgently required." He says hopefully, after wishing that I could "get to know" when your report will be out, "*so that what changes are necessary may be at once adopted,*" that it, the report, will have the greatest influence.

I was honestly unwilling to put myself forward to urge and trouble you. But when another letter comes from Sir J. Lawrence, I cannot do otherwise, can I?

Should you think well to expedite the work by calling in all the copies of the report sent to the members of the commission, so that a revise might be made, in which either all their views are represented or their objections met? If you thought well to send the copies to me here, we would set about it at once.

If Lord de Grey could be Sir G. Lewis's successor [it was to be the case], he, though not a very able man, would be the making of us in carrying out *administrative* (sanitary) reforms for the men.

27 April 1863

It is of great importance, as you say, to get out the report as soon as possible. But we have never yet received the copies sent out so as to put everything into a consistent shape. As it was sent to you, the report was an arrangement only of the matter, requiring very careful consideration to see that it was, after all, logically accurate. The references have also all to be revised, and fresh references (to facts) put in. There are two or three days' work of mere editing to do.

If you will send all the papers, we will return a copy to you with the corrections in manuscript, together with all the copies thus returned from the members. You will then be able to judge of the whole.

Source: From an incomplete letter to Sir Charles Trevelyan, Newcastle University Library 35/19

[20 May 1863]

As there will be many questions of water supply and drainage and sewerage of cities and stations, which did not come before our War Office commission (our home stations *being* drained, sewered and water supplied), Mr Rawlinson, engineer to the Local Government Act Office and the best water and sewerage engineer we have, will be added. Should the India Office name the commission, it will still consist of Sir P. Cautley, Sir R. Martin, Dr Sutherland, Captain Galton, Mr Rawlinson, C.E. They would advise in either case on all plans, collect and publish information, and be useful in all matters connected with barracks, hospitals, stations, towns, etc. The object is to have a temporary connecting link between the sanitary science and experience of England and the insanitary ignorance of India. Whichever form of (home) commission is appointed, it should draw up and lay before Parliament an annual report on the whole Indian subject. This is the only effectual check against carelessness and backwardness. It should bring before the eyes, or rather the nose, of the secretary of state for India the state and progress of things *every year.* (I did not make!! the present connection of India with England. But if we retain any power over India in London, let it be for good.)

The report was signed yesterday [19 May 1863] after four years' heavy work. I shall send you out my proof by this mail. You will then have the whole case and will be able to judge of what is required. . . .

What a work it would be to bring sanitary civilization not only to our men in India but to the native cities, a work worthy of *the old Roman power, Christianized* if that combination be possible.

Believe me, dear Sir Charles Trevelyan,
ever yours with the truest affection and gratitude
Florence Nightingale

Source: From a letter to Sir James Ranald Martin, in Joseph Fayrer, *Inspector General Sir James Ranald Martin* 173

20 May 1863

After the Saturday's discussion, I certainly did feel very deeply on the subject of the home and presidency commission[s] proposed in the Indian reports. They are the very central points, I believe, of the vast reform which your report will initiate. This is the dawn of a new day for India—not only for our army there, but for the poor natives—a day when the representations of men such as you will at length be carried out. Had I been able to see you, as I much desired, I believe that you and I could have agreed entirely and found on explanation that we had the same view. Now that the question is settled, I feel as if the first lease of joy had come to me since Sidney Herbert's death.

Source: From a copy of a letter to Sir James Clark,[74] Wellcome RAMC 1139/S4/23, Add Mss 45772 f173

Oakhill Park
Hampstead, N.W.
7 October 1863

*Confidential.* I wrote you my candid opinion about the commission proposed for the medical officers' grievances. I would gladly also give you some private reasons against the men chosen, altogether conclusive to my mind.

Catch Lord Stanley soiling the tip of one of his fingers to help out of the mire anybody! If we could have put Hamlet's ghost into the chair of the India commission, he would have served us better! And Lord S. has done NOTHING for us neither then nor since. Besides, *were* he to urge anything on our government, it would rather set them *against* it. He is so disliked! But the first royal sanitary commission, backed as it was by the whole country, would have served us nothing, had not Sidney Herbert undertaken and drawn up the warrant himself. He was a great man going out of his way to help many little men. If they expect anything of the kind of Lord S. they are woefully mistaken.

*I* could tell you how, as far as he has done *any*thing, he has stood in the way of *every*thing, in re India commission. Again, who is to write the report? General Eyre can't write. Lord S. won't. Confidential. In every single instance it has been Sutherland and I who have written the reports. . . .

Believe me, the Army Medical Department knows little what it is about, if it thinks that the commissions, headed by Sidney Herbert, which *had* the elements of success, could be reproduced (without him and without any of the elements of success) to do the same thing.

## *Observations by Miss Nightingale on the Evidence Contained in Stational Returns*, 1863

**Editor:** These *Observations* had been requested from Nightingale in October 1861 by the royal commission with a view to reaching a wider public than the report could. Formally they are addressed to Lord Stanley, chair of the commission. A first draft was completed in April

74 Sir James Clark (1788-1870), physician to Queen Victoria and a friend. Nightingale stayed with the Clarks at Birk Hall in 1856 when pressing Queen Victoria, Lord Panmure and others for the first royal commission.

1862, a second one in August. The final draft, dated 21 November 1862, was to be included in the official report of 1863. Nightingale's remarks here were concerned first of all with the conditions of the British soldiers; in further writings she devoted more attention to the situation of the native soldiers (sepoys). Essentially the *Observations* show that the main obstacles to the soldiers' health in India were "camp disease" and "liver disease" (see p 133 below), not wounds inflicted by combat. Camp diseases were due to unsuitable sites, bad living conditions and wide neglect of sanitary measures, liver diseases to overdrinking. Causes are itemized; a scathing review of daily life uncovers the barracks' bad habits that have to be corrected; significant and apt suggestions are made to improve the life of soldiers in India. The state of native towns was particularly appalling, which occasioned the cry: "Can it be possible that such a state of things exists after all these years of possession and unlimited authority?" (see p 174 below).

Nightingale's text, referred to as her "little red book" when reprinted as a book, was interspersed with graphic illustrations based on sketches of barracks and hospitals provided by Indian officers and touched up by her cousin Hilary Bonham Carter, who also provided woodcuts. One print, "Daily Means of Occupation and Amusement," which shows the deplorable idleness of barrack life, was sent to her by a Colonel Young. It is reproduced in the Illustrations section.

The royal commission report called for betterment in the conditions of the army in India, British soldiers and sepoys. Improvements were brought to barrack construction, while hospitals received more attention as regards buildings and the care of the sick. Nightingale was regularly asked for advice concerning the state of barracks and hospitals, as well as the maintenance of prisons and police stations. Moreover, the report itself insisted that "the habits of the natives are such that, unless they are closely watched, they cover the whole neighbouring surface with filth." Those topics received priority in Nightingale's involvement with India. In the course of her career such involvement grew and addressed larger problems of public health and societal evolution.

Source: "Observations by Miss Nightingale on the Evidence Contained in Stational Returns Sent to Her by the Royal Commission on the Sanitary State of the Army in India," *Report of the Royal Commission on the Sanitary State of the Army in India 1863*, 2 vols., Blue Book, Vol. 1:347-70, reprinted separately as *Observations on the Evidence Contained in the Stational Reports Submitted to the Royal Commission on the Sanitary State of the Army in India*, by Florence Nightingale (London: Edward Stanford 1863)

Right Hon Lord Stanley, MP
President of the Royal Commission on the
Sanitary State of the Indian Army

21 November 1862

My Lord

In compliance with the request sent to me by the Royal Commission on the Sanitary State of the Army in India, in Mr Baker's letter of 11 October 1861, that I would make on the contents of certain manuscript replies to queries addressed to all Indian military stations any observations which might occur to me as bearing on the sanitary condition of cantonments and hospitals, I beg to transmit the following. In doing this, the difficulty of giving what everyone might consider a fair representation of questions of such extent by stating specific cases has been great. Some will see no importance to health in the facts. Some will think the facts given the exception and not the rule. If there be an exception, i.e., if there be a single station in India with a good system of drainage, water supply and cleansing for itself and its bazaars, with properly planned and constructed barracks and hospitals, provided with what is necessary for occupation and health—a station where the men are not encouraged to drink and where they are provided with rational means for employing their time—to such a station these remarks do not apply. But I have not found it. Everywhere there are grievous sanitary defects which, wherever they exist, can lead only to sickness and loss of life to the degree in which they exist. And let those who doubt whether this representation is true, taken as a whole, look at the stational reports themselves.

In the papers sent me I find an amount of evidence showing the causes of disease in the Indian Army, such as perhaps was never before brought together on any similar subject. It is shown in these papers that:

### Indian stations are subject to the diseases of camps

The prevailing diseases at Indian stations are zymotic diseases connected with camps—such as I myself have seen—all of them, cholera, fevers, diarrhea, dysentery, together with hepatic disease. The main point of the Indian sanitary question is, indeed, camp disease, the causes of which are rendered more intense by climate; and liver disease, occasioned to a great extent by overeating and overdrinking and sedentary habits, the result of these habits being, as in the former case, intensified by climate.

Stations have been chosen with as little regard to health as camps often have been. Many are in positions which the mere verbal description proves to be unsuitable. Or, at all events, little or nothing appears to have been done to render them suitable. They are low, damp or even wet, often mixed up with unhealthy native towns and bazaars abounding with nuisances.

### INDIAN STATIONS PRESENT THE SAME SANITARY DEFECTS AS CAMPS

At all or nearly all the stations the usual causes of camp disease appear to exist. I will give examples of the more important of these as shortly as I can, as they exist at the larger British stations. These are:

1. Bad water;
2. Bad drainage;
3. Filthy bazaars;
4. Want of ventilation;
5. Surface overcrowding in barrack huts and sick wards.

1. *Bad Water.* Hyderabad (in Sind) says, "No doubt it (the water) *swarms* with animal life."

Where tests have been used, the composition of the water reads like a very intricate prescription, containing nearly all the chlorides, sulphates, nitrates and carbonates in the pharmacopoeia, besides silica and large quantities of organic matter (animal and vegetable), which the reports apparently consider nutritive, for few of them but "consider" the water "good" and "wholesome"; e.g., Fort William, Calcutta, says that the water for cooking, drinking, etc., is carried from a tank *filled by surface drainage,* which tank is kept "perfectly clean" and is "generally free" from "surface impurities." Many "*city* tanks are in a most filthy condition, producing malaria." Sealkote calls its water "decidedly good" while containing a considerable portion of sulphate of lime. Ghazipur calls its water "good and sweet" and says that it "does not seem contaminated by the amount of leaves that necessarily fall into open structures." Chunar says that its water is clear, sweet and inodorous "if allowed to settle before it is drunk." Agra's water is "laxative" and "apt to disagree *at first.*" Dinapore admits that its wells have been poisoned by infiltration from barrack privies. Nusseerabad says, "The flavour (of the water) varies according to the quantity of the salts." At Murri the quality is "considered inferior by native visitors, and to cause colic." "Boiling" and filtration through sand and charcoal are necessary to "render it wholesome." At Hazarybaugh tank water, "on standing, copiously deposits" and contains "organic matter in considerable quantity." Its well water for domestic use contains silicic, phosphoric, hydrochloric and carbonic acids. But it is satisfactory to know that "persons *particular* about the quality of their drinking water" can "obtain their supply" from "several good wells."

At Bangalore, the Ulsoor tank, used for drinking, is the outlet for the whole drainage of a most filthy bazaar (125,000 inhabitants), for that of our cavalry, infantry and horse artillery barracks, and of the greater proportion of the station. The commander-in-chief says, "The disgustingly filthy nature of the source, from which the water used at Bangalore is taken, has been brought to notice scores of times by me within the last 4½ years; but, as usual, nothing has been done to remedy this most crying evil." Even the wells from which drinking water is taken are impure from sewage. They are open and, "when they get dirty, are cleaned."

At Secunderabad, as much as 119 grams of solid matter and, as it would appear, 30 grams of organic matter per gallon are found in some of the well and tank water. (Secunderabad and Pune are almost the only stations which give a chemical analysis.)

At Surat "no one thinks of drinking the camp water." At Asseerghur the same tank is used for drinking and bathing. "For the former the natives slightly clear away the surface." Asseerghur thinks that its water "*smells* good." The application of chemical science to water supply appears hardly to be in its infancy in India.

The arrangements for raising and distributing water are everywhere, as Bombay presidency remarks, the same as what they might have been "1000 years or more ago." Belgaum has attained the maximum of civilization under this antique system. The water is there "raised in leather skins by bullocks, emptied into "troughs and thence conveyed by water carriers." At Kirkee "no such a thing as a pump is known"; government pays 617 rupees per (hot) month to water carriers.

Everywhere "each individual has his bheestie and each regiment its set of bheesties." (Words convey such an imperfect idea of the actual state of things that I obtained, by the great kindness of an Indian friend, illustrations taken from the life, which I have had cut in wood and transmit with this paper. I have also had woodcuts prepared of barrack and hospital plans from drawings contained in the papers sent me.)[75]

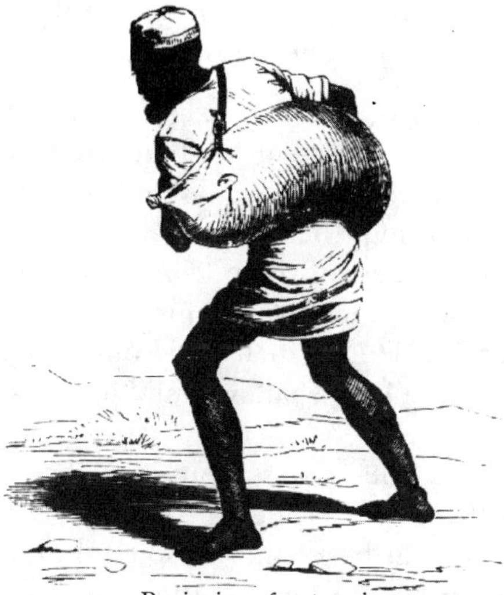

Beginning of water pipe

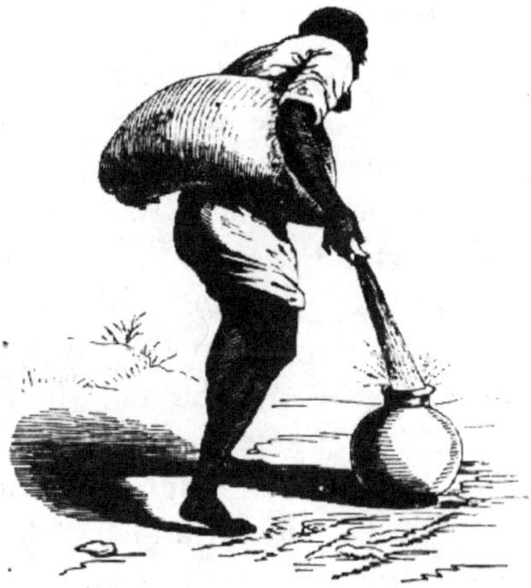

End of water pipe

The reason usually assigned for employing these human water pipes in barracks is that they are indispensable on field service. But so are tents; and yet nobody proposes to barrack men in tents in time of peace. Barracks are built for peace and ought to be supplied with reasonable and decent conveniences. Why should the bheestie and waterskin be preserved when the tent is abandoned? Let the bheestie be for field service if no better device can be discovered, but let some civilized method be adopted of supplying barracks, garrisons and towns with this prime element of health and cleanliness. Besides, human labour is daily becoming of higher value in India and it may be actually more expensive to use men as beasts of burden now than to use the appliances of civilization.

These water pipes with a will are not always found to answer, for Fort William (which pays them £134 per annum) admits that they sometimes take the water from "nearer and impurer sources." Would it not be better to try water pipes without a will?

It is singular that, while describing water sources, qualities and modes of distribution which civilized cities have ceased to use, most of

75 The small woodcuts are incorporated in the text and the large one is in the Illustrations section.

the reporters consider the water as good and fit for use. The practical result of this part of the evidence is that safe water supplies are yet to be found both for Indian cities and for British cantonments, and that many sources, as described in the returns, would in England be scouted as infallible causes of cholera in epidemic seasons.

*Lavatories.* As for all means of cleanliness, bathing, except in a few cases where there are plunge baths, seems to mean washing the face or throwing water over the body, for where there are lavatories there are no or few fittings; where there are fittings there is no water.

At Lucknow a small canal runs along the bathroom from which the bathers draw the water and throw it over themselves, being prevented by iron bars across from "lying at full length in it and soiling the whole supply." The bath at Mian Mir is a long shallow tank "in which the man can lie down and bathe."

Madras and Wellington are literally the only stations where anything like lavatories and baths, with proper laying on of water and proper draining it off, is known, either in barrack or hospital. But at St Thomas' Mount and at many other stations, each lavatory is a tub filled by a bheestie, in which all the men wash, there being no basins.

Figure 1 gives a plan, elevation and section of a lavatory at Aden, which affords rather a favourable specimen of the kind of accommodation provided. It will be observed that all the refuse water is conveyed into a built cesspit, 8 feet deep, from which it is expected to "make away with itself" as it best can. Why cannot civilized basins be provided for men to wash in and the foul water be properly drained away?

Washing and bathing in barracks and hospitals will have to be conducted on quite a different scale from the present in India if health and cleanliness are aimed at. If the facilities for washing were as great as those for drink, our Indian Army would be the cleanest body of men in the world.

2. *Bad Drainage.* This may be rendered NO drainage whatever, in any sense in which we understand drainage. The reports speak of cesspits as if they were dressing rooms. As at Nusseerabad and Kolhapur, "a small cesspit is attached to each bathing room, urinal or privy" and "to each married man's quarter there is a bathing room with cesspit."

At the capital of the Bombay presidency, where civilization has introduced a "main drain" two feet square with a "flat bottom," this "main drain" is a "great nuisance" and the "stench at times scarcely to be endured." At Fort George, in Bombay, the "latrines are not drained except into an open ditch which is always in a foul state."

**FIGURE 1**
**Lavatory in Aden**

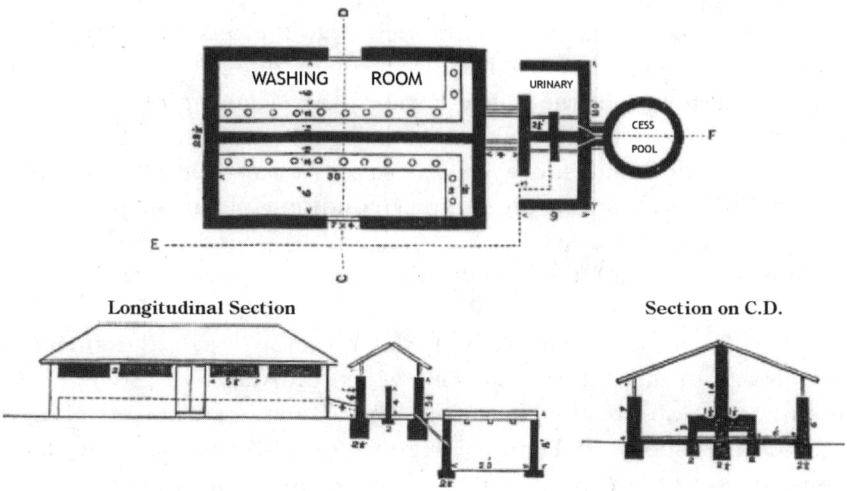


Indeed, Bombay would gladly say, as the London woman said when asked to point out the drains, in the days when London drainage was in a similar state, "No, thank God, sir, we have none of them foul stinking things here."

At Madras (Fort St George) the drainage hitherto is stated to be worse than useless. The main drain of the town is 80 yards distant from the European fort; the effluvia from it very offensive. The arrangements at the native lines, as described in the reports, are simply abominable. The old privies in Fort St George are "as bad as they well could be."

At Bellary, a large station, there is no drainage except the fall of the ground.

At Secunderabad (Trimulgherry) there is no drainage of any kind. The fluid refuse evaporates or sinks into the subsoil. A nullah [dry riverbed or ravine] which intersects the cantonment stinks. The extent of the cantonment is so enormous that it is said "to preclude any general surface draining," a statement which, if true, would amount to this, that the occupation of ground by human beings must inevitably lead to disease, a statement as applicable, or rather much more applicable to the area of London than to that of Secunderabad, and yet London is drained both on the surface and below it.

Everywhere the system of "drainage" is that "cesspits" are "emptied" when "filled" or "when necessary," and their contents carried away by hand, as at Deesa and Belgaum. Generally they are close to the buildings.

At Hyderabad, in Sind, in the native lines, the contents of the cesspits are "thrown about in close vicinity to the cesspits." "Anything edible is immediately picked up by birds or dogs." There is "great room for reform" in the native latrines, the cleansing of which consists mainly in the liquid "sinking into the subsoil, so that the earth is thoroughly saturated and a *noisome odour pervades* the atmosphere." And yet it is added that the sanitary condition of the station is, "in every respect, satisfactory."

At Neemuch the "drainage of privies and urinals is only on the surface."

Often, as at Aden, it is expressly stated that it (viz., "all drainage") is "allowed to sink into the subsoil" which (at Aden) we are told is so useful as to "absorb the contents." The arrangement for enabling it to do this is shown in Figure 1. Figures 2 and 3 represent the usual construction of latrines. In Figure 2 the contents are intended to be swept up and removed daily by hand—a noisome and dangerous process, especially during epidemics. Figure 3 shows the cesspool system of "cleansing," which means saturating the subsoil with filth and endangering all the wells in the neighbourhood.

At Neemuch, which has attained the high pitch of civilization of building latrines for its bazaar, the "latrines are too close to the houses and are not used at present *for lack of a proper establishment to keep them clean.*" Therefore the people at Neemuch do like their neighbours in this respect, a proceeding which it is impossible to describe farther. At Asseerghur a similar abomination appears to be practised on an "open space of ground near the main guard and parade," which is "always offensive" and "ready to nurture epidemic disease."

At Asseerghur the "construction of sewers and drains has not as yet been considered." They "consider," on the contrary, that the sewage "will probably be removed by hand." "The refuse, in all cases, is thrown over the fort wall." "One of the tanks" is called "unsavoury."

Almost everywhere it is said, as at Nusseerabad, Kirkee and Pune and Dinapore, all of them large and important stations, "barracks and hospitals" are "only wet" or "damp" during the "rainy months," as if it were a proof of great and unusual precaution in construction which builds buildings to be dry in dry weather.

**FIGURE 2**
**Latrine in Pune**

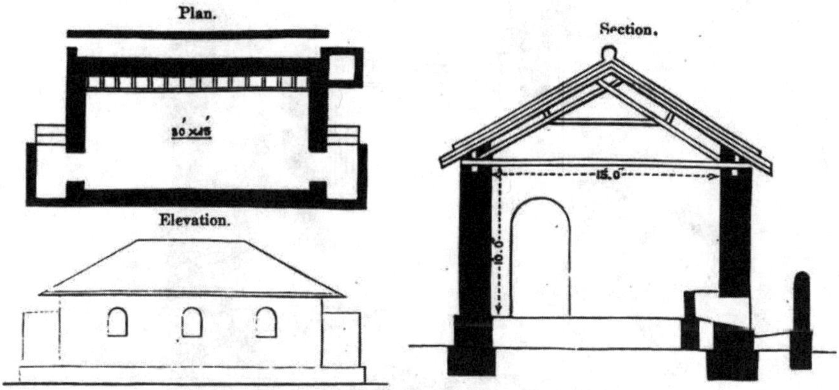


**FIGURE 3**
**Infantry Barracks Latrine in Belgaum**

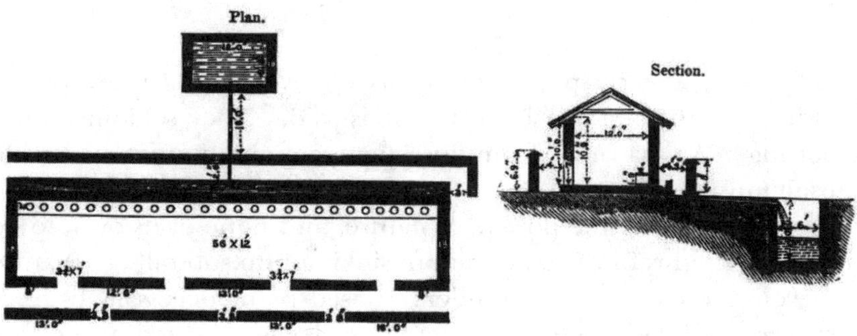


At Fort William it is stated that the fluid refuse is swept away by garrison sweepers and water carriers with the *aid of a fire engine*; that much of it evaporates; that the outlet is a foul ditch. Dinapore also boasts of a foul ditch, often very offensive. At Poonamallee the "foul ditch" surrounds the fort and encloses the hospital; and "all fluid refuse sinks into the subsoil where it falls."

At Kanpur is the singular statement that the drains are "not intended" for draining cookhouses, privies, etc. Here, as elsewhere, the drainage is effected *by hand*; that is, everything that will not evaporate or sink into the ground is carried away to a distance in pails, skins or carts, and emptied out.

**Indian Drainage System**

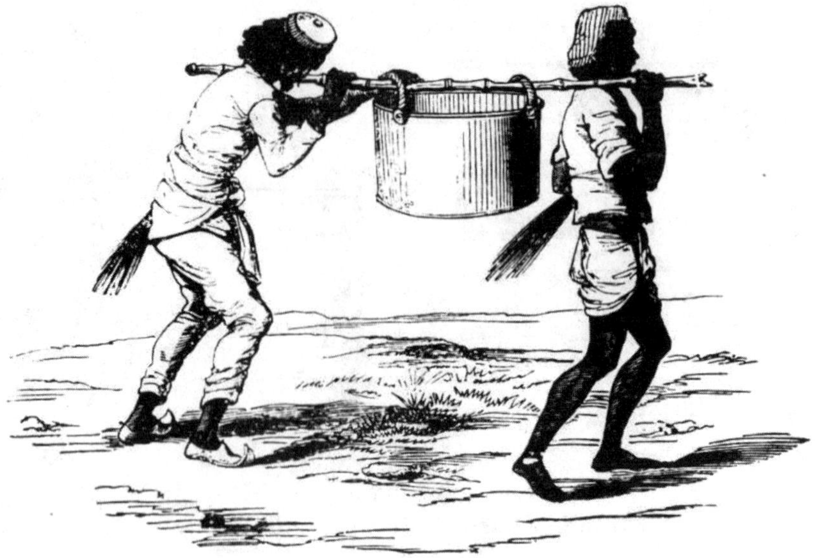

At Meerut the cesspools are cleansed "by opening the tops and drawing out the fluid in buckets." It is said, "They seldom require cleansing." We may infer from this what a condition of saturation the subsoil must be in!

Agra employs all the powers of nature, and none of its own, to get rid of its "fluid refuse": evaporation, sinking into subsoil, etc. Nature, however, is dilatory, which renders "raised paths necessary between the barracks." The water from the lavatories is collected in an open cesspool from which it is *spread over the ground.* The hospital cesspits are deep wells, *never cleaned.* It is "tried to keep them sweet by lime, *but in vain*" (probably).

At Umballa the surface water "disappears with tolerable rapidity."

Mian Mir, the new station for Lahore, has no drains about the barracks. The water lies for hours. The lavatory cesspools sometimes overflow, saturate the ground and taint the atmosphere.

These cesspools, as in Figure 3, were intended for saturating the ground with foul matter, and out of the same ground the well water is taken.

Is not the whole history here of the late frightful cholera at Lahore?

And why cannot the refuse, which does so much mischief by remaining, be used to do good and raise any amount of vegetables in soldiers' gardens?

Firozpur tells the same story of no sewerage or drainage. Also at Firozpur the lavatories *are* brick and mortar floors, "adapted for receiving and draining off the water into the subsoil outside, so that the men may freely bathe themselves!" There is no bath except the aforesaid floor. So at Peshawar and Sealkote is the same want of all sewerage or drainage.

At Berhampore, with its square mile of cantonment, only one cart is allowed to remove the contents of the privies to "holes a mile from barracks." The vicinity abounds in jheels [reaches of old river channel beds] and foul ditches with putrid water.

Allahabad, one of our largest and most important stations, in one of the worst positions, as if that position were not unhealthy enough by itself, trusts to nature again, has no drainage nor sewerage, and leaves its surface water to "evaporate," "percolate" and "run off."

Banaras follows in the train. At Rangoon the drainage is supposed to run uphill. For we are told that all sewerage and drainage are merely "trenches made without reference to slope."

Landour, which is a hill station, has every house damp for three months in the year. Yet their "spacious lavatory with brass basins" is not much used "from the scanty supply of water in the dry season."

It is evidently quite possible to locate the whole army on hill stations and leave it more unhealthy than on the plains.

Nynee Täl, also a hill station, lets all its fluid refuse flow down to plains below.

It is impossible to pursue this subject further. There are such much worse things in the stational reports than what I have chosen to give that I must say to those who call my "bonnet ugly," "There are much uglier bonnets to be had."

The system of water supply and drainage in India may be briefly defined as follows: they draw water from a well, not knowing whence it comes, and if there be any means to drain off water it is into a cesspit or into long, open, pervious drains, not knowing whither it goes. Where this is not done, all the fluid refuse is collected in open cesspits and carried away by hand labour or carts. Or else it is allowed to dispose of itself in the air or earth as best it can.

Drainage, in the sense in which we have found it necessary for health in this colder climate, is by no means considered necessary for health in the hot climate of India; for, as in the case of the water supply, most of the reporters consider *no drainage* a sufficient guarantee for health.

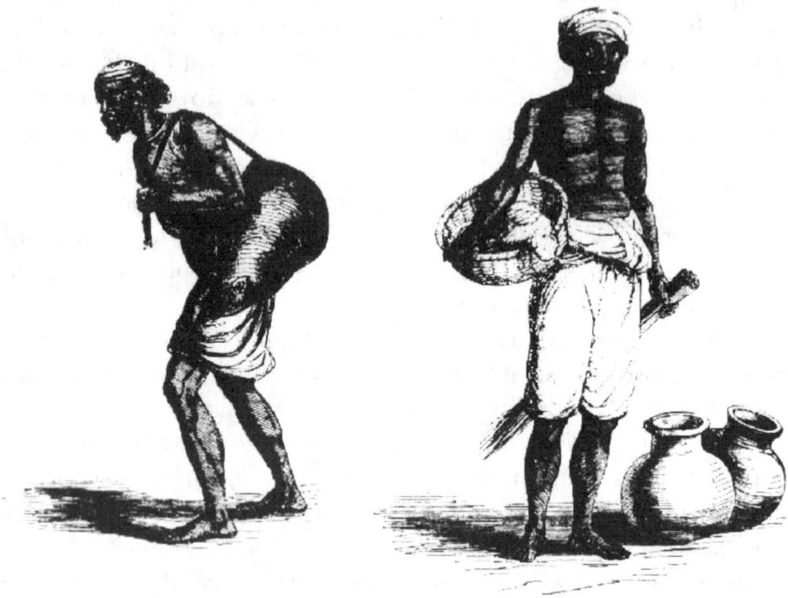

Bheestie Mehter

These two officials represent the system of water supply and drainage in India for garrisons and towns

3. *Filthy Bazaars.* It is almost impossible to describe these. But one description will do for all. Except where the two Lawrences [Henry in Oudh, John in the Punjab] have been—there one can always recognize their traces—the bazaars are simply in the first savage stage of social savage life.

No regular system of drainage, no public latrines, or if there are any, no sufficient establishment to keep them clean, no regular laying out of houses, overcrowding, bad ventilation, bad water supply, filth, foul ditches, stagnant water, jungle and nuisances, this is the account of all. The country round some is stated to be "one immense privy."

At Neemuch, the bazaar superintendent maintains "strict supervision" and "punishes the inhabitants," although the latrines cannot be used. The native houses are all more or less dirty, with dung heaps close to them. The "disagreeable emanations" from the bazaar are felt in barracks.

In Dinapore some streets were impassable dunghills "last year" "until cleared." The elephant sheds and all the south of the station in a state disgraceful to any cantonment. The drains, deep holes of festering mud. No latrines, although "the population is as thick as can be"; until lately, only one filth cart, now three. At a neighbouring village the dead are buried within the huts.

At Agra it is a proof of "respectability" to have cesspools. The inhabitants (152,000) generally "resort to the fields."

English works, treating of sanitary improvement, insert sections of the bad drainage arrangements. But none contains such an illustration as this of how a woman is made to supply the place of a drain tile.

At Berhampore "nothing can be worse than the sanitary condition of bazaars." The native houses are dirty in the extreme. Dung heaps or deep holes full of stagnant water, the common cesspit of the houses, are close to them. The nuisance is felt even at barracks. The "conservancy" establishment is quite unequal to its work.

At Muttur the bazaar is an accumulation of huts without order. "Drainage bad; ventilation worse; water supply execrable." "All the wells brackish, from nitre," the earth being contaminated with all sorts of impurities. Latrines "hardly known." "In short, the bazaar is a mass of filth."

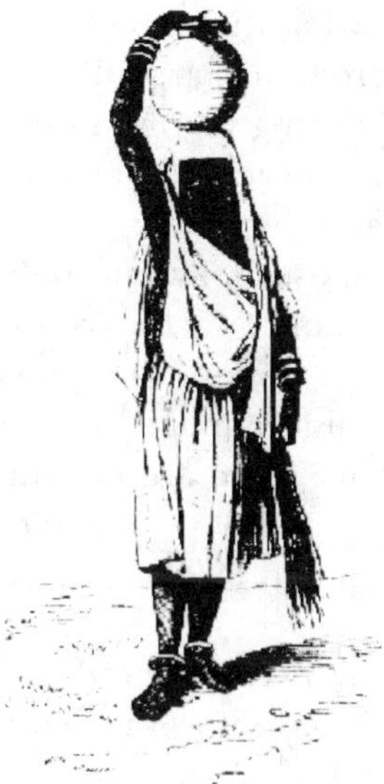

Female Sweeper

At one hill station, Nynee Täl, where *men are sent for their health (!) the stench is at times overpowering,* from both bazaars being in a filthy and crowded state, no proper drainage or latrines, no means of preserving cleanliness, which causes nuisance even in the barracks. At another, Darjeeling, among other defects, the native villages, writes the medical officer, "are the most filthy" he has "ever entered, and it is quite sickening to walk through them."

At Jubbulpore, where every hut is crowded, where there are no latrines, there cleanliness is almost impossible, the same causes produce the same results.

At Cannanore the native houses have dung heaps and cesspits within the compounds. Owing to the want of latrines, the "filth and indecency" are described to be what it is impossible to repeat. The dead are buried within the compounds of houses.

At Trichinopoly the water supply is bad, scanty and brackish. The bazaar is said to be "clean," while the open cesspits are described as an "intolerable nuisance," when the wind blows over them. The native houses are ruinous and not ventilated. Levelling, filling up, pulling down deserted huts, etc., is urgently required but not done.

Those who think I have given anecdotes and not fair illustration, I refer again to the stational reports for further and fouler evidence.

These instances are enough to illustrate the subject. Bazaars are the real hotbeds of disease and require sweeping reforms as much as or even more than the stations. Native regimental bazaars, from which the soldiers procure supplies, are within military limits and as much under military control as the ground on which the barracks stand, and *ought* to be kept in as good a sanitary state as the barracks will be when thoroughly improved.

4. *Want of Ventilation.* The reports generally say, ventilation good, if barracks not overcrowded. But as the barracks are almost always overcrowded, we must conclude ventilation is bad. Or they say, ventilation sufficient, because doors are kept open during day, which is as much as to say, ventilation is sufficient because it is not.

At Kirkee there can scarcely be said to be *any* ventilation in barracks. There are pigeonholes in the roof, but during the rains, when ventilation is most wanted, these have to be covered with tarpaulin. At Pune the weather side has to be "dammed up" during the monsoon. At Bombay it is said that ventilation is generally sufficient; "at least there are no complaints" although "improvement is imperative."

At Kamptee the ventilation is described as "most faulty and deficient" although there are three openings in the roof of each barrack. The windows are unglazed. At Ramandroog, a hill station, the doors are venetianed in the upper half, "a great disadvantage in wet weather." Half glass doors are required. At Bellary there are no windows. The doors are half venetian, half panel. At Trichinopoly, one of the very hot stations, the old artillery barrack is stifled by having only doors.

At Dinapore, where the ventilation is entirely by doors and skylights, "which latter, however, do not open," one may safely say, ventilation not sufficient when doors are shut (at night). In the "permanent hospital" at Dinapore, placed so that the "wind does not blow across" it, the ventilation is only "sufficient" when the doors are open.

At Allahabad the doors have to be closed in high winds, dust storms, etc., and the ventilation, although there are roof ventilators and small windows over the doors, is generally insufficient. The hospitals of Allahabad, although they "face the wind," have "in most instances no windows except openings over the doors and in the roof." And the ventilation is pronounced to be "very defective," especially when the doors have to be closed.

So at Dum Dum.

At Agra ventilation is said to be sufficient, provided the verandahs are not occupied for sleeping. But the verandahs are occupied for sleeping.

At Landour, where sick men are sent to get well, there is both overcrowding and bad ventilation. There is no roof ventilation.

At Nynee Täl the air is said to be "pure" inside the huts, which means that they are always full of "smoke."

The cooling by tatties, i.e., air passing through damp vegetable matter, often tends to produce ague.

External ventilation is often also bad, not giving the barracks the benefit of the prevailing winds, as at Dinapore, Allahabad and Berhampore. This is a point of primary importance in India. At Muttur, although there is abundant ridge ventilation the entire length, it is insufficient at night simply because the barrack is in a position which the wind cannot reach.

At Allahabad one third of the station is below the level of the river.

Generally, very little attention appears to have been paid to independent ventilation as a cardinal point of barrack construction. Doors and windows have been trusted to; yet they are so placed that men are often exposed in bed to hurtful draughts and, if shut, the fresh air is also shut out. Sometimes there is no glass in the windows and when these are shut there is darkness as well as foul air.

A knowledge of the proper application of sanitary appliances to building in India appears to be as yet in its infancy.

5. *Surface Overcrowding.* The structure of Indian barracks varies much. But in one thing they almost all agree, viz., in crowding the men upon the floor.

Figure 4 represents a plan and section of a hut room at Deesa, no less than 200 feet long, intended for eighty men, at 1116 cubic feet per man. It is well constructed for ventilation and is altogether one of the best plans in India. But for its 80 men, which is just four times too many for any room, it allows less than 59 square feet per man.

**Figure 4**
**European Barrack at Deese**

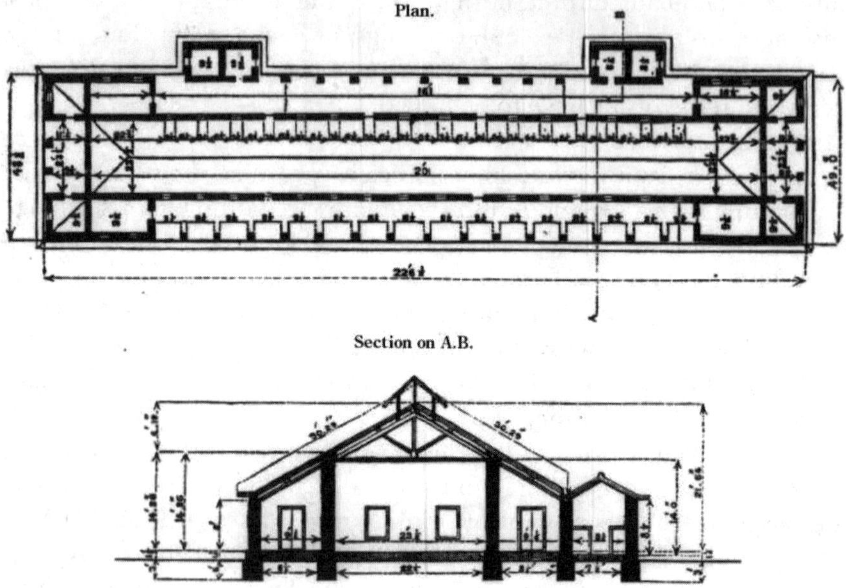


Even in the most recent barrack plans there is the same defect.

Figure 5 gives a plan, elevation and section of the new barrack, either erected or about to be erected, at Mhow. The elevation shows a magnificent and costly structure. But it is on two floors; it has double verandahs, the inner ones occupied by beds, so that there are four rows of beds and 53 feet between the opposite windows; the ventilation of the whole interior is interrupted in a rather ingenious way by cross walls and the men have 65 square feet of space each.

But even this is not the worst. At Fort William, the Dalhousie Barracks, which are said to be "perfect," have *six* rows of beds between the opposite windows, 216 beds by regulation in each room and three floors of such rooms. While it is added "900 men" (300 men per room) "are generally accommodated in the barrack without inconvenient overcrowding." What is *convenient* "overcrowding?"

The cubic space generally looks large in India but, the height of the rooms being enormous, often greater than their width, the superficial area is comparatively small. At Kanpur the barrack rooms are from 25 to 30 feet high. The superficial area for 1000 men in 10 rooms is only 41 square feet per man, for 140 men in two rooms 61 square feet per man, and for 240 men in two rooms 88 square feet.

**Figure 5**
**Infantry Barrack at Mhow**

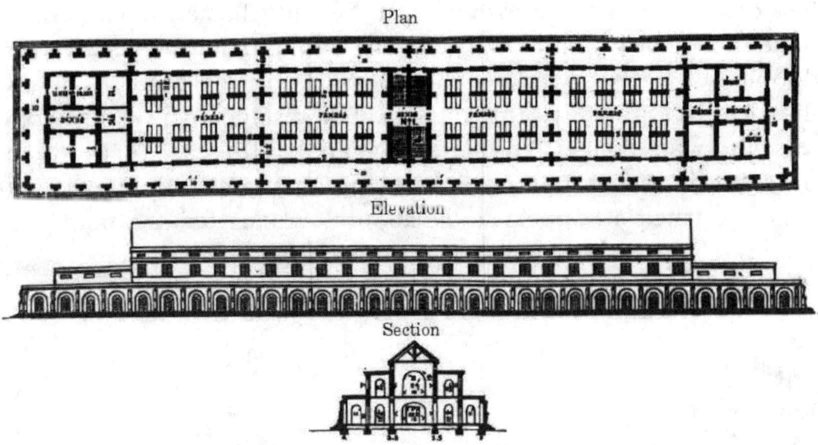


Also, the cubic space presupposes the inner verandahs not to be occupied. But in some places, as at Kanpur, they are invariably occupied from influx of troops beyond the accommodation; there are then four rows of beds between opposite windows.

In all the five barracks of Fort William the men put their cots in the verandahs in hot weather. Perhaps the wisest thing they can do.

At Dinapore again are two of these enormous barrack rooms (827 feet long, for 308 men). The superficial area in these rooms is 94 square feet per man. But one may safely say that 120 would be barely enough under such circumstances. Madras has two storeys, of one room each, for 1030 men, the upper of which rooms is stated in the return as nearly 2125 feet long (probably the longest room in the world), for more than 600 men, and the other, 1483 feet. The superficial area per man is only between 60 and 70 feet in these overgrown monsters of barrack rooms. Secunderabad has ten rooms, for 104 men each, with only from 40 to 60 square feet per man. At Poonamallee there are two long rooms, with 300 men in each, of which the space given by the dimensions is so incredibly small (112 cubic feet and 8½ square feet per man) that it is scarcely possible to believe them given correctly. The verandah, it is said, is frequently used as sleeping quarters. (No wonder!)

At Meerut, for upwards of 4000 men, the superficial area is only from 52 to 79 square feet per man, and the verandahs are occasionally used for sleeping on sudden influx of troops.

At Agra it is the same. So at Jullundur.

There is one barrack at Fort Govindgarth, at Umritsar, in the Punjab, a plan and elevation of which are given at Figure 6, which is a perfect nest of rooms one within the other and has an open verandah besides. The elevation looks promising enough; but the inside, with its double defences of windows and doors against the outer air, is about the last place to put seventy men in. The distance between the opposite windows is 86 feet. The superficial area in this case (better than in the other instances, but more than counterbalanced by the extraordinary construction) appears to be about 85 square feet per man.

**Figure 6**
**Infantry Barrack at Fort Govindgarth (Umritsar)**

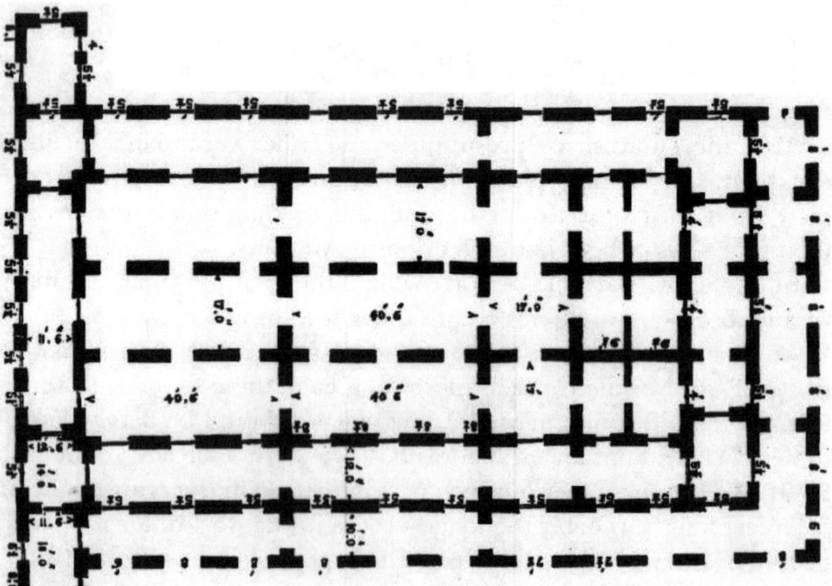

The men are far too crowded in their Indian barracks. In almost every case there are too many men in the rooms for health. The floors in most barracks are merely the ground bricked over, or they are of stone or of a kind of plaster.

At some stations the floors are of earth, varnished over periodically with *cow dung!* A practice borrowed from the natives. Like Muhammad and the mountain, if men won't go to the dunghill the dunghill, it appears, comes to them.

To sum up: it is not economical for government to make the soldiers as uncivilized as possible. Nature sends in her bill—a bill which always has to be paid—and at a pretty high rate of interest too.

### INTEMPERANCE

There is a good deal of intemperance among soldiers everywhere, but I very much doubt whether the same amount of tippling ever goes on in the British Army in this country as appears to be encouraged by the canteen system in India.

A soldier in India may buy at the canteen no less than a gallon of spirits in twenty days or he may have a quart of strong beer every day *and* one or two drams of rum or arrack. It is easy to see what must be the effect of this on health in such a climate.

The gist of the stational returns amounts to this: Men all "temperate." The maximum daily allowance per man is three quarts porter or two drams spirits *and* one quart porter, or one dram spirits and two quarts porter. This as at Mhow, the largest of our stations in the Bombay presidency. Agra too issues to each man per diem, during the "cold season," two drams of rum *and* one quart of beer. But "no more than" two drams spirits, or "one quart (32 ounces) porter and one dram (3 ounces) spirits" per man per diem is the common allowance.

Sale of spirits "strictly forbidden" in bazaar to soldiers; every man can nevertheless get as much as he likes in bazaar, *besides* the above quantity. For, as might be expected, it is practically impossible to encourage and restrict an evil at the same time. Government sells the licence to sell drink in the bazaar and orders the men not to profit by it. The present law is like lighting a fire and charging it not to burn anything.

"No confirmed drunkards"; cases admitted into hospital directly from intemperance, numerous; *indirectly*, innumerable. Average of habitual drunkards in some European regiments not less than 15 percent.

At Fort William seven trials for habitual drunkenness in 8th Regiment in three months; in the 5th Fusiliers admissions into hospital *indirectly* for intemperance, 17 in 100; *directly*, 2 in 100. Spirits, it is said by more than one report, are the curse of the European soldier in

India; also, that the evil effect of spirit drinking was manifest during the last field service. In seven regiments in Madras in 1849 the percentage among different classes was (roughly) as follows:

| | *Punished* | *Admitted* | *Died* |
|---|---|---|---|
| Teetotallers | 23.5 | 131 | 1.1 |
| Temperate | 58.5 | 141.5 | 2.3 |
| Intemperate | 171 | 215 | 4.5 |

Again, it is said (Hazarybaugh), "soldiers as a body temperate," *and* one third of disease and one half of crime produced directly or indirectly by drink.

The long-cherished idea as to the necessity of spirits for the British soldier is, it is stated, thoroughly exploded. A man who drinks tea or coffee will do more work than a dram drinker, though considered sober. And why? Because we now know that tea and coffee prevent waste of the system under exertion; while spirits afford no more than temporary stimulus followed by exhaustion or collapse, both of which conditions are powerful predisposing causes of disease, especially in an exhausting climate. It is an error to sell spirits in canteens to prevent men obtaining worse spirits in bazaars. It creates craving, to be satisfied elsewhere. Again and again it is said that selling rum in canteens is an unmitigated curse to a regiment, destructive alike to health and discipline; that it will be a "happy day" when nothing but beer, light wines, coffee, tea, lemonade, etc., are to be sold. Colonel Greathed, than whom we have no better authority, says that he "should wish beyond everything to see the practice of supplying spirits in canteens abolished."

In one year (1859), at Allahabad, there were thirty-six cases of delirium tremens, of which five were fatal. At Umritsar one sixth of the admissions are directly, and one half indirectly, from drink. Its effect is "injurious to the last degree." At Chunar, though the men are "mostly temperate," yet, on a ten years' average, *one man in three* (!) was admitted into hospital directly from drink, besides those indirectly, out of the admissions. The deaths were just twice, the crimes just ten times as many among the intemperate as among the temperate.

It is a comfort to hear that at Secunderabad the "average number of confirmed drunkards varies." But twenty-five out of twenty-six cases admitted into hospital indirectly from drink (Secunderabad's statement) is really too bad. Though when it is added that in this large station, occupied by nearly 3000 men, there is so little for them to do that they "go out in search of liquor," it is the less surprising. And the immense amount of epidemic dysentery that sweeps over the place occasionally, under such a system, is still less surprising.

At Bangalore, one of the largest of our Madras stations, where numerous acute attacks of disease are brought on by the quantity of spirits drunk, notwithstanding its fine, healthy, temperate climate, 3000 feet above the sea, it is stated that probably "not three men out of five go to bed perfectly sober," and when pay is issued not two in five. That, of one-year soldiers, 1 percent is a drunkard; after two years, 2 percent; and so the proportion increases with length of residence, owing to their "idle, listless, objectless lives." In India temperance is the exception and intemperance the rule. "But government is to blame." It "bids them drink freely" and when the habit is confirmed "denounces them as a disgrace to their country." "The habitual daily two drams ruin the health and habits of the soldier who thinks that as long as he takes only what government allow him, he cannot go wrong." The taste for spirits, it is said, is "not easily acquired by young soldiers." "The habit of spirits is maintained by their authorized use."

The temperate men, it is stated, all drink occasionally; impossible to say how much spirit is sold in the bazaars. At present the collectors encourage the sale as much as they can for the sake of the revenue. Under no circumstances, except extraordinary fatigue, almost all agree, should any drink but beer, tea or coffee be allowed, and the loss of revenue should be otherwise compensated for. Acquiring a taste for spirits should be discouraged in men by every means. It should be absolutely interdicted on the passage out, and malt liquor given instead with good food, good water and good accommodation. For want of these, about 10 percent of the recruits arriving from England at Karachi have in certain years suffered from scurvy.

"All spirit drinking is injurious to health." "Nine tenths of all the crime is caused by it." "It is directly or indirectly the root of all evil in the army." Such is the testimony borne in these reports.

In Burma, when malt liquor could be had, health always improved. A marked change for the worse took place when spirit was issued instead. Where beer was introduced, the "tremulous, yellow-skinned, emaciated" spirit drinker was rarely met with.

Madras presidency says that "health, efficiency and discipline would be materially improved by tea and coffee in preference to spirits and malt liquor," "as has been proved when neither spirits nor malt liquor could be had."

Barrackpore says that, if spirits were abolished and dietary improved, the mortality among our men would be "extraordinarily diminished." Fatal cases (in sickness) mostly occur among intemperate men.

There is hardly a difference of opinion as to the necessity of abolishing the use of spirits in the Indian Army. Men would be blind, indeed, to the most glaring facts who would justify its continuance. The only plea on the other side in the reports is a very old one, which has been used to justify other vices besides dram drinking, viz., that "if we do not give spirits in the canteen, which we all believe to be bad for health and discipline, the men will get worse spirits in the bazaar." Thus the men are killed by liver disease on canteen spirits to save them from being killed by liver disease on bazaar spirits, government in either case benefiting pecuniarily, as is supposed, by the transaction. May there not be some middle course whereby the men may be killed by neither bazaar nor canteen spirits?

### Diet: *Excess of Food*

It appears extraordinary to give the soldier the same amount and quality of diet in all seasons, in tropical as in temperate climates. And yet every day the soldier has 1 lb. animal food, 1 lb. bread, 1 lb. vegetables, 4 ounces rice, tea or coffee, and sugar, besides his spirits and beer and any amount of extra animal food he may buy for breakfast and tea. Of all countries India is the one where men cannot be dieted the whole year round by the same rule without mischief. But only a few enlightened men appear to have any idea of what effect this extraordinary system of dietetics has on the soldier's health.

Surely we have sufficient knowledge of dietetics to be able nowadays to vary our diet to suit climates and seasons, and to know that we cannot eat everything everywhere. Sir John Lawrence says, in his evidence, that government "might try to induce the men, by varying the ration with reference to hot or cold weather, to take more to vegetable diet."

The means of cooking are of the rudest order—a small square outhouse, sometimes without a chimney, often far from clean, is the regimental kitchen. As for boilers and ovens, considered indispensable at home, there are none. A few holes to put the fire in, and moveable utensils to hold over them, are all that India thinks it wants. There is of course no water laid on and no drainage. Here as elsewhere is the inevitable cesspit and sometimes there are two.

Figure 7 is a plan of a double kitchen at Hazarybaugh. Figure 8 is a by no means bad example at Belgaum. Both show the total want of civilized appliances. And although the cooking is not often complained of by the stations, there is very good authority for stating that the food is imperfectly cooked or served up in a way which destroys the digestive organs and leads to the use of stimulants to promote digestion.

**FIGURE 7**
**Cookhouse in Hazarybaugh**

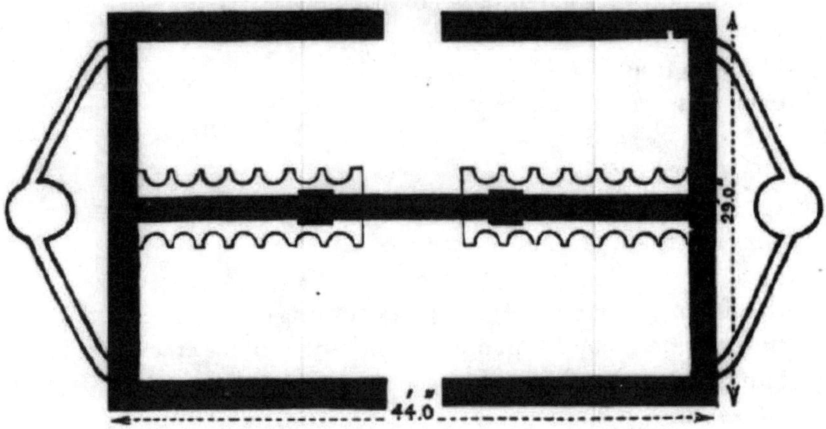


**FIGURE 8**
**Artillery Cookhouse in Belgaum**

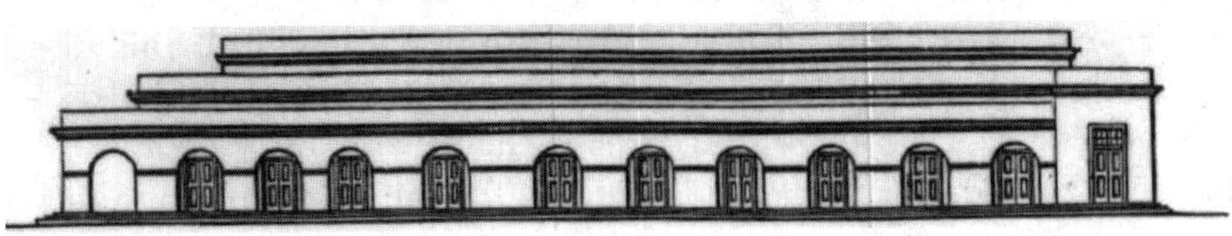

### WANT OF OCCUPATION AND EXERCISE

To understand the influence of this system of dieting and drinking, it must be remembered that, except morning and evening parades, and the man's turn on duty, he has nothing in the world to do. He can neither amuse himself, take exercise nor turn his time to profit for himself, for there are no means of doing any of these things. All the spare time people usually give to active occupations he spends lounging in his hot barrack room, most of it on his bed.

The graphic woodcut of the manner in which a soldier spends his day is from a drawing kindly sent me by an Indian officer of rank [Colonel Young]. [*See* the Illustrations section of this volume.]

India actually reverses the ordinary human day, for the men spend eighteen hours of the twenty-four in or on their beds, and six hours only up or out. Indeed, Kamptee says that "for many months of the year the men are confined to barracks for twenty out of twenty-four hours." And your imagination must fancy 100 to 600 men or more packed into the same room for eating and sleeping away these twenty hours.

This is an account of a soldier's day:
bed till daybreak;
drill for an hour;
breakfast, served to him by native servants;
bed;
dinner, served to him by native servants;
bed;
tea, served to him by native servants;
drink;
bed; and *da capo* [repeat from the beginning].

So that the Briton exactly spends his spare time between eating, drinking, lounging or sleeping; and he eats meat always twice and sometimes three times a day.

All his meals are condensed into the hot hours of the day. And just when he wants one most, viz., *before* he goes out to his early morning work, he does not get it. Why not give him hot coffee before morning parade and beer, if he must have it, at dinner and at night? Not one report except Tonghoo but prays for the abolition of all this dram drinking; and it is said that the *abstinent* man is more enduring of fatigue and less obnoxious to disease than even the *temperate* man. Spirits, it is said, should never be offered for sale, as men are induced to take spirits who never would if they were not so "handy." Trichinopoly says that the sale of spirits should be abolished in canteens, bazaars and within a circle of ten miles round barracks.

### Daily means of occupation and amusement in India

If the men had employment, recreation, good tea, coffee, milk, more variety of food and of cooking, spirit drinking might be abolished. A good hot cup of coffee is the best stimulant for a soldier. As it is, the old soldiers often take a dram before morning parade and nobody can prevent them.

The following piece of information is curious (the scene lies in the Madras presidency), viz., that "the canteen funds" (the profits derived out of the soldiers' drunkenness) "are insufficient to provide amusements to keep the men from drinking." Also that where there is no library there are "plenty of books which can be read till 8 P.M. when all lights are put out." Berhampore has a library and reading room, but "neither lighted at night."

That want of occupation, leading to drink, lays the seeds of disease among the troops is acknowledged. "Alcohol and unrefreshing day sleep," says Bangalore, "contribute to engender disease and accelerate mental and physical decay." Ahmadnagar says that, for one man occupied in a barrack there are six idle. Also, that when men are actively engaged in the field in hot weather, there is little sickness or epidemic disease among them. So unaccustomed is the soldier to ordinary exertion that, as might be expected, the short parades are talked of as injurious, as if they were long harassing marches; while, curiously enough, it is admitted that the soldier is never better than when he is exposed to the harass and fatigue of field service.

Kolhapur and Belgaum say that, the more varied and agreeable a soldier's occupations, the better his health; that the troops require means of occupation and amusement to keep them out of the bazaars.

All the sensible reporters say that too much stress cannot be laid on the importance of using the utmost exertion to provide legitimate amusement and occupation for the men—workshops, shelter for athletic games, etc. We must always remember that, in hot weather, the men, save those who can read, "have positively nothing to do." Employment on public works "would be a great boon"; "the work would be as cheaply done as now; it would occupy the soldier and he would feel he was doing good." Savings banks would answer, "if workshops for trades were established." The usual account from a station is, no library, nor reading nor day room, no club, no garden, no workshops, no theatre, no gymnasia, no means of instruction or recreation whatever, no skittle grounds, or if there are any, not covered, no sufficient shade for exercise. And the men are generally confined to barracks from 8 A.M. to 5 P.M. in hot weather.

Kanpur actually orders the men to be confined to barracks for 10½ hours a day in hot weather; but the order "is often disobeyed." At Chunar there is no restriction as to exposure to the sun. The "men go about at all times and, except when under the influence of liquor, do not appear to suffer from exposure." Yet Chunar's mean temperature is 65° in December and 92° in June, its sun temperature as high as 120° in June. And yet the men do not "suffer from exposure."

Agra, Firozpur and Umballa say that a large covered building for gymnastics, workshops, games, with a library, reading and coffee room, a theatre and plunge baths, "would draw many men from their cots where they idle and sleep all day." And Peshawar recommends that this building should be separate from barracks.

Dinapore recommends a farmyard to employ the men: an excellent idea.

Mian Mir (Lahore) suggests photography, modelling and drawing as occupations for the men.

Sealkote (1200 men) and Ghazipur (850 men) may be offered as examples of the two opposite types of rational occupation and idleness.

Sealkote, indeed, is the only station, except Rangoon, which has anything like completeness. It has ball courts and skittle grounds. It has schools and regimental libraries. It has a well-lighted reading room with chess, backgammon, dominoes and sixteen newspapers, etc. It has a soldiers' garden with seeds and tools provided by government, who grant prizes for the best cultivation (soldiers' gardens, when they exist at all, are elsewhere worked by natives). It has armourers', saddlers', tailors', shoemakers' and one watchmaker's shops. It has theatres; it has cricket and regimental clubs; it has football and it is particularly fond of quoits. The savings bank of one of its regiments has £8000. It has sufficient shade for exercise. Yet Sealkote does not think it has done enough. And while other stations, whose men "lie in their cots all day," seem unaware that anything else is desirable, Sealkote wishes that "workshops for every trade" were instituted, as they might be, and "strongly recommends" a gymnasium. It is noteworthy that the health of the troops at Sealkote seems to require but little amendment and that no complaint is made of its climate.

Rangoon has a ball court and skittle grounds; schools, three libraries and day rooms; soldiers' gardens; shops for trades; two theatres. But Rangoon says it requires lofty open sheds for gymnasia and that government should afford every aid in establishing good coffee rooms, *independent of canteens*, all amusements to be as near as possible, all canteens to be as far as possible from the coffee rooms.

Now take Ghazipur. Its whole means of occupation, instruction and recreation are one ball court and two skittle grounds. Its whole shade consists of the verandahs, under water during the rains. "Almost everything has yet to be done."

The large station of Allahabad (with accommodation for upwards of 4000 men) is almost as ill off. Tonghoo, the only station which considers the quantity of spirits drawn as "conducive to health," and the amount of "sickness, mortality and crime occasioned by intemperance" as "trifling," has, as might be expected from this statement, absolutely no means of occupation and amusement for its men, and few of instruction. It appears to consider drinking and idleness the normal state of things. At Bangalore (1700 men) "day rooms, soldiers' clubs, workshops, theatre, gymnasia and gardens are things unheard of." The "regimental library has no attraction for men who read with difficulty." This is the place where, as soon as "the noonday gun announces that the canteen is open, a rush is made for the raw spirit dram"; where "the canteen and the cot divide the hours unoccupied by the daily routine of petty duties." What else can be expected? There is, of course, plenty of liver complaint here.

But amusements are not all that is required. In conformity with all reason and experience, Sir Charles Trevelyan observes that, however necessary and useful chess and backgammon, ball courts and skittle grounds, and even books and newspapers may be, they only furnish some present diversion and do not supply any strong pervading motive, such as induces men to submit to sacrifices and to make persistent exertions in other lines of life. This motive is to be found only in the hope of rising to a higher and better position. He advocates a system by which every soldier who conducts himself well and cultivates himself so as to acquire a knowledge of the native languages and other necessary attainments should be able to look forward to promotion as a matter of course, either in the army or in the commissariat, ordnance or other military departments, or in the department of public works or police. The British soldier in India would then feel himself engaged in the serious business of life, at least as much as any of his countrymen of the same class at home. The army would take its tone from the active influential portion of the men. The amusements of various kinds provided for the soldiers would be more appreciated and would have a more wholesome effect, because they would take their proper place in subordination to higher interests.

This is no theory. It was actually carried out by Sir C. Trevelyan at Madras. Men were first selected by competitive examination within the regiment. There was a second examination at Madras and the result was the obtaining "of twenty men who were the pick of the whole army for the administrative service of the government in the civil and military departments."

One element essential to placing soldiers in positions of civil usefulness is, of course, their learning the language of the country, necessarily part of that voluntary education which they must have for competitive examination. Teaching the native languages in regimental schools would at once provide the men with interesting occupation and the prospect of future advantage. The War Office has already sent to all European regiments in the Madras presidency a cheap edition of the New Testament and Psalms with a clavis [key or glossary] in Hindustani, in furtherance of this object.

Sir C. Trevelyan would also encourage trades and handicrafts to the full extent consistent with the means of profitably disposing of the produce. And this is the more necessary because all are not equal to the intellectual acquirements to which the previous remarks refer.

All officers who give an opinion on the subject concur in recommending workshops.

Dum Dum, in the total absence of all means for occupying the men, opens a small museum with lectures, to which the men crowd, showing "that soldiers are ready to avail themselves of any means of rational amusement in the evening in preference to spending all their time in the canteen."

Muttur again has no means of instruction, occupation or amusement whatever, except a soldiers' garden for which there are no tools, although indented for a year ago. Carpentry, saddlery and coopers' work are in great demand and would benefit the men, as regards health, morals and finance.

Lucknow is building everything that is required, except workshops. Rawalpindi has nothing but schools. Barrackpore petitions for fives courts, a theatre, gymnasia, swimming baths, public reading of good biographies, travels and novels; for trades, such as clothing, accoutrements, barrack furniture, watch making, printing, paper making, baking. It says that savings banks should be connected with workshops.

Darjeeling has a hospital reading room and reader: a very good plan. But for its men out of hospital, at a hill station where the rains fall incessantly for five months, there are no means under cover provided and the men are pent up in barrack rooms to the great injury of their health. Darjeeling says, "there should be restaurants where men could get coffee, tea, newspapers, magazines, *and mix with men of other regiments* instead of the discomfort of the everlasting barrack room."

Hazarybaugh has a government library, *not* lighted at night, a temperance reading room, well lighted, with upwards of 200 members (out of 1080 men, for which number the station has accommodation) and, although it has armourers', shoemakers' and tailors' shops, it strongly recommends further means of occupation and amusement "as the long days of the Indian hot weather hang heavily on the soldiers' hands."

This part of the subject is by no means exhausted but these examples and illustrations are quite sufficient to show the small amount, indeed, of physiological knowledge which has been practically applied to the British Army in India.

Suppose anyone wanted to try the effect of full diet, tippling and want of exercise, in a hot climate, on the health of men in the prime of life, the Indian Army method would be the process to adopt, in the certain expectation that every man exposed to it will be damaged in health.

While all this scientific "turkey stuffing" is practised, the men are carefully kept in barracks and not allowed to exercise themselves. And everybody seems to believe that the way of making diseased livers in geese for Strasbourg pies is the best way of keeping men's livers sound and of making efficient healthy soldiers for India. Wherever the régime is otherwise, as in the case of cavalry and artillery, who have some exercise, or where an enlightened officer allows his men to go shooting, there is, of course, improved health. But nobody learns the lesson.

People seem to consider that health is a natural production of India, instead of being the result of rational management. At the same time everybody says that India is "so unhealthy." Under this system of diet, regimen, drink and idleness, it is indeed to be expected that cases sent to the hospital will be much more numerous, much more severe and much less amenable to treatment and management than under a sensible system.

## HOSPITALS

The Indian hospitals, though planned on simple principles, admitting of admirable details, are, as a rule, exceedingly bad as regards points considered essential to health and administration, even in this country. What would be, e.g., thought in this country of a hospital without a water closet or bath or means of personal cleanliness? Such a hospital would be considered as a mere makeshift till accommodation fitter for recovery could be provided.

The "means of ablution" in Indian hospitals are often "a tin pot with which the sick pour the water over themselves." Or, as at Bombay, they "take water to bathe themselves from a trough." Elsewhere they have "one tub, one basin, to one hundred men." The means of washing, as at Ramandroog, a convalescent station, are "two shallow earthenware pie dishes" "on a form in a room" ("very chilly in damp" weather), "adjoining where the night stools are."

At Rangoon the "bathing accommodation" is "hitherto nothing but a tub of water, without basin, soap or towel."

There may be a bathroom. But "all apparatus is entirely wanting." The sick "can always, if they please, get a skinful of water thrown over them by the water carriers," as at Hazarybaugh.

One may safely say that when the sick are able to bathe in India, it is a sufficient test of their being able to leave hospital, as has indeed been discovered to be the case at some home stations.

At Nynee Täl the sick bathe in the lake. Darjeeling says, "In fact the inducements to remain dirty are, especially in the case of sickly men, greater than those to be clean."

There does not appear to be a single well-placed orderlies' or nurses' room in any of the hospitals from which the sick can be seen at all times and where the nurses themselves can be inspected. The surgeon's and "nurses'" quarters are sometimes three quarters of a mile or a mile off, so that they (the medical and nursing attendants) are represented as spending their whole day in going backwards and forwards on the road.

The hospital is generally surrounded by a "high prison-like wall." At Ghazipur it is said "of course all the buildings generally are most unsuitable for hospital purposes." Proper ventilation is represented, as at Baroda, as "next to impossible." At Kolhapur the rain beats in through the cowls [hood-shaped coverings for ventilation shafts] and "makes the wards so damp that charcoal has to be used to dry them." The water for drinking may be brought, as at Bangalore, from a tank which receives the whole sewage of the cantonment and which "just now is not very clean," from which "hundreds of bullock loads of impure matter are removed year after year when the tank is low and the smell from it most offensive." Or the water may be brought (cholera also being brought with it) from wells into which the said tank drains. The drainage may be by an open ditch into the tank, whence the hospital derives its water. Or the water supply may, perhaps, have to be carried from half a mile off or even from two miles off, as at Madras. But "no improvement is required in this respect."(!) The privies are everywhere either "highly offensive" or "not more offensive than the best of such places usually are in this country." Or the privies are "without seats" and are "kept pure by burning salt in them." "Arrangements admit of improvement."

Scarcely ever is there any provision of separate wards for convalescents, although in a country whose scourge is dysentery, to leave men convalescent from dysentery in the same place and under the same circumstances as those suffering from dysentery is just to ensure as far as possible their *not* convalescing. The same may be said of fever and of bowel diseases generally. Convalescents pass their whole twenty-four hours in bed, except during their time of exercise (*where* they have means of exercise) on elephants, in sick carts or doolies. They have not even a room to take their meals in but eat their food upon their knees, sitting on their beds, "possibly with dying men around," or they are sent to barracks and put on barrack rations and "marched out under a non-commissioned officer morning and evening for exercise."

Where there is no guard house the "men on guard occupy a corner of the hospital verandah where they eat, drink and smoke at their discretion." No hospitals have dining rooms, although all ought to have them because of the pest of flies in India. Not one has a day room for men who can leave their beds.

The "sanitary state" is generally represented as "good" although at the same time we are told as in certain cases that the hospital is "unfit for accommodation of European patients"; or that "epidemic disease has appeared in it"; that "sores become erysipelatous" [inflamed]; that, as at Bangalore, "one of the flags" in the floor being removed, "the smell from the opening was so offensive that" the surgeon was "obliged to run"; that "gangrene and phagedaena [ulceration] have appeared when the hospital was crowded"; that the "privy is a nuisance to one ward"; that the "cesspools are always more or less offensive"; or that the "outhouses are in a very dirty and unwashed condition." At Muttur the contents of the latrines are "carted away every morning for combustion in one of the many brick kilns which surround the station and help to poison the air." At Madras the "sanitary state" is called "good" and the commander-in-chief himself adds, "if the vile stinking river Cooum were not under the very noses of the patients." Both cholera and gangrene have appeared at times in the hospital. The latrines are placed to windward "unfortunately"; "tubs only are used." The privy is washed daily and charcoal "burned in it." It is called "not offensive," the commander-in-chief again adding, "a year ago it was odiously offensive."

No wonder that it is stated, as at Bangalore, that "sick men are reluctant to come into hospital from barracks" and that the medical officer does not want "convalescent wards" because he finds it better to send his convalescents to barracks, where they recover faster.

From some hospitals the "impurities" are removed by hand carriage to thirty yards from the hospital. In another, the privy is said to be a "disgrace to the nineteenth century." One wonders to what century it would be a credit.

At most hospitals the bedsteads are of wood instead of iron and the men break them to pieces in their "efforts to expel the vermin." As at Ramandroog, where men are sent for their health, "the building swarms with bugs." And so of every barrack and hospital where these wooden bedsteads are used. One surgeon complains of the serious injury to his sick occasioned by want of sleep from vermin. The bedding is of hemp or straw, instead of hair, which latter it ought always to be in hospitals and which is now the regulation in all queen's hospitals. It appears from several reports that sheets are not provided except for dysentery and fever: and certainly in no hospital deserving the name should the inspector general feel himself called on to recommend that "a good mattress, a blanket, *sheets* and pillow cases should be provided for every bed," as does the excellent inspector general of the Madras presidency.

Figures 9 [and] 11 are illustrations of the smaller class of regimental (British) hospitals. Figure 9 shows the simpler form of construction, a single large ward partially enclosed by other rooms for sick, all communicating and having a common ventilation, the arrangement good and simple up to a certain point, and then marred in the details. There are privies in place of water closets, with covered passages, to conduct foul air to the sick in certain states of the wind. Bangalore gives a reason for "the covered way to the latrines" which we never should have thought of. It is a "covered place for exercise."

It will be seen that the hospital is entirely destitute of proper ward offices.

Figure 10 shows the privy arrangements in plan and section. There is no drainage; the contents are carried away by hand.

## Figure 9
## Horse Artillery Hospital in Bangalore

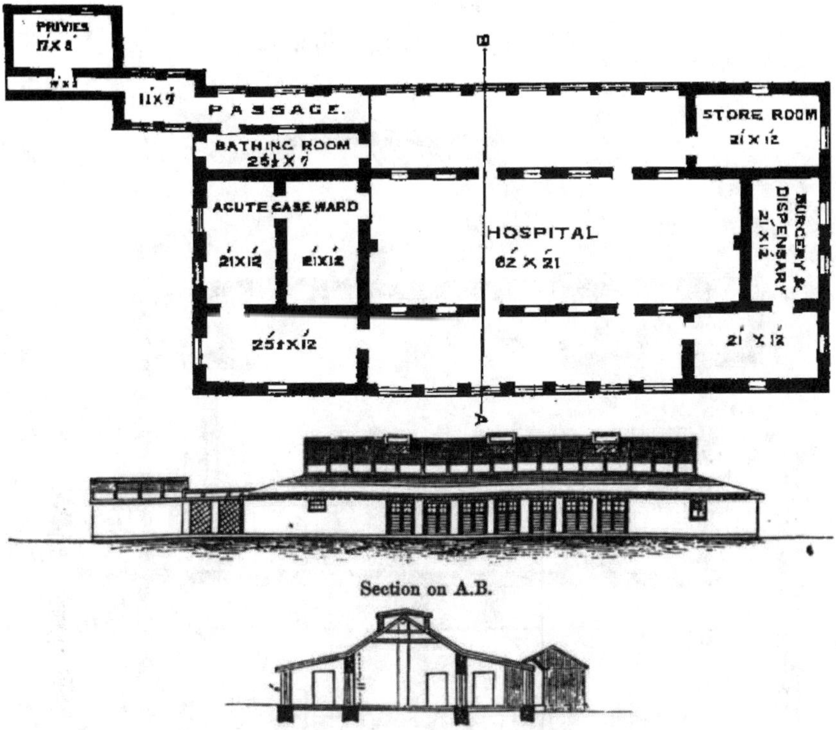


## Figure 10
## European Infantry Hospital Privy, Belgaum

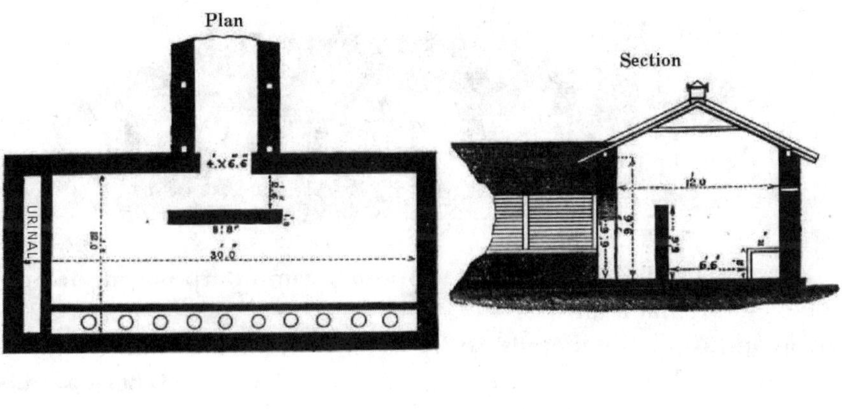

Figure 11 shows a somewhat better construction of hospital but there is the same defect in detail.

**FIGURE 11**
**Artillery Hospital, Belgaum**

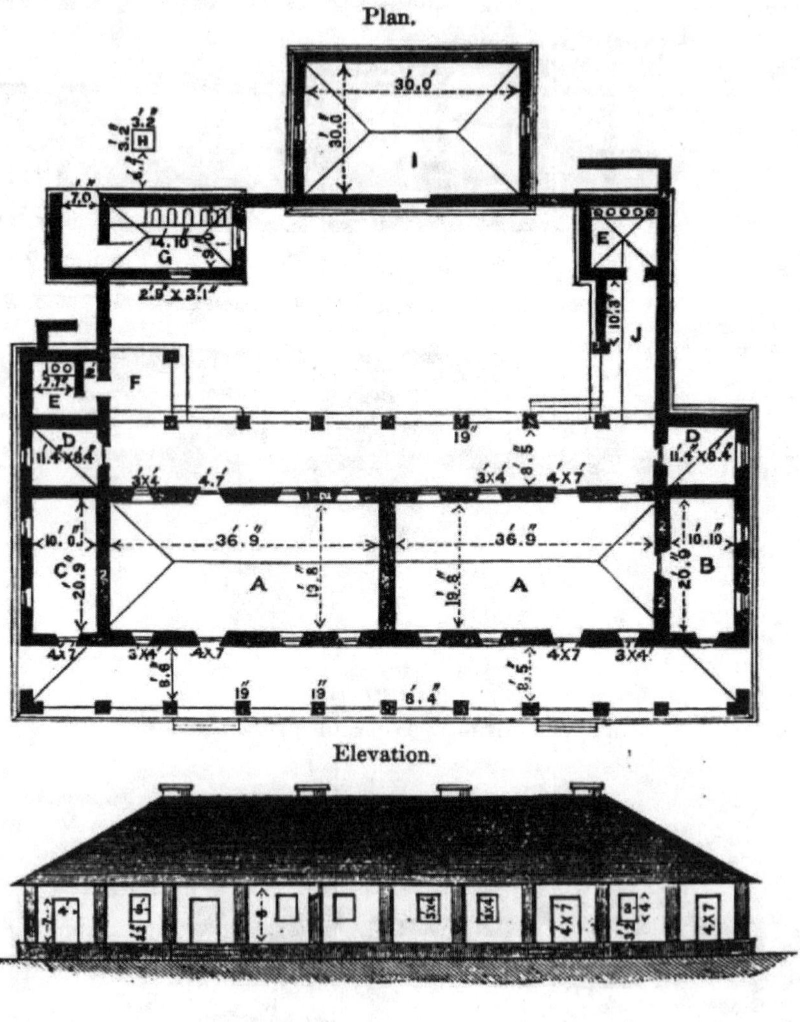


Either plan might answer for temporary camp purposes, in default of better, but that is all.

Indian hospitals generally, so far as all conveniences and comforts are concerned, appear to be simply camp hospitals; good, because the best possible for field service, but by no means good or the best possible for permanent stations.

There is no instance, except at Wellington, where the hospital, if on one floor, as is usual, is raised from the ground with any current of air beneath. These hospitals are stated, as at Bangalore, to be "always damp in wet weather." And often the floor is merely the ground bricked over. Rangoon and Tonghoo live like the beavers and raise their barracks and hospitals on piles, with free passage for air underneath. The consequence is that in those jungly swamps they are more healthy than at most other Indian stations where the men sleep close to the ground.

As at Allahabad, Barrackpore, Dinapore, Meerut, Karachi and Secunderabad, vast wards of from 100 to 150 beds, and even up to more than 200 beds, exactly the same as the barrack rooms, are in use.

The wards can never be said to be light or airy; "as a general rule, hospitals are badly lighted and gloomy"; doors are more common than windows. And these doors, when closed, leave the ward, if not absolutely dark, yet absolutely dismal and close. Indeed a dark ward must always be a close ward. Or "light enters from a couple of panes in the doors near the top and when closed darkness is almost complete." There is in Indian hospitals hardly a room light enough to perform a surgical operation. And operations, it is stated, have to be performed in verandahs.

The inner verandahs are generally used for sick wherever more room is wanted: the outer ones sometimes cut up for lavatories, destroying what ventilation there is.

The superficial area per bed is almost invariably too small and the wards almost as invariably too high; the result to the sick being that, with an apparently sufficient cubic space, the surface overcrowding is excessive. One of the worst examples of this is the recently constructed hospital at Trimulgherry (Secunderabad) which consists of three wards, two of which contain no fewer than 228 beds each; the wards are 42 ft. high and afford 1001 cubic feet per bed, but the surface area per bed is only 24 square feet. This surface overcrowding is greater than I have ever seen it in the smallest or the largest temporary war hospitals. Such facts strike one very forcibly in connexion with the high mortality among sick entering these and similar hospitals.

All the defects of barracks re-appear and with worse consequences in the hospitals: viz., bad water supply, bad ventilation, no drainage (Firozpur says, "drainage not necessary"), offensive latrines, so offensive indeed that the patients have sometimes to leave a particular ward, no means of bathing and hardly any of cleanliness. There are besides, however, two grave defects not felt in barracks but peculiar and fatal to hospitals.

These are the cooking and the attendance. It is in several reports complained that under the present system the cooks (natives or Portuguese) are nothing but "miserable pretenders" because the pay is so small; that the kitchens are no better than, but just the same as, the barrack kitchens. They are often small open sheds without chimneys, the smoke finding its way out as it can, and with but few utensils; sometimes the food is prepared on the ground. "But we are accustomed to this in India." It is added that though common food is tolerably well prepared, there is nothing whatever that can be called sick cookery, nothing whatever to tempt the appetite or spare the digestion of the sick man whom the hospital is for.

In hospitals at home, trained cooks of the army hospital corps are now in charge of the cooking under the direction of the purveyor, who is responsible that the diets are properly cooked. In India the chief quality in native cooks appears to be the "pursuit of cooking under difficulties"; their ingenuity in bringing about an *apparently* good result, in a rude and often bad way, is frequently admired by the reporters, as if the end of cooking were "to make a pair of old boots look like a beefsteak."

In England where the grass-fed meat is so much better than in India, it is found necessary to put the purveying of meat for hospitals under the charge of the purveyor for the sake of always obtaining the best quality. There does not appear to be any provision of this kind in India, where all is under the commissariat.

As to the attendants, they are just the same as would be supplied to idle healthy men. Quantity, it would seem, is supposed to supply quality. In serious cases a "waiting man" is supplied "from the battalion who is relieved daily." That is, he goes on guard for 24 hours, as in the guard room, so in the sickroom. It appears that mounting guard in the sickroom is disliked and the guard sometimes neglects his patient.

As to supposing that any nursing is required, the thing is totally out of the question. There are neither trained orderlies nor female nurses.

A matron is sometimes "sanctioned" but "only for a complete battalion." If there are fewer sick they must do without. Every severe case, as has been stated, is allowed to have its comrade to itself in from the ranks, i.e., the case which requires the best nursing is to have the worst nurse. Something more is needed to make a nurse, as well as a surgeon, than mere kindness. Wherever the above comrade-practice is found, we know beforehand that there can be no nursing, no discipline in that hospital and any amount of drink.

There is generally one hospital sergeant and a "plentiful supply of ward coolies." The hospital sergeant is for discipline and under him are seventy-nine coolies and bheesties in cold weather, 240 in hot weather. This for an European corps. The general impression, as regards the native attendants, is that they are in some sense kind but "as a rule very inattentive," and when there is any pressure of sick they are "lazy" and "apathetic," and the sick, it need hardly be said, neglected and "averse to be waited on by them." When at a hill station, as Landour, the hospital sergeant is taken at random from the sick men themselves, sent up for convalescence, it is needless to point out the consequences. This grievance has been repeatedly represented, but in vain.

(And here comes in again the difficulty of difference in language. Our men dislike and despise the natives and are regarded by them in return more as wild beasts than fellow creatures. The native, however, makes much more effort to learn the Briton's language than does the Briton to learn the native's. It is difficult to give an idea of the evil effects of the gross ignorance of all that relates to the country in the ranks of our army in India. The commonest attempt at conversation gives rise to feelings of impatience and irritation, too often followed by personal ill-treatment. Where the Briton is sick, it is of course worse.

To enable our soldiers to hold ordinary intercourse with the people among whom their lot is cast is the first element of an useful and happy life for them in India. Every soldier should be required to learn something of the native language. And a somewhat higher voluntary standard should be fixed, the inducement to attain which should be: 1. A specific pecuniary reward. 2. Eligibility for employment in the various departments of the public service.)

Nynee Täl has one hospital sergeant, one barber, one orderly, for its attendance.

Lady Canning introduced female nurses at Allahabad, who are mentioned (in the stational return of Allahabad) as being a great comfort to the sick. Wherever there are general hospitals there should be female nurses, but only under the organization laid down by the Medical Regulations of October 1859. It is a great mistake to put down a few women among a parcel of men (orderlies and patients) without exactly defining the women's duties and place.

Lastly there appears nowhere in India to be provided any means of drying hospital linen, even during the rains. It is often complained that the washing is very bad and that the native washermen tear the linen, and at one cavalry hospital this keeps two tailors constantly employed in repairing the rents and injuries; for native washing is done by beating the linen against large flat stones or wooden boards.

If the British military hospitals are such, what must be said of those for our native troops? Here the patients "diet *themselves.*"

As regards construction, where native hospitals have been specially built, they resemble the smaller class of British hospital. One of the most complete of these is shown in Figure 12. There are wards within wards, completely enclosed by other rooms, of which, although there are plenty, not one is suited for ward offices.

**Figure 12**
**Kurnool Fort Hospital (Native)**

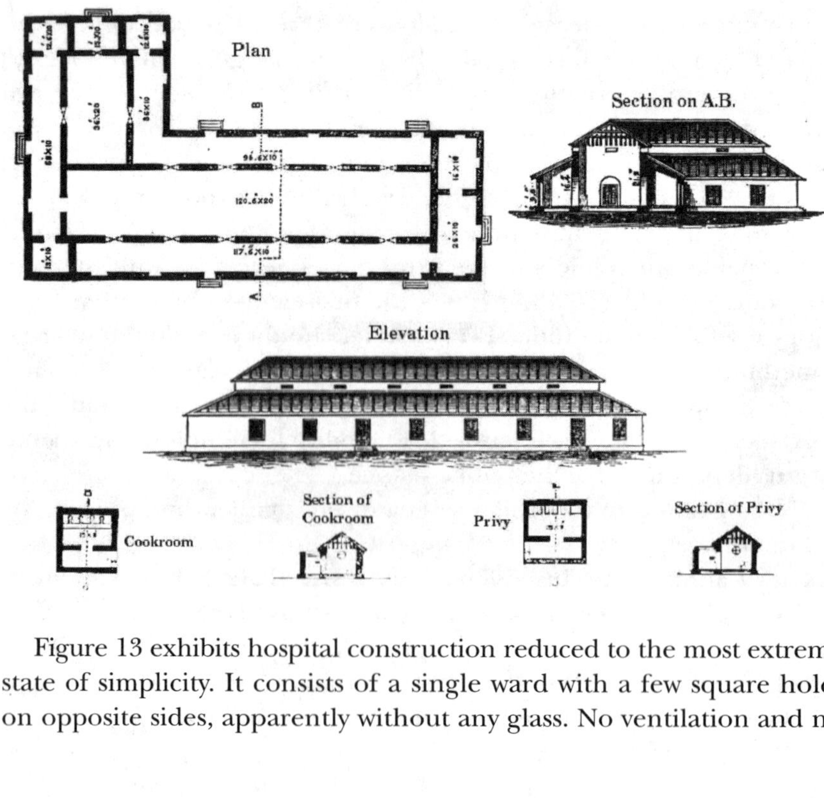


Figure 13 exhibits hospital construction reduced to the most extreme state of simplicity. It consists of a single ward with a few square holes on opposite sides, apparently without any glass. No ventilation and no ward offices whatever. But there is a dispensary and storeroom exactly where they ought not to be.

**FIGURE 13**
**Native Infantry Hospital, Kulladghee**

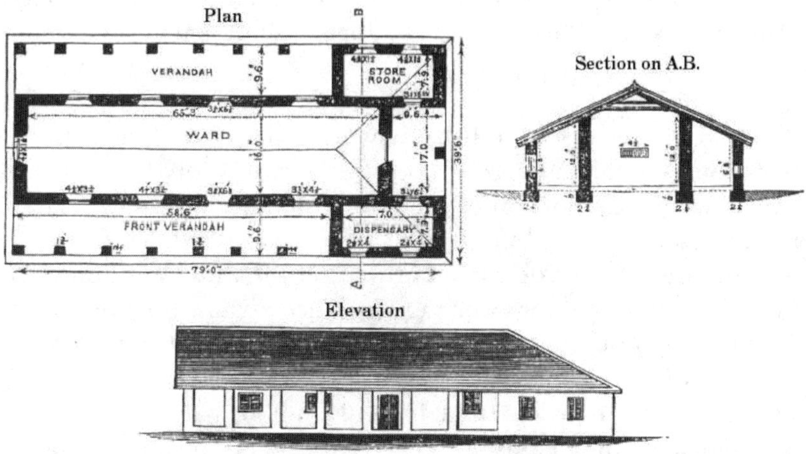


But it must not be supposed that native hospitals are all as good as these. They are generally nothing but a shed, perhaps a "gun shed" or a "cattle shed," as at Kolhapur, converted into a hospital, where the sick receive nothing but medicine. The patients cook their own diets, eating and drinking what they please. Or when too ill to cook for themselves, an orderly friend is detailed for the purpose. There are no conveniences; sometimes the sick go home to wash or bathe themselves in a tank. Such are the "ward offices usually provided for these establishments." In one native infantry hospital at Secunderabad it is stated that hospital gangrene frequently occurs from overcrowding, from the cachectic [debilitated] state of the patients, *owing to the unhealthy character of their lines,* and from a cesspool in the hospital enclosure, which last is, however, being remedied.

At Rangoon it is stated that the privies, for native regiments, are built of matting "which is most objectionable as allowing the escape of noxious effluvia." Is it then desired to keep the "noxious effluvia" *in?*

It is supposed that "caste" prejudices are such as to prevent native hospitals being properly built and supplied with requisites for sick. But this has to be proved by giving natives a properly constructed and provided hospital. There are plenty of "caste prejudices" in this country against good hospital construction; but good hospital construction advances nevertheless.

At Ludhiana one native doctor, one coolie, one water carrier, one sweeper are the attendants "sufficient for the ordinary wants of the sick." The present arrangements for the female hospital are said to be "sufficient" (which means *none*) (Ludhiana is now a native station).

### HILL STATIONS

Sir Ranald Martin wisely and strongly urges that the whole subject of hill stations should undergo a thorough revision for the purpose of deciding whether a portion of the army could not be always taking its turn as a reserve on the hills, thus to preserve its stamina.

Children too might be reared as well on the hills as at home. One of the native chiefs going over the Lawrence asylum (of five hundred children) at Sunnawur, said to Sir John Lawrence that they looked like lion's cubs.

It strikes one, however, that it would not be safe to depend for improvement of the health of troops solely on occupying hill stations, with such an overwhelming amount of evidence as to the bad sanitary state of the stations on the plains and even of not a few of the hill stations themselves, such as Darjeeling, Landour, Nynee Täl.

"At some hill stations there is malarious fever; others predispose to diarrhea." The barracks and hospitals at Mussoorie and Sabathu are defective both in plan and in structure. At Mount Aboo they are "bad barracks," built in a "malarious gully," and the men return suffering from intermittent fever and from scorbutic disease [scurvy], the result of want of vegetables. Will it be credited that, at one of the two hill stations of the Madras presidency, the privies are built on the edge of the hill in order that the natural slope may save us all the trouble of sewerage, the lavatories the same, which are emptied by "upsetting the tubs" down the hill; and that, at the other, with more than nine hundred men, the barrack square was an immense swamp for want of drainage. Low fever, from March to May, from which the men have suffered who were sent there for health, is attributed to this as if it were a meteorological observation. This refers to Wellington on the Neilgherries. Indeed the Neilgherry stations, the best in India, are in great danger of being permanently injured by sanitary neglects.

In fact, all that the hill station evidence proves is that healthy men, put under healthy conditions, will remain healthy, and *vice versa.*

Hill stations, it is said, are highly favourable to troops arriving *in health,* IF lodged in good barracks; are unfavourable in some states of disease. Dry, spacious, well-ventilated barracks, in well-chosen positions, drained, supplied with wholesome water and out of the way of nuisance and malaria, have been the great want of hill stations. And want of fresh vegetables and of pure water has produced much mischief. In the rains, the water is often loaded with "rotten vegetable matter causing diarrhea." (Is this supposed to supplement the *want* of vegetables?)

High authorities advocate sending certain invalids to seaside sanitaria.

Hospitals at hill stations appear to be very much on a par with hospitals at plain stations, as far as can be learnt from Figure 14 which represents the hospital at Darjeeling used for sick of the depôt. The arrangement is much that of a field hospital with fireplaces to suit the climate. At this hospital an open privy was placed in one corner of the verandah, which compelled the sick to evacuate the ward and it took five years' writing to get it removed.

**FIGURE 14**
**Julla Puhar Hospital, Darjeeling**

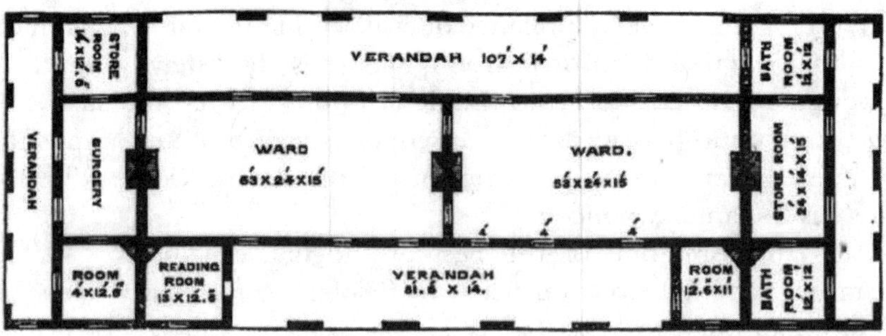


Hill climates, judiciously used, would no doubt be of great value. But they are by no means all that is required for the salvation of the Indian Army. This must by brought about by sanitary measures everywhere, of which hill stations, if kept in a good sanitary condition (but not if kept in a bad condition) are one. This is the unquestionable result of the evidence.

When our troops went into a notoriously unhealthy district in China, they were not placed on hill stations. They were properly managed and their sanitary condition provided for; and they had no larger proportion of "constantly sick" than the troops at home.

### Native lines

Native troops have no barrack accommodation, no doubt a most excellent thing for their health. They have hutting money (very little) and make their own huts which are so badly built as to ensure thorough ventilation, being often indeed only open sheds in compartments. But little or no pains are taken to make them put up these huts in any regular order; they are crowded, or rather huddled, together and without drainage of any kind. They are always damp and the men always sleep in malaria. When they have families the huts are too small because the hutting money is too small.

Native troops have no rations and stint themselves of proper food in order to hoard their pay. They are almost invariably temperate and have little or no liver disease, whilst the British troops are decimated with it. So far as can be learned from disease statistics, native troops are far more moral than British.

Except schools, no means whatever of instruction, occupation or amusement are provided for them. They are, in fact, stipendiaries receiving a day's pay for a day's work with their uniform, but they are not what we should understand by troops provided for by the State.

With regard to every appliance of civilized life the tale is even more absolutely *nil* than for British troops. There is absolutely no drainage or sewerage, no latrines. And the descriptions of what the surrounding country and bazaars are in consequence are absolutely impossible to repeat. There are no lavatories nor baths. There are no kitchens. There is no sanitary police.

At Mangalore, one of the best of the native stations, "surface cleansing has hitherto been performed solely by the heavy rains." At Quillon, another, there is (as usual) no drainage but ruinous buildings, harbouring the dead carcasses of animals and, "on one occasion, of an old woman."

The water supply is of course as bad as, or worse than at European stations. At Kherwarrah, in Bengal, the water "has not unfrequently a filthy taste and disagreeable organic smell."

The degree to which native troops almost everywhere suffer from guinea worm would alone tell us what the water is. At the same Kherwarrah, one in every six has suffered (for seventeen years) from guinea worm.

There is no "conservancy" establishment or cleanliness. At this same large station of Kherwarrah "this is left very much to the jackal, vulture and carrion crow" (beyond the lines). There are patrols to prevent nuisances "except in specified localities." The lines are kept clean but the "sweepings are deposited thirty yards to windward."

The most ordinary sanitary precautions are not taken. "Every family has its own cesspool; dung heaps close to every hut," also holes for ordure. Animals are slaughtered to windward. The offal is thrown to dogs, jackals and vultures. During the rains the stench from the offal, the increasing accumulation of years, is sometimes dreadful.

The native population is "decidedly unhealthy" from jungle, swampy ground, cramped, damp dwellings (which shelter sheep, goats and cattle as well as men), bad food and water, neglected cesspools, middens, exuviae [bodily excretions] of men and animals, absence of drainage, opium eating, etc. What wonder if native troops suffer from quotidian, tertian, quartan, remittent and typhoid fevers (which alone constitute two fifths of the sickness and cause one fourth of the deaths in some places), from acute and chronic dysentery, from sporadic and epidemic cholera, from simple and confluent smallpox and from acute and chronic rheumatism.

The intelligent medical officer of Kherwarrah imparts a very important secret as to the unhealthiness of Indian stations when he says that none of them have had "fair play" (not even such large British stations as Dum Dum, Barrackpore and Dinapore), owing to the "utter disregard of the commonest sanitary precautions."

At Cochin, in the Madras presidency, the water is unfit for use from privy infiltration. Drinking water is brought daily 18 miles. One tank is used for bathing and drinking. The sanitary condition of the bazaar is "as bad as it can possibly be." "Cleanliness is unknown." There is "no drainage." The "streets are used as privies without hindrance." No regulation for cleanliness is attempted. The old rampart was converted into a ditch, now used as a public privy. Every odd corner is "in the most disgusting condition." Rajeote, in the Bombay presidency, might give similar instances of more or less neglect. But it is needless to follow this subject further. Everywhere there is the same ignoring of natural laws and the same penalties of disease and death.

The hospitals, again, combine all the disadvantages of civilization without any of its advantages. In one place the hospital was so overcrowded that for two years "gangrenous and spreading sores" were "frequent." (Labuan says that its hospital is much larger than "the strength is entitled to" but that "frequently the number of patients far exceeds the number of beds" and the "extra" sick—60 in a strength of 161!—"have slept on the floor between each bed and some in the verandahs.") Another hospital was so much out of repair that "it would before long be a ruin" (the best thing that could happen to it). If there is a privy it is a "small room with no place in which the excrement can go to be cleared away." If there is a lavatory or bath, it is "two tubs out of repair" (does that mean that they cannot hold water?). If there is a kitchen, as at Mercara, it is under the same shed as a privy and cannot be used for the stench. Indeed the medical officer proposes that it should be turned into a privy. The sick generally cook under the nearest tree and, if unable to do so, a comrade cooks for them under the tree. Linen is washed and dried by caste comrades or by the patients when not too ill. Each patient brings in his own bedding; generally his own bedstead. "Each patient defers bathing according to custom till he is cured, when he retires to the nearest well, draws water and undergoes the bath of cure," i.e., when he no longer wants it. Every report begs for a bathroom.

The general construction of native hospitals has been described under the head of "Hospitals."

## Native towns

The description given of the native towns is astonishing. Can it be possible that such a state of things exists after all these years of possession and unlimited authority?

So far as one can judge from the evidence, the sanitary state of entire large cities is as bad as, if not much worse than, was the state of the worst parts of our worst towns before there was any sanitary knowledge in the modern world at all. What, for instance, is to be thought of the following?

At Bangalore, a station 3000 feet above the sea, with the climate of a hill station indeed and quite as healthy as any in Europe where we have 1700 men, we have allowed to grow up within our cantonment a native population of half a quarter of a million without any of the arrangements of civilization whatever. Houses, tanneries and slaughterhouses are crowded together without any plan. There are no public necessaries. The natives resort to open spaces. The Ulsoor tank, which may be said to be the receptacle of the sewage of the whole place, including our barracks and hospitals, is used for drinking. In dry seasons the tank itself is a great nuisance. Even the wells are poisoned "owing to the amount of filth percolating into them from bad drainage." There is a dirt heap at almost every door. In the better houses where latrines exist, they are wells sunk in the ground within the house, which are closed up when filled and others opened. The filth from the cow-houses flows into open drains. There are no arrangements for stabling the bazaar horses, which with other domestic animals are kept *in the houses.* This bazaar is all close to our own barracks; and it is said that now nothing short of removal of the one or the other will remedy the evil. There is nothing, therefore, to astonish us in the fact that, in this, one of the healthiest stations and climates in the world, the mortality of our European soldiers should have been 129 per 1000 (including cholera) in one year. (Dr Macpherson's Report on Madras presidency, 27 December 1860.)

In Hyderabad, not far from our largest Madras station (Secunderabad) all the promoters of zymotic [infectious] diseases are at work and cholera, smallpox, diarrhea and dysentery are, it is stated, the most common of these.

But the capital of the Madras presidency is, perhaps, the most astounding. Its river Kooum is a Styx of most offensive effluvia. The air in Black Town and Triplecane is "loaded with mephitic [poisonous] effluvia at night." The atmosphere around Perambore and Vepery is "perfectly poisoned."

At Kamptee, with its 70,000 souls, "all filth is thrown into pits in the streets (!) of the cantonment." The poorer houses are huddled together without order on ground intersected by nullahs, making the houses difficult of access. The cesspits, "where accessible," are cleansed every 24 hours. The next information is curious. "Persons committing nuisances are closely watched and taken up daily." At Jaulnah there are no dung heaps nor cesspits "outside at least."

The native population around Fort William, Calcutta, is peculiarly unhealthy; fevers of all kinds, cholera and fatal diarrhea are "remarkably prevalent." The causes are "bad overcrowding," "bad drainage," foul drains, rank jungle, stagnant water, bad unwholesome drinking water, filth.

At Ahmadnagar it is acknowledged that almost every epidemic in the cantonment has its origin in the crowded, ill-ventilated and dirty village of Bhinga (of 3000 souls). The town itself of Ahmadnagar, with its 36,000 people *and no latrines,* uses "the very boundary of our camp" for this purpose and "the smell of ordure is very perceptible." At Pune, where is a city of 80,000 people, three quarters of a mile off, a bazaar of 27,000 quite close, a village (Wanowrie) 100 yards from officers' lines, where cholera first arose, there is the same story about "no latrines," "conservancy" establishment far too small for the daily removal of filth, and nuisance experienced in barracks from this cause. Belgaum says of its bazaar that there is "no want of cleanliness" *and* "that the public privies and cesspools are at times very offensive." The town, with 18,000 people, is between the fort and the camp. It affects the general health of our station from its "bad conservancy." But, again, we are told there is "no want of cleanliness!"

At Kolhapur "*one* sweeper is maintained by government" (for the bazaar), who collects the filth and throws it into a nullah, 400 yards from camp, which is also the public necessary; "two peons" prevent nuisance being committed in camp "from 4 to 10 A.M. daily." At Bombay, with a town of from 400,000 to 600,000 souls, there is a municipal commission with sanitary powers and the result of its practical labours is as follows: Native houses generally in a filthy condition; much ordure within precincts of buildings where it has been accumulating *for years*; native town proverbially unhealthy; nuisance from wind blowing over it, experienced in Fort George and town barracks; washermen's tanks particularly obnoxious; site of slaughterhouse as bad as can well be; sea breeze cut off by bazaars, etc.

Dung heaps are a "never-failing condition of native life in India." At Baroda the military hospital is close to a nullah used as a "necessary" by the natives and as a "receptacle for the filth of the whole station." When cholera occurred, the hospital had to be evacuated. And yet it is added, with great *naïveté*, "the sanitary recommendations of the medical officers are always attended to."

At Dinapore the native towns are "disgracefully filthy" with "holes near all native houses." At Kanpur there is overcrowding and want of ventilation with all manner of filth.

At Peshawar the streets are dirty, the houses densely crowded and ill-ventilated. The population suffers from a "severe and fatal" typhoid remittent fever, which rises to an "epidemic" in certain districts, also from epidemic smallpox, etc. At Ghazipur, in the latter months of 1859, there was a "fearful" fatality from "fever" due to a total want of sanitary arrangements.

At Berhampore there seems to be scarcely any epidemic which the native population has *not*. Among the causes, "holes full of stagnant foul water, close to almost every house, forming the usual cesspool of the neighbourhood. Utter neglect of ventilation and of all sanitary measures.

At Hazarybaugh cholera and smallpox are the "most common and fatal epidemics."

Only the presentable flowers are here. The stational reports are a garden to which those who doubt the truth of this representation, taken as a whole, and think it merely true as to particular facts, are again referred.

The stational reports generally state the native populations to be "healthy" or "remarkably healthy," and then give a list of every disease that flesh, *under defective civilization,* is heir to, to which they are subject endemically or epidemically. What must be the state of health of the natives when "unhealthy"?

One remark or rather inference, viz., native "caste" prejudices appear to have been made the excuse for European laziness, as far as regards our sanitary and hospital neglects of the natives. Recent railroad experience is a striking proof that "caste," in their minds, is no bar to intercommunication in arrangements tending to their benefit.

Sir C. Trevelyan justly says that a good sanitary state of the military force cannot be secured without making similar arrangements for the populations settled in and around the military cantonments; that sanitary reform must be generally introduced into India for the civil as well as the military portion of the community; that now is the time, for not only has the subject been worked out by actual experiment in England, but the improved financial stage of India, the increased influx of Europeans, especially of engineers and mechanics, and the powers of local legislation lately conferred upon the subordinate governments, have given facilities which never existed before. The sanitary arrangements for towns will be conducted by municipal bodies, for the creation of which there is already a very good act of the Government of India.

The mere passing of such an act presupposes the impotence of "caste" prejudices; and nobody who understands the relation of bazaars and native town to garrisons and cantonments can fail to see that the sanitary improvement of the Indian Army involves the sanitary improvement and the advance of civilization in India, a work before which "caste" prejudices and many other prejudices will have to give way.

### Absolute perfection of causes of disease

Our experience at home as to the results of sanitary improvement on the health of the army affords every reason to expect a very great improvement in the health of the Indian Army if proper sanitary measures be carried out. And it would require very strong evidence indeed to convince the people of this country that the epidemics which have devastated India arise from any other causes than those which the stational returns and the evidence prove to exist in what one may call a state of absolute perfection in the Indian towns, but which have been removed with entire success in this country.

### Soldiers' wives

"Leave to marry" in the British Army means that those only who marry with consent of the commanding officer have a claim to quarters in barracks. The proportion of quarters allowed by regulation at home is six married men per company of 100, in addition to married sergeants. When going to India, twelve married couples per 100 men, together with a proportionate increase of wives of sergeants, are allowed to go with the regiment, a number which high authorities consider too small. There is a general opinion that the proportion of married people allowed to go to India should be raised. The question is mainly one of sea transport and barrack accommodation, neither of which would be very costly as compared with the benefits to health and discipline which all agree would result from increasing the number of married men, always the steadiest, most temperate and best behaved in the regiment.

Throughout India, however, there is better provision of "married quarters" generally than on home stations. At most places they are reported as "sufficient," at some "insufficient," at others "very bad" and at a few there are none. Where they are insufficient or non-existent, the "married quarters" are men's barrack rooms or huts, divided off by curtains or partitions. Only at a few places are married people placed in barrack rooms with unmarried soldiers, still this practice does exist. One of the consequences of "allowing" marriage in the army is certainly that decent healthy quarters should be "allowed" too. No time should be lost, for this is especially necessary in India.

In the matter of soldiers' wives there are two instances of striking contrasts (each happened during the Mutiny); one, the destruction by dysentery of sixty-four wives and 166 children of British soldiers at Dum Dum; the other, a request made to and complied with by Sir John Lawrence from an officer of a native regiment of guides regarding the native wives. "Mind you look after these women carefully and do not let them be in distress; several of their husbands, men of rank, have been killed." The request was loyally fulfilled and as loyally appreciated by the men.

At Dum Dum 554 women and 770 children were crowded together without care or supervision, and the proportion which fell victims to intemperance, immorality, filth and foul air was more than six times, in either case, the ordinary mortality of women and children in Bengal. The fathers and husbands were fighting or dead in our battles. This massacre killed as many as it is supposed fell by the hands of the mutineers.

It is singular that in no one part of the Dum Dum report does the slightest allusion occur to this tragedy, making one think that it cannot be an isolated case. And it appears to have arisen solely from the absence of any regulation as to the care of soldiers' wives and children in the husbands' and fathers' absence. Families go to India and as long as the regiment remains fixed things may go on pretty well, provided there are decent separate quarters and a careful kindly commanding officer. But send the regiment on active service and there is no way of caring for the families. They take their chance under circumstances where they *cannot* help themselves. Or they are all huddled together, as at Dum Dum, with this result that, while the husbands were punishing the murderers of English women and children in the upper provinces, their own wives and children were being destroyed in vast numbers for want of care. Why? Could it not be made a necessary part of army arrangements to appoint a "picked" married officer to act as guardian over these women and children, to see to their comfort and conduct, to their being properly lodged and cared for? The manner of providing for them out of their husbands' pay is a matter of detail easily settled. If only anyone will take the trouble to do it the thing can be done. But more than this, it should be made matter of regulation throughout the whole service. There should be personal responsibility somewhere. At Dum Dum nobody was held responsible and nobody was punished for the result. If one tenth of the calamity had happened in England, there would have been coroners' inquests over and over again, and public opinion, if not law, would have punished someone. At Dum Dum the inquiry took place after the destruction of human life had been going on for months.

Sir John Lawrence expresses forcibly his practical opinion that there should be a "system," treating the "men as so many children," in binding them to "remit" money for their families, but also providing guardianship for those families when the "regiment is going on service" and so averting the "terrible results" of "abandoning the wives." Why cannot what was done for the Sikhs by Sir John Lawrence be done by regulation and on system for our own country people?

There are shocking illustrations of how soldiers' wives and children fare when the men are on foreign service and how a man does not become a better soldier for knowing that his country does not care for his wife and children while he is risking his life for his country. To the extent to which marriage is allowed in the army should all its necessary consequences be acted out.

But so far from this being done, the principle everywhere has been the reverse. Even as regards illness, in some notorious instances soldiers' wives have expressed (and justly) the strongest indignation that government took more care of prostitutes in illness than it did of honest wives; the government will pay to cure the prostitute to go on with her horrid trade which destroys their husbands, and will not pay to cure the wives and children or to make the married quarters more comfortable; and it is true, although not applicable to India, where there are female hospitals.

Some of these hospitals, as at Karachi and Deesa, Lucknow, Raneegunge and Firozpur, appear to be very complete with female attendants. In the Madras presidency they are too often, as at Bangalore, Trichinopoly and Kamptee, merely men's wards appropriated to women and justly stated to be "objectionable in every way." Elsewhere they are rather bare. Indeed, as at Baroda, Kirkee, Pune, Darjeeling, the sick women and children "have to be attended at their own quarters," either because "there is no matron" or because the "ward is too small," or etc. Curiously enough, it is generally stated that the "present arrangement is conducive to comfort." What arrangement? Of having no matron? While it is added that a lying-in ward and a matron are "much wanted." At Darjeeling the women and children are treated in their own quarters which "would be satisfactory enough if the married quarters were not so dark and damp as they are." Sometimes it is said that "the arrangements are quite equal to those for the men."

The construction of these hospitals appears to be the same as that of small regimental hospitals.

The following plan and section of a female hospital at Mian Mir (Figure 15) (one of the most recently built in India) shows that they require quite as much structural improvement. It is a nest of rooms within rooms; and the same may be said of it that one of our engineers said of the Pacha's new fort on the Dardanelles, that "he would be much safer outside of it."

But whatever defects there may be in the hospital accommodation for soldiers' wives and families in India, at least prostitution is not encouraged and its immorality systematically palliated by lock hospitals on any large scale, although recent attempts have been made to extend them. Lock hospitals, alas! exist—exist, I mean, and are advocated and supported on the principle of restoring the vicious to go on with their vice, the only institution I am aware of for this purpose. (Prisons and lock hospitals in England at least aspire to reclaim the vicious.) And lock hospitals and police regulation are, alas! sometimes recommended, just as if they could do any good. At Secunderabad, it is said, a lock hospital has been long in existence with these "excellent results," viz., that 20 percent of admissions into (military) hospital are from the disease engendered by vice, which is five times as much as exists among the native troops. On the other hand, the enlightened medical officer at Karachi has entered a striking protest against the present lock hospitals and has shown how utterly incompatible at once they are with morality and how utterly useless in practice. Indeed common sense is the same as moral sense in these as in other things. As in the kindred vice of drunkenness, government licenses in order to control vice and the soldier is more drunken than before.

**FIGURE 15**
**Female Hospital at Mian Mir**

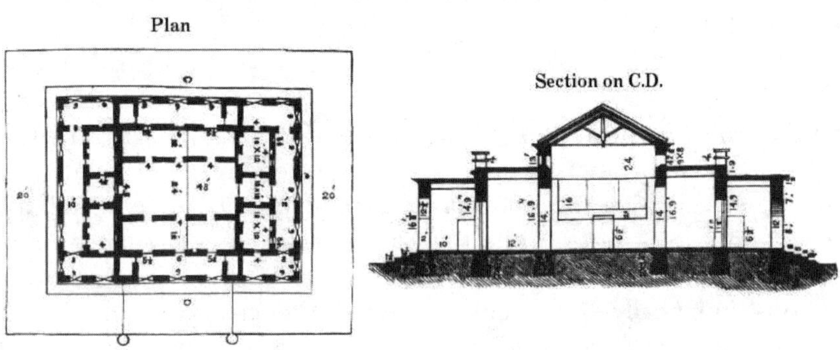


Lately in one of our own largest seaport towns—and I understand it is not the only place where such a measure is contemplated—I was consulted as to the structure of a hospital where government was going to pay for fifteen and for ten beds for fallen women for the army and for the navy. These are called the "War Office prostitutes" and the "Admiralty prostitutes." The title is just and therefore the less agreeable. In this same town a hospital for soldiers' wives only lately exists, although it had been long corresponded about, although several women had been confined in barrack rooms, several had had fever in consequence and one, at least, upon testimony of the army medical officer, had died from it, as well as children.

With two or at most three exceptions, there is no accommodation for sick women and children at any home station. As regards army prostitution, there is, as I have said, the same helplessness as with army drunkenness. It is apparently never considered that they are both parts of the same vice and that, so far as human agency is concerned, they both spring from the same causes.

India has its licensed "lal bazaars" [brothels] and its licensed spirit selling. And both are encouraged to the utmost by leaving the men utterly without rational employment for their time. The "lal bazaar" and the canteen both send men into hospital in abundance. While, instead of confronting both evils with the strong arm and providing men with useful occupations and manly amusements, government sets up lock hospitals under its authority and makes ineffectual attempts to stop drunkenness by keeping the supply of drink, as far as it can, in its own hands, and so encouraging the evil by its own authority. The authority of government is avouched for both evils. So long as this is the case, they will extend and flourish and the taxpayers in India and England will have to bear the cost.

### Statistics

All that can be said under this head is that the statistical abstracts of sickness and mortality for the European troops of the Indian Army afford no data of sufficient accuracy to enable us to judge of the sanitary state of the troops, while they are defective in some most important data required for estimating the exact sanitary condition of the stations. Practically, these statistics are very much in the same condition as were those for queen's troops before recent improvements were introduced. The facts may be in existence, but there are no means of rendering them easily accessible. The question of mortality and efficiency is one of even greater importance now than it was formerly, seeing that the whole British Army must pass through India in the course of its service.

The only way to keep a proper check over the sanitary condition of stations is to lay their sickness and mortality statistics annually before Parliament. This can be easily done by adopting the new statistical methods and forms at present in use for queen's troops at home and on foreign service. These should be introduced over the whole of India and the results published every year, together with those of the army at home.

### SANITARY SERVICE

In times past there has been no proper sanitary service in India. No doubt there has been more or less of cleanliness, because wherever Englishmen go they attend to this in one way or other. Otherwise there is just the same neglect of civilized appliances, of water supply, drainage, etc., as used to exist in unimproved towns at home, notwithstanding repeated representations made by Sir Ranald Martin and by other enlightened professional men. In India, as at home, no good will be done unless it be made some competent person's express business to look to these things.

Even with our habits of self-government, it has been found necessary for the central government to step in and assist local progress. It is certainly of far greater importance for the Government of India to do so, seeing that there is no local self-government at all.

There is, it is true, a kind of local sanitary government at the seats of the three presidencies, the result of whose labours has hitherto been that no one of those three large and populous cities has as yet arrived at the degree of civilization in their sanitary arrangements at which the worst parts of our worst towns had arrived, before sanitary reform sprung up in England at all. Bombay, it is true, has a better water supply; but it has no drainage. Calcutta is being drained; but it has no water supply. Two of the seats of government have thus each one half of a sanitary improvement, which halves ought never to be separated. Madras has neither. As to barracks and cantonments, it is quite evident that both sanitary medical officer and sanitary engineer need to "be abroad."

I am, my Lord,
your faithful servant
Florence Nightingale

## "How People May Live and Not Die in India," 1863

**Editor:** Nightingale's paper, "How People May Live and Not Die in India," was first read by Dr Scoresby Jackson at the Edinburgh meeting of the National Association for the Promotion of Social Science in October 1863, and was highly praised. The paper presented a summary of the facts contained in the report of the second royal commission and in her *Observations*; it was included in the *Transactions* of the Association. Nightingale had it published again in November 1864 with a new preface dated August 1864. The new preface described the work done in India by Sir John Lawrence and the measures already taken by the army to remedy the abuses uncovered by the inquiry. The paper emphasized a key point of the royal commission report, that now was the time to stop blaming all the diseases of British soldiers in India on the climate. The conclusion of the royal commission, it says, was clear: disease is caused by sanitary neglect; "all that the climate requires is that men shall adapt their social habits and customs to it" (see p 189 below). This paper can be seen as Nightingale's first attempt to get the core findings and recommendations of the royal commission out to opinion leaders.

Source: Florence Nightingale, "How People May Live and Not Die in India," a paper read at the meeting of the National Association for the Promotion of Social Science held at Edinburgh October 1863, in *Transactions of the National Association for the Promotion of Social Science* (London: Longmans 1864), published again separately with a new preface (London: Longmans 1864)

A meeting of the Social Science Association is surely the place to discuss one of the most important of social questions, viz., how the British race is to hold possession of India and to bestow upon its vast populations the benefit of a higher civilization. The first part of the question is for the present the most important. For if it be impossible to keep possession of the country, there is an end of the problem.

The Royal Commission on the Sanitary State of the Army in India, whose two-folio volumes of report and appendix constitute a new social starting point for Indian civilization, has shown that, unless the health of British troops in India can be improved, and the enormous death rate reduced, this country will never be able to hold India with a British Army. (It is a pity that by mistake the complete report and evidence of this Commission, in two-folio volumes, was not presented to Parliament, not distributed, not sold at the Parliamentary Depôts. This Report, unlike other reports, was based on two kinds of evidence: (1) The usual oral evidence of witnesses; (2) Reports from every station in India, in answer to printed questions sent out, the answers being signed by the commanding officer, the engineer officer and the medical officer of each station. It was truly said that such a complete picture of the life in India, both British and native, is contained in no other book in existence.)

The time has not yet arrived for the pressure of the death rate it discloses to be fully experienced because the present large army is comparatively new to the country. But unless active measures are taken by the India government and by the military authorities to give effect to the recommendations of the commission, it is unhappily certain that the mortality will increase with the length of service. And then will be felt the difficulty stated by Sir Alexander Tulloch, viz., of filling up the ranks of those, prematurely slain by preventible disease, from the recruiting depôts at home. Few men have had so much experience in this department of the Service. And he tells us that he very much doubts whether an army of seventy thousand men can be kept up in India with the present death rate.

In former times, when the Company's troops bore but a small proportion to the resources (in men) of this country, the death rate was not so much felt. The small army was swept away; and its place supplied, as often as necessary, from the recruiting offices at home. But now that a large proportion of the whole British Army is stationed in India, the question whether we shall hold or lose India will depend very much on the steps taken to protect it from disease.

The statement that the average death rate of troops serving in India was no less than 69 per 1000 per annum took the country by surprise. The accuracy of the average could not be denied because the statement was made on the authority of Sir Alexander Tulloch and confirmed by a separate inquiry made with the help of the Registrar-General's Office, at the request of the commission.

But it was endeavoured to explain away the obvious result of the figures by showing that the average was not constant; that, in certain years and groups of years, the death rate was much greater than in others; that the mortality in the years of excess was due to wars or other causes; that peace, and not sanitary measures, was therefore the remedy. In short, that the statement of a death rate averaging 69 per 1000 per annum was not a fair representation of the case.

To this there is the simple reply that, during this present century, there has been an average loss, from death alone, of 69 men out of every 1000 per annum—it matters not how the mortality has been distributed; that there is every reason to believe that, if things go on as they have done in this present century, we shall go on losing our troops at the rate of 30, 50, 70, 90, 100 and upwards, per 1000. And all the arithmetic in the world cannot conceal the fact that the law, by which men perish in India under existing sanitary negligence, is 69 per 1000 per annum; this death rate is in fact understated for it says nothing of the invalids sent home from India who die at sea or within a short time of their arrival at home; nor of the loss to service by destroyed health; nor of the Mutiny years. It takes into account only those who die in India and in the ordinary course of service.

Few people have an idea of what a death rate of 69 per 1000 represents—the amount of inefficiency from sickness—of invaliding. Assuming the strength of the Indian Army at 73,000 British troops, and taking the death rate at present alone, without the sickness and invaliding, such an army, with this present death rate, will lose, on an average of years, an entire brigade of 5037 men per annum. It may lose, some years, half that number. But in other years, it will lose two such brigades. And where are we to find 10,000 recruits to fill up the gap of deaths of a single unhealthy year?

It is said that the death rates of the war years being the highest (not from wounds), peace, and not sanitary measures, is the remedy. As well might it be said that the British Army, having nearly perished before Sevastopol, not from wounds but from want of every supply of civilized life, peace, and not the supply of the wants of civilized life, was the remedy.

The royal commission has shown that, if the death rate were reduced to even 20 per 1000 per annum (which is too high), i.e., double that of home stations since these stations were improved, to India would be saved a tax equal to £1000 sterling per diem; and this represents the mere cost of replacing the men cut off by excess of premature and preventible mortality.

1. Unofficial people are everywhere asking the question, how this great death rate has arisen, how it happens that one of the most civilized and healthy nations in the world no sooner lands the pick of its working population in tropical climates (for similar losses occur in all tropical climates among us) than they begin to die off at this enormous rate.

I am afraid the reply must be that British civilization is insular and local and that it takes small account of how the world goes on out of its own island. There is a certain aptitude amongst other nations which enables them to adapt themselves, more or less, to foreign climates and countries. But wherever you place your Briton, you may feel quite satisfied that he will care nothing about climates.

If he has been a large eater and a hard drinker at home, ten to one he will be, to say the least of it, as large an eater and as hard a drinker in the burning plains of Hindustan. Enlist an Irish or a Scotch labourer who has done many a hard day's work, almost entirely on farinaceous or vegetable diet, with an occasional dose of whiskey, place him at some Indian station where the thermometer ranges at between 90° and 100° and he will make no difficulty in disposing of three or four times the quantity of animal food he ever ate under the hardest labour during winters at home, if indeed he ever ate any at all.

Now the ordinary system of dieting British soldiers in India is more adapted to a cold climate than that of outdoor farm servants doing work in England.

More than this, the occasional dram at home is commuted, by regulation, in India into a permission to drink two drams, i.e., 6 ounces of raw spirits every day. And be it remembered that, at the same time, the men have little or nothing to do. The craving for spirits, induced by this regulation-habit of tippling, leads to increase of drunkenness, so that, what with overeating, overdrinking, total idleness and vice springing directly from these, the British soldier in India has small chance indeed of coping with the climate, so-called. The regulation allowance of raw spirit which a man may obtain at the canteen is no less than 18½ gallons per annum, which is, I believe, three times the amount per individual which has raised Scotland, in the estimation of economists, to the rank of being the most spirit-consuming nation in Europe. Of late years, malt liquor has been partly substituted for spirits. But up to the present time every man, if he thinks fit, may draw his 18½ gallons a year of spirits, besides what he gets surreptitiously at the bazaar. (Tippling is unfortunately not confined to common soldiers. Officers also use spirits, generally brandy with water or with soda water. It relieves exhaustion for the time at the expense of the constitution and is a prime agent in sending officers to the hills to recover their health, and home on sick furlough. The practice is at some stations called "pegging," alluding to putting pegs in one's coffin. Is not this practice of "pegging" one reason why officers are less healthy in India than civilians?)

So much for intemperance. But not to this alone, nor to this mainly, nor to this and its kindred vice together, is to be laid the soldier mortality in India.

The diseases from which the soldier mainly suffers there are miasmatic: now intemperance never produced miasmatic diseases yet. They are foul-air diseases and foul-water diseases: fevers, dysenteries and so on. But intemperance may cause liver disease and it may put the man into a state of health which prevents him from resisting miasmatic causes.

2. What are these causes? We have not far to look.

The Briton leaves his national civilization behind him and brings his personal vices with him. At home there have been great improvements everywhere in agricultural and in town drainage, and in providing plentiful and pure water supplies. There is nothing of the kind in India. There is no drainage either in town or in country. There is not a single station drained. If such a state of things existed at home, we should know that we have fevers, cholera and epidemics to expect. But hitherto only a few enlightened people have expected anything of the kind from these same causes in India (although they are always happening).

As regards water, there is certainly not a single barrack in India which is supplied, in our sense of the term, at all. There are neither water pipes nor drainpipes. Water is to be had from tanks into which all the filth on the neighbouring surface may at any time be washed by the rains, or from shallow wells dug in unwholesome or doubtful soil. So simple a piece of mechanism as a pump is unknown. Water is drawn in skins, carried in skins on the backs of men or bullocks, and poured into any sort of vessels in the barracks for use. The quantity of water is utterly insufficient for health. And as to the quality, the less said about that, the better. There is no reason to hope that any station has what in this country would be called a pure water supply. And at some it is to be feared that, when men drink water, they drink cholera with it.

The construction of barracks, where men have to pass their whole period of service, is another illustration of how completely home civilization is reversed in India. All our best soldiers have been brought up in country cottages. And when in barracks at home, there are rarely more than from twelve to twenty men in a room. But as soon as the soldier comes to India he is put into a room with 100 or 300 and, in one case, with as many as 600 men. Just when the principle of subdivision into a number of detached barracks becomes of, literally, vital importance, the proceeding is reversed. And the men are crowded together under circumstances certain, even in England, to destroy their health.

To take another illustration. Our home British population is about the most active in the world. In fact we in this country consider exercise and health inseparable; but as soon as the same men go to India, they are shut up all day in their hot, close barrack rooms, where they also eat and sleep; they are not allowed to take exercise; all their meals are eaten in the hottest part of the day and served to them by native servants; and they lie on their beds idle and partly sleeping till sunset! "Unrefreshing day-sleep" is indeed alleged as one of the causes for the soldier's ill-health in India—the soldier, the type of endurance and activity, who now becomes the type of sloth!

3. The Indian social state of the British soldier is not only the reverse of the social state of the soldier at home, and of the class from which he is taken, but there is a great exaggeration in the wrong direction. Yet people are surprised that British soldiers die in India; and they lay the whole blame on the climate.

It is natural to us to seek a scapegoat for every neglect and climate has been made to play this part ever since we set foot in India. Sir Charles Napier[76] says "that every evil from which British troops have suffered has been laid at its door." "The effects of man's imprudence are attributed to climate; if a man gets drunk, the sun has given him a headache, and so on." In regard to Delhi, he says: "Every garden, if not kept clean, becomes a morass; weeds flourish, filth runs riot and the grandest city in India has the name of being insalubrious, although there is nothing evil about it that does not appear to be of man's own creation."

One most important result of the inquiry of the royal commission has been to destroy this bugbear. They have reduced "climate" to its proper dimensions and influence, and they have shown that, just as hot, moist weather at home calls people to account for sanitary neglects and acts of intemperance, so does the climate of India call to account the same people there. There is not a shadow of proof that India was created to be the grave of the British race. The evidence, on the contrary, is rather in the other direction and shows that all that the climate requires is that men shall adapt their social habits and customs to it; as indeed they must do to the requirements of every other climate under heaven.

This necessity includes all the recommendations made by the royal commission for improving the health and reducing to one sixth the death rate of the British Army in India. They all amount to this: You have in India such and such a climate; if you wish to keep your health in it:

76 Sir Charles James Napier (1782-1853) general, conqueror and governor of Sind (now Pakistan).

Be moderate in eating and drinking; eat very little animal food, let your diet be chiefly farinaceous and vegetable.

Spirits are a poison, to be used only (like other poisons) for any good purpose, under medical advice.

Use beer or light wine, but sparingly.

Drink coffee or tea.

Clothe yourself lightly to suit the climate, wearing thin flannel always next the skin.

Take plenty of exercise and use prudence and common sense as to the times of it.

So far for personal habits. But a man cannot drain and sewer his own city, nor lay a water supply on to his own station, nor build his own barracks. What follows pertains to government: Let it be the first care to have a plentiful supply of pure water laid on for every purpose.

Drain all dwellings.

Have no cesspits.

Attend rigidly to cleansing, not only to surface cleansing.

Never build in a wet hollow nor on a sludgy river bank, which would be avoided by sensible people even at home.

Never crowd large numbers into the same room.

Build separate barrack rooms, instead of large barracks.

Place these so that the air plays freely round them.

Raise them above the ground with a current of air beneath.

Do these things and the climate may be let to take care of itself.

But if we would make India about as healthy as England, only somewhat hotter, let us have improved agriculture and agricultural drainage.

If all these improvements were carried out, the normal death rate of the British soldier would be not 69 per 1000, but 10 per 1000, say the commissioners.

But it is not for the soldier alone we speak. The report has a much deeper meaning and intent than this: it aims at nothing less than to bring the appliances of a higher civilization to the natives of India. Such revelations are made, especially in the reports from the stations, with regard to the sanitary condition of these, as to be almost incredible. Everywhere the people are suffering from epidemic diseases; fevers, dysenteries, cholera: constant epidemics we may call them, and constant high death rates (how high can never be known, because there is no registration).

The plague and pestilence is the ordinary state of things. The extraordinary is when these sweep over large tracts, gathering strength in their course, to pass over gigantic mountain ranges and to spread their ravages over Western Asia and Europe. And all this might be saved!

We know the causes of epidemic outbreaks here. Take the worst condition of the worst and most neglected town district at home; and this is, to say the least of it, much better than the normal condition of nearly the whole surface of every city and town in India.

Not one city or town is drained. Domestic filth round the people's houses is beyond description. Water supply is from wells or tanks, in ground saturated with filth. No domestic conveniences. Every spare plot of ground is therefore in a condition defying us to mention it farther.

Rains of the rainy season wash the filth of the past dry season into the wells and tanks. The air in, and for some distance round, native towns is as foul as sewer air. (At Madras a wall has actually been built to keep this from the British towns.) No sanitary administration. No sanitary police.

Here then we have, upon a gigantic scale, the very conditions which invariably precede epidemics at home. India is the focus of epidemics. Had India not been such, cholera might never have been. Even now, the Sunderbuns, where every sanitary evil is to be found in its perfection, are nursing a form of plague increasing yearly in intensity, covering a larger and larger area and drawing slowly round the capital of India itself. Are we to learn our lesson in time?

Some say: What have we to do with the natives or their habits? Others find an excuse for doing nothing in the questions arising out of caste. But caste has not interfered with railways. The people of themselves have no power to prevent or remove these evils, which now stand as an impassable barrier against all progress. Government is everything in India.

The time has gone past when India was considered a mere appanage of British commerce. In holding India, we must be able to show the moral right of our tenure. Much is being done, no doubt, to improve the country: by railways, canals and means of communication; to improve the people: by education, including under this work, European literature and science.

But what at home can be done in education, if we neglect physical laws? How does education progress here without means of cleanliness, of decency or health? The school lessons of a month are sapped in an hour. If the people are left a prey to epidemics and to immoral agencies in their homes, it is not much good sending them to school. Where should we be now with all our schools if London were like Calcutta, Madras or Bombay?—the three seats of government in India. The next great work then is sanitary reform in India. There is not a town which does not want:

Water supply,
Draining,
Paving,
Cleansing,
Healthy plans for arranging and construction buildings,

Together with agricultural drainage and improved cultivation all round.

These things the people cannot do for themselves. But the India government can do them. And in order to do them, three health departments (one for each of the presidencies) have been recommended by the royal commission together with a home commission to help these departments in bringing the appliances of a better civilization to India.

The work is urgent. Every day it is left undone adds its quota of inefficiency to the British Army and its thousands of deaths to the native population. Danger is common to European and to native. Many of the best men this country ever had have fallen victims to the same causes of disease which have decimated the population of Hindustan. And so it will be till the India government has fulfilled its vast responsibility towards those great multitudes who are no longer strangers and foreigners, but as much the subjects of our beloved queen as any one of us.

The real, the main point in the report of the royal commission is this:

Look to the state of your stations first, then look to the hills for help. Your stations and cities are in a condition which, in the finest temperate climate in Europe, would be and have been the cause of the Great Plague, of half the population being swept off by disease. And on the other hand, no climate in the world, certainly not that of India, could kill us if we did not kill ourselves by our neglects. We complain of the climate when the wonder is that there is one of us left, under a sky which certainly intensifies causes of disease: so much so indeed that, one would have thought, it might set men to work to remove these causes and twice as vigorously as in a temperate climate, instead of not at all. But no: our cities are not those of civilized men.

It cannot now be said, as Burke[77] did: "England has built no bridges, made no high roads, cut no navigations." But in all that regards the social improvement of cities, still it must be said, as he did (how many years ago?): "Were we driven out of India this day, nothing would remain to tell that it had been possessed, during the inglorious period of our dominion, by anything better than the ouran-outang or the tiger."

For how much is it better now? Bring your cities and stations within the pale of civilization. As they are, they are the life destroyers, not the climate. The hills, those very climates to which you look for succour, are becoming so pestiferous from your neglects that they bear out this indictment. They cry to you as we do: reform your stations, thence comes the deadly influence.

The question is no less a one than this: How to create a public health department for India, how to bring a higher civilization into India. What a work, what a noble task for a government—no "inglorious period of our dominion" that, but a most glorious one! That would be creating India anew. For God places His own power, His own life-giving laws in the hands of man. He permits man to create mankind by those laws, even as He permits man to destroy mankind by neglect of those laws.

## Postscript

Since this paper was read, the lower death rate of troops new to the country has actually been put forward as a proof that India is becoming healthy, and the 69 per 1000 is an old antiquated average! But more than this, the diminution of mortality arising from the short duration of service is ascribed to improvements carried out at Indian stations since the royal commissioners began their inquiry. The leading authorities on the subject ascribe the main causes of disease to

77 Edmund Burke (1729-97), MP, writer and critic who opposed English colonialist policy in America and in India at the end of the eighteenth century. Burke's actual text says: "England has erected no churches, no hospitals, no palaces, no schools; England has built no bridges, made no high roads, cut no navigations, dug out no reservoirs. Every other conqueror of every other description has left some monument, either of state or beneficence, behind him. Were we to be driven out of India this day, nothing would remain to tell that it had been possessed during the inglorious period of our dominion by anything better than the ouran-outang or the tiger" (Edmund Burke, *The Works of the Rt Hon Edmund Burke* 2:354).

want of drainage, bad sites, bad water badly distributed, wretched sanitary condition of native bazaars and towns, bad barrack and bad hospital construction, surface overcrowding from want of barrack accommodation, want of occupation for the men, intemperance in eating and drinking, want of proper barrack and hospital conveniences; it is difficult to see how India could have been freed from these causes of disease in three short years, which is about the average time since the stational reports were signed.

That something may have been done in the way of cleansing, ventilation, ablution arrangements, means of recreation, is possible. But as to ventilation, it may almost be said that it is better to keep the foul air out than to let it in, at least at certain stations of which we have reports up to nearly the latest date from India.

As to cleansing we have the report of a government commission on the last cholera, dated 21 July 1862, which tells us that, at a large station where cholera was fatal, the filth from the latrines was thrown down at places 100 yards from the barracks; that dead animals and every kind of refuse are accumulated in the same places without burial; that, before the cholera appeared, there were abominable cesspools poisoning the whole atmosphere; that neglect of the commonest principles of sanitary science favoured the epidemic; that the filth from the native latrines was used for feeding sheep! that, for all this, the local military authorities had not neglected "conservancy in any unusual degree," the reporters state; and that, bad as they considered it, the station was kept in much better order than many that they had visited.

We have also two printed documents of the public works department, dated Calcutta, 26 June and 9 September 1863, proving that the capital of India was in a much worse state than appeared from the stational report sent to the royal commission in June 1860.

## Role of Sir John Lawrence up to 1864

**Editor:** As Sidney Herbert was Nightingale's "master," so was Sir John Lawrence her "hero" (see p 208 below). Among all the officials involved with her India work Nightingale assigned a very special place to John Lawrence and, throughout her active life, expressed enormous admiration for his work. They had met in March 1860 at the time Lawrence was serving on the Council of India (1858-63) and when he gave evidence to the second royal commission. John Lawrence was appointed viceroy 30 November 1863; he saw Nightingale 4 December

1863 and reached India 12 January 1864. Prior to 4 December Nightingale and Lawrence had corresponded. He had commented on her *Observations.* She was impressed by his previous career in India in the days of the Company, especially the years 1843-59: he was celebrated as "the saviour of the Punjab" mainly for his work as chief commissioner of the Punjab (1853-59) at the time of the Mutiny. Because of the centrality of John Lawrence in Nightingale's India work, we give special attention to their correspondence at this point, although much of their relationship has already been highlighted in the introductory section on "Nightingale's India Work" and in the previous pages. Numerous references to Lawrence are found in Nightingale material from 1860 on. The excerpts presented here cover John Lawrence's time leading to his departure for India to take up his post as viceroy and to his first year's work. Respected for his rich Indian experience, he served as consultant to Nightingale's cause. Collaboration with other officials, which offered some analogy to her relation to Lawrence, is also reported in the present section. A further section relates Nightingale's relationship to Lawrence as viceroy, introducing in India the measures recommended by the royal commission.

Source: From three letters to Sir Harry Verney, Wellcome (Claydon copy) Ms 8998/19, 21 and 8999/23

29 February 1860

I should indeed like to see Sir John Lawrence, whom of all men I, with all Europe, revere and admire. I am very glad to hear that present ministers, if they stop in till December, wish *him* to be the next governor general. But I should not think of troubling him to call upon me for the mere pleasure of seeing him, did I not believe that it might materially help forward the "Indian sanitary commission" (which intends, of course, to take his evidence), if he would be so good as to give me some of his instruction as to Indian sanitary affairs.

The worst of it is that I am getting more and more helpless as to seeing people. I have such bad nights now and am so drenched with morphia that I am sometimes unable even to get up to see Mr Herbert on business when he comes. And I feel so unwilling to take up the time of a man like Sir J. Lawrence.

If you would say something of this kind to him tonight (as you so kindly propose) and say, too, that if he would allow me, through you, to make an appointment with him some few days hence, *ad* HIS *libitum* [at HIS *pleasure*], I should indeed think it a privilege.

5 March 1860

I am sure you will be glad to hear that Sir John Lawrence was so good as to come here to give a very important direction to the Indian inquiry. And I trust that the information he was kind enough to give in other ways and the views (in which as far as I can agree with "Hercules" I entirely agree) will be of real use in stronger hands than mine. I trust he will live to see the good of his exertions for human (Indian) nature in all ways.

9 June 1861

I think that you will like to see our return from Umballa, as your son is there, although in manuscript only. The abstract, made as the other printed Returns I have sent you, is not come back from "*revise.*" I must ask you to send me back this return immediately, as, being an important Station, we mean to have the plans lithographed for our report. You will see by a glance at the "cantonments" plan that it comprises the best (the echelon) and the worst arrangement of barracks. . . .

I should indeed like to see Sir Hope Grant. But on the eve of his departure can hardly hope that so great a man will give me a few minutes of his time. And I [am] such a poor creature that I can hardly name a time. I should like to be allowed to give him the printed abstracts of all such stations within his presidency as we have ready. . . .

We meet constantly with this remark: "These queries apply only to Europeans. No reply." It is not the least necessary for natives to have any of the requisites for life, or for exercising.

Source: From a letter to Sir John Lawrence, Add Mss 45777 ff10-12

5 December 1862

I have kept your Punjab report an unwarrantable time. I thank you very much for it. It shows two things: (1) that it is impossible to exaggerate the sanitary defects of Indian stations; (2) that Indian medical officers (if this report fairly represents their intelligence on such subjects) are the best possible agents for increasing the high death rate of the Indian Army.

Anything more hopeless than the infinite hiatus between the mischief described and the remedies recommended I have never seen. (It is greater than that in the Crimea.) The point where sanitary engineering touches medical disclosures is entirely missed. . . . What has produced endless choleras in Europe in temperate climates, what killed Lord Raglan in the Crimea, what is the curse of India they advocate. Men like Mackinnon, Green, Gordon, Chevers, all good men, advocate what we know to be pestilence and death. The medical officers have proved themselves quite and entirely able to point out the evils. But they have no more clue to the remedies than my cats have (who, by the way, advocate just the same system of dry drainage, only they cover it up, which the Indian doctors don't propose to do—at least not for natives).

Source: From an undated letter to Sir John Lawrence, in Reginald Bosworth Smith, *Life of Lord Lawrence* 2:394-95

[1863]

Among the multitude of affairs and congratulations [for his appointment as viceroy], which will be pouring in upon you, there is no more fervent joy, there are no stronger good wishes, than those of one of the humblest of your servants. For there is no greater position for usefulness under heaven than that of governing the vast empire you saved for us. And you are the only man to fill it. So thought a statesman with whom I worked not daily, but hourly, for five years, Sidney Herbert, when the last appointment was made. In the midst of your pressure pray think of us and of our sanitary things on which such millions of lives and health depend.

Source: From two letters to Sir Harry Verney, Wellcome (Claydon copy) Ms 9000/148 and 149

4 December 1863

Lord Stanley has twice repeated his wish that I should see Sir John Lawrence in order to "explain to him the proposals of the royal commission" which, Lord S. adds, I could do so much better than he can.

Were it not for this and for your kind wish, I should never have had the audacity to wish to take up even an hour of the time of so great a man. You said something about coming up to London to settle it with Sir J. Lawrence. If you are coming up to wish him goodbye, it certainly would forward it very much, if you could do so in time to give him time to make a vacant half hour to see me. He starts on Thursday and must be overwhelmed with business. But so great a man is never overwhelmed.

I should have not the least objection to show him Lord Stanley's letter, which indeed appears to be written for that purpose. But I don't like to send it him. It looks too urgent. Also, it would be very desirable if he could see me in time to see Sir C. Wood afterwards, supposing he thinks well to do anything with Sir C.W. before he starts.

Sir C.W. has finally refused *any* instructions whatever to our home commission. But *that* is of minor importance now.

I need not say that any hour I would see Sir J. Lawrence, if he will see me.

4 December 1863

Since I wrote to you my letter of this morning, Sir John Lawrence has made an appointment to see me. I hope therefore this will reach you by the same post as my first. I hope you still will come up and see him on your own account. He goes on *Wednesday*.

Source: From a letter to Frances Nightingale, Wellcome (Claydon copy) Ms 9000/150

6 December 1863

I am quite overdone with India business as you may suppose, but so glad to have it to do. I have seen Sir J. Lawrence [4 December], God bless him! and Lord Stanley. And these are the only two hours I have been up since I came here. I am to see Sir J. Lawrence's private secretary tomorrow. They start on Wednesday.

Source: From a letter to William Farr, Wellcome Ms 5474/64, copy Add Mss 43399 ff159-60

10 December 1863

*Confidential.* You may be sure that I have thought of nothing else but our India business during the last busy ten days. . . . I have had the great joy of being in constant communication with Sir John Lawrence, and of receiving his commands to do what I had almost lost the hope of being allowed to do, viz., of sending out full statements and schemes of what we want the presidency commissions to do.

I should be glad to submit to you copies of papers of mine, which he desired me to write and which he took out with him as to the constitution of the presidency commissions, if you care to see them. They are, of course, confidential.

His is the greatest government under God's. And he is the only man to fill it.

I have also seen Lord Stanley more than once during these busy days. And, with Sir J. Lawrence's command, we feel ourselves empowered to begin the "home commission," and to father our plans upon it. Sir J. Lawrence, so far from considering our report exaggerated, considers it under the mark.

And, though I have not seen Colonel Norman's[78] furious attack upon us, I have (now in my possession) the Cholera Commission report, dated July 1862, Public Works Department papers, dated August and September of *this* year, which give an idea of a state of things of which we had no idea, *have given no* idea. I send you an extract of the former. (The India Office, wise in its generation, (?) keep these a dead secret. And I am indebted to Sir J. Lawrence and Sir C. Trevelyan for them.)

Please return me all these papers, and consider them really "confidential."

ever yours sincerely

Florence Nightingale

Remember we shall want you in February when we are all to be blown into atoms.[79]

Source: From a letter to Mary Clare Moore,[80] Convent of Mercy, Bermondsey, copy ADD Mss 45789 ff13-16

15 December 1863

Just now things look a little better. Perhaps you may have heard that the governor general in India is dead [Lord Elgin[81]] and that Sir John Lawrence has been appointed governor general. He goes out with very bad health and for two years only. He was so good as to come here before he went and I had the great joy of receiving his commands to do what I had almost lost the hope of our being allowed to do (namely as to sanitary work in India). The men at home still thwart it in every possible way, and just as much since he went as before. But his appointment is a great thing for our work.

Source: From a letter to Lord de Grey, ADD Mss 43546 ff86-95

16 December 1863

*Confidential.* I was in constant communication with Sir John Lawrence during the ten busy days before his departure. What he said ought to be placed before you as minister. But you will see it is for yourself *alone.*

---

78 Henry Wylie Norman (1826-1904), later Sir, member of the Council for India 1878-83.

79 Nightingale was referring to the tabling of the objections to the royal commission report that were expected from India at that time.

80 Mary Clare Moore (1814-74), "Reverend Mother." See the biographical sketch in *Theology* (3:648-49).

81 James Bruce, 8th earl Elgin (1811-63), governor general of Canada 1847-54, viceroy and governor general of India 1862-63.

He was so good as to go very fully with me into the questions of the constitution of the presidency commissions of health, of how they are to work by sending out inspectors, of what the local authorities in each town, both native and stational, were to be, for the same sanitary purpose. And I had the great joy of receiving his commands to do what I had almost lost the hope of our being allowed to do, viz., prepare a scheme of the sanitary work to be carried out in India.

He then went into the questions of what the government in India alone could do, and of what the War Office and Horse Guards alone can do. And this it is which should have been placed before you. But I could have wished to have given the force of all that he said. But that would be writing not a letter, but a book.

The idea that the report of the royal sanitary commission was overstated, or that the defects printed out were remedied, was quite scouted. Especially about questions of "conservancy," much that India has been *given the credit* of doing (in the report) is really done only *on paper*. And I was laughed at for believing it. "Conservancy" is in a *much worse* state (than we have represented it) now at this very moment, 1863. He was most strongly of opinion that your "home" commission should begin operations at once in sending out plans of barracks and hospitals, with complete "instructions"—this was his own word—in drawing up a "direct statement and description of the kind of sanitary works, improvements and appliances applicable to Indian stations to meet the requirements described in the stational reports," in drawing up heads of a sanitary code. I urged repeatedly that it would be much less offensive (to India authorities) if this were done by the home commission under a direct instruction from the S. of S. for India. And he answered repeatedly, Just the reverse. You have lost time. You should *volunteer* all this. He told me, in the strictest confidence, that the I.O. thought the W.O. had "snubbed" *them*, when asking for this assistance, rather than that the W.O. had been too forward. (This, of course, had no reference to the secretaries of state.) This was the main point of his discourse, that the "home" commission should send out *at once*, acting under a general sanction *from you*, all plans, schemes, codes it thought applicable to India, to be rejected or accepted, of course according to the opinion of the India authorities.[82] He then entered a good deal into detail points of the report.

82 This request was to result at long last in the *Suggestions* of 1864.

That India was a hundred years *behind* England in sanitary things was especially dwelt upon.

The one single point in which he differed (even seemed a little annoyed) was that he thought we had implied that government in India had encouraged drinking among the soldiers for the sake of the revenue. I said, No, but government in England does the things out of its estimates for the soldiers, which are done in India out of *their* canteen fund. Yes, he said, but none but the Horse Guards can put a stop to the drinking. The government supply the spirit on the requirement of the regiment. A temperance regiment would not be obliged to take any spirit. Over and over again he repeated as if it quite haunted his mind, No good will be done till the Horse Guards discontinue the sale of spirits in the canteens. The government in India must suppress the sale of spirits in the bazaars, under the control of the magistrate. But the W.O. must make the same law (which exists in England, that no spirit can be sold within barrack boundaries) be in India that no spirit can be sold within *cantonment* boundaries.

He also dwelt on how desirable it would be to increase marriages among the men and said, None but the Horse Guards can do this. But it will be an actual *saving* in time. Everything that raises the *man* is an actual saving. It was implied that there would *not* be the difficulty in introducing sanitary reform among the natives that there will be among the India military authorities! (This I can believe.)

You are aware, of course, that the "defence" (this is not my word) of the India military authorities is to be brought before the House of Commons. This is a very good thing for us. For ours is the strongest case ever S. of S. had to stand upon. But I hope we shall be in readiness for them.

The gist of what Sir John Lawrence asks is this:

1. We have told the Indian engineers that *they* "know nothing" in sanitary matters; we must not imply that *we* "know everything"; it is too much to expect the I.O. to *instruct* the Barrack and Hospital Commission to tell them that they "know nothing." They will never ask for help, but whatever help is offered they will accept. They will cry out that they are "vastly ill-used" but they will take help and never acknowledge it.

If Lord de Grey then, either in concurrence with Sir C. Wood or alone, will give such a general instruction to the home commission as would include the India work, the sooner they are called together the better. I told Sir J. Lawrence, and I may tell you, that we have *not* "lost time." In private, we have prepared the sanitary heads of a code (this we had been instructed to do by Sir C. Wood); we are drawing up directions about sanitary works and measures, etc. The W.O. is preparing barrack and hospital plans (though I wish it would get on a little faster with them). And for these we are writing "instructions." Before long then, we shall have some useful matter to submit to you (and which will, of course, be then submitted to the S. of S. for India) to send to India.

It is an immense thing to have a governor general at the other end who will take up these things. His is the greatest government under God's. And he the only man to fill it, I think.

2. I have separated (in the two sheets enclosed) what can only be done by the W.O. from what can only be done by the governor general. What is suggested is that Lord de Grey should draw up a minute, including all that is proposed to be done by the W.O. and Horse Guards, and have it discussed with the H.G. On certain points, they must consent, e.g., in the disuse of spirits in Indian canteens, as has been done at home, also in introducing gymnastics and workshops. . . .

I have put this crudely. A telegram always sounds crude, because a telegram cannot go down on its knees. And that is much my position (morally) at this moment to you. You will see that this letter could not be for Sir C. Wood and that it must be for yourself *alone.* Also, I was almost unable to write so long a statement a few days ago. And yet it ought to be much longer to give Sir John Lawrence's arguments. . . .

I understand that, in February, we are all to be blown into the smallest atoms Dalton[83] ever invented or discovered (I don't know which) by the "defence" of the India military authorities in Parliament. If we survive this, we shall be in a better position than ever we were before.

Source: From four letters to Douglas Galton, ADD Mss 45762 ff69-70, 78-80, 81 and 83-84

7 March 1864

*Confidential.* Of all the papers, I am most glad to have Sir C. Wood's No. 297. But I think you have utterly forgotten that, in December, you asked us to draft a letter to the India Office, consequent on a conversation I had with Lord de Grey; that, about the middle of January, you

83 John Dalton (1766-1844), British physicist and chemist, formulated the first practical atomic theory and table of atomic weights.

wrote to me that you had a reply from *General Pears*[84] as to some points in the respective jurisdictions (without knowing which the letter could not be drafted), which reply of *General Pears* we have never seen.

You will all be "out" this session, after which I shall be able to get what I like from Lord Stanley; but you won't be able to get what you like from General Peel. It is therefore very desirable that this letter should be written now at once, while you are still "in"; besides that Sir John Lawrence will be greatly disappointed at the (*three months'*) unnecessary delay, which has not forwarded the desired letter one bit. *Please burn.*

12 March 1864

I am sorry if I have been a "turbulent fellow." But I must recall to you how the matter stands: after my conversation with Lord de Grey, it was I who was asked (*not* I who proposed) to draft a letter to the India Office. Although I do not see Lord Stanley as I used to see S. Herbert, yet of course I render an account to him, as our chairman, of all the steps taken to carry out his "recommendations"; indeed it was he who insisted in *writing* upon my seeing Sir J. Lawrence, when he was appointed governor general, otherwise I should never have dared to take up so much of his time as I did.

I think we might make it a "grievance" that, all this being as we have stated, we were never told two months ago that the War Office could not do anything, IF it cannot (for nothing has been discovered between your receipt of General Pears's letter in January and your letter to me in March).

Of course, if this is the *final* answer of the War Office, I shall now communicate with Lord Stanley (who will take such measures as he thinks fit in the House of Commons, or personally with Sir C. Wood, to carry out his recommendations) and with Sir John Lawrence, who will do the same as he thinks fit with Sir Hugh Rose.[85] (I must mention that Sir J. Lawrence came to me straight from the commander-in-chief one day. And the account that functionary gave him was quite different.) But as I say, of course the War Office has a right to manage its own affairs. All I venture to complain of is that, after having *asked* me to do a thing, it should have left me, *and* our chairman, *and* our

84 Thomas Townsend Pears (1809-92), later Sir, Madras Engineers.

85 Sir Hugh Rose (1801-85), later Lord Strathnairn, commander-in-chief in India.

governor general, for three months in ignorance that *it was not to be done*, consequently in powerlessness to do anything else. . . .

I had written thus far on Saturday, when I received a letter from Lord Stanley (the first time he has taken the initiative) asking what has been done and where the delay has arisen? asking whether he shall go to Lord de Grey? and asking to call upon me to hear the answer. He says that Sir C. Wood will not stand in the way, if urged from Calcutta to proceed, and safe from Parliamentary attack. I have kept this letter since Saturday. And I must give Lord Stanley an answer.

Believe me, it was through no desire of my own that I acted, instead of Lord Stanley acting. (It would be infinitely better if he managed his own affairs.) I believed honestly when I was told that Lord de Grey would prefer my "interference" to Lord Stanley's. I now write honestly to ask your advice as to what Lord Stanley should do, as to what I should do, as to what I should say to Lord Stanley and as to what you mean to do. I don't want to be rude and I don't want to be civil, I only want the thing done. . . .

We hear that the whole art of government offices is to give "snubs." We hear of the "artistic snub" in which Mr *Lugard* and Mr Lowe[86] are of the "clumping unscientific" snub, of which Lord Palmerston[87] is a professor, of the "coarse and bungling" snub of Lord Granville.[88] What are we to call the "snub" I receive? The "snub indifferent"?

15 March 1864

When I saw Dr Sutherland yesterday, he told me that you now proposed to bring under the notice of the Horse Guards the regimental improvements in India (proposed by the royal commission) with a view to the Horse Guards communicating with the authorities in India on the subject. In a conversation with Lord de Grey three months ago, I understood him to say (when I proposed this very thing) that that would be the very way to balk the whole matter, as Sir H. Rose would take nothing from the commander-in-chief here. I am not advising. You know your own affairs best, I am only asking, and honestly asking what you think best to do. The present position of the question does

86 Robert Lowe (1811-92), later Viscount Sherbrooke, MP and vice-president of the council of the Education Office.

87 The 3rd Viscount Palmerston (1784-1865), prime minister, family friend and supporter on liberal causes.

88 George Leveson-Gower, 2nd Earl Granville (1815-91), Liberal leader in the House of Lords, later to serve as foreign secretary on two separate occasions.

not seem to be altered from what it was on Saturday, when I wrote the previous sheets. Would you be so very good as to give me an answer as soon as possible that I may know what to reply to Lord Stanley, as also to Sir John Lawrence by the mail of the 18th?

28 March 1864

*Private.* In going through (by letter) with Sir J. Lawrence all the recommendations of the report on the India Army sanitary commission and latterly the *regimental* recommendations, I told him that possibly we might be able to manage the application of the new "medical regulations" to regiments in India through the director general here. We have communicated with him on the subject. He says that part of the code for hospitals could not be applied because the India government undertake all the hospitals. All the rest, however, might be applied. If you will call his attention to the subject, he will report on the matter to you.

Would you therefore be so good as to *request the director general to report on the application of the new medical regulations to her majesty's regiments serving in India,* and to point out for your information, *what sections of the regulations might be applied with advantage and without interfering with the Indian government?* Already all the reporting comes direct to the director general.

Source: From a letter to Sir John McNeill, Florence Nightingale Museum (LMA) H1/ST/NC3/SU152, typed copy Add Mss 45768 ff183-84

17 May 1864

You will wish to hear how our sanitary affairs are going on. Sir John Lawrence's appointment gave us a most unexpected hold on India. He was so good as to see me during the short time between his appointment and departure. And he has carried out everything then suggested—a commission of health appointed for each presidency, etc. But few have had such extraordinary chances as I have had twice—a secretary of state and a governor general delivered, as it were, into my hand. And few have seen such disappointment as I have.

I remember well your saying that no man had even had so noble a game to play as Sidney Herbert, and had not played it. It was true. And now, no War Office has ever had such an opportunity with such a governor general actually asking, what would you have me to do? The instructions for his health commissions, which he positively solicited, are still pending, as they were five months ago. And, except my private suggestions, he has had nothing.

I am entirely a sick prisoner now.

Source: From a letter to Douglas Galton, ADD MSS 45762 ff132-34

6 June 1864

I had a letter from Sir John Lawrence (God bless him!) by this mail, dated Simla, 6 May. He is extremely indignant at the non-arrival of our plans and suggestions. After graciously and contemptuously (like a great man) accepting the Mediterranean report, out of which he has "no doubt of gaining some" thing, but not much (you remember clause 2 of General Pears's letter, enclosing Mr Strachey's minute!!),[89] Sir J. Lawrence goes on to say "but our great want is your standard plans and rules, without which we are quite at sea, and *so far from doing better* than formerly, *shall be in danger of doing worse.* As it is now, the reconstruction of some of our worst barracks is at a standstill, until we get these documents."

(It would have been a broad farce, if it had not been something of a tragedy, to hear Sir P. Cautley's and others' assurances of the deadly jealousy of the government in India, when I was hearing by nearly every mail from the head of that government (personally or by a secretary) all the permutations and combinations which could be rung on these expressions, that they were "at a standstill" "quite at sea" "in danger of doing worse, instead of better," etc., because *we* WOULD *NOT* do as they asked. Are all official assurances of the nature of Sir P. Cautley's and company's?)

I don't want to make a grievance now that the plans are so nearly ready. But I certainly ought to put you "au fait" of the real state of things. And I don't suppose Sir J. Lawrence writes to me in order "by a song to conceal his purposes."[90] He goes on to describe his inspections of diverse stations and barracks. He also writes of soldiers' libraries, says they are much improved. Also of workshops. Says that Sir H. Rose has brought them quite into fashion (soldiers'). Also of drinking, that Sir H. Rose has issued a g[eneral] o[rder] reducing the dram of spirits "to one half." (You know Sir J. Lawrence wishes for its total abolition.)

I sing for joy every day at Sir J. Lawrence's government. I have little enough to sing for besides (and much to howl for).

---

89 John Strachey (1823-1907), president of the Bengal Sanitary Commission from 1864.

90 Perhaps Horace and James Smith, *Rejected Addresses*, 1812, a collection of parodies of Byron, Scott, Southey and other famous writers; on page 225 the conspirators say, "Let us by a song conceal our purposes. . . . "

Lord de Grey would probably wish to be informed as to these matters, as they strictly concern the War Office.

Source: From a letter to Sir Harry Verney, Wellcome (Claydon copy) Ms 9001/36

18 June 1864

I must give you an instance of the cool impertinence of the Horse Guards. Their answer to me (to a complaint as to delay in our sanitary affairs) was that "Sir John Lawrence had nothing else to do (sic) but think of India sanitary affairs, whereas we have so much to do." (This referred to sending out something he had asked for.) *Pray tell this.* I really could break those jackasses' heads.

Source: From a letter to Douglas Galton, ADD Mss 45762 f141

23 June 1864

The Horse Guards say that "they were quite aware of Sir J. Lawrence's application and of the delay," but "that it is Sir J. Lawrence's *one only object of interest*" (sic) "while it is only one *out of a thousand* of the War Office's." They ought to have the Victoria Cross for their cool intrepidity in the face of truth.

I have told Sir J. Lawrence of the opinion of these dining-out *freluquets* [whipper-snappers] as to his hard work. And I think I shall publish it after my death.

Source: From a letter to Caroline Clive,[91] ADD Mss 45798 ff241-45

25 June 1864

It is not, as Colonel W. Greathed supposes, because the overworked War Office has not time to attend to the underworked viceroy that the delay has arisen. Not one moment of time or work has been required from any single member of the India or War Offices to do what Sir J. Lawrence desired. All has been done by other hands. All that was required was to sign the initials: de G. [de Grey], C.W. [Charles Wood] on two minutes' conversation between "de G." and "C.W."

It is not that the War Office "has 1000 interests pressing on it," while Sir J. Lawrence "has only one." It is that Sir J. Lawrence was so idiotic as to believe (in December 1863) that the habitual jealousy, supposed to be entertained of the India government at home by the

---

91 Née Caroline Meysey Wigley (1801-73), poet and novelist, friend. See *Women* for a brief discussion of their correspondence (8:648-49) and for photographs of a letter to Clive (8:523-24). Further letters to Clive are published in *Crimean War.*

India government in India, and alleged as an excuse by Sir C. Wood for not sending out the required plans and schemes, alleged not once but nearly every week during the last six months . . . it is that the viceroy, who cleared off half the arrears of eighteen months of his predecessors at one sitting, was so weak as to believe that his written word would be taken, without a printed minute.

At last I wrote out to him for the printed minute. And it is come. But this took four months. "Hence the delay."

I have taken effectual means that all my papers shall be destroyed after my death. But I would gladly have left, as a lesson to the nation, the record of how the greatest living administrator, who rules over one tenth of the human race, not by courtesy but absolutely, who organizes/governs the financial, territorial, judicial, international affairs of 120 millions, compared with whose sway that of the three absolute monarchs, France, Austria, Russia, is a sham where it is not a tyranny and a tyranny where it is not a sham in endeavouring to bestow upon these 120 millions health and civilized life, has been foiled by the torpor and the self-sufficiency of a petty, peddling office, which rules over at most half a million. . . .

And then he is to be told that the War Office has no time to attend to him! Was there ever anything like it since the treatment of the duke of Wellington in the Peninsula by the home government?

If I am told that I know not what the War Office has to do, I say, no man knows it better. I have done the work of an under secretary of state for five years, up to the time of Sidney Herbert's death. But I shame to speak of myself in the same hour as of that great man, Sir John Lawrence. Had I known what a government office was, I fear I should rather have shot myself than entered it.

Did it ever strike you how, if Christ had had to work through Pilate, how would he have done? I have often had to think of it.

Source: From a letter to Frances Nightingale, Wellcome (Claydon copy) Ms 9001/41

Wednesday [June 1864]

My heart bleeds for great John Lawrence, and for my own troubles (of which Sutherland is the greatest), mainly or only as they affect him. And I am his only help in some things.

Sidney Herbert was a knight of the chivalrous times. But great John Lawrence is a hero of the old Roman times, the last of the heroes.

Source: From a letter to Charles Hathaway,[92] Florence Nightingale Museum, typed copy ADD Mss 45782 ff156-57

27 June 1864

*Private.* I hoped to have told you by this mail of the completion of the standard plans, etc., required by Sir John Lawrence. But the lithographs only came from the lithographers on Saturday night last.

I scarcely know whether it is worthwhile to trouble you with the following little incident. I hear from the Horse Guards that they "were perfectly aware of Sir J. Lawrence's application (for these plans, etc.) and of the delay, but that it is Sir J. Lawrence's only interest (sic) while the War Office is pressed by a thousand." (sic)

To which I responded that it is not because the overworked War Office has not time to attend to the underworked viceroy that the delay has arisen, it is because the India Office has used, not once but every week for six months, the pretexted jealousy of the India government in India, supposed to be entertained of the India government at home, as an excuse for not sending out what the head of that very government in India asked for; that all might have been settled (but was not) by a verbal understanding between the war secretary and India secretary in two minutes; but that nothing was done, nor would ever have been done, had it not been for a printed minute from India (5 April) (Mr Strachey's); that the greatest living administrator, who rules one tenth the human race, in whose hands are the destinies of 120 millions—territorial, judicial, legislative, international, communicational—in endeavouring to bestow upon his 120 millions, for the first time, civilization and health, has been foiled by the torpor and self-sufficiency of a petty War Office, which rules over at most half a million. . . . That then he is to be told that the War Office has no time to attend to him! and his "one only interest"!!

You will use your own judgment as to telling this little story to Sir J. Lawrence. Great men smile at what is "aggravating" to little ones. Otherwise it is no use giving him one moment's useless irritation. Did it ever occur to you—what would Christ have done, if Christ had had to work through Pilate!

---

92 Dr Charles Hathaway, sanitary commissioner and John Lawrence's secretary.

Source: From an incomplete letter to Douglas Galton, Add Mss 45762 ff162-63

[July 1864]

He [doubtless Sir J. Lawrence] then alludes to the "good folks of England really believing that I had sanctioned an attack on the religion of the Hindus, because I desired to improve the health of the people in Calcutta."

(Now this last he rather exaggerates to himself.) They did not "believe" it. But I am sure it would do him good, if he knew that statesmen appreciated him. He is doing such great things. What a pity heroes are but flesh and blood like us. You will see that I ought scarcely to have betrayed his confidence, even to you. But you know better than anyone else what he has to do. Please burn this note.

Source: From a letter to Lord Stanley, Liverpool Record Office, Derby Collection 920/15/50

28 July 1864

*Private and Confidential.* I do not know whether you correspond with Sir John Lawrence. I sometimes think that he would be strengthened if he knew that you and others capable of appreciating the greatness of his charge did feel his difficulties. What a charge, what a government, great and glorious. I do not think the old Roman Empire came near it in its greatness.

I sometimes fear (but what follows is strictly for yourself alone) that his fine heroic temper is rather worn by the constant jags and back thrusts it receives. In his last letter to me, dated 12 June, Simla, he says, "I am doing what I can to put things in order out here, but it is a very uphill work and many influences have to be managed and overcome. I often think of the last visit I paid you before leaving England, and of your conversation on that occasion. You will recollect how much I dwelt on the difficulties which met one on every side. These have been exemplified in a way I could scarcely understand or anticipate." He then alludes to the "good folks of England really believing that I had sanctioned an attack on the religion of the Hindus, because I desired to improve the health of the people in Calcutta." (Now this he overrates to himself. They did not "believe" it. But) I am sure it would do him good if he knew that *statesmen* appreciated the greatness of his administration and of its difficulties. What a pity heroes are but flesh and blood, as we are. You will see I ought scarcely to betray his confidence, even to you. But you know better than anyone else what he has to do.

Pray burn this note.

Source: From a letter to Sir John McNeill, Florence Nightingale Museum (LMA) H1/ST/NC1/64/155, copy ADD Mss 45768 ff188-89

Hampstead, N.W.
4 August 1864

*Private.* You have no idea how heartbreaking much of my work is. Sidney Herbert has been dead three years on the 2nd. And these three years have been nothing but a slow undermining of all he has done. Sir J. Lawrence writes discouraged—"difficulties," he says to me (but this is quite confidential), he "could scarcely understand or anticipate." This, I think, breaks my heart more than anything.

At the same time. I bear in mind how extraordinary are the chances I have had. To have met with three men like yourself, Sir John Lawrence and Sidney Herbert, while so many people, wiser and better than I, have gone through life without ever anyone listening to their plans.

I think Sir J. Lawrence is a really great administrator—do not you?

Source: From two letters to Douglas Galton, ADD Mss 45762 ff179 and 186 (both written from Hampstead, N.W.)

11 August 1864

Confidential. In the very last letter I had from him [Sir J. Lawrence] . . . he says: "I often think of the last visit I paid you before leaving England and of your conversation on that occasion. You will recollect how much I dwelt on the difficulties which met one on every side. These have been exemplified in a way I could scarcely understand or anticipate," etc. No one could have "anticipated" that Lord de Grey would not have lent one helping hand to the Indian sanitary reform.

You know that, if we had not insisted on that letter to the Horse Guards at the point of the sword—also on the victualling troops on board ship—and if *you* had not been at the War Office, *nothing* would have been done. You know that, if Lord [in another hand] de Grey would have said the words to Sir C. Wood, the India Office would never have tabled that stuff about not sending out the *Suggestions.*

22 August 1864

I am requested to inform you that Sir John Lawrence has ordered your Indian *Suggestions* to be reprinted and lithographed in India, and that you and the India Office will receive copies in England with the utmost possible despatch. It is suggested that it might be as well to hurry your 200 copies for the India Office, who will otherwise receive them first from India.

Source: From a letter to Sir John Lawrence, Florence Nightingale Museum, typed copy Add Mss 45777 ff49-53

26 September 1864

I always feel it a kind of presumption in me to write to you—and a kind of wonder at your permitting it. I always feel that you are the greatest figure in history, and yours the greatest work in history, in modern times. But that is my very reason. We have but one Sir John Lawrence. Your Bengal Sanitary Commission is doing its work, like men—like martyrs, in fact—and what a work it is! all we have in Europe is mere child's play to it. Health is the product of civilization, i.e., of real civilization. In Europe we have a kind of civilization to proceed upon. In India your work represents, not only diminished mortality as with us, but increase of energy, increase of power of the populations. I always feel as if God had said: mankind is to create mankind.[93] In this sense you are the greatest creator of mankind in modern history. Your Bengal commission must be the model for the other presidency sanitary commissions. . . .

It seems to me so base to be writing while you are doing. Oh that I could come out to Calcutta and organize at least the hospital accommodation for the poor wretches in the streets. There is nothing I should like so much. But it is nonsense to wish for what is an impossibility. I am sure you will be glad to hear that one of my lifelong wishes, viz., the nursing of workhouse infirmaries by proper nurses, is about to be fulfilled.

God bless you. I am,
yours devotedly
Florence Nightingale

P.S. I think with the greatest satisfaction upon your reunion with Lady Lawrence and (some of) your children. The Calcutta municipality does not seen[m] yet to have wakened up to a sense of its existence. It does not know that it exists: much less, what it exists for. Still, you are conquering India anew by civilization, taking possession of the empire for the first time by knowledge instead of by the sword.

F.N.

93 In her essay "In Memoriam" for Quetelet, Nightingale emphasized this idea of self-creation. See *Society and Politics* (5:55).

Source: From a letter to Douglas Galton, ADD Mss 45762 ff221-23

Hampstead

3 October 1864 [archivist's date 3 August 1864]

*Private.* Dr Sutherland wants to go to Bermuda with Captain [Edward] Belfield about this yellow fever. I offer no opinion for or against. I only offer this consideration: Sir J. Lawrence is so willing to do everything, the Colonial Office so unwilling to do anything, soon we may expect from India their answers to the *Suggestions* asking for fresh *Suggestions.* It seems a pity that, when we have a man who will do anything for us, and a man who may not last long, and a field like India to do for, to waste ourselves upon a petty place like Bermuda, when perhaps nothing will come of it, and where perhaps a man like Mr Roberts would do quite as well. But all I write this for is to say that, if Captain Belfield and Dr Sutherland do go, it had better be *as soon as possible.* For, after Sir John Lawrence's return to Calcutta (in November), I expect his applications to us will be incessant. And six weeks would be the very shortest time, I suppose, for a Bermuda trip. (Even now I hear by most mails from the Bengal Sanitary Commission.)

Source: From two letters to Frances Nightingale, the second incomplete, Wellcome (Claydon copy) Ms 9001/83 and 96

23 November 1864

Don't despise me for reading with tears of joy Sir J. Lawrence's (Lahore Durbar). *There* is reality. I am not given much to pomps but the "great viceroy" (the little Londonderry boy), the man "feared and loved throughout India," no lord but in whom the maharajahs, less flunkeys than we are, recognize one of God's lords, and come to do him honour as they would come to no Lord Canning, although it was prophesied by us flunkeys at home that the want of the "noble" would be a great drawback to plain John Lawrence.

[12 December 1864]

Sir C. Trevelyan is NOT out of danger and will not be while he remains at Calcutta. Much of India's salvation and Sir John Lawrence's depends upon Sir C. Trevelyan being able to remain in India, of which there is not a chance *after* this winter, and *during* this winter there will be constant danger of a relapse. And this foolish unthinking boy writes of his father in this way.

Source: From a letter to Sir John Lawrence, Florence Nightingale Museum, typed copy Add Mss 45777 ff58-61

26 December 1864

*Private.* Thank you a thousand times for your great kindness in writing to me—you, whose hands and head are fuller than those of anyone on earth. I rejoice to think that, by this time, Lady Lawrence and your daughters are with you, to take care of you. And I do not at all agree with you (nor, I am sure, do they) that it will be "a sad sacrifice to them." It is anything but a "sacrifice" to be with you. It must have been a great sacrifice to keep away.

There is only just time to write by this mail to ask you a question. And, if it is an impertinent one, you must lay the impertinence entirely on me. I believe Lord Stanley is at this moment asking the same question of Sir Charles Wood.

Would you not think it well that papers which involve sanitary principles of permanent importance (and which involve also expenditure of money)—such as, e.g., Colonel Crommelin's[94] paper on the construction of hospitals, dated Simla, 15 August 1864, his former paper on similar things as to barracks, many, perhaps all of the papers emanating from the most able and energetic Bengal Sanitary Commission, and still more, the papers of the less-skilled other presidency sanitary commissions—should be sent home officially through Sir Charles Wood, to the home ("Barrack and Hospital Improvement") commission? . . .

My reasons are as follows for this request: Everybody here who knows anything about the matter knows that what is to be done (in sanitary matters, as in many others) must be done in your time, that, but for you, but for your strong personal view of the importance of sanitary measures, the sanitary commissions would be—nowhere, that Mr Strachey, e.g., in spite of his great abilities, knowledge and energy in these things, depends upon you for his support. . . .

For such things as the bond of connection between the presidency and home sanitary commissions, it does not do to depend upon the life of one person, the good will of another, upon, etc. They should be done, if at all, regularly, officially.

No undue control (by us upon you) *could* be entailed by a regular, official sending home of all such papers as I have described, before being sanctioned, to the home sanitary commission for revisal. On the contrary, I believe, as so much of the control, in *money* matters, is vested in the *home* India government, we might materially assist you in obtaining authority for expenditure in these matters. Still more will this be the case, when present authorities and influence have changed hands.

94 Henry Blyth Crommelin, (1806-83), R.E., Bengal Medical Service.

# IMPLEMENTATION OF THE ROYAL COMMISSION'S RECOMMENDATIONS

The Indian royal commission's report, signed by the commission's members 19 May 1863 and by Lord Stanley, Lord de Grey and Sir Charles Wood in June, was issued 8 July. The first task toward its implementation was to set in motion the War Office and the India Office work in London while securing the co-operation of British officials in India. To that effect, lobbying and agitation had to be deployed and consistently sustained. Nightingale's conviction was firm, and she kept repeating that "a report is not self-executive" (see p 220 below).

Parliamentary interest in Indian affairs had to be stimulated. Lord Stanley sadly remarked on the "empty state of the House when Indian discussions had taken place within the last two years or eighteen months. . . . "[1] At times Lord Stanley himself had to be prodded and spurred to action; compared with Sidney Herbert, Nightingale felt, doubtless unjustly, that he was somewhat less committed to the cause she had espoused. At any rate she kept stressing to Lord Stanley that, if the needed practical reforms were not done, "the four years' labours of your royal commission are as bad as lost" (see p 265 below).

The report had first to be disseminated and brought to the knowledge of friends, media, politicians and British officials; it also had to be constantly recalled to the attention of Parliament. Nightingale was in almost daily communication with Sir Charles Wood, secretary of state for India, as well as Lord Stanley, who was now involved in setting up the home sanitary commission. Lord Stanley kept responsibility for the implementation of the report until he was named secretary of state for foreign affairs in 1866. Sir Harry Verney gave Nightingale a further privileged link to Parliament. She was also in close contact with Lord de Grey, secretary of state for war, and with the members of

1 Remark made 13 June 1861, cited by Donovan Williams, *The India Office 1858-1869* 25.

the Barrack and Hospital Improvement Commission, John Sutherland, Douglas Galton, Robert Rawlinson and William Farr, among others. She sought to convey the necessary information to the decision makers and to keep the pressure on the administrative machine.

In India she made full use of her friendship with John Lawrence. Important British officials and most of the successive viceroys paid her a personal visit on being appointed to their post, kept correspondence with her and "reported" to her. She would most diffidently offer to provide information, emphasizing that previous governors general had granted her that privilege. She also had precious contacts in India to see to the realization of sanitary changes in the army and in the population at large. She knew who was committed to the cause.

In London, the Barrack and Hospital Improvement Commission, appointed in October 1857, became a permanent body in 1862. It proposed in 1864 the important *Suggestions in Regard to Sanitary Works Required for Improving Indian Stations,* mainly written by Nightingale; it is reproduced below. The commission was renamed "Army Sanitary Commission" in 1865 and was expected to co-operate with the India Office Sanitary Committee formed in 1867—Nightingale consistently preferred the term "commission" to "committee" (see p 514 below). Obviously both commissions or committees were directly involved in the implementation of the reforms. Nightingale knew that, if the home commission were not put in place and established, "we are on the brink of ruin . . . , the royal commission had better not have been" (see p 227 below). She had no confidence that officials in India would act on key reforms without pressure from London. She quoted Douglas Galton to Lord Stanley that "they will spend the money so as to do harm, not good, if they are not advised by home experience" (see p 228 below). She pointed out further to Lord Stanley that the halving of the mortality rate at stations other than the ones in India had been achieved by sanitary works being carefully examined in London at the War Office and then returned. "This is what is wanted for India" (see p 229 below). Still better, all plans and proposals for sanitary improvements should be sent directly to the India Office itself for examination and then sent back to India.

In India each of the three presidencies (Bengal, Madras, Bombay) formed a sanitary commission as early as 1864 to relay the "suggestions" from London and apply them to the concrete situation. Already in 1863 the report of the royal commission considered the formation of the presidency commissions essential to the implementation of its resolutions. John Lawrence's Bengal Sanitary Commission, being located in the capital, Calcutta, served as a model for the other commissions and for the carrying out of changes in the field.

The letters and notes here cover all these (simultaneously occurring) aspects: dissemination, review and the early steps toward actual implementation. Interspersed are items dealing with administrative problems, such as payment of active members, and new issues brought to the fore by fresh material (e.g., the report of the Cholera Commission).

## Dissemination and Review of the Report

**Editor:** Ensuring good distribution of the report and favourable reviews as early as possible was a crucial intermediary step. The report was issued in three forms: (1) in two volumes, called here the two-folio volumes or Blue Book; volume 1 included Nightingale's *Observations* and an "abstract" of the stational reports prepared by her and Dr Sutherland, volume 2 the entire evidence from the Indian stations; (2) an octavo (8vo) book made of printer's sheets folded into eight leaves, abridged edition, without the *Observations* and the "abstract"; (3) a revised abridged edition issued by the War Office, prepared by Nightingale and including her *Observations* and a new "abstract of the evidence."

Nightingale was concerned that the persons who would determine the acceptance and implementation of the royal commission's recommendations receive the full report and not a mere summary of it (as was done in the presentation of the report to Parliament). She went to considerable lengths to promote this, asking people to send for the full report, sending out copies herself, sometimes with a covering letter, and making sure that certain people (e.g., Sir John McNeill) received advance copies of the report.

Since favourable reviews in the press would help encourage acceptance of the proposed measures, she made concerted efforts to get reviews in the most relevant journals by the most eminent people who could be counted on to say the right things. But when the reviews appeared, she was "greatly disappointed that not one single review article has seized our main point, viz., reform your stations first—it is not your climate, it is not even mainly your sites—it is your living like beasts, not civilized men, without water supply, without drainage, etc., heightened by climate and by sites, which kills you" (see pp 232-33 below).

Not everybody was pleased with the depiction of Indian conditions found in the report. Criticisms were expressed in India (especially by Dr Leith, but also Colonels Henry Norman and Henry Crommelin), at the India Office and in the British press. Replies were necessary and came in various forms, above all in the *Remarks* on Dr Leith's attacks, as is seen below. Much time and effort had to be devoted to defending the facts presented in the report, questioned by people at home (even by Sir Charles Wood) as well as in India. Throughout those debates Nightingale remained constant in her assessment of the beneficial impact of the royal commission; with confidence she could tell Lord Stanley that it had "hastened the political growth of India by half a century in self-government" (see p 375 below).

Much energy was also spent and time wasted to answer viceroy John Lawrence's request for directions as to the practical translation of the royal commission's recommendations to improve the Indian stations. Nightingale's patience was exhausted by the official negligence in responding to the viceroy's demands. The answer finally came in the form of the important *Suggestions* of 1864, written mainly by Nightingale with the important participation of Robert Rawlinson.

The letters and notes that follow give an idea of Nightingale's concerns, frustrations and actions mainly in the months following the publication of the report on 8 July 1863; they also show that the mechanism for new sanitary measures was being put into place.

Source: From a letter to Lord de Grey, Add Mss 43546 f28

21 March 1863

*Confidential.* I send you the first (unrevised) proof of this long delayed report. If you could just glance through it and return it to me, I should be much obliged. And I will send you a more respectable copy to keep for your "very own," as the children say as soon as the *vero ultimo* proof is out.

Source: From a letter to the duke of Newcastle, University of Nottingham NeC 10,938

23 May 1863

You will perhaps remember that, three or four years ago, under your authority, and with your assistance, I began (at the instance of Sir George Grey of New Zealand), an inquiry into colonial school and hospital mortality. It has been a very unsatisfactory one, from the incomplete nature of the materials. . . .

(Quite different has been another inquiry on which I have been engaged for the last four years, the "Indian Army Sanitary Commission," where the materials were so complete, the returns received so full, that the conclusions were clear and complete also. I would, if permitted, send you my paper on the Indian subject.)

Source: From two letters to Lord Stanley, Liverpool Record Office, Derby Collection 920/15/14 and 15

25 June 1863

*Private.* I have made some arrangements for having your India sanitary report reviewed by some papers and reviews (I wish you would write one for the *Westminster* or *Quarterly* yourself). But I must send early copies to the people who will take the trouble.

I have inquired of Mr Spottiswoode what state the printing is in. All the letter press is printed off, Vol. 2 is binding as fast as it can. So will Vol. 1, as soon as the plans come, hourly expected. Everything will be ready in a day or two.

Do you think you would be so good as to write a line to Messrs Eyre and Spottiswoode, directing them to send twelve early copies to me, and enclose this note to me to forward? It often makes all the difference (especially in the case of the *Times*) in the good feeling of the writers whether one sends them a copy early and personally, or not. And I am particularly requested in this case to be *early*.

8 July 1863

I see, in the copies of your India Army Sanitary Report, which I have just received, that Mr Baker signs himself "Secretary" (p LXXXIV). He never was secretary. Had he your authority to append his name as such? If not, the page should be cancelled.

Source: From a typed copy of a letter to Edwin Chadwick, Add Mss 45771 f28

8 July 1863

By dint of sending three times a day to the printers and almost every half hour to the lithographers, I have got a few copies of our India Army sanitary report, *before* it is issued. Can you do anything for us in the way of *publicizing* it? and if so, where shall I send a copy?

Source: From a letter to Harriet Martineau, Add Mss 45788 ff188-89

8 July 1863

We have lost five precious months of the session in getting it [the report] out, and I am now canvassing Lord de Grey and Sir C. Wood with all my might for the working commission. . . . But without a chairman, for Lord Stanley does nothing for us, and without a secretary, what can a poor invalid woman do?

Source: From a letter to Sir John McNeill, Florence Nightingale Museum (LMA) H1/ST/NC3/SU149, typed copy Add Mss 45768 ff180-81

9 July 1863

I am distributing a few copies of our Indian Army sanitary report to newspapers and ministers, before the general issue. And I cannot forbear sending you a copy. You will see that your advice about a working organization has not been neglected. And I am now busy in pressing it upon India Office and War Office. No one knows better than yourself that a report is not self-executive and when the report is ended, the work begins.

Our object is to obtain the immediate appointment of three commissions in India, one for each presidency; and a home working commission, to be attached to India Office or War Office, as they prefer, on the basis of the Barrack and Hospital Improvement Commission, and simply consultative, of course, consisting of Sir Proby Cautley, Sir Ranald Martin, Captain Galton, Dr Sutherland, Mr Rawlinson, C.E. It is to advise till the presidency commissions can walk alone.

Sir C. Trevelyan has provided £300,000 for us in his budget, which he thinks is as much as we can spend in the *first* year. But if more is wanted, he says it shall be forthcoming. I am sure if you can do anything for us in reviewing or pressing this report on the public, you will.

Source: From a copy of a letter to General Clark-Kennedy, Wellcome RAMC 801/9/18

9 July 1863

*Private.* I have a few copies of our Indian Army sanitary report, to distribute (before the general issue takes place) to newspapers and ministers and people of that kind. I should like to send a copy to you for *his* [Sidney Herbert's] sake, with whom I began this commission, and to forward whose views you did so much. Poor fellow, he would have liked to have seen this, his work, finished.

Where shall I send it to you? It is, I am sorry to say, two very bulky volumes. If you can do anything for us in the way of urging it on the public, either through reviews or by personal influence, I am sure you will.

It is needless for me to tell *you* that a report is not self-executive. And that, when the reporting is finished, the work begins. I am now busy in urging upon the India Office and the War Office the appointment of the three presidency commissions, recommended in the report, and of the *home* commission, also therein recommended, on the basis of the War Office Barrack and Hospital Commission, to advise until the presidency commissions can walk alone.

Source: From three letters to Lord Stanley, Liverpool Record Office, Derby Collection 920/15, 16 and 17

10 July 1863

*Private.* Perhaps I ought not to be sorry about Mr Baker's peccadillo, since it compels me to lay the whole case before you. I begin by apologizing to you and to myself for the time and strength it will take.

When you have all the facts of the case you will know best how to do justice. Mr Baker knows perfectly well he is *not* "secretary." Four years ago, when Lord Herbert first began this commission after you had issued it, he wished to have the same secretary who served him in the first Royal Army Sanitary Commission. But this man [Dr Thomas Graham Balfour], having just been made head of the Army Statistical Branch, was too busy. As the real work of the commission would fall upon Dr Sutherland, Lord Herbert finally decided that *he* should act as secretary *and be paid* as secretary, but *not* be called "secretary," because he was wanted as member of the commission; that he must have a clerk to issue the letters to call the meetings, to see the evidence through the press, etc., but *not* to correct the proofs, the whole of which, as well as the writing and sending out the printed questions, was to be done by Dr Sutherland and by myself. The *clerkship* was offered to Mr Baker, at Dr Sutherland's recommendation and accepted by him, on condition that he should be not clerk but called *assistant* secretary. (This he would not deny, if he were asked the question.)

I am exceedingly sorry that I cannot furnish you with written proof of all this. It was the fault of my dear chief not to require such, because he thought all men as honourable as himself. But he told me himself, about the beginning of 1861, that he had himself informed you of the whole of this and of the conditions under which Dr Sutherland was acting.

2. If I have ever called Mr Baker "secretary" to you in any of my letters, I must have been dreaming. But I cannot believe it. For at that very time I was warning Dr Sutherland that I had seen Mr Baker's signature as "secretary." (He would not believe it.) Mr Spottiswoode could show you letters of mine in which I call Mr Baker assistant secretary.

3. As for Mr Baker having "acted as secretary," the only things he has done as secretary have been calling the meetings and arranging the printing with the printers, so far as my cognizance goes, which, of course, relates only to the *domestic* part of the commission. You are probably cognizant of other things, relating to the *public* part of the commission, in which he has acted as such. The things in which he has NOT acted as secretary, but which *were all done by the secretary* of the first royal army sanitary commission are as follows:

Vol. II: The whole of these stational reports were not only corrected by Dr Sutherland and myself, but we began copying them ourselves with condensations from the original replies. Finding this took up too much time, a good deal of the copying was done by Vacher's clerks. But even the whole of *this* work was actually given out from my house to Vacher's. And I have the whole of the books at this moment in my house "to witness if I lie," as Lord Macaulay sings.[2] The only thing that Mr Baker did of which I am cognizant was *certifying* the work of Vacher's clerks. The whole of these (condensed) copies was afterwards compared with the originals, and verified by Dr Sutherland and by myself; the whole of the proofs were corrected by Dr Sutherland and by me. (And very tough and dreary work it was.)

The maps and plans were selected and corrected by Dr Sutherland and by me. And all that Mr Baker did was to hinder us with McCulloch. Nay, the very diagrams (Vol. I) he pretended to have corrected we found out the errors—he pretended to send our renewed corrections to Day's—and they were actually put up *un*corrected in the bound volumes which I have received. And I, *after* the volumes were bound, sent back the corrections, which were important, to Messrs Spottiswoode's to beg them to put them in (by hand) into those copies I have given away. I must beg you to remember that, had we intended to have a secretary to do our work, a very different kind of secretary would have been selected from Mr Baker. And that it was only on the express stipulation that the secretarial work was to be done by Dr Sutherland and by me, and that Mr Baker was only to act as clerk, that Lord Herbert arranged the commission thus.

You cannot pay *me*. You must therefore pay Dr Sutherland. And certainly it was not to spare Mr Baker's labour that I undertook all this.

Vol. I: The whole of the abstracts of stational reports, pp 371 to 528, were done by Dr Sutherland and me, written out in my hand (of which I have fortunately proof, as by some lucky oversight the manuscript have been preserved), the whole of them were proof-corrected and revised by us two. I have not these proofs and revises. For unfortunately Mr Baker said they were to be destroyed. But I conclude you will take this on my word.

The whole of the report was written by Drs Farr, Sutherland, a great deal of it in my hand. The whole of it was shaken together, revised

---

2 Thomas Babington Macaulay (1800-59), poet, historian and politician. Quotation from "Horatius," in *Lays of Ancient Rome* LXV.

and corrected by Dr Sutherland and myself. Of this I have the proofs. I have been accustomed to see these correctings done by the secretary. If Mr Baker were secretary he should have done this.

Dr Farr. The mortality and actuarial tables were prepared by him and it was understood for an actuarial fee. On Lord Herbert's statistical sub-commission, Dr Farr worked thus on a verbal understanding for an actuarial fee, and received it.

Mr Glaisher. The meteorological tables were done by him, on a similar understanding (and very bad they are).

In short, the only thing that I know of which Mr Baker has done is the Précis before the evidence, which he has chosen to put in in large letters, but which was so badly done that it had to be done again. The whole of the queries sent out to stations were written by Dr Sutherland and myself, in my hand, revised and corrected by us, sent out through the War Office, received back by us, lists of them kept by us. Surely this is secretary's work, if anything is.

I beg Lord Stanley's pardon for being so lengthy about a matter which will seem to him of little importance. I do not wish to be sentimental. But it has been a most painful thing to me to go over these four years' doings begun with my dear master, whose last words were, It is unfinished. I have done so for the sake of justice to Dr Sutherland and to Dr Farr, whose interests are, as it were, laid in my hand by him, from his habit of not requiring written proof—I being now almost the only witness left. I trust you will excuse me. The words he used were (his last), "Poor Florence, our work unfinished."

Please burn this last sheet.

11 July 1863

*Private.* I am deeply obliged to you for your very kind note. And indeed I have no fear but that justice will be done, now that you have taken the case in hand. I am afraid no "communication was made by Lord Herbert to the Treasury." It was not his habit. And I know, on a previous occasion, it was not done.

At the last, the years he had promised himself were shortened into hours. And claims much more important were left unrecorded and unfulfilled. Pray "make it public" that "to Dr Sutherland," and pray do *not* make it public that "to me" is due the work of this report. I do not wish that should be at all. Indeed I wish that that should *not* be. It is obvious what my only reason was in giving to you (privately) a full statement of the work.

I am greatly comforted by your assurance that the work of improving sanitary administration is going on. But I wish it interested *you* more. Perhaps I do not know you enough to say that it does not. But, if you could forward your own report by reviewing it and, what is much more important, by forcing it upon the War Office and the India Office, both personally and in the House of Commons, then indeed the progress thereof would be safe.

Lord Herbert did not think it beneath him to work for and upon an administration of which he was not minister. Perhaps no one (but I) knows how much work he did for General Peel in the W.O. And you know, when you yourself were at the I.O., he willingly and earnestly entered upon this India Sanitary Commission. And he would have worked just as hard at bringing out the (working) commissions afterwards, as he did, under Lord Panmure and General Peel successively, at organizing and heading the four sub-commissions, which really carried into effect the whole of the first royal sanitary commission's recommendations.

Excuse me: I did not mean to be suggesting to *you*. But I hear that Mr Cunningham[3] is going to take up your report in the House of Commons. Is that desirable? And every day lost in appointing these three presidency commissions and in arranging the home I.O. or W.O. commission recommended by the report is worth ten times its weight to India. Who will press these upon the India and War Offices?

I have heard that you disapproved of the decision of the W.O. against the amalgamation scheme of the two medical services. I think I could submit to you what might modify that opinion. But I should not like to intrude my "turbulencies" upon you unasked.

11 July 1863

*Confidential.* Sir John Lawrence writes to me, in confidence, "One word from Lord Stanley" will "move Sir Charles Wood to action" "as regards the commission at home." He says that Sir C. Wood "will not be backward in the matter." Lord de Grey is also using his weight on our side.

Sir John Lawrence thinks that it would be better to attach the home commission to the India Office (though I believe Sir P. Cautley would

3 Henry Stewart Cunningham (1832-1920), later Sir, India expert in Madras and Calcutta, member of the Famine Commission 1878-80; he was married to Harry Verney's sister and, on her death, was engaged to Emily Lawrence, daughter of Lord Lawrence.

rather graft it on the War Office commission). Either would do for us. In the former case, Sir Proby Cautley, Sir Ranald Martin, Captain Galton, Dr Sutherland and Mr Rawlinson, C.E. (of the Local Government Act Office) for the great drainage and water supply questions which are after all the most pressing in India, should be the members.

Would that this home commission could be arranged this month, before you all of you go out of London. For God knows what may happen in India if all these things are left unsettled!

"As regards the nomination" of the presidency commissions, Sir John Lawrence thinks "that they should be nominated by the local governments out there." I am too ignorant of India administration to know whether the best possible be the best feasible. But the question concerns nothing less than the creation of a Public Health Department for India, i.e., a department of government, with consultative commissions of health, each with a responsible administrative head. I hope this will not be left to the "local governments out there" to do, or not to do, or to do anyhow.

Please not in any way to quote Sir John Lawrence. He always seems to me like a great fish out of water, where he is, or like a great Roman dictator returned for Marylebone, to serve as an MP.

Source: From a letter to Sir Harry Verney, Wellcome (Claydon copy) Ms 9000/111

10 July 1863

I have been druv, druv, druv [driven], these last three days with bringing out the India Army sanitary report. Copies have now been sent to the newspapers and ministers. But it is not yet presented. I hear that the report is to be taken up in the House of Commons by Mr Conyngham[4] (or Mr Cunningham, which is it?) Is he a proper man for so great a subject? And if it is to be taken up, ought not some one of weight to do it and not a member whose influence is doubtful. Could you help to a solution of this difficulty? I am afraid that Mr Conyngham is going to give notice of a motion directly. . . .

I find it a very bad thing to have to do with highly honourable men because they always think everyone else as honourable as themselves

4 Probably William Coningham (b. 1815), Liberal MP for Brighton in 1863, "a general and independent supporter of Lord Palmerston," according to Dod's *Parliamentary Companion.* There were also, but less likely meant, George Henry Conyngham, later marquess, who sat in the House of Lords, and Lord Francis Nathaniel Conyngham, who sat in the House of Commons.

and leave no written agreements about anything, or depend upon others acting honourably. Here am I in a peck of troubles, because Lord Stanley will not carry out Sidney Herbert's verbal understandings as to the pay of the two members of the India sanitary commission who did all the work.

And Colonel Brown, whom you thought to move, writes a blackguard letter, the sense of which is "Miss N. is *not* dying and therefore she can move. But if she *is* dying, I take advantage of it to claim twenty-five guineas a week in August."

Source: From a letter to Robert Rawlinson, Boston University 1/2/33

13 July 1863

*Private.* I hasten to send you a copy of our India sanitary report. It is not yet presented. And the House of Commons will only have the 8vo edition.

If you can do anything to publicize it for us, I am sure you will. It is always necessary to use much pressure. Lord de Grey and Lord Stanley are arranging with Sir C. Wood the home commission, consisting of yourself, Dr Sutherland, Captain Galton, Sir P. Cautley, Sir R. Martin. I only hope and pray that it may be done this month before London disperses. As to the India administrative arrangements, we are putting what pressure we can upon authorities out there to have them carried out. The question is nothing less than the creation of a Public Health Department for India. The report proposes commissions of health, one for each presidency. Possibly a fourth will be necessary for the Punjab: a consultative commission, with a responsible administrative head, would appear to be the best. And the whole might possibly be raised into a department of government.

If you can do anything for us in the newspapers, urge these things. Every day's delay is a loss.

Source: From three letters to Lord Stanley, Liverpool Record Office, Derby Collection 920/15, 18 and 19

17 July 1863

I have just received the 8vo form of your India sanitary report and can scarcely recover from my surprise at seeing it. Is this all the fruit of four years' labour, all the result of the India commission, which is to be presented to Parliament? viz., the report and a précis of evidence which is simply ludicrous, as being so incomplete and incorrect, that it weakens the report, by not bearing it out. We speak with "connaissance de cause" [full knowledge of the facts], for we found it entirely useless as any guide to the evidence.

I understood from you that the abstract of stational returns (prepared with great care, in order to get into a short compass the whole of the valuable evidence of those stational returns, upon which the report is based *quite as much* as upon the oral evidence, and of which not a vestige of a trace appears) I understood from you that my own paper [*Observations*] prepared with the same view, and as short as anything could possibly be made were to be presented to Parliament with the report. Certainly it has not been worth our four years to give to the House of Commons this.

yours faithfully

Florence Nightingale

I see the fatal error in the first diagram, by which you are made to say that the mortality in Bengal is 6.7 instead of 67 per 1000, is repeated everywhere.

22 July 1863

*Most Private.* I understand from Lord de Grey that Sir C. Wood has consented to the home commission in the following form. He proposes to add two India members on to the War Office Barrack and Hospital Commission (existing). If this is your doing, as I have no doubt, receive the most fervent thanks of all your fellow workers in the India cause. . . .

It is the greatest work that a secretary of state could do for India. Equal in importance to the decision itself are the men that may be appointed on the commission. To carry out the recommendations of the first army sanitary commission, it was wisely determined to have a large sprinkling of the men who had studied the subject on the royal commission upon the four sub-commissions. Sir P. Cautley and Sir R. Martin answer to this description, being the only India men upon the royal commission, and having had the unspeakable advantage of following the whole inquiry from first to last. If new men are put on, they will have all to learn. Mr Rawlinson, as our first water and drainage engineer, is indispensable, as water supply and drainage are of paramount importance in India.

22 July 1863

I think we are on the brink of ruin if this home commission does not pass. If India is to be left to work out its own sanitary salvation, the royal commission had better not have been. Nothing is of any importance compared with the (home) commission. I heard Captain Galton, the assistant under secretary of state at the War Office, say, "they will spend the money so as to do harm, not good, if they are not advised by home experience." I have tried to draw up shortly the reasons, which I venture to enclose. Compared with this, the question of the presentation or non-presentation of parts of the report sinks into nothing. Still I cannot but repeat my conviction that the curious blunder by which Sir C. Wood presented the 8vo, while he thought he was presenting the whole, is very fatal to us, for this reason: not one single soul has as yet grasped our main point, viz., reform your stations first and then look to the hills. Your stations as to drainage, water supply, etc. are the main cause of your death rate, not your climate.

Had we known that the report was all that was to be presented, we should certainly have brought out this point more strongly, so that every ass might see it. . . .

The objection made to the home commission is that at present there is no direct reference of plans from India to England. Such a reference as regards sanitary works is what is required. It would work as follows: suppose that the Madras presidency commission of health were to draw up, at the request of the Madras government, a plan for the sanitary improvement of Secunderabad or of Madras itself. They would do this without any practical experience of how such cases had been dealt with at home. If such a plan were carried out, it would be mere matter of choice whether the whole did not prove a failure. The only way to prevent this as far as practicable would be to refer the plan home, without loss of time, to the India government here. It would then come before its special commission; the details of the plan would be minutely canvassed by men of home experience; and, after the best practicable decision had been arrived at, the plan would be sent back with all needful information as to matters of detail in water supply, drainage, latrines, construction and improvement of buildings, etc. And then, after the Madras commission had profited as much as possible by the criticisms and information, the plan would be put forwards for sanction in the usual way.

As to the proposition to send out ready formed commissions of practical men to deal with the India question, it is quite certain that for some time the men will not be forthcoming. There are as yet very few men practically conversant with this class of works. And all we have are occupied on duties here. To send out inferior men would be to misspend money. The medical school at Netley is now training young men in sanitary knowledge, but it will be some years before any number will be available. Cadets of engineers for Indian service will, it is hoped, before long be trained in this branch of knowledge. But as yet nothing has been done.

As regards India, your latest barrack (at Fort William) is one of your worst. And Calcutta is being now drained, apparently without a water supply. There is then no reasonable hope of progress, unless some arrangement be made, whereby you *here in the India Office* may by good advice prevent such mistakes. All plans or proposals for sanitary improvements should be sent voluntarily from India, direct and without circumlocution to the India Office here. There need be no jealousy. For all wish to help India. And there need be no interference with freedom of action. The interests, though by no means the sole interests at stake, are those of our queen's regiments.

And we cannot understand why, after the War Office has had a commission of practical men at work to improve our home and Mediterranean and colonial barracks and hospitals, with a result of half the former death rate at home (the latter stations have not been tried long enough) the troops which have had such care bestowed on them here should go to India and be there decimated and deteriorated, because there is no authority sufficiently informed to deal with these health questions. The India Office plan might be similar to the War Office plan. At present all sanitary works are sent from every station, from the West Indies to China, to the War Office.

The plans are carefully examined and corrected by the special commission and then returned to the station. This is what is wanted for India. And there is no reason why it should not work as well. If not in strict accordance with existing system, surely the system should bend to the greater necessity, not the necessity to the system. . . .

P.S. Of course all the sanitary work must be done in India. It cannot be done in England. All we can do or propose to do is to give to the commissions in India the benefit of English experience, and to prevent the mishaps and failures quite certain to ensue if the Indian commissions are left to gain their own experience. The report of the royal commission only states the most general principles. But the question really lies in the application of these principles to suit specific cases.

Source: From a letter to Harriet Martineau, ADD Mss 45788 ff190-91

22 July 1863

I am so anxious about the results of the Indian sanitary report. No one but I who have been trying for seven years "come" August to work a War Office without being secretary of state can tell how much cause for anxiety there is. Had Sidney Herbert been alive the thing would have been done directly. He never wanted anything but a reason to go himself straight to any minister and get it done. Lord Stanley wants a great deal besides a reason. He told me that he would not offer his services—but he would like to be asked. So I got Lord de Grey to ask Sir C. Wood to ask him. And on Monday there was a meeting of Sir C. Wood, Lord Stanley and Dr Sutherland at the India Office. But there is a most unfortunate hitch about the appointment of the home commission on the ground that there is no direct reference of plans from India to England, at present. Now such a reference is just what we want, as regards sanitary works. and without it the royal commission had better never have been.

Source: From a letter to Mary Jones,[5] Florence Nightingale Museum (LMA) H1/ST/NC1/63/7

26 July 1863

Since Wednesday fortnight when the India sanitary report's first copy saw the light, I have had every moment taken up with pressing it and distributing it, for the sake of getting our home and presidency commissions appointed before the session is over.

I have had the most discouraging contradictions and disappointments. Such as one must expect, working as I do, without a chairman and without a secretary, sometimes I think I must be mad to attempt such a work as this alone from my bed. But they say I am not.

After the first week in August this great press will be over. And I hope we shall then see each other very often at Hampstead and talk over many things.

**Editor:** In July 1863 Nightingale sent a letter with a copy of her *Observations* to Sir George Grey, who had prompted her study of mortality in the colonial hospitals and schools (*Public Health Care* 6:196-97). Sir George Grey (1812-98) was made governor of New Zealand for a second term in 1861, elected to the New Zealand Parliament in 1875 and later prime minister. Nightingale had met him in 1859, when he expressed concerns about losses in the Maori population in New Zealand. Her covering letter called the materials collected "as full as they were meagre in the colonial case." She noted that her *Observations* enabled one "to judge of the extent to which British soldiers and British people

---

5 Mary Jones (1812-87), Anglican sister and superintendent of nurses at King's College Hospital. See the biographical sketch in *Theology* (3:649-50).

ignore the laws of nature in warm climates, and then blame everything and everybody but themselves for the result."[6]

Source: From a letter to Harriet Martineau, ADD Mss 45788 ff194-97

29 July 1863

*Private.* I think it is of the highest importance that you should write to Lady Elgin. But you know the points quite as well as I do. I do not know either her or Lord Elgin at all. To mention a few heads: The report has made a great impression and all England is expecting to see it carried out. The first thing to do is to select good men for the presidency commissions *and to make them cordially and voluntarily co-operate with the home commission.* That energetic steps should at once be taken for draining, paving, cleansing and supplying with water the seats of government, *and well-digested schemes of improvement should be sent home for consideration on matters of detail not yet known in India.* (All here are desirous of co-operating in the good work of civilizing India and saving the army.)

I have only two points, not for Lady Elgin but for you. (1) Not one single soul has really laid hold of our main, our essential point, viz., Reform your stations first. Your climate is not essentially in fault. Your situations are not necessarily or always in fault. It is your own habits of beasts and not of civilized men which are primarily the cause, only heightened by site and climate. I am sure I hope to live to see the seat of government removed from Calcutta. But for all that, they have contrived to make some of the healthiest positions in India nearly as unhealthy as Calcutta. Calcutta, if it were situated in the healthiest position in Europe, would be unhealthy with its want of paving, want of water supply and of other things too shocking to mention.

(2) We are going on extremely well at home. Sir J. Lawrence, Lord de Grey and even cool Lord Stanley have worked well at Sir C. Wood for us. The home commission is to be a conjoint commission with the present War Office barrack and hospital ditto. I have been bid to write instructions for it and also for the presidency commissions, but I don't know how Lord de Grey thinks these can be enforced or accepted. So I hope it [the joint commission] will be appointed immediately. I am sorry to say they have conceded the point, that the initiative is to remain with the presidency commissions. I had rather we had kept it ourselves, because they are quite sure to send home stupid schemes.

6 Letter 28 July 1863, Auckland Public Library GL N8 (4).

There will really be more interference with their action than if we had had the initiative. But I can't help it.

I find that the blocks (woodcuts) are mine, but that members of the commission are negotiating with a publisher to reprint my paper with the woodcuts of course at his own expense. I do not know the result. I did not know this when I wrote 1000 thanks for the photograph. It makes me feel almost there.

Source: From a copy of a letter to Sir James Clark, Wellcome RAMC 1139/S4/22, typed copy Add Mss 45772 ff168-69

29 July 1863

I sent today, according to your desire (at least I understood it so) one two-folio copy of our report for the king of the Belgians, two 8vo copies for yourself and the queen. I also enclose a letter for the queen which please send or burn as you like.

Mind, I am not responsible for the 8vo copy, which I never give, unless I am asked for it. There has been a perfect outcry (and, as I think, a legitimate one) that the two-folio book is not to be sold, not to be had, not to be published, not to be presented to Parliament, and that the 8vo makes references *passim* to a work which is not to be had. Officers, of all men those one most wants to interest, will not look at the 8vo copy, and say the government is keeping something back. And officials say, we don't want opinions (in the report), we want the facts (in the Blue Book).

Might I not at least send the queen my own paper (which you have and which is only printed in the two-folio book, fast becoming a very rare work)? She might look at that, because it has pictures. And she certainly will not look at the report. I have sent some copies of my paper separately, like the one I gave you. Ought I to bind the 8vo for the queen? If so, I can send you a bound copy almost immediately. And one for your copies will do for Prince Louis of Hesse.[7] You mentioned that he might like one. Perhaps I ought to bind the two folios for the king of the Belgians. If so, please tell me.

We are getting on very well in having our home (working) commission appointed. Sir C. Wood is much more amenable. But I am greatly disappointed that not one single review article has seized our main point, viz., reform your stations first—it is not your climate, it is not

7 Frederick William Louis, grand duke of Hesse-Darmstadt (1837-92), married to the daughter of Queen Victoria, Princess Alice (1844-1900).

even mainly your sites—it is your living like beasts, not civilized men, without water supply, without drainage, etc., heightened by climate and by sites, which kills you.

Source: From a letter to Dr Robert Christison,[8] Wellcome Ms 5482/54

Hampstead, N.W.
29 July 1863

I confess I had some faint hope that you might write one review yourself. But I scarcely expected it. I knew you had no time. If you will ask the editor of the *Edinburgh Medical and Surgical Journal* to give us a good review of the India sanitary report, we shall be very much obliged. And I will, as soon as you have been so good as to ascertain that point, send the two-folio copy, which is not published, I am sorry to say, and not to be sold, to my great disappointment, for officers (whom of all men one most wants to interest) and people of all descriptions are asking for it and even complaining that the government is keeping something back from the press and the public. It will soon be a very rare book.

It was a great relief to me to hear *no* bad news of Sir John McNeill.

Source: From a letter to Douglas Galton, ADD Mss 45761 ff55-57

Hampstead, N.W.
1 August 1863

*Private.* I am rather in tribulation about the India Office, which I think is going against us. But, if Lord de Grey is for us, we shall be all right at last.

Lord Stanley has had an extremely foolish letter from Colonel Baker, of the India Office, attacking our statistics. This, from an extremely clever man and a very good man of business, is provoking. It is true we had just the same kind of attacks after the first royal sanitary commission and weathered them all, and did what we wanted. But then Lord Stanley is not Sidney Herbert, dead two years tomorrow—two years!!

Colonel Baker will be our enemy. And when we have proved him wrong, still more our enemy. And he primes Sir C. Wood.

They say that the death rate in the report is exaggerated (it is in fact *under*stated). The *Times* has reproduced this blunder. And Parlia-

8 Robert Christison (1797-1882), later Sir, professor of medicine, Edinburgh University.

ment being up, it is most unfortunate. For it cannot be contradicted by Lord Stanley. And so the error continues in circulation.

Their argument is that the war years produced the high death rate (*not* from wounds) and that these ought to be left out in the averages, that peace and not sanitary measures are the remedy. As well might they say when the British Army was destroyed before Sevastopol, *not* from wounds but from want of every necessary of civilized life, that withdrawing the troops from before Sevastopol and not supplying them with the necessaries of life, was the remedy.

It is astonishing how careless and superficial the views of even very clever men are on this subject. Colonel Baker's attack is, as Lord Stanley says, "extremely courteous" and therefore the more dangerous, say I.

Source: Letter to Professor Christison, National Library of Scotland Ms 10335 ff161-64

Hampstead
3 August 1863

My dear Sir

I send you by post today a copy of the two-folio Blue Book of the India Army sanitary report. Will you allow me to make two remarks?

1. The India Office is attacking our statistics, as being exaggerated, whereas they are in fact *under*stated, i.e., the death rate is understated, because it does not bring into account the invaliding from the army for disease, including the men who died on their passage home. (b) The India Office says the war years which yield the highest death rates *not* from wounds (ought not to be taken into the averages), and that therefore peace and not sanitary measures is the remedy.

As well might it say that, because the army nearly perished before Sebastopol, *not* from wounds but from the want of every appliance of civilized life, therefore peace and not the supply of the appliances of civilized life, should have been the remedy. Please tell Sir John McNeill this. It is astonishing how easily the India Office is satisfied of the truth of anything it is thought desirable to assert.

2. Not one single soul has laid hold of our chief, our main, point, viz., reform your stations first—the state of your stations is such as to account for any mortality, even in the finest climate of Europe, and the finest climate of Europe could never make your stations healthy in their present state, viz., that of dwellings and of beasts, not of civilized men. What must they be then under a tropical sun?

3. Please let the reviewers press the sanitary organization recommended, viz., the presidency commissions, *and the home commission* to

set them going with some experience. The question is nothing less than to create a public health department for India.

Many thanks for interesting yourself about the review. I wish you could have looked it over with Sir John McNeill. Believe me,

ever yours very faithfully
Florence Nightingale

Source: From a letter to Harriet Martineau, Add Mss 45788 ff202-07

Hampstead, N.W.
4 August 1863

1. About the two-folio volumes: There were 1000 copies printed (which number we obtained with difficulty). Of these were sent 350 to India, 100 to House of Commons, fifty to House of Lords (for any members of either house who would *ask* for them. And I write to as many of my friends as I can, of either House *to ask for them*). 100 more copies are to be sent to the Houses of Parliament, *if* they are asked for.

Another *attempt* made to have them sent for sale to the Parliamentary Depots has been suppressed, with this concession, "orders have been given at the sale offices of Parliamentary papers to refer anyone who wants a copy to (the self-styled secretary) Mr Baker!!" (The notes of admiration are not mine.)

The remaining copies, not distributed, are in the possession of the I.O., who will therefore, I suppose, refer the applicants to Mr Baker. . . .

The government actually made a profit by selling the first army sanitary report. And it is said that they would make a much larger one upon this, because civilians go so much to India now that scarcely a family in England but has some connection either in India or in the army. (It is therefore certain, it is said, that their economical excuse is humbug.)

Some copies are said to have been sent to W.O. and Horse Guards. But these have been not received. And thirty-five to permanent libraries.

2. The 8vo copy contains the report, the actuarial tables at the end of report in folio Vol. I and the Précis of Evidence (following these) in folio Vol. I. This Précis, drawn up by (the self-styled secretary) Mr Baker, is simply ludicrous from its imperfection and incompleteness. If people read it, it weakens the report by not bearing it out. If they don't, why take up so many pages with printing it?

The 8vo contains of course all the marginal references to the report. And what people (justly) say is, can a report be trustworthy based upon documents (which we have inquired about and) which are not to be had? But the public must only look at the Précis of one of the documents, viz., the oral evidence (said Précis said to be very imperfect), all the rest is ignored. Vast labour, vast expense, four years' time, have been spent on collecting the stational returns (replies to questions), and this the public is to hear nothing of. Vol. II is invaluable (these are the stational reports in extenso) to commanding and other officers. The Abstract of these in Vol. I, prepared by me and Dr Sutherland with the utmost brevity (and which took me six months' work), *on the express understanding* that *that*, as well as my "Observations," should be presented to Parliament and included on the 8vo (this understanding was not asked for but offered) is necessary for the public.

The attacks of the I.O. upon us are vexatious. For example, the death rate is *under*stated, because it takes no account of the men invalided from the army for disease nor of those who died on the passage home (no inconsiderable number). Yet we are said to have exaggerated. So with everything.

3. I have sent for Macmillan. I hear that your articles in *Daily News* have produced a great impression, as also that for Lord de Grey's appointment at Easter did. I feel I have never thanked you for these as I ought. I have a great deal more to say, but must put it off. . . .

It is amazing how easily Sir C. Wood is satisfied of the truth of anything it is held desirable to assert. The answers to Colonel Baker's statements through Lord Stanley do not reach the public (the only way of reaching ministers), you see. But you have reached the public.

I must say for poor Sidney Herbert never, never would he have burked evidence, as Sir C. Wood tries to do. Lord de Grey is honest. He has written me a satisfactory letter in answer to my appeal. He will do his best. But Sir C. Wood's imputation was public. And our answer is not public (my appeal to Lord de G. was of course *qua* the home commission).

Source: From four letters to Douglas Galton, Add Mss 45761 ff58-61, 62-63, 63-66 and 67-68 (all written from Hampstead, N.W.)

4 August 1863

*Private.* We are quite sure of ultimate success, if Lord de Grey is with us. But nonetheless is the India Office trying to destroy our statistics. Colonel Baker's points may all be proved not only no points at all, but absolutely to tell on our side. *But then* our answer does not receive circulation. Sir C. Wood stated in the House (and the *Times* reproduced it in a leading article) that our death rate was exaggerated. Now e.g., it is *under*stated, because it does not bring into account the men invalided from the army for disease, nor those who die on the passage home (no inconsiderable number). For example, Colonel Baker's point about the war years is no point at all because the death rate in barracks in the peace provinces was as high in those years as in the campaigning troops. For example, Colonel Baker appears entirely to have forgotten, since he was secretary, the real nature of the reductions in the army in India. For he gives the death rate of Her Majesty's troops alone, where certainly the reductions of all the weakly men, *when* reductions for peace took place, reduced *temporarily and sometimes* the death rate. But the mortality of the E.I.C.'s [East India Company's] troops, where no such reductions took place, continued steadily rising during the last years. I could not give any more e.g.s without giving the whole of Colonel Baker's letter, and the answer to it, and the whole of Sir C. Wood's speech and what ought to have been the answer to it.

The suppression of the circulation of the two-folio volumes has been of great disservice to us. A last effort has been made to have it sold at the Parliamentary depots *and has failed.* The answer positively was that only this could be granted, viz., "orders have been given at the sale offices of Parliamentary papers to refer anyone who wants a copy to (the self-styled secretary) Mr Baker!!" . . .

*Tear off.* I am not sorry I wrote to you, nor to see Lord de Grey's letter, which is burnt. The India Office ARE trying to burke our evidence.

If you like to show the other pages of this note to Lord de Grey, pray do. Pray all your MP friends (as I have done) to order from Mr Varden, librarian of the House of Commons, copies *for themselves* of the *two-folio* volumes. He has a certain number to send *only* to those members who ask for it.

F.N.

5 August 1863

If you put any of this in the *Times*, only put the parts between the red brackets. It might be introduced by saying that the writer had had no opportunity of seeing the India Army sanitary report, but that he fully bears out, to say the least of it, what they have stated about barrack construction. It is a capital letter.

This fellow would make a capital officer of health. He has it in him; if he could but contain himself and not abuse everybody. This letter is too overflowing. They had much better, for their own peace, have made him a pathologist, and let him overflow into dead bodies, than a regiment surgeon. He will give them some [breaks off]

7 August 1863

As to the enclosed proposition, I can only say that it would do no harm to circulate the 8vo among the officers. It would not do the least good. The report is a report (*per se*) like any other report. And the numerous reviews which have appeared upon it, *especially* the medical ones, are only another proof that no understanding, especially *not* the medical understanding, is sufficiently informed to take the main, the practical, the essential points out of it.

As for the précis, at the end, it is simply ludicrous. So inaccurate and incomplete is it that it weakens the report, by not bearing it out, if people read it. And if they don't, what is the good of wasting all those pages? Therefore I think it is simply money thrown away distributing *the 8vo* among "commanding medical and engineer officers."

But you have here a good opportunity of circulating the really practical and popular parts. Sidney Herbert would have done it directly. Make up one good 8vo volume, with the report, a *good* abstract of evidence, *which we will do for you* if you like it, the abstracts of stational returns, already done and with the utmost brevity, and my papers.[9]

This would make a really good useful India manual. And surplus copies would sell. Of this we have undoubted evidence. We would see it through the press for you. We would also put in a few useful scraps, which are scattered about among the addenda of the first volume and the stational returns of the second volume (folio). I would get from Mr Spottiswoode what the cost would be. And if there is any demur to it, I would pay it.

I paid £700 in the same way for the circulation of parts of the *first* army sanitary report. This will cost nothing like that. And done, in some way or other, I am determined it shall be. Only give the word. For it must be issued *by the War Office* with a circular letter from you, *ordering* them to read it. Your officers can neither read *nor understand,* unless *you order* them to do it. I think I told you that people (and officers too) have expressed the most unbounded disgust at finding that they *could not buy* the two-folio volumes.

13 August 1863

We send you the enclosed notes on the proposed India scheme. They raise questions rather than answer them. For it is better that the whole question should be thoroughly understood rather than incur any risk of throwing away advantages which could not be recovered.

---

9 This seems to be the third form in which the report was published.

If the new scheme be properly guarded it can be made the basis of immense good to India. For besides providing first-class medical attendance, it will enable the home commission, *when appointed*, to assist effectually in providing the India government with the new class of medical *officers of health* necessary for giving effect to many important recommendations of the royal commission.

After you have had time to go over these notes, will you return them again with any observations or additional information upon the points raised? It would be very desirable to have the opportunity of reconsidering them, after you at the War Office have done so. . . .

Pray, am I to have my Presbyterian chaplain, or not? (2) And pray, what about the printing (India Army Sanitary Report)? Am I to ask Mr Spottiswoode for an estimate or not? Don't let us be another four years about it. As for Sir C. Wood, he *wrote* that he had presented the 8vo *by mistake.* He ought to be very much obliged to *us* for remedying *his* "mistake," *if we do.*

Source: From a letter to William Farr, Wellcome Ms 5474/61, typed copy Add Mss 43399 ff131-32

Hampstead, N.W.
7 August 1863

One thing he [Engel] says, is perfectly certain, viz., that all this vexatious opposition [around the Berlin Congress] has the effect of advertising the thing much more than our own utmost efforts could do. So it will be with the attacks upon our India report at Newcastle and elsewhere. But why are you not there to answer them? There will be no one else to do so.

Source: From a letter to Sir Charles Trevelyan, Newcastle University Library 35/26

9 August 1863

Of course we are undergoing the invariable persecution which is a simple conformity with the traditions of a government office, viz., that the lamentable exposures made in our Blue Book should be denounced as exaggerated and extravagant by the India Office. Now our death rate is *under*stated, because it does not take into account the men invalided from the army for disease, nor those who died on the passage home (no inconsiderable addition). What is worse, the India Office says that, because the mortality is highest in the war years, *not* from wounds, therefore peace, and not sanitary measures, is the remedy. As well might they say that, because the army nearly perished before Sevastopol, *not* from wounds but from want of all the supplies of civilized life, therefore peace, not supplying the wants of civilized life, was the remedy. But this is not all. Even in those war years, the death rate was quite as high among the troops in barracks in the peace districts as among the campaigning troops. The temporary and occasional reductions in the death rate, for a year or two afterwards, were brought about by getting rid of the weakly men, in reducing the numbers for peace establishments. This in H.M.'s troops. In the E.I.C. [East India Company] troops, where no such reductions were made, the death rate continued steadily rising every year during the last years.

Source: Letter, Boston University 1/2/34

Hampstead, N.W.
15 August 1863

Dear Lord Shaftesbury[10]

Always remembering that to you first we owe the giving of sanitary hope to our poor army, I should have ventured to solicit your acceptance of a copy of the complete report and evidence of our "India Army Sanitary Commission." It was however understood by us that it was to be *of course* presented to Parliament. "By mistake" Sir C. Wood presented (so he writes) a paltry 8vo containing only the report and a précis of evidence simply ludicrous from its incompleteness. "By mistake" the type of the *two-folio Blue Books* is broken up. "By mistake" it is not to be sold at the Parliamentary depots. "By mistake" it is not to be published—not to be had—not to be distributed to Parliament.

A small number, however (fifty only to the House of Lords and 100 to the House of Commons), have been sent to Parliament, to be given to those members only who *apply* for them. Would you apply for the *two-folio Blue Books* for a copy for yourself?

We want immediate pressure made to obtain the working commissions, three in India, one for each presidency, and one at home, attached to the India and War Offices (to advise), which have been recommended in the report. I should be proud indeed to be called upon at any time for information by you.

your faithful servant
Florence Nightingale

---

10 Antony Ashley Cooper Ashley, Lord Shaftesbury (1801-85), urged the appointment of a sanitary commission for the Scutari hospitals, supported Nightingale in her India work.

Source: Letter, Columbia University, Presbyterian Hospital School of Nursing C67

Hampstead, N.W.
15 August 1863

Dear Lady Monteagle[11]

Knowing how often and how kindly you have interested yourself for me and mine, I venture to send you a paper of mine, printed in our India Army sanitary report, which is out at last. Would you ask Lord Monteagle to order for himself (from the clerk of the House of Lords) a copy of the *two-folio Blue Books* of the said *India Army Sanitary Commission*?

By mistake" Sir C. Wood (so he writes) presented to the House of Commons, not this which is the complete report and evidence, but a paltry 8vo containing nothing but the report and a précis of evidence, "simply ludicrous from its incompleteness. "By mistake" the type of the complete work has been broken up. "By mistake" it is not to be sold at the Parliamentary depots. We have obtained that 150 of the two-folio Blue Books (100 to the House of Commons, fifty to the House of Lords) should be sent to the Houses of Parliament. But they are to be given to those members only who apply for them. We have also obtained, and with great difficulty, that orders be given at the sale offices of Parliamentary papers to refer anyone who wants a copy to a Mr [Thomas] Baker (Burial Acts Office, 4 Old Palace Yard, S.W.). It is of course of the greatest importance to us that the few copies, of what is already a very rare book, should be in the hands of good men for future reference.

Even before the session was up, Sir C. Wood attacked our statistics in the House of Commons. Now our death rate is actually *under*stated. What we venture to hope is that Lord Monteagle will give us his support, if he thinks fit, in pressing upon government the immediate carrying out of the recommendations of the royal commission, especially and principally the appointment of the three commissions in India, one for each presidency, and of the home advising commission, attached to the India and War Offices, to bring our home experience of sanitary works to help the presidency commissions. Any MPs or others, whom you could induce to get the complete report, (in the respective ways indicated,) would strengthen our cause. Believe me, dear Lady Monteagle,

ever yours gratefully
F. Nightingale

11 Lady Ellen Mary Monteagle, née Frere (d. 1869), member of the board of the Harley Street establishment.

Source: From a letter to Mrs Gaskell,[12] Manchester University, John Rylands Library Eng Ms 731

17 August 1863

I have been entirely absorbed, since the beginning of the year, in bringing out the report of our commission on the state of our army in India and in acting upon it. I mean to do myself the honour of sending you a reprint of one of my papers on the subject.

"By mistake" Sir C. Wood (so he *writes*) has not presented our *whole* report and its documents to the Houses of Parliament. "By mistake" the type has been broken up. Should the subject excite the least interest in you, I should be "proud" to furnish you with all the information possible.

Source: From a letter to Lord Stanley, Liverpool Record Office, Derby Collection 920/15/20

Hampstead, N.W.
20 August 1863

I had promised myself never again to mention a matter to you, about which I had already given you such lengthened explanations, as fully to lay the case before you. But I understand that Mr Baker has obtained £1000 from the India Office for his services. And also that Dr Sutherland has been offered £1000 (one thousand pounds) and Dr Farr £600 (six hundred).

What Mr Baker's services can have been to warrant the giving such a sum as a thousand pounds to a clerk in the Home Office, at I believe £250 a year, I am totally at a loss to imagine. Yet I know the circumstances of the case from beginning to end.

Mr Baker is perfectly aware that he was engaged by Dr Sutherland four years ago, with Lord Herbert's sanction, to do clerk's work at clerk's pay; and because he objected to clerk's name, he was allowed to style himself "secretarial *assistant*." He was to keep the minutes, attend the meetings and pass through the press the corrections, made by others, of the printed matter. Whatever he has done more than this, has been on his own authority to others' great inconvenience, and has all had to be undone by those others as far as it could be undone. The précis of evidence is simply ludicrous from its incompleteness and inaccuracy (as I know to my cost).

12 Elizabeth Cleghorn Gaskell, née Stevenson (1810-65), author, correspondent, visitor and family friend.

The whole of the real secretarial work was done at my house. The very work to Vacher's clerks was given out at my house. And the whole of it compared with the originals and corrected in my house. The whole of the corrections in the two-folio volumes were done in my house, excepting those in the evidence, which were done by the witnesses themselves.

I was perfectly well aware that the bungling literal corrections (in names), put in so clumsily that they were not even uniform in any two pages—producing inextricable confusion—were put in *afterwards* and without our knowledge, simply in order that Mr Baker might say that *he* had "corrected" the work.

Now for Dr Sutherland's work. It has been constant and daily for four years, with the exception of two months. The very least they could have offered him would have been £1.1 a day (or assistant surgeon's pay) for four years. And this merely as an acknowledgment. The whole work of secretary, *besides* the whole *creation* of the sanitary work, has been done by him. It is very easy afterwards to say of a creation what was said of Columbus's egg.[13]

Dr Farr's work was definite, though I am not seeking to undervalue it by any means. Putting it at £600, as it has been put, Mr Baker's work would be *over*paid at £250, and Dr Sutherland's *under*paid at £1500. But I am unwilling to make this a mere matter of £ s.d.; the whole case is so flagrant that I cannot but hope some inquiry will be made.

It is not that my peace is affected by Mr Baker being enabled to keep a pony carriage, any more than it was by Sir John Hall being allowed extra retiring pay, because he destroyed the hospitals in the Crimea. But it is that I cannot but feel it a matter of public duty to try once more to represent the case to you. Believe me, it cannot be more disagreeable to you than it is to me. I would fain write about the consequences to India, not those to Mr Baker. It has taken the very heart out of me. I hope I have not said any ungentle word, but I must be quite firm in saying that I have never met with a parallel case in educated life.

If the India Office is so liberal as to give such a sum to Mr Baker for such work, then all I can say is that never was pay so disproportionate to service as that allotted to Dr Sutherland and Dr Farr. I cannot but

---

13 The legend has it that Christopher Columbus, using his practical judgment, made an egg stand on end by striking its smaller end on the table; once done, it is the easiest thing in the world.

believe that there is some great mistake, which a word from you would set right. To interfere in this matter has been more repugnant to me than I can tell. . . .

May I add, in answer to a former objection of yours, that the name of "secretarial *assistant*" was expressly conceded, because it would lead to the question, "Who then did the *secretary's* work?"

Source: From a letter to William Farr, Wellcome (Claydon copy) Ms 5474/63, typed copy ADD Mss 43399 f148

Hampstead, N.W.
28 August 1863

I cannot tell you how vexed and mortified I have been with all this. It has quite knocked me up. You say, they "must have been singularly misled by somebody." We know very well who that somebody is. He [Colonel Baker] has been at it for more than two years. If you wonder that an "ill-conditioned beggar," as he was justly called, *not* by me, could prevail against several persons of much more than ordinary ability, industry and honesty, I answer, falsehood does give a man such an immense advantage (over truth). Did not the one traitor prevail against the eleven faithful[14] in the greatest tragedy in history? Yet there is no sign of his having been a clever traitor. An old Irishwoman once warned me to have no doings with a certain person because "he can lie and you cannot." Was not that profound?

I have been warning them against this swindler any time these two years. But he was always on the spot. I was not. I cannot tell you the grief this affair has caused me.

Source: From four letters to Douglas Galton, ADD Mss 45761 ff69, 72-73, 99-100 and 102 (all written from Hampstead, N.W.)

15 August 1863

Would you tell Lord Stanley of Alderley[15] and Mr Lowe [chairman of the board, Chelsea military hospital] (and tell Mr Lowe to tell Lord Granville when he comes back from Germany) to apply to the respective librarian and clerk of their respective houses for a copy, each for himself, of the *two-folio Blue Book* of the "India Army sanitary commission," and tell them the reason why?

---

14 An allusion to Matt 26:25.

15 Edward John Stanley, 2nd Baron Stanley of Alderley (1802-69), entered the House of Commons as a Whig MP in 1831 and served in various capacities until 1866.

19 August 1863

I send you for Mr Greg[16] the pamphlet in question. Please send it *as from yourself.* I will return his note tomorrow. It occurred to me that I might be able to send him other papers through you, as he has written to you for information. He is writing a review (for the *National,* I believe) on the India Army sanitary report. And I sent him the two folios through Mr Spottiswoode. . . .

Your two notes of the 17th I received one only this morning (19th) and one late last night. I mention this, because it might happen that things of importance might be thus delayed. This often happened, while I was at Cleveland Row.

21 August 1863

In returning Mr Greg's letter, I had thought of sending some of the reports, etc., referred to in my lilac pamphlet [*Observations,* also called the "red book"]. But I don't think he has a passion for Blue Books. All the official facts Mr Greg wishes to know are in said pamphlet, and the margin gives a list of references to all the reports of the respective commissions. To use them intelligently the documents must be compared.

Should he write to you for them, I will put them together.

The report of the royal commission on the sanitary state of the army gives the death rates, as they were *before* the improvements. The last two annual reports (and there is another in the press) of the army medical department give the annual death rates *since* the improvements. But the lilac pamphlet gives the facts.

26 August 1863

Colonel Wilberforce Greathed, younger brother of the Colonel Greathed, says that he "knows personally at the Horse Guards that 300 copies of the royal (India sanitary) commission report have been ordered by government for distribution." What does this mean? will you put it in my power to contradict or confirm it? Is it that that wretched 8vo is, after all, to be the one "for distribution"? Or is it that these men cannot be accurate to save their lives?

16 William Rathbone Greg (1809-81), essayist.

Source: From a letter to Dr Robert Christison, Wellcome Ms 5482/56

Hampstead, N.W.
30 September 1863

I have sent a paper in the India sanitary subject to your section of the Social Science meeting. Will you be so good as to get someone *who can read* to read it? In making this request, my object is rather to make another, which is, would you, in your introductory address, draw public attention strongly to the India sanitary question? It would be the making of us, if you would.

My paper is quite general and enters into no details. A powerful notice, on your part, of the report would have great influence in hastening the government's tardy steps and enabling us to get our working commissions to carry out the practical measures in India, which is the main point now.

The *home* advising commission we carried yesterday. The India Office appointed its two members, Sir Proby Cautley and Sir Ranald Martin on the Barrack and Hospital (War Office) Commission (Mr Rawlinson, C.E. is to be added), which consists of the quartermaster general, Dr Sutherland, the assistant under secretary of state, the director of works and a member of the Army Medical Council. Also, after a great deal of fighting, we passed the instructions we wanted, which were written by us at Lord de Grey's desire.

So far so good. But what we want now is the appointment of the three commissions of health in India, one for each presidency, to be put in connection with the home (advising) commission.

2. Any remarks of yours about the personal hygiene of the soldier in India, the dieting, the drinking, the want of exercise—a subject which you have made so peculiarly your own—would tell with the military authorities both here and in India. They are very difficult to convince and we require whatever help we can have, viz., as to the need of more vegetable and farinaceous diet to suit the climate, of disuse of all spirits, except under medical advise, of more exercise, occupation, gymnastics, etc.

I venture to send you a pamphlet of my own on the popular part of the subject, reprinted (not by me) out of the big Blue Book. It is at all events light reading, though it leaves a smell in the imagination.

Source: From a letter to Lord Stanley, Liverpool Archives, Derby Collection 920/15/21

Hampstead, N.W.
2 October 1863

*Private.* I have been so "turbulent" (vide Lord Panmure on F.N.) when there was anything to be had by it, that it is right I should be thankful, when that something *is* had. On Tuesday we got at last, thanks to you, our home India (sanitary) advising commission and carried our instructions, after a hard fight. But they have *not* yet been before Sir C. Wood. He appointed Sir P. Cautley and Sir R. Martin "unofficially," at first (I don't quite know what that means but am afraid it meant, "I give you my two men, and now I wash my hands of you" on the "Barrack and Hospital Improvement Commission" of the *War Office*). Mr Rawlinson is, I believe, to be appointed by Lord de Grey.

We wrote the instructions, at Lord de Grey's desire. And I trust these tie them up to real work, and that their decisions will be "official" and *not* to be "reconsidered."

The India members are to attend—for all, not only Indian, purposes—the Barrack and Hospital (War Office) Commission. This was not our doing. We should have felt safer, if the India Office had constituted the commission, so as to be more peculiarly its own. But we have done our best. It is by no means the best theoretical plan possible.

Of course this is only one step. Till the presidency commissions of health (or departments of health) are constituted in India, it is little we can do at this end. But all we have heard, as yet, is that they are "very much wanted" "out there."

Perhaps you are furthering the object "out there." Perhaps you will be glad to hear that we are preparing, by desire of the War Office, an 8vo manual from your big Indian Blue Books, consisting of the report, an abstract of the evidence, any useful bits out of the addenda, an abstract of the stational returns, etc., to be sent by the War Office to all commanding and some other officers, with orders to them to read *and to understand* it (without which orders they will not). . . .

The next step for this commission, IF the instructions are approved, will be for it to form itself into a sub-committee and make a scheme for the work of the presidency commissions. Sir P. Cautley is so honourable a man that I have no fear but that he will press any decisions he comes to on our commission before the India Council. Pray burn this note. And pray help us farther with Sir C. Wood, if you can and think right.

Source: From a copy of a letter to P. Davies, British Library RP 3133 (i)

7 October 1863

I am extremely obliged to you for your valuable paper on points in the sanitary condition of the British soldier in India. They are important, being just the points which a careful N.C. officer would note in his daily life. It would be well if all N.C. officers would do, as you have done. I have kept the paper and I will take care that it shall be made use of.

I wish that we could have had your evidence before the Commission on the Sanitary State of the Army in India. I send you a paper of mine, reprinted (not by me) which was laid before that commission. Should you wish to look over the two Blue Books, comprising the report and evidence, I would gladly send them you for perusal. But I could not give them to you, as the work is already becoming a very rare one. Otherwise I would most willingly.

Source: Letter, Liverpool Record Office, Derby Collection 920/15/22

27 October 1863

*Confidential*

Dear Lord Stanley

We have not yet got our instructions for the home India sanitary commission, and our affairs are not prosperous. As you are aware, Sir C. Wood named Sir P. Cautley and Sir R. Martin on the War Office Barrack and Hospital Improvement Commission some weeks ago. But the instructions (which I wrote, by Lord de Grey's desire) which were submitted to and approved by the commissioners, have not yet been approved by Sir C. Wood, who is, I understand, "averse" to them. And Lord de Grey proposes to compromise the matter and to let the commission act for India on the same instructions on which it acts for home.

I remonstrated and showed that it is on quite a different state of things we have to work. For example, in England sanitary improvement *outside*, by local and general acts, has been going on for years. And not a local administrative body but has its sanitary powers. In India no such progress has been made and no such powers exist. It was on this state of progress *outside* in England that we began our barrack and hospital improvements, i.e., we had little to do *outside* though everything *inside*. In India everything has to be done *outside*. And it will be little or no use to rebuild, ventilate, etc., *inside* the barracks, if no powers are to be given to remedy the deplorable state of stations, bazaars, cities and towns; or rather, I should say, to plan, to propose a scheme for such remedies.

Our home instructions are therefore totally inadequate to meet the case. They do not cover a tenth of the ground. Nothing can result but failure and disappointment. Failure, I mean, in improving Indian health if it is supposed that, while *outside* drainage, sewerage and water supply are left in their present state, which is NO state at all (or left for India authorities to do, or not to do, as they choose), all that has to be done here for India is to do what we have been doing at home, viz., reform the buildings.

I represented a good deal more of this kind, which I may spare you because you know it better than I do. And I urged that Sidney Herbert had, in the case of the first royal sanitary commission, taken himself to and pressed upon Lord Panmure and General Peel (successively) the working schemes of the four sub-commissions (which carried out his recommendations subsequently). And that thus everything was done that was done.

I was told that, "if Lord Stanley would have done this, the thing would have been carried," or words to that effect; that Sidney Herbert "had the power to say to the minister, Do this, and he did it"; and that "Lord Stanley could have done the same thing"; that "Lord de Grey is in a different position and could not step in to advise Sir C. Wood how to carry into effect the report"; that he "did say all he could."

Here the matter hangs now. Of course this is for yourself alone. No human being has the least idea that I should state these things to you.

2. As you are aware, Sir C. Wood's despatch to India on your report (1) sent out a summary of your commission's recommendations, (2) authorized the formation of the presidency commissions, (3) pointed out that all plans for sanitary improvements should, before being carried into execution, be sent to him for reference to the sanitary commission *here*, (4) directed that the Calcutta, in communication with the Madras and Bombay, commissions, be charged with the preparation of a draft code of sanitary regulations, such as is referred to in 37th clause of your " recommendations," that this draft code is to be transmitted to him for revision in this country and the completed code will then be sent to India for promulgation.

There is enough to give one very great uneasiness in (2) and (4). With regard to (2), I have a letter from Colonel Strachey,[17] the head of the Public Works Department in India, as you know, proposing that these

17 Colonel, later Lieutenant General Richard Strachey (1817-1908), later Sir, brother of John Strachey.

presidency commissions should consist of an "officer of health" and—he does not know what. Now, while fully sharing the "horror" of Colonel Strachey "for deliberative boards," your commission never contemplated this; officers of health and engineers must be employed, to inspect and report, by the presidency commissions. But the officer of health should *do* no more than he does at home, viz., report on causes of disease. The presidency commissions will have to decide on all sorts of sanitary engineering works. How can an "officer of health" do this? It should have a good civilian administrator as an *administrative* head. And its *consulting* members should represent all the scientific elements which have to do with health. There is no man living who could be recommended as an "officer of health" to do what Colonel Strachey imposes upon him.

I am sadly afraid the Indians [i.e., the British administrators in India] will mismanage their presidency commissions.

As to (4), I ventured to remonstrate and to show that, had Sidney Herbert left *our* "codes" to the Horse Guards "to draw up," we should have been just where we were before. It is a very different thing drawing up one's own code and having it accepted by the Horse Guards, which was our case, and letting the Horse Guards draw it up, to be "approved" by the war minister.

This point was carried so far as this: that we have been instructed privately by Sir C. Wood "to draw up a memorandum of the heads of a code to be submitted" to him for transcription to the presidency commissions. But this is not of such *immediate* importance as the instructions to the home commission. It is very little use making a regulation to prevent the chimney from smoking, while nothing is being done to cure smoky chimneys. The very first thing is to put the stations to rights. Afterwards we may make a "code" for them. The very first thing for the home commission to do is to report on, and to draw up a scheme for the best sanitary arrangements applicable to India, merely to save time and to keep the presidency commissions in the right path. (We are not so wild as to think that we are to draw up their administrative rules and forms of procedure for them.)

I have often apologized for troubling you about things. But I make no apology now. For the very existence is at stake, as it seems to me, of the practical good to be derived from your report. You were once so good as to tell me that almost all the India Office measures passed through your hands. Help us now.

yours very faithfully<br>
Florence Nightingale

I do not forget to thank you for the successful trouble you have taken in making the India Office give Dr Sutherland his due. Please to burn this letter out of the world and out of your memory. It is for yourself alone. If you think well to act, you will act as from yourself, of course. Sir C. Wood was with Lord de Grey at Studley Royal [Estate, Ripon, North Yorkshire]. Perhaps he is not gone.

F.N.

Source: From an incomplete letter to Edwin Chadwick, Woodward Biomedical Library A.8

[October 1863]

*India sanitary question.* I have sent a paper on this to the Edinburgh meeting, but I am afraid it will be read in the sanitary section. I have answered generally Sir C. Wood's accusation about the statistics. He did not say that our "69 per 1000" annual death rate was exaggerated. He only said that it vibrated round that number in different years and that, in some years, it was much less. This was in fact admitting it. And then he said, war was the cause of the excess, *not* from wounds but from disease, which was, in fact, again admitting our statement, provided his averment were correct, which still has to be proved, as you will see by a statement of mine which I enclose. Part of its substance, not all, is in my paper. But if you take a part in the discussion, which I hope you will, you may like to have these facts before you.

I have ceased to take in the *Examiner* because (1) it has done its little all to help to ruin St Thomas' Hospital's chance of a good site; (2) it never took any notice of India sanitary matters till Saturday week when, after Crawfu[o]rd had been much poked by M Mohl, he gave an article reproducing all the old fallacies, which, if they were true, the royal commission might as well not have been.

Source: From a letter to Sir Charles Trevelyan, Newcastle University Library 35/29-30

26 October 1863

*In re Colonel Strachey's letter.* 2. As to the statement that a "good deal" of the recommendations is "quite unpractical and visionary," such an opinion was to have been expected. It is nothing new and cannot be argued down. It will be corrected by success. The mental process from which it arises is perfectly well known in this country.

The charge of "exaggeration" (in regard to the statement in the report that there are barracks in India intended to hold from a quarter to a half of a regiment in a room) may be rebutted at once by going into the Dalhousie Barracks, which contain 306 men in a room, Dinapore barracks, which contain 308 men per room, and Fort St George barracks (Madras), one room which contains above 600 men and the other about 500. Very likely Colonel Strachey has been unaware of the facts.

3. As regards the statement that, if you in India do all the royal commission wants, you will have to spend the whole surplus revenue for some years to come upon soldiers—why not, if it be necessary? They have so misspent the public money on barracks that the Public Works Department ought to be the last to raise such an objection. If you intend to hold India with British troops, the stations must be made healthy at whatever cost.

Colonel Strachey's averment that he does not much mind killing a few men if efficiency is gained, shows, I am afraid, that he has hardly considered the subject, because it is a law in these matters that you can't do both of these things. The number of men you kill is the best sign of the INefficiency of the remainder. No army that did not show a low death rate was ever, or ever will be, an efficient army.

4. The only remaining point in his letter is the *workshops.* We entirely agree with Colonel Strachey that a cardinal defect and cause of unhealthiness in the Indian Army is want of work. But if India looks to diminishing the mortality by workshops *only*, she will be disappointed. The soldier's diseases in India are foul air and foul water diseases. This is so well known that the question does not admit of a discussion, although Indian officials seem not hitherto to have realized the fact. Whenever they do so and are able to conceive a complete idea of what constitutes the conditions of health in India, the question of workshops will take up its proper place. Give them this emphatic caution: not to nibble at the recommendations, they must be taken in their totality and applied in their totality, or very little good will be done. We can help and will help in England in getting gymnastics made a parade and in obtaining the recognition of work as part of the soldier's duty. This has all been already considered. But repeat the caution: not to trust to workshops *alone* to save the British Army in India.

Source: From a letter to Lord Stanley, Liverpool Record Office, Derby Collection 920/15/23

31 October 1863

*Private.* I beg to enclose to you the whole of a packet I have just received from Sir C. Trevelyan. But the part I would particularly call your attention to is the two "Public Works Department" sheets, Nos. 2919, 4007. They give an idea of the state of Calcutta which nothing, no evidence in your Blue Books, comes near.

The fact is, the ground of the maidan[18] is used up. And Calcutta, already nearly uninhabitable, is fast becoming quite so. The only thing, in those papers, which equals the state of things they reveal to an experienced sanitary eye, is the utter helplessness they betray. And while this is the state of things out there, they are *chaffering* here *as to the powers they shall give us to help* them.

I would fain ask you, if you have half an hour to spare when you come to London "on the 10th or 12th," to let me see you in regard to your interview with Sir C. Wood any day, any hour; only let me know beforehand.

Source: From handwritten notes, Add Mss 45781 ff101-02

[November 1863]

Course of proceeding recommended by your [Lord Stanley's] royal commission for carrying out the sanitary improvement of Indian stations and towns:

1. to vest the executive in a local authority, or commission of health, for each presidency;

2. to give to these Indian authorities the advantage of home experience in the details of sanitary improvement, leaving to the Indian authorities the sole responsibility of accepting or rejecting any information or advice sent to them;

3. as a commission already existed at the W.O., *advising* not only at home but at all foreign stations, e.g., Ceylon, close to India itself the royal commission proposed, if the secretary of state for India did not appoint a special commission, that Indian members should be added to the W.O. commission and that the joint commission should advise and transmit information to the India authorities.

18 The Indian term maidan designated any open plain; here it refers to the name of the park in Calcutta surrounding Fort William, or the Calcutta commons.

This was done. England is now constantly consulted by foreign governments who send commissions to obtain information as to nearly all existing practical experience of sanitary works both as regards civil and military improvements. Why should not her own Indian Empire do the same? Neither interference nor control is proposed in any case, but simply to offer to the India commissions our OWN accumulated experience.

The constitution of the presidency commissions comes first in importance. Next would follow the question of local authorities already discussed in India. Each presidency commission should present a report to the government once a year.

According to present understanding, the connection between the presidency commissions and the home commission would be:

1. The W.O. has been already asked to prepare model plans of barracks and hospitals, these are now considerably advanced. . . .

2. The presidency commissions are to send home to the S. of S. for India any plans or proposals of their own which, before being sanctioned, will be sent to the home commission for advice and information.

Besides this, however, which is good so far as it goes, the home commission should help the presidency commission by a direct statement and description of the kind of sanitary works, improvements, etc., applicable to Indian stations, as described in the stational reports.

If the home commission were authorized to draw up such a statement, it would clear away at once most of the presumed difficulty in applying improved sanitary methods to India.

Source: From a letter to Lord Stanley, Liverpool Record Office, Derby Collection 920/15/24

2 November 1863

*Confidential.* I saw yesterday the whole of Sir C. Wood's correspondence relating to the India home commission. And in a despatch to India, dated 15 August (and not communicated to the War Office till the end of October), regarding the recommendations of your royal commission, he commits himself in a way that renders it hopeless to think of our obtaining the (home) instructions we thought necessary. For we proposed that the (home) commission should draw up a scheme for carrying out the recommendations in India; this despatch has actually sent out such a scheme, drawn up in its own way, on 15 August.

They cannot stultify themselves by sending another. And I have therefore given way, as far as I am concerned, and written a short instruction (at the War Office desire) for the barrack and hospital commission merely to enable them to be asked to prepare plans and descriptions of new barracks and hospitals, methods for improving existing ditto and to give their advice on all proposals of a sanitary nature sent from India.

As we have been asked by Sir C. Wood (privately) to draw up the "heads" of a code, we may introduce such explanatory matter, by way of note, as will cover a good deal of the ground which the commission now can't touch, in the absence of the specific instruction which Sir C. Wood declines giving.

You will have seen (by the Calcutta minutes I sent) that, though Calcutta has a municipal council, they don't know how to begin and are actually sending their engineer to England to learn. Now, of whom is he to learn? Would not the wisest thing be to put him into relation with the home (India) commission? The *very case has arisen.* And yet they have no power whatever to deal with it at home.

2. Two of the points in the original draft instructions for home, relating to the training of officers of health and of cadets of engineers in sanitary principles for India, are now omitted in the present short Instruction. Yet they are of great importance.

I have thought it but honest to tell you exactly how things stand now. Yet, if you still could do anything to help us, pray do not neglect us. An almost fatal step has been made at first starting. But much may still be retrieved. And I trust that you will still allow me to consult you personally about it, as you were so good as to mention in your note of 31 October, just received. Although the state of things is different from what we supposed it to be, and from what I stated to you somewhat.

Source: From three letters to Douglas Galton, Add Mss 45761 ff215-16, 219-20 and 221

10 November 1863

This (of Sir C. Trevelyan's) is of a mail posterior to the one which brought the papers (about the maidan), which I did so want you to see and which Lord Stanley has kept. Please return me the whole of these. You will see that, though we shall disagree with him on some points, there is no talk of our report being "exaggerated" on the Indian side. On the contrary, they tell us things which make our hair stand on end and which I wish we had put into the report.

As to the "cholera commission" report,[19] it is obvious they are ashamed to send it.

Pray show these papers to Lord de Grey, if you wish it.

10 November 1863

I return No. 297 with great reluctance. I think Lord de Grey might get me a copy. As for the report being "exaggerated," there is nothing in it which gives at all any idea of the state of things *compared* with this account (their own) of the maidan at Calcutta. I sent you Sir C. Trevelyan's letter on purpose and will send you the papers, as soon as Lord Stanley returns them.

As for the cholera commission report, it has never reached us, though we have applied for it scores of times. But we know its history. We know that they were evils which accumulated under McClelland,[20] that it is a divided report—part of the commission refused to sign it—and that they are ashamed of the state of things and keep it close. Please get us a copy.

17 November 1863

*Private.* The enclosed was sent to me by Lady Monteagle [packet of correspondence concerning the suppression of the folio volumes of the report on the India Army commission]. And I thought it so shocking that I send it on to you, as I should have done to Sidney Herbert. Please return it to me.

Source: From a letter to Lord de Grey, Add Mss 43546 ff82-83

18 November 1863

*Private.* Could you send me the Cholera Commission report (from India) of which Sir C. Wood has lent you one of his two copies? and allow me to keep it as many days as you will grant permission for?

Sir C. Wood, through Sir Proby Cautley, has, as of course you are aware, desired us to draw up the heads of a sanitary code for India, to be submitted to him and transmitted to the presidency commissions of health in India. We have already made some way. But, to go further, it would be necessary for us to see this cholera commission report.

---

19 *Report of the Commissioners Appointed to Inquire into the Cholera Epidemic of 1861 in Northern India* (Calcutta 1862).

20 Dr John McClelland, principal inspector general, Medical Department, wrote "Notes on the Recommendations Contained in the Report of the [Indian] Sanitary Commission," 10 October 1863. Nightingale briefly commented on these notes, Newcastle University Library 35/15.

I had already been promised it from the I.O. But now they say that two copies only were sent to England, of which Sir C. Wood keeps one himself and lent you the other.

Source: From two letters to Lord Stanley, Liverpool Record Office, Derby Collection 920/15/25 and 26

22 November 1863

I have been waiting patiently (or impatiently) to hear from you. You were so good as to say that you would make an appointment with me "at the close of the week beginning 9 November."

We are just where we were (as to the "instructions") four months ago. Sir C. Wood will not approve *any* instructions now for the home (India) commission to act upon. And all that he will say is that your report is "exaggerated." I think he must act or *not* act thus from want of information. And there is no one to press such information on him but you.

I received, by yesterday's mail, printed documents from the Bengal Army Medical Department approving of all the recommendations and differing only on certain engineering details, with which they are less familiar than we are. This printed letter, so far from stating that all the recommendations had been "anticipated," states that one only had been anticipated. The India Office sent me the Cholera Commission's report of 1862, giving such an account of the stations in Upper India, as we gave no idea of. I have seen a similar report for the Punjab. All this does not look as if India thought your report "exaggerated." But the strongest of all is the document (of Sir C. Trevelyan's) about Calcutta, which you have still. Would you have the kindness to return me that and his commissariat minutes which you have? I have many subsequent documents of his, if you would like to see them. Some I have sent to the War Office.

Meanwhile all our time is being wasted. The Calcutta municipality have actually sent their officer to England for information. And we have no means of entering into relation with him.

If you would like Dr Sutherland to wait upon you, he would doubtless give the necessary information (as to the present state of things, with regard to the instructions) better than I should.

23 November 1863

*Private.* I understand that "a paper has been received" (by the India Office) from Colonel Norman, "in which he positively declares that the grievances and abuses complained of" (by you in your report) "have long been remedied and that in fact the report attempts to slay the slain." (I presume that this Colonel Norman is the military secretary of the Government of India.)

Of course you, as the chairman of that commission, are the only person who can claim and answer Colonel Norman's "paper." I will only say that, of all things, I desire to see it and to assist in answering it.

I enclose an extract from the Cholera Commission report, dated last year, received by the India Office on 2 November only (*this* month) and lent me for forty-eight hours (I must therefore beg that you will return me this extract, which I cannot reproduce). I only remark that to this very Colonel Norman this report is addressed, that your report gives no idea of anything half so shocking as his and that the account of the other stations in North India is, if possible, worse.

I add an extract from a *private* letter of Lady Elgin's [wife of the viceroy]: "*People who know*" (how much mischief that phrase has authorized) "have detected *serious* mistakes in the report, tending to exaggerate *much* the *real* rate of mortality," etc.

Napoleon's pope [Pius VII] saw nothing more wonderful in Paris than to see himself there. I see nothing so wonderful in all these letters as to see how "people who know" are shaken by them.

Source: Note to William Farr, Add Mss 43399 f153

23 November 1863

The Government of India, as well as the different presidency authorities, state that they "have detected *serious* mistakes in the report" (royal sanitary) "tending to exaggerate *much* the *real* state of mortality." These words come from the very highest source in India though they are in a private letter.

Besides this, Colonel Norman, military secretary to the Government of India, has sent home a "paper" to the same effect, stating that *all* the "recommendations" had been "anticipated." So is it not, then, incumbent to bring out a statement, showing the truth of the figures impugned? Please to return Dr Crommelin's letter.

Source: From a letter to Harriet Martineau, Add Mss 45788 f229

25 November 1863

I was in hopes to have written yesterday about Lady Elgin's letter, but could not. I had to see Lord Stanley and to get sight of the official papers of denial sent home against us from India.

I enclose a letter from Dr Farr, which please return to me. But nothing can give you an idea of the horrors of the disclosures as to the state of the stations which these Indians make themselves while declaring themselves "to be 100 years before England." I mean to send you some extracts. But it is poor work refuting them, instead of helping them.

Could you ask Lady Elgin to look at the *Cholera Commission* Report for Northern India dated Calcutta, July 1862, received at home 2 November 1863. *We* have no disclosure like that. It is appalling.

Source: From two letters to Lord Stanley, Liverpool Record Office, Derby Collection 920/15/27 and 28

25 November 1863

*Private.* Of course the papers, here sent by your permission, are for yourself alone, and to *be returned to me* please, without being mentioned to Sir C. Wood.

It occurred to me, would it not be well if you would take the trouble to see Lord de Grey before Sir C. Wood, as the home commission is partly War Office? Lord de Grey would then be acting in concert with you. But whether you think well to do this or not, do not let me be mentioned in it.

1. As to the "inspections" in India, what I meant by inspections was this: I did not mean that inspectors must be sent from this country, but that, in following out the principles laid down by your royal commission, all duties of inspection should be carried out by officers of the presidency commissions. They should be done by a sanitary and an engineering officer, who should report defects and proposals for improvement to the presidency commissions. In this work, all that the home commission could do would be to aid the presidency commissions by their advice as to points of detail, such as laying on of water, etc.

2. The Calcutta people have themselves anticipated the supposed objection to interference by sending home an officer on purpose to gain information about drainage. And yet we must not put ourselves in connection with him.

29 November 1863

As to one of the three subjects of our conversation, Sir John Lawrence has "only just ascertained that the copies (of your report) were sent round the Cape and not overland. Hence the delay. It was ordered that a certain number of copies were to go overland also, but by some mistake this was not done. Some have since been ordered off."

("By mistake" also Sir C. Wood did not present to the House of Commons your whole report and evidence.)

There remain the other two topics of our conversation (of much more importance), viz., (1) to get some kind of instructions for your home (advising) commission, and (2) to get "Colonel Norman's paper" denying the facts of your report, for answer. It seemed to me that your three principal objections to me were (1) the "impossibility of water drainage in a country *with dry* seasons." To this I now venture to enclose an answer. (2) About "inspections," to which I have sent you an answer, as to what I meant by "inspections"; as it is of incomparably more importance to know what to do with the old barracks than to build new [ones], which will be comparatively few in number. (3) About the "unwillingness" (and "uselessness") to "refer home such questions as those of drainage and water supply," to which I answered that they HAVE *done it.* The Calcutta municipality has actually sent home an officer for this very purpose. And we have no powers to meet him.

Poor Lady Elgin![21]

Source: From a letter to Sir Charles Trevelyan, Newcastle University Library 35/35-36

26 November 1863

I have communicated the fact (both to Lord Stanley and to the I.O.) that on the 14th of last month, the "450 copies" of the royal sanitary report had not arrived. I hope you received a copy I sent you by the first mail after 8 July. Mrs Holland was herself good enough to take it (for transmission) to the I.O.

Do you think you could be kind enough to send me a copy of the Cholera Commission Report (Dr McClelland's and Mr Strachey's) with Appendix, in N. India, dated Calcutta 21 July 1862. Two copies only were received by the I.O. and only on the 2nd of this month. I was lent one for forty-eight hours only. It contains disclosures which nothing that we have said in our report as to the bad sanitary state of stations approaches. I return a copy of Dr McClelland's "Notes" with a few remarks. His objections to certain engineering details would certainly not have been made if he had been aware of the great improvements which are being introduced with success both in warm and cold climate stations of the British Army and which are just as applicable to India. These are precisely the point on which the home commission (which I am rejoiced to see Dr McC. advocates) *can* send to the presi-

21 Lord Elgin died on 20 November 1863.

dency commissions a large amount of experience in a class of works new to India. Could you also send me Mr John Strachey's remarks on sanitary administration, founded on the cholera report? (The I.O. cannot "lay their hands" on a copy.)

Let me add that, when I said what was thought of the "cholera report" by the medical officials here (in my last) it was merely as such. The forty-eight hours' reading of it, which I have had since, show me that it contains an amount of valuable *information* and makes disclosures such as we have never had, nor made, in our report. But its *recommendations* are not equal to what we in this country should consider necessary from experience. However it is a great step in advance to have had such a report, although I can easily understand why it should offend army medical officials. . . .

You have no doubt heard that the mortality statistics in the royal sanitary report have been fiercely disputed in India. So far as we know, this is mainly on the question of the years since the Mutiny. They say: "The report alleges that the mortality is 69 per 1000 while, if you take the mortality for 1859, 1860, 1861, 1862 it is nothing like this amount. It is indeed so much below 69 that it argues greatly improved health in consequence of improvements carried out at stations. And hence the commission is altogether wrong."

In answer to this,

1. If you will look at the last para. of p X of the folio report, you will find the difficulties stated of arriving at correct statistics for India. At p XI you will find the 69 per thousand set down as the probable mortality from the data since the occupation of India.

2. You will find in the same page that an annual variation in the mortality is distinctly stated.

3. If you will now turn to p LXXXVIII, Table 10, you will find the mortality for all India and for each presidency grouped according to periodical series with the view of enabling readers to arrive at a correct idea of what was the real rate up to the year preceding the Mutiny. As a mean term, the report assumes the years 1800 to 1856 as the mortality rate 6.86 per *cent.*

4. If you now turn to Sir A. Tulloch's evidence, p 319, you will find a table showing the mortality from 1817 to 1855, the result of which is that, for this term, the mortality was 70 per 1000.

5. In addition to this evidence, the commission applied for the mortality statistics from Bengal and Madras in the summer of 1861, with a view of bringing their information down to the latest point.

They actually sent printed forms with instructions in order to save trouble. But no notice whatever was taken of the application. It was not until the application was again renewed, without the slightest notice being taken of it, that they deemed it their duty to insert a clause in their report, p 1, line 13 from top, pointing out the inattention with which their request had been treated. And now these are the very people who turn round and adduce the mortality of the years we wanted as an argument against the correctness of the estimate made from the only data at the disposal of the royal commission.

6. Even admitting the accuracy of their statement, which we in this country would *not* do without further inquiry, it is really no proof of a lower mortality rate. No one who knows anything of Indian sanitary statistics would dream of adducing three or four years as any proof of what the death rate has been, except for the three or four years.

7. The objectors appear to have overlooked the fact that, since the Mutiny, a large army, new to India, has been poured into the country, a proceeding which will always be attended by a lower death rate than that incident to the country and its present defective or bad sanitary conditions. This lower rate will rule until the bulk of the army has been located for a sufficient time in India to receive the full impress of these conditions. It appears to require about 6 (six) years' residence for health to be seriously affected. And thenceforward, supposing the strength to be kept up so as to compensate for losses and time expired then [?], the Indian Army will begin to show what its mortality rate really is to be.

8. Take any group of years in Table 10 you choose (for a *group* of years you must take) and you will find that all past experience points out a rate far exceeding that from the three or four years, now adduced to show what the rate is. You will find periods of years exceptionally healthy, for instance, 1770 to 1800, 1830 to 1840, 1830 to 1856. You will find also periods of more unhealthy years. Now the true way to have dealt with the four exceptional years since the Mutiny would have been to have added them on to a longer group with an explanation that these four (4) years applied to a large new army, exposed for the first time to Indian influences.

9. Taken by themselves, these four years prove nothing more than that new regiments are more healthy than old ones. The years would have been noticed in the report, if the returns had been sent. But as they were not sent, the commissioners cannot be blamed for not noticing them.

The whole of the mortality records available were worked out by the most practised statistical staff in Europe, that belonging to the Registrar-General's Office, under the superintendence of Dr Farr. If the Indian statisticians have any "mistakes" to point out, by all means let them do it. Those who worked out the statistics have expressed their earnest desire for this. They say "they will answer for or acknowledge their 'mistakes.' But, if the Indian men have nothing further to adduce than the years since the Mutiny, they will certainly lay themselves open to the charge of keeping back evidence, which was asked for by the royal commission, and of misunderstanding it at the same time."

Source: From three letters to Douglas Galton, Add Mss 45761 ff222-24, 225 and 226-27

30 November 1863

*Confidential.* I know that you are particularly busy about estimates just now. And therefore my cry shall be short.

We have never received any kind of instructions (for India) for the barrack commission. *In confidence* I may tell you that I have sent for Lord Stanley and seen him. And he is going today or tomorrow to Sir C. Wood about them. I have done the same by Sir John Lawrence. I asked Lord Stanley to see Lord de Grey too. But I don't know that he will.

I think that Lord de Grey could not have done LESS for us than he has.

Please return me Sir C. Trevelyan's letters and papers. I want them for Sir J. Lawrence.

Lord Stanley has returned me what he had of Sir C. Trevelyan's. But I suppose you are too busy to look at them now.

We have long since finished the "heads of sanitary code" asked for by Sir P. Cautley. Through Sir John Lawrence I got a sight of the cholera report, which I asked Lord de Grey for in vain. It is *far, far,* stronger than anything *we* have written *against* Indian stations. It is incredible. They "feed sheep in latrines" !!!! No attempt is made "to bury, or otherwise dispose of, the filth removed daily from" these!!!! Lord Stanley has a copy, which he showed me, of Sir C. Wood's despatch (No. 297, 15 August); Lord de Grey might therefore have got me a copy. It would have been of great use to us.

Poor Lady Elgin!

30 November 1863

I am desired to ask whether, now that the plans of barracks and hospitals for India are in hand, we should not prepare a description of them to be ready *to send to press*? This description will enable many questions to be discussed with reference to water supply, drainage, etc., which must be settled, before the plans can be of use in India.

1 December 1863

I send an abstract of the evidence taken before the royal India sanitary commission, in which everything has been cut out but what it will be practically useful for officers to know. We shall have to revise it carefully; and after the text of the evidence is settled, we shall then make such additions from the other documents as will be in conformity with Lord de Grey's minute. Please direct that two proofs with the copy be sent *here* as soon as possible.

Source: From three letters to Lord Stanley, the last one incomplete, Liverpool Record Office, Derby Collection 920/15/29, 30 and 31

1 December 1863

*Confidential.* You were saying that the India government at home and the India government in India were jealous. Now you have a governor general in your hand.[22] He is not at all jealous. On the contrary. He could settle all we want with Sir C. Wood in five minutes, if you would tell him, as chairman of the royal sanitary commission, what you want. He is a man never *too busy* for business. In these few last days of pressure, he has actually found time to let me know several matters of detail in the India Office.

No doubt you have much hand in his appointment. His is the greatest government now under God's. And he is the only man to fill it.

Here is an opportunity where what might take months of correspondence may be settled in a few minutes, such as

1. the constitution of the presidency commissions, to consist of (1) an able civilian to be responsible administrative head advised by (2) an engineer of "Public Works Department," a medical sanitary officer, a military officer, an army medical officer.

This board to proceed (a) to direct local inquiries, or "inspections," best carried out by an engineering officer and an officer of

22 Sir John Lawrence was appointed governor general and viceroy on 30 November 1863.

health in concert, (b) to receive reports, prepare plans, direct and see to execution of works. It is the opportunity.

2. to establish a proper connection between the presidency commissions and the home commission, i.e., an *entente cordiale.*

3. to enable the home commission to help the presidency commissions by a direct statement and description of the kind of sanitary works, improvements and appliances applicable to Indian stations, to meet the requirements described in the Indian stational reports.

Sir John Lawrence, governor general, could do what the secretary of state for India might feel a reluctance in doing, viz., he might desire the home commission to send all the information and suggestions they can as to the best means of initiating and carrying out sanitary improvements at the stations, together with the most improved appliances for barracks and hospitals.

If something practical of this kind is not done, the four years' labours of your royal commission are as bad as lost. The enclosed statement anticipates some objections.

3 December 1863

I will try and see Sir John Lawrence. But I never convinced anyone yet but Sidney Herbert. And I could have wished you had done it.

I cannot leave what you give "as the substance of *their* case" unanswered. I could wish that you would bring the substance of my answer before Sir C. Wood.

As to the home commission, instead of there being "nothing for it to do," there is everything for it to do. But I let that drop.

Would you have the goodness to return me a manuscript of the heads of a sanitary code; also two printed papers of the principal inspector general of Bengal and one or two other papers, I *think*, which you have of mine. The heads of code we were directed to draw up by Sir C. Wood. And I have no other copy.

3 December 1863

So far as the main causes of disease are concerned . . . it is difficult to see how India could have been freed from these causes of disease in three short years, which is about the average time since the stational reports were signed. That they may have done something in the way of cleansing, ventilation, ablution arrangements is probable, seeing that they could hardly escape the consequences of the printed queries put to them and the replies which they made. Besides which, they have had the general report of the Barrack and Hospital Improvement Commission before them (but the measures recommended in this report are only applicable to cool climates, like England).

But even on the subject of cleansing, we have, as you know, the report of a government commission on the last cholera, dated partly 21 July 1862 and partly in the last months of 1862 (an extract of which I sent you), which conclusively proves that, *up to these dates,* nothing whatever had been done in the country to which the report refers.

I also sent you two printed documents of the Public Works Department, one dated Fort William, 26 June 186*3*, one 9 September 186*3*, having reference to the sanitary condition of Calcutta and giving *at these dates* a worse account of the city than the report sent to your royal commission in June 1860.

There is also another document from the principal inspector general of Bengal (which you still have in your possession) dated 16 October 186*3* in which the recommendations of the commission are virtually accepted as necessary.

The danger will be that partial improvements will be put forwards in proof that a great deal has been done and that little requires to be done. The recommendations of your royal commission must be carried out entirely. The Indian sanitary problem consists of many factors and it will not do, in dealing with it, to leave out any one of the factors. India can be cured neither by engineers, nor by doctors, nor by sanitary officers, nor by military authorities, but by a concurrence of all of these. And the end aimed at is:

1. healthy barrack and hospital accommodation,
2. enough of good water, properly laid on,
3. good drainage,
4. a proper sanitary police over bazaars and towns,
5. abolishing spirit drinking,
6. providing means of occupation and other things indicated in your report.

A moment's consideration will show that no engineer, *and no adjutant general,* and no inspector general can bring about this reform. Your report asserts this, in asking for the appointment of presidency commissions, to deal with the questions. There is indeed no other way of reaching them. They will never *permanently* lower the army death rate by any other course of proceeding. The death rate of the new soldiers poured into the country since the Mutiny is, of course, considerably lower than past averages. You will hardly believe it, but I have actually seen this fact adduced by Indian *engineering* officers in proof of the statement that the small improvements they have carried out at a few stations have made the army healthy.

Source: From a letter to Sir Charles Trevelyan, Newcastle University Library 35/[44?]

3 December 1863

Sir John Lawrence, who is never too busy for business, has, in the midst of his overwhelming occupations of the last few days, obtained for me the following information, in answer to yours of last mail. "The copies of the sanitary report were sent round the Cape and not overland. Hence the delay. It was ordered that a certain number of copies were to go overland also, but by some mistake this was not done. Some have since been ordered off." ("By mistake" also Sir C. Wood did not present the whole report and evidence to the House of Commons.) Sir John Lawrence will himself go out to you by next mail.

Source: From a letter to Sir Harry Verney, Bodleian Library, Ms Acland f2

5 December 1863

I know how busy a man Dr Acland[23] is. But he seemed to take kindly to this review [of the report of the India sanitary commission for the *Quarterly Review*] which would be an invaluable assistance to us. And I cannot think of any other way which would be *less* inconvenient to him.

Source: From a letter to Lord de Grey, ADD Mss 43546 ff84-85

10 December 1863

*Confidential.* For the last ten busy days, I have been in constant communication with Sir John Lawrence. And I have had the great joy of receiving his commands to do what I had almost despaired of ever seeing done, viz., to send him out such schemes and statements of sanitary work as we want done by the "presidency commissions" (proposed in the royal India Army sanitary report). (I have also seen Lord Stanley, its chairman, more than once.) I believe I ought to submit to you yourself what was said with regard to the "home" Barrack and Hospital (India) Commission, which Sir John Lawrence wishes to see at work as soon as possible under *your* sanction.

If you would grant me an interview, I believe I could tell you this more shortly. But if, as is probable, you are too busy to spare me half

23 Henry Wentworth Dyke Acland (1815-1900), later Sir, professor of medicine at Oxford.

an hour before you go out of London this Christmas, I will do my best to put it on paper for you, provided it is considered *for yourself alone.*

**Editor:** In his reply of 11 December 1863 (ADD MSS 45778 f27), Lord de Grey expressed his inability to see Nightingale, but affirmed his willingness to attend to anything pertaining to India she might write. He met with her later in the month, as letters to Dr Farr and her sister indicate.

Source: From two letters to William Farr, Wellcome Ms 5474/64 and 65, copy ADD MSS 43399 ff159-60 and 163-64

10 December 1863

*Confidential.* You may be sure that I have thought of nothing else but our India business during the last busy ten days. And, in order to put you *au courant* [up to date], I send you (1) a letter of Lord Stanley's, and (2) part of my answer. We shall not get Colonel Norman's paper. But never mind. The best thing that can happen to us is that they should produce their complaints against us in the House of Commons. And Lord Stanley has already engaged my services in person to prompt him in February. He has also engaged to produce in the House of Commons the scheme of instructions which we wished the "home commission" to send out to India.

Since then, I have had the great joy of being in constant communication with Sir John Lawrence, and of receiving his commands to do what I had almost lost the hope of being allowed to do, viz., of sending out full statements and schemes of what we want the presidency commissions to do.

I should be glad to submit to you copies of papers of mine, which he desired me to write and which he took out with him as to the constitution of the presidency commissions, if you care to see them. They are, of course, confidential.

His is the greatest government under God's. And he is the only man to fill it.

I have also seen Lord Stanley more than once during these busy days. And, with Sir J. Lawrence's command, we feel ourselves empowered to begin the "home commission," and to father our plans upon it.

Sir J. Lawrence, so far from considering our report exaggerated, considers it under the mark.

And though I have not seen Colonel Norman's furious attack upon us, I have (now in my possession) the cholera commission report, dated July 1862, Public Works Department papers, dated August and

September of *this* year, which give an idea of a state of things, of which *we had no* idea, *have given no idea.* I send you an extract of the former. (The India Office, wise in its generation (?), keeps these a dead secret. And I am indebted to Sir J. Lawrence and Sir C. Trevelyan for them.)

Please return me all these papers, and consider them really "confidential." . . . Remember we shall want you in February [session of Parliament] when we are all to be blown into atoms.

22 December 1863

*Private.* I was busy all Saturday, Sunday and Monday with and for Lord de Grey, to screw up the War Office to accede to Sir J. Lawrence's sanitary wishes.

With regard to your question: there is no civil hospital of a large size in England which can be called "a model." The Herbert Hospital is a model for a military hospital, i.e., having respect to the character of the ground, the pavilion system is there applied in a model manner.

Source: From a letter to Parthenope Verney, complete in *Life and Family* (1:330), Wellcome (Claydon copy) Ms 9000/76

Christmas Day [1863]

I am not what I was this time last year. Sir John Lawrence says that we ought to have been at least five months forwarder with our work. And Dr Sutherland has scarcely done a stroke since 8 July. I have had Lord de Grey here and we have concerted a plan for helping Sir J. Lawrence. . . .

The India military authorities are coming round, i.e., the blow is struck; they declare themselves vastly "ill-used," but they do what we want. Sir C. Trevelyan has just sent me a printed paper from a Colonel Crommelin, R.E., who has the supervision of barracks in Bengal, which has adopted nearly all our principles. Now I saw a few weeks ago a private letter from this Colonel Crommelin full of foul-mouthed violent abuse against us. We ought to be and I hope are very thankful. For this adoption of our principles, without thanking us, is all we want.

Source: From two letters to Sir Charles Trevelyan, Newcastle University Library 35/40 and 41

26 December 1863

*Private.* I write in haste merely a few words to say that, from the paper on designing barracks, 29 October 1863, you have been kind enough to send me, of Colonel Crommelin's, it is obvious that they, the royal engineers, are thoroughly imbued with right principles. The blow is struck. They will consider themselves "vastly ill-used." But they will adopt all the right principles. And we are most thankful. Your letter and its enclosure are indeed cause for gratitude.

I have only had time to glance at Colonel Crommelin's draft report. There will be little difficulty in coming to an agreement about the sanitary improvement of Indian stations.

By Sir John Lawrence's desire, whose commands I had the great joy of receiving before he went, we are getting on as fast as possible with the draft plans and the sanitary descriptions, which the joint W.O. and I.O. commission is to send out to India, through Sir Charles Wood. The plans very nearly correspond to the description given in Colonel Crommelin's report. But as there are no plans attached to his report, we can of course judge only from the description.

There ought indeed to be no disagreement. Sanitary principles are the same everywhere. They only need to be applied to suit local circumstances. And when the joint commission sends its plans and statements to India, it will be found that all have been approximating to a very similar, if not to *the same* solution of the Indian problem.

I saw a private letter of this very Colonel Crommelin, abusing our commission in the most unmeasured terms. This is what makes me so thankful that sound principles are displayed by him, however violent he may be against us.

Lord de Grey said to me on Sunday, with two such men as Sir C. Trevelyan and Sir John Lawrence at the other end (in India), all the good we want to see will ultimately be done. God bless you.

ever yours gratefully

Florence Nightingale

You will see that this letter is strictly confidential, save the general appreciation of Colonel Crommelin's paper on barracks.

26 December 1863

*Private.* Allusion is made in Dr McClelland's paper to the report of the Cholera Commission. This report never reached us here. All we have heard is that it is the report of a minority and that one of the ablest sanitary men in the British service, who was a member, refused to sign it. For some cause it has given offence. We trust, however, that their methods of dealing with the causes of unhealthiness are not like those proposed by the "sanitary commissioner" in the Punjab, which virtually amount to denying the necessity of sanitary works altogether.

Source: From a letter to William Farr, Wellcome Ms 5474/66, copy ADD Mss 43399 ff167-68

2 January 1864

*Private.* I have not laid aside (out of my heart) what you said in your note of 22 December about the "weekly table" in Calcutta, etc. It is so very important.

We have been engaged, without intermission, since Sir John Lawrence went, and by his desire, in drawing up a kind of general scheme of what is wanted in Indian stations: water supply, drainage, construction of barracks, means of employment for soldiers, etc. This is now gone to press. On Tuesday the joint War Office and India Office commission, for which I have toiled and moiled, holds its first meeting, to discuss the proposed barrack plans for India and the general scheme above alluded to.

Dr Sutherland will propose the "weekly table." And, if carried, you will be applied to for a *form.* I hope, if there is anything different from the English form necessary, you will be ready with your scheme.

Sir John Lawrence's presence at the other end is an immense thing for us. And I shall moil and toil at him and his private secretary [Dr Hathaway], whom he sent here to me as well as coming himself before starting. . . .

I think I told you that we can't get "copies of (any of) the Indian attacks," although I sent Lord Stanley to Sir C. Wood for them. They are venomous. (I have seen some of them.) But when Parliament meets, Sir C. Wood is to lay them before the House, in a *civiller* form, and we are to answer them.

Source: From a letter to Sir Harry Verney, Wellcome (Claydon copy) Ms 9001/1

2 January 1864

I hope you will be able to do something for us in this session in the way of soldiers' trades and in supporting Lord Stanley against the attack of the India military authorities to be laid before the House by Sir C. Wood.

Source: From two letters to William Farr, Wellcome Ms 5474/67 and 68, copies ADD Mss 43399 ff169 and 170

7 January 1864

*Private.* On Tuesday the proposal to have your weekly table for Calcutta, Madras and Bombay, with an ultimate view to its extension throughout India, was carried at the joint India Office and War Office commission as the best means of carrying out the recommendation as to registration of your royal commission.

And I am told that (with unusual promptitude) the War Office drafted an official letter the same day to the Registrar-General, requesting a form for the purpose, with the view of assimilating the registration of India to that of England.

If you could send us a copy (of what you propose) here, with your instructions for carrying it into effect, also what you wish to have said in the section (to be devoted to statistics) of the "recommendation," which, in accordance with Sir John Lawrence's desire, we are preparing for the press to be sent to India, it would greatly expedite matters—as Sir John Lawrence begged that we would use the greatest despatch in forwarding to India all that we wanted his help in.

9 January 1864

As I have not heard from Your Holiness, will this section on the registration [the "weekly table"] do as a basis? Please let Your Infallibility give your decision, so that it may be embodied in a bull and send us all the forms referred to in it.

Source: From a letter to Robert Rawlinson, Boston University 1/3/37

8 January 1864

Dr Sutherland and I have been preparing the India drainage subject for the commission. And I have written down the result, for the purpose of sending it to you. The peculiarities of the India drainage question are

1. want of sufficient fall,
2. difficulties of outlet,
3. the long dry season,
4. excessive rain floods,
5. peculiar habits of the people.

In some places, it might be necessary to obtain a fall by pumping the sewage. But then fuel is scarce and dear, and steam unavailable. Would you be good enough to look over the enclosed, which has reference only to cities, and return it to me after you have had time to consider it and improve it ?

The Public Works Department, which would carry out the works, contains the cream of all the Indo-European engineering talent. But what they require is mainly information as to what has been done in solving drainage questions similar to theirs in Europe. The paper therefore should have this aspect. You will see what use we have made of your "Instructions and Suggestions."

Source: From a typed copy of a letter to Charles Hathaway, ADD Mss 45782 ff124-25

11 January 1864

As you are so kind as to offer it, I send a copy of the last edition of my *Notes on Hospitals*, just out, for Sir C. Trevelyan, the finance member of Council at Calcutta. If it will amuse you to cut it open on the voyage, pray do. But (except the recommendations at the end of the section on Indian hospitals) its principles of construction are adapted only for temperate climates.

I send you half a dozen of my India paper read at Edinburgh, if you can make any use of them in India. But pray remember not to take them unless convenient, nor the book [her *Notes on Hospitals*] for Sir C. Trevelyan, which can be sent by post if returned to me.

I wish you Godspeed on your voyage to India. I look upon the sanitary work there now as the true missionary work, as you see.

Source: From a letter to Lord Stanley, Liverpool Record Office, Derby Collection 920/15/32

13 January 1864

*Private.* We are in tribulation about our reviews. The *Quarterly*, after having accepted a review by Dr Acland (of your India Army sanitary report), has sneaked shabbily round to the enemy and is about to insert a review *by the enemy* with all the Norman (Colonel) and Crommelin and India military "information," stating just what you told me was the "India military authorities" case.

Lady Herbert, when she left England, left in my hands a note from you to her, saying that you would see the editor of the *Westminster*[24] about a review of the said report. If you will write one yourself, so much the better for us. If not, will you ask the editor of the *Westminster* whether he will have Dr Acland's (of Oxford) for his next number?

I have had a furious correspondence with the editor of the *Edinburgh*,[25] who was altogether taken in by the "India military authorities," in which I was *not quite* so uncivil (but nearly so) as these same "authorities" are and which ended in my being engaged to write a review (in my own sense, of course) for the next number of the *Edinburgh*.

This is of course private, as I should not wish it to be known that the "turbulent fellow"—vide Lord Panmure—was "at it" again.

---

24 Dr John Chapman (1822-94) was the editor of the *Westminster Review*.

25 Henry Reeve (1813-95), with Harriet Martineau initiating it; see correspondence with him in ADD Mss 45798.

Source: From a letter to Douglas Galton, ADD Mss 45762 ff4-5

14 January 1864

We shall want for the East Indian *Suggestions* the following illustrations:

1. Reduced barrack and hospital plans.
2. Ventilating arrangements.
3. Latrines, urinals and water closets.
4. Lavatory and bath arrangements for barracks and hospitals.
5. Several forms of improved cooking apparatus.
6. Plans of the respective outbuildings for these.
7. A good water filter.
8. A good sewage filter.

Mr Rawlinson has kindly undertaken to prepare drainage illustrations, sections of sewers, etc., also waterworks ditto. Pray let us see the draft of the letter to the India Office (about the recommendations of the royal commission) as soon as it is *in egg*.

Source: From a letter to William Farr, Wellcome Ms 5474/69, ADD Mss 43399 f182

4 February 1864

I send two letters of your friend Dr Mühry anent the India Army sanitary report (I sent him a copy of the two-folio volumes). Please to return the letters to me.

Source: From a letter to Lord Stanley, Liverpool Record Office, Derby Collection 920/15/33

9 February 1864

*Confidential.* The editor of the *Edinburgh Review* has written to me to urge the performance of my promise to write an article on your India sanitary report for his April number, also to say that the manuscript must be in his hands by 10 March at latest. But the promise was expressly made on condition that it was to be a fair discussion of the two sides. And for this it is necessary that the other side shall have spoken out. A discussion cannot be made upon one side only.

May I ask whether you know, or whether you will ascertain, if Sir C. Wood has received the "defence" of the India military authorities, for which he wrote to Lord Elgin [viceroy], and which he intended to lay on the table of the House of Commons? Or whether he would let you have any documents which might be made public use of? Of private ones I have seen plenty (from India). But, for the life of me, I cannot make out what their "defence" is—nor in what their contradictions (of the truth of your report) consist. On the contrary: as in

*Rejected Addresses* the conspirators say, "Let us by a song conceal our purposes," I am sure the conspirators (against our truth) most effectually conceal their "defence" by alleging facts ten times worse than yours. I don't feel in the least inclined to write a réchauffé [rehash] of your report. And, if you cannot furnish me with something to contradict or answer, I shall beg off from writing the said article.

2. Have you heard whether the *Westminster Review* will take in Dr Acland's article, as you were so good as to ask them?

3. We have nearly done what Sir John Lawrence bade us do: (1) the general scheme of sanitary works for stations in India, with plans and diagrams, to be sent in the name of the joint I.O. and W.O. commission; (2) the draft of the letter from W.O. to I.O., embodying those recommendations of your commission, which can only be car ried out by W.O. and I.O. But this last has been most untowardly delayed, first by nobody knowing what the respective jurisdictions were, second by the discovery of a committee which had been worked by Sir E. Lugard in the W.O., unknown to Lord de Grey, ever since August 1861 (i.e., the month of Sidney Herbert's death) on the victualling of troops on board ship going out to India, and which would infallibly end by consigning half the troops who land in India upon such diet to scurvy. As this was a very important item, delay has arisen till Lord de Grey can take steps *to undo this mischief.*

And they say that the W.O. is reorganized !!!

We have also almost done a manual (8vo) from your report and evidence (the two-folio volumes) which the Horse Guards is to give a copy of to every officer in the service.

If I have told you anything about the W.O., which you have not heard from other sources, pray consider it really "confidential."

Source: From a letter to Henry Acland, Florence Nightingale Museum (LMA) H1/ST/NC1/64/3

13 February 1864

*Private.* Immediately after receiving news of the untoward behaviours of the *Quarterly* from Sir Harry Verney, I communicated with Lord Stanley, and again upon his arrival in London, with a view of inserting your article on the sanitary state of the Indian Army in the *Westminster.* I have only this day received the final answer. Lord Stanley says: "I have settled for its insertion, though I suppose Dr Chapman (the editor) will claim the usual editorial right of review." He farther asks you kindly to send your article as soon as possible to the editor of the *Westminster*, Dr Chapman. . . .

I am afraid you will be less glad to hear this than we are. Still I trust you will not desert us; and that the article will come forth triumphant. The enemy has not yet appeared in any public way. I wish he would!

Source: From a letter to Douglas Galton, Add Mss 45762 f46

19 February 1864

We send a proof for revise, also some more of the copy, for the 8vo abstract [the "manual"] of the India Army sanitary report. Please forward it to printer and please let the result come to me here.

Source: From a letter to Lord Stanley, Liverpool Record Office, Derby Collection 920/15/34

20 February 1864

*Confidential.* After much "speering" [inquiring] at the India Office, I find, as regards the correspondence about your sanitary report:

1. that they "now expect a full report from Colonel Norman";
2. that they are "pretty sure that Sir C. Wood will not present anything to Parliament until that report has arrived and then been considered";
3. that they "have not heard that anyone is likely to move for papers."

Would you not ask a question in the House? I wish you would. However, you probably know more from Sir C. Wood than I do.

I wrote to Dr Acland immediately to send his review to the *Westminster.* I have put off mine in the *Edinburgh* till July [her review was not done]. It is no use entering the lists till the enemy has appeared.

Our abstract in 8vo, or "manual," for the W.O., of your two-folio volumes is finished. The sanitary scheme, asked for by Sir John Lawrence, would be finished (including the scheme for registration and a weekly table, as for London), if only the engineering people would send us in their part. It is most vexatious to have to wait for this, for all is done but the engineering part.

Much more vexatious is the delay brought to drafting the letter from W.O. to I.O., embodying some of your recommendations, by the vagueness about respective jurisdictions. (1) M. General Pears has been applied to and has answered. But little has come of it. (2) A reference has been made *from* the W.O. committee, of which Lord de Grey was not cognizant, by him to the joint W.O. and I.O. sanitary committee, about the victualling of troops on their passage to India. (3) The Horse Guards have managed so to discontent medical officers that we positively can't get candidates to supply the Army Medical

Department, now that it has to furnish doctors to both British and Indian troops, the best thing that could have happened to us as now the W.O. must go into the market and buy their doctors. But all this has provokingly delayed the drafting of said letter to I.O., which we were asked to draft for the W.O.

Source: From two letters to Douglas Galton, ADD Mss 45762 ff55 and 56

25 February 1864

*India Army Sanitary Abstract.* We send you the rest of the abstract; this is *all,* as far as the stational returns go. (We will send you the report as soon as we can.) Please forward to printer and send us two proofs *here as soon as you can.* . . . Where is M. General Pears's letter? where?

27 February 1864

We return the proof of the *Suggestions for India Sanitary Works,* with a quantity of new matter, partly from Mr Rawlinson, referring to the principles of drainage and water supply for towns. I believe we have now all the matter. And, after it is in type, we will revise it. Pray send us three revises *here* as soon as possible. . . .

Where is M[ajor] General Pears's letter? where?

Source: From two letters to Lord Stanley, Liverpool Record Office, Derby Collection 920/15/35 and 37

4 March 1864

*Private.* Probably you have forgotten a correspondence we had (in December) as to the difficulty of a proper system of sewerage and drainage in a country with dry seasons. I stated that we had established such at drier stations than any in India. And I proposed to send you our report on the Mediterranean stations (it possesses a great interest for me, for it was the last request made by me and granted by Sidney Herbert before his death).

Of course you will have this report in the regular manner. But you may not take notice of it. So I venture to send you my copy, which I get rather sooner than the House of Commons. Will it be giving you too much trouble to ask you to return it?

If you have time, in the midst of your hard duties, to look at it, you will find the gist of the whole matter, both defects and remedies, in the first twenty-two pages. These, with the "pictures," give a very fair idea of the *Indian* subject, except that all the improvements for *India* need to be on a greater scale, with more water, more cubic space in barracks and hospitals, more complete ventilating arrangements, more constant attention to sanitary police. (By the way, we hear there is to be a debate on the cession of the Ionian Islands [to Greece]. If England has done so little for them, as shown by this report, I think the sooner we give them up, the better.)

Pray let me take this opportunity of saying, with regard to your not moving in the House for our Indian enemies, that I not only submit to your judgment, but do so with my head in the dust, like a Roman Catholic before his superior. It is a matter upon which I have (and can have) absolutely no opinion. And I was almost sorry I expressed a wish.

Also let me say I did not mean to complain of Lord de Grey [secretary of state for war], in the matter desired by Sir John Lawrence. Lord de Grey does everything he can for us. It is not likely he should have the weight with crown, Cabinet, commander-in-chief and Parliament that S. Herbert had. But he is willing (Sir G. Lewis was not). It would be most ungrateful of me to complain of Lord de Grey, especially as this is such a new matter, that the respective jurisdictions are all uncertain and confused. But we are getting on.

15 March 1864

*Confidential.* In answer to your very kind note of 12 March: the "delay" I am sorry to say, arises from Lord de Grey's inability, I will not say unwillingness, to be *snubbed* by Sir C. Wood. The "exact thing waiting to be done" is to make the Horse Guards and the India Office carry out certain of your recommendations, which do not belong to the War Office to do. Of this more presently.

## John Lawrence's Early Viceroyalty

**Editor:** When he assumed the viceroyalty in January 1864, Sir John Lawrence was clearly Nightingale's best chance for substantial reform in India, practically through the implementation of the royal commission recommendations. Nightingale's high hopes were generally fulfilled. She was pleased with his early measures, as the first items in this section show. That is why she was bitterly disappointed when the India Office let him down in the events surrounding the sending of *Suggestions.*

It seems that already before leaving England he had asked for guidance concerning the precise functions of the presidency sanitary commissions. On 5 February 1864 he wrote: "I hope that you will expedite the transmission to India of the codes and rules and plans which have been approved of for home and the colonies."[26] He was therefore waiting for a "guide" to determine the kind of sanitary work the presidency commissions should do. Because of negligence at the India and War Offices he was to wait a long while, many times renewing his request. Nightingale's correspondence in the next months is full of impatient reminders that the delay in helping Lawrence was totally irresponsible. She told Sir James Clark that Sir John Lawrence was "mad with our delay."[27] She pressed the issue all the more eagerly since she herself seemed to have been at the origin of Lawrence's request for guidance, which might be implied in her statement of 2 November 1863 to C. Trevelyan: "First among the home commission's duties should be to draw up a scheme for carrying out the recommendations of the royal commission, i.e., the laying down of principles in regard to details of sanitary works for India" (see p 471 below), and in her further statement of 1 December 1863 to Lord Stanley: "He [Lawrence] might desire the home commission to send all the information and suggestions . . . " (see p 265 above), both statements made prior to Lawrence's visit to her. Moreover, for many weeks prior to December 1863, Nightingale had been involved in devising and drafting a "sanitary code for India" (see p 256 above), which can be viewed as the first stage of the *Suggestions.* At last the process started for good some time in June, and resulted in the final writing and sending of the *Suggestions* in July.

Thereafter, again at Lawrence's request, she wrote her scheme for female nursing (1865). Communication went on during and after his viceroyalty and his return to England. Those further items are covered below, the present section being limited to 1864 and early 1865.

In her enthusiasm for Lawrence she was to declare: "We have but one Sir John Lawrence" (see p 212 above). "He is the Ramesses II of Egypt. . . . All the ministers are rats and weasels by his side" (see p 622 below). She called him "Hercules" (see p 196 above). On Lawrence's death she told W.E. Gladstone that she had been "privileged to know and serve with two such men as Sidney Herbert and John Lawrence."[28]

---

26 Letter 5 February 1864, Add Mss 45777 ff31-32. See Cook, *The Life of Florence Nightingale* 2:46-48.

27 Copy of a letter 7 April 1864, Wellcome RAMC 1139/S4/26.

28 Letter 6 July 1879, *Society and Politics* (5:479).

Of Sir Bartle Frere, whom she admired, she said: "He impressed me wonderfully—more than any Indian I have ever seen except Sir John Lawrence" (see p 571 below).

Source: From a letter to Robert Rawlinson, Boston University 1/3/41

16 February 1864

*Private.* We are very anxious not to hurry you, knowing how laden with a weight of work you are already. This is only a reminder that, when you can let us have your "water supply," the work of the War Office/Indian commission can go on. And Sir John Lawrence was very urgent that their general scheme for sanitary works should be sent out as soon as possible.

Source: From two letters to Douglas Galton, Add Mss 45762 ff73-74 and 76-77

10 March 1864

*Private.* In the enclosed little tidy bag came a letter from Sir John Lawrence, dated 6 February. He has done all we asked, and more than we asked, and in our way, not in his, about the presidency commissions of health. But he is greatly disappointed that there are no signs yet of *our* having done what *he* asked. Poor man! he really expects despatch, he thinks we can write a letter in three months!! (He must be more fit for a lunatic asylum than for a governor generalship.)

Do pray get those plans and "suggestions" ready, as soon as ever you can. And do pray do something about General Pears's letter. (*I* had a letter from General Pears this morning—an unexpected pleasure.) I shall write to Lord de Grey in the course of today about Sir J. Lawrence's matters. But I suppose he is now at the christening.

2. The following list of books is wanted for India. I have written to Mr Rawlinson to have the Local Government Act Office part put up ready for you. Sir J. Lawrence took these all out with him (to look at during the voyage) from me. Dr Sutherland thinks the best way will be for the next meeting of the Barrack and Hospital Improvement Commission to send out these reports in its name, if you will be so good as to have them ready.

11 March 1864

I am entirely miserable about Sir John Lawrence. He is very much surprised that our "views" have not arrived on *6 February*!! This is 11 March, and our "views" are not on the way. It will be three months from this time, at least, before he receives them. And it may be *six months* from the time he appointed our Bengal commission of health, which, he says, is prepared to go the whole extent of our "views," that they may sit without them. Pray urge forward the plans and printing as much as you can.

As to the other: I refer to the list of points I drew up for Lord de Grey. There was some doubt as to who was responsible for carrying out each. And you asked General Pears. General Pears's answer is not relevant, according to yours of yesterday. He says that *they* have written out to India about the sale of spirits, day and recreation rooms and workshops. This was in the first letter sent out with the India commission report. But how much remains to be done before the recommendations are complied with! And we have still to find out who is responsible for dealing with them.

You have double government throughout. The India government provides (say) workshops; you must provide that the men are encouraged to use them. The India government discourages the sale of spirits. You must see that the regimental regulations do the same, so of other points. Of course it does not matter how the improvements are carried out, provided they are carried out.

Source: From three letters to Lord Stanley, Liverpool Record Office, Derby Collection 920/15/36-38

12 March 1864

*Private and Confidential.* I heard from your great man and mine, Sir John Lawrence, by last mail. His letter was dated 5 February. He has done all you asked, and in your way, not in his. He has appointed the Bengal Commission of Health: capital men—three of them I know—representing the five different interests you recommended. He has made a civilian [J. Strachey] the president and the responsible executive, and this is to be his sole work—quite enough, one would think, for one man (even were he Hercules with his twelve labours). He has also made a *secretary* [J.P. Walker] with this as his sole work. Nothing can be more in conformity with your recommendations than the whole proceeding, as far as Sir John Lawrence is concerned. He says that he would have created the commission of health for Bengal immediately on his arrival, but that your two-folio report did not arrive till February (you know he ascertained, before he left, that the copies had been sent round by the Cape "by mistake"). The two-folio copy seems to have taken the Indians aback, from the (too) intimate knowledge it betrays that you had as to the state of their stations.

At least I augur this from the fact that Mr Strachey,[29] C.S., who is the author of that India cholera report which has been suppressed in

29 John Strachey, president of the Bengal Sanitary Commission from 1864.

England, and from which I sent you a most astounding extract, containing revelations as to the state of the stations which we had no idea of (I have since received a "confidential" copy from India, which is much at your service, but it is very *nasty*), this Mr Strachey, when Sir J. Lawrence did me the honour to discuss with me the appointments to your "commission of health" in Bengal, I suggested. And Sir J. Lawrence answered that nothing would induce Mr Strachey to accept such an appointment for any money, as he had been worried out of his life about his cholera report. I conclude, from his accepting the appointment, that the reception of the two-folio report has considerably modified Indian opinion and quickened their wits as to the desirableness of doing something.

If the governor general is for us, as you said, I do not mind, however, who is against us![30]

But Sir John Lawrence is grievously disappointed that, whereas he has done all we asked, we have not yet done what he asked. He implies that his health commission is quite ready to go the whole length of our "views." And he asks why we don't send our "views." He asks this on 5 February. On 12 March our "views" are not on the way. And I very much fear that his commission may have been sitting six months waiting for our "views" before they come. (Poor man! he really expected dispatch! he really thought the War Office could get ready a document in three months! he must be fitter for a lunatic asylum than for a governor generalship.)

This part of the matter is very distressing. *Our* part of the work was ready almost as soon as Sir J. Lawrence started. But the double, nay treble jurisdiction there is in everything concerning the Indian Army, also the delays of the plan—designers and the printers—*I* am *fit* for a lunatic asylum with them all. The matter has turned out the very reverse of what we expected. India has done its part at the other end. And at our end it has *not.*

Sir J. Lawrence winds up with saying, "without such a guide" (our "codes" and "rules" and "plans") "we shall often be perhaps working in direct opposition to your views. Where we differ, it will become our duty to set forth the grounds for so doing, in sending our plans and reports home."[31]

---

30 An allusion to Luke 9:50.
31 Add Mss 45777 ff31-32.

Sir John Lawrence has certainly brought in a new day for India, as in sanitary things, so in others. . . .

Pray consider whatever may come through me (about this) really "confidential." Of course Sir J.L. tells the I.O. himself what he thinks fit. You have perhaps forgotten that you gave me a hint to give Sir J.L. before he started, as to conciliating the "*millingtary*" [military]. I did so.

15 March, continued 17 March 1864

The War Office mind appears to have been stirred up, like the Indian mind, during the last four days. And during this time, the proofs from the printers and the plans from the designers—for barracks and stations and sanitary schemes—have been pouring in. This was what Sir John Lawrence more particularly insisted upon, viz., the "delay" which the joint War Office and India Office commission has been guilty of in sending out its plans to his (Bengal) commission, when they are so good as to wish to be taught.

I am sorry to say we cannot have a meeting of the said (home) commission till after the 26th owing to Sir Proby Cautley's absence from the I.O. Sir P. Cautley writes, "It is most desirable that they the (papers) should reach India as soon as possible, so as to be in the hands of the (Bengal) commission in their early sittings." But meanwhile he does not come back. However, I dare say we shall hardly be ready before the 26th, as we have had to correct both plans and papers, and I have only today sent to Mr Rawlinson, the Local Government Act Office engineer (who did the water supply and drainage part) *his* part to correct. If we can send the plans and papers in to the I.O. soon after the 26th (and they will forward the whole immediately to India), although *this* is too bad of us, still it is better than I had dared to expect.

But *this* is comparatively straightforward, though aggravating from its blundering delays, when Sir John Lawrence had made such virtuous haste on his side. The rest (the "exact things waiting to be done") is the real difficulty. Here please glance at the enclosed lists.

Here is the difficulty. And, except that everybody has been using the most violent language to everybody, we are just where we were three months ago. And Sir J. Lawrence complains that we *are* so, while his part is quite and completely done, as far as Bengal.

Three months ago, Lord de Grey asked me to draft a letter for him to Sir C. Wood, embodying those of your recommendations, out of Nos. 1 to 13, which the India Office must carry out. "For," he says, "the Indian Army is under Sir C. Wood and Sir C. Wood must write out to general officers in India, as the W.O. writes out to general officers in colonies. The W.O. has no direct communication with the Indian Army." (This is not quite true. But that is not my business.)

Two months ago, a meek little letter was written by W.O. to General Pears, inquiring some preliminaries, in order to draft the great letter to Sir C. Wood. A very terrible letter came back from General Pears, saying that Sir C. Wood HAD recommended what he thought fit and did not want any interference from the W.O. The poor W.O. shut up directly—or rather not directly, but went shilly-shallying on, doing nothing, till 10 March, Lord de Grey sounding Sir C. Wood, Sir C. Wood *snubbing* Lord de Grey and telling him to mind his own business (Lord de Grey is a humble and a vain man, and that makes a man pedantic and that gives a man a mortal dislike of being snubbed and makes him think a great deal about his "influence." Sidney Herbert had influence, without ever thinking about it. Lord de Grey has none, by thinking too much about it. Besides, it is no doubt difficult for a man to act as colleague to a minister whose under secretary he has been. But, as I am not making a psychological study of Lord de Grey, I had better go on to facts). Therefore.

We have besides another difficulty, which is that, whatever the commander-in-chief in England [the duke of Cambridge[32]] recommends to the commander-in-chief in India [Sir Hugh Rose], *he* does *all the* LESS for being recommended. Also, it appears that when her majesty makes regulations for her troops, the Queen's Regulations do not obtain when her troops are in India. (I can hardly believe it.)

However, when I proposed three months ago (by Sir J. Lawrence's desire) that Lord de Grey should write to the duke of Cambridge about those of your recommendations which are purely Horse Guards and War Office, Lord de Grey told me the above. The reason I don't quite believe it is that this is the very act to which they now have determined themselves after three months' delay.

I was to have received a copy of this letter to the Horse Guards, that I might communicate with Sir John Lawrence by this day's mail. And I also waited for this in order to show it to you, before writing to you. But as it was only three *days* ago since the W.O. made up its noble mind to this manoeuvre, it is not to be supposed that the letter can be written in three days. And it is not.

32 Prince George, duke of Cambridge (1819-1904), the longest serving head of the British Army, commander-in-chief for thirty-nine years.

I have now written the exact state of things with regard to each one of your recommendations. Pray excuse me that it is so long. I believe I could have *told* it so as to be less tiresome. But (1) I have been quite laid up. (2) I did not like to *waste* your kind offer of a visit, hoping to turn it to account soon, when we really see our way. With regard to your kind offer of acting for us yourself, I see that Lord de Grey would rather you did *not* urge *him*, would rather you *did* urge Sir C. Wood. Because he, Lord de Grey, *is* willing, even anxious, but not able. Sir C. Wood *is* able but not willing. It is awkward for Lord de Grey to have to tell you he would, but he can't. Of course I have nothing to advise with regard to your speaking to Sir C. Wood, although you are so kind as to ask the question. I am afraid he will say, "*I* have done all I can. We must wait till we hear from India." In that case, we are just where we were, viz., to act through Sir John Lawrence and to make him act on Sir Hugh Rose. (But there is no occasion to *make him act*, as I have incorrectly put it.) I saw him, however, once, immediately after he had seen the duke of Cambridge. And he was eager in wishing that the *Horse Guards* should put down the canteen system, at least, from here and in saying that no way else could it be done. Please to remember that the whole of this is "confidential." If you act, you will of course act from yourself. Sir J. Lawrence, of course, writes to India Office himself what he thinks fit. . . . Did I mention that Sir J. Lawrence asks us to write a sanitary code for his commissions, as well as the work we are doing for him? I think *we* had better write the duties, and *they* codify. He also asks for all old reports and manuals for his commissions. I have sent out three sets, one for each presidency commission, of all board of health reports, etc., and all W.O. sanitary ditto. There *is no* manual. . . . I shall write again, with your permission, in a day or two because your offer to act for us is too good to be wasted.

19 March 1864

*Confidential.* The War Office have really written a letter, not, of course, in time for the Indian mail of yesterday. But it is really written, and sent to the Horse Guards with "Immediate" over it, dated 15 March 1864 (when it ought to be 15 August 1863, the date of Sir C. Wood's despatch).

This letter contains the following points out of your recommendations:

1. the discontinuance or limitation of the sale of spirits in regimental canteens, and the more extended use of beer, coffee, etc.,

2. the suppression as far as possible of the sale of spirits in bazaars,

3. the superintendence of cooking by (European) regimental cooks (even the regimental cooks, already gone out with their regiments to India, complain that they are not employed and have no control over the cooking),

4. making gymnastics a parade,

5. employing men in trades where workshops have been provided, and promoting soldiers' gardens.

The letter proposes that Sir Hugh Rose be requested to consider these various points in conference with the India government, and to report what measures are most applicable for meeting the recommendations of your commission. The letter treats of regimental points only, with which the military authorities in India must deal by means of the commanding officers.

I am to write to Sir J. Lawrence on the 26th and expound the doings of the War Office (very difficult) and send him some very good practical experience we have just had on trades. He is very strong on the point.

It is a very odd thing that nobody knows even now who are responsible for *regimental* reforms, nor who are to carry out your *regimental* recommendations.

We are going to try now how far the new army medical regulations of 1859 (sanitary and statistical) can be introduced into India by the director general here, before any other step is taken.

I am going to send you a proof of the paper of "Suggestions" which included the duties of the officer of health, to be sent out by the (home) commission to the presidency commissions at Sir J. Lawrence's desire. If the War Office has not sent you one, it is because it is not ready.

Source: From a letter to Robert Rawlinson, Boston University 1/3/42

26 March 1864

*Confidential.* We are getting on (about India) although by no means so fast as I could have wished. For Sir John Lawrence writes to urge haste and his own health is so uncertain that he has only accepted India for two years. Perhaps he may not even live as long.

Sir Proby Cautley has seen your paper. He acquiesces in everything except one or two points, which are the very ones you yourself have doubted, viz., those where you will find a pencil mark thus (?) and which might seem like teaching Indian engineers, who are particularly touchy. He proposes not to destroy the type but to transfer it to an appendix.

Would you be so very good as to look over the engineering detail and mark passages which an engineer of ordinary education ought to know? All *strictly sanitary* points should be kept in text. *General engineering* principles only might be divided as proposed, between text and appendix.

Sir P. Cautley says they don't make tanks in India as in England (*as you say too*). He says all material for embankments is more or less plastic. It is carried by coolies in baskets on their heads and the whole mass trodden down solid by incessant walking of hosts of labourers, each carrying a few lbs. of earth and treading it down. They never use puddle walls, as the entire mass is solidified and made watertight.

I dare say you know all this as well as he does. Will you be good enough to return the proof to me after you have marked the passages which may be taken out? (The last page is gone to press, as we have considerably enlarged the registration part.)

We hope to have a meeting of commission on Monday week. I wish we could have had it before!

Source: From a letter to Douglas Galton, ADD Mss 45762 f88

5 April 1864

*India Army Sanitary Report (Abstract).* We send you back the (confounded) proof of the volume. We want it made up in the 8vo form, to correct it before printing off. Please tell them to send two proofs *here.*

Source: From a letter to Charles Hathaway, Florence Nightingale Museum, typed copy ADD Mss 45782 f142

11 April 1864

As regards the dead of Calcutta: they should either be disposed of below the city at high tide or in another branch of the river as suggested. There must be plenty of wood in the Sunderbuns for cremation. And if you have to supply it to the poor, it would be nothing more than is done in England, where the parishes bury the dead poor at the public expense. Could you not contrive some machinery for stopping the dead descending from the Ganges, and either burning or burying them above Calcutta? Under a general system whereby the state found wood for the poor, the evils might perhaps best be remedied.

Source: From two letters to Lord Stanley, Liverpool Record Office, Derby Collection 920/15/39 and 40

14 April 1864

*Private.* I bear in mind that you said you could not look at any more of our papers after 18 April. And I am very sorry for it, for our sakes, not yours.

I think you will like to see the first minute of our first commission, as Sir John Lawrence calls it, sent me by him. It has made a great disturbance at Calcutta. It is strictly private. Please return it to me, that I may answer it by the mail of the 18th. Their great difficulty now is that the police is under the government, the officer of health under the municipality. We have settled this difficulty satisfactorily in England. And Sir John Lawrence asks me to send him out all the information on the subject.

There is no doubt that this minute is an immense step. And the reform has begun.

I shall venture to send you some other papers before *your* "18th." Sir John Lawrence scarce lets a mail pass without sending me something. I have his minute on the commissariat report. But as the India Office has not yet received the commissariat report, it is not of much use to us.

India is now far ahead of us in carrying out your sanitary things. It is we who are hanging back, not they, in forwarding your "recommendations."

15 April 1864

*Private.* I send you three documents all sent me by Sir J. Lawrence. Please be so good as to return them all to me, at your convenience.

1. Sir J. Lawrence's minute about the commissariat report, which very likely you have and about which I sent you Sir C. Trevelyan's minute of 22 September 1863. Please consider this really private, as (29 March at least) the India Council here had neither commissariat report nor Sir J. Lawrence's nor Sir C. Trevelyan's minutes.

2. A pamphlet about officer of health's duties.

3. A newspaper article by (as I understand) Sir J. Lawrence's private secretary.

What comes out of all this is:

1. that your commission by no means overstated the case,

2. that the Bengal commission is beginning in the right direction and vigorously.

Lord de Grey *says* that *he* is "in a right course" too. He says that he "called" (4 April) "on the director general to report on the best mode of applying the medical regulations to India." He referred the question of victualling on board ship to the joint I.O. and W.O. (home) commission. (And they adopted the scale obediently, just as we told them.) And he has sent in the letter for Sir Hugh Rose to the Horse Guards about the regimental reforms.

The joint (home) commission passed the building plans for India last Monday. But (unfortunately) Garibaldi's[33] entry distracted the attention of our enthusiastic chairman, Sir Richard Airey. And he rushed off, without finishing the business. I shall not fail to send you a copy, when it is done, as also, having your kind permission, anything Sir J. Lawrence sends me.

As to the mistake of the Calcutta spasmodic effort about dead bodies in the Hugli,[34] it first allowed the law to remain in abeyance, *without* making any provision for otherwise disposing of the dead; then it spasmodically puts an end to the present system and that too in the height of an epidemic. What they want is either a public burning establishment, or else to carry the dead to another branch of the river. The first the best; it could be done by retorts (like gas making) without nuisance, as was done 1800 years ago at Pompeii.

Source: From a letter to Robert Rawlinson, Boston University 1/3/43

19 April 1864

*Private.* We are almost in despair at the loss of time inflicted on Sir John Lawrence. To expedite matters, as you said you would wish to make some additions in drainage and water supply, I send you back that part and will ask you, to save time to make your additions on this proof. . . .

If the plans had been passed, we could have completed the proof. But as there will still be a delay of some days in passing them, it would save time to have all the matter ready to proceed to press with, immediately after the next meeting of the commission. This is why I trouble you.

33 Giuseppe de Garibaldi (1807-82), made a triumphant visit to London in April 1864, speaking in Parliament and being widely feted. His meeting with Nightingale is described in *European Travels* (7:335-36).

34 Dead bodies were routinely disposed of in Bengal by throwing them into the river Hugli.

Source: From two letters to Douglas Galton, Add Mss 45762 ff116 and 120-21

3 May 1864

We have detained your director general's draft of medical regulations for India, which seems to have been very well considered, because we want to abstract from it into our proof of Indian "Suggestions" the sanitary duties of inspecting and regimental officers. We shall then return you the director general's draft with our comments.

4 May 1864

This proposal of the director general to substitute a quarterly for a monthly report from foreign stations is another illustration of the way in which regulations and warrants are rendered nugatory in the army from not bringing common sense to bear on their administration. 7.(2). p 93 states that the monthly reports are to be sufficiently detailed to enable the principal medical officer and director general "to ascertain that every necessary precaution for protecting health of troops has been in use." The obvious method of administering this regulation, so as to prevent unnecessary repetition, is simply at all ordinary times to state whether the circumstances remain the same as during preceding period reported on, or whether any change, and if so what, has occurred. If nothing has occurred, the monthly report may go into a line. If epidemic disease has occurred, it may require twenty pages.

The evil of the director general's proposal is that at tropical stations the health of a regiment might be deteriorating for "a quarter," and yet the director general knows nothing about it. Tell him to draft a note for principal medical officers allowing them to administer the regulation, as pointed out. And let us see it before he sends it out.

Source: From a letter to Lord Stanley, Liverpool Record Office, Derby Collection 920/15/41

14 May 1864

You wished to see any papers sent by Sir John Lawrence, which showed the practical working of your royal commission.

One of the three I send I think you have seen before (in a different form). It shows that we have been abused, and I particularly for my little paper, for telling in a very mild form the half of what they themselves tell in a very strong form.

The two others (discussion and minute), inasfar as they relate to vice-disease,[35] would be good, were the facts reliable. But in the absence of

35 Vice was a code word for prostitution, hence syphilis, the disease of vice.

any correct posology of the disease, and in the absence of any statement of data on which the foreign facts rest, there is nothing, absolutely nothing, in the papers to alter the position of the question, as laid down in your report. And much to regret in that they did not state your conclusion as to this matter, viz., that occupation and such like are the best remedy for vice.

If you could return me these papers by Monday, you would much oblige me, as Tuesday is the India mail. . . .

I wrote some time ago to India all our methods in England as to connection between magistrates, police, municipalities and officers of health in sanitary matters.

Source: From a letter to Douglas Galton, Add Mss 45762 ff128-29

18 May 1864

I think the director general's proposal to issue "drinks" to patients on "low diet" is an improvement. Not so the purveyor's to remove the *butter* from the "diets" and make it an extra. When the diet table was drawn up, *butter* was one of the substances required to complete the elements. To withdraw the butter would involve the rearrangement of the entire scale, the finding a substitute for the butter and increasing the cost.

And let me tell you that when you want butter, it is not a substitute to give you a "drink," though I perceive that is the way you treat me, for when I want the butter of the Indian "Suggestions," which Sir J. Lawrence is crying out for *for five months*, yes, for five months, you give me the wishy-washy barley water of the abstract.

Source: From a letter to Robert Rawlinson, Columbia University, Presbyterian Hospital School of Nursing C69

19 May 1864

We are precluded by our instructions from entering on the subject of your memorandum. We have indeed been obliged to alter materially in principle the proof of the "Suggestions" (which you saw) on account of feeling shown at the I.O. In all matters relating to temporary means of dealing with epidemics, the Indian code is very good, and in some respects in advance of anything we have here. The great thing is to make them carry out what they have.

Sir A. Tulloch's almost sudden death and grievous loss will I am sure be felt by you.

Source: From four letters to Lord Stanley, Liverpool Record Office, Derby Collection 920/15/42, 43 and 45

21 May 1864

*Private.* With pardonable exultation (as if a patient escaped out of a lunatic asylum) I send you the enclosed. For six months Sir John Lawrence has been expecting *in vain* the scheme of sanitary suggestions, which he asked for before his departure and which was then all but ready. Now, never weary in serving us against our will, he desires Mr Strachey, the president of his Bengal health commission, to write us the enclosed. Now we are all in activity. I told Sir J. Lawrence that nothing but a blue foolscap printed minute, with a (very high) printed No. in the left-hand top corner, would "do it." Poor man! he did not see the virtues of the blue minute. But he does now.

The W.O. aggravates me, as usual, by telling me "that our delay has lost us nothing," that "we now are *asked* for plans for India," "which puts us in a good position." It is because "our delay" had lost us everything that Sir J. Lawrence gives us another chance, by trying the blue minute and *summonsing* us officially.

The W.O. might as well say, when the bailiffs are at the door and in execution, that they have "lost no time" in paying their debts. However, all's well that ends well. We have lost six months of Sir J. Lawrence's two years (you know he has only gone out for two years). And I had begun to think that we had lost the noblest game ever W.O. had to play, with a governor general, as it were, delivered into its hands. For it is not every governor general who will ask of a W.O., What would you have me to do? Sir J. Lawrence said as plainly as so modest a man could say it: "This is a thing" (viz., forcing our sanitary plans upon India) "I must do by my own personal influence. Regimental reforms you must do from your Horse Guards in England." He has repeated this in nearly every letter.

However, I will not enter into a detailed panorama of my grievances and disappointments. I write this only because you wished to be kept "au courant" of the workings of your commission. Indeed you were right when you said, if Sir John Lawrence were for us, no man could be against us. God bless him.

Please return me the enclosed as soon as possible. I ought to return it to the War Office on Monday. (Perhaps the concentrated essence of a blue minute evaporates.)

28 May 1832 [1864]

The enclosed is from the *secretary* of the Bengal commission of health; you perhaps may like to see it. Pray return it to me. You will see how great are the practical consequences of your royal commission. Of course we think this man is wrong in certain points. But that can't be helped. And Sir J. Lawrence has repeatedly used this very argument to induce us to hasten that sanitary scheme and plans which I should believe a fate was against, if there were fate. But the strongest power in the whole world is *want of* power—inertia—the only thing which cannot be overcome.

28 May 1864

I have not heard one word from Sir John Lawrence about his health since he left England.

It is clearly the duty of Sir C. Wood to act upon what he hears from Sir J. Lawrence alone and not upon anything which comes to him through a third and a fourth person. I fancied I had made a general preface (to all my letters to you) that nothing in them was to go farther than yourself, unless you found it was otherwise known. But, in this case, there is nothing to know, i.e., since Sir J. Lawrence left England.

No one knows better than Sir C. Wood that *he* would be the first to hear of it from Sir J. Lawrence himself, if a private estimate were to become of public importance. My reference (to what had passed *before* Sir J. Lawrence left England) was simply made in regard to the time lost by the W.O. and I.O. commission in sending out what Sir J. Lawrence had asked for *so urgently and repeatedly*. It would be black ingratitude on my part towards Sir J. Lawrence, who can, of course, communicate what he pleases to the India Office directly, to make difficulties in his path.

Pray throw any blame you please upon me to Sir C. Wood. I do not feel in the least *deprecatory* but, rather than bring any difficulty in Sir J. Lawrence's way, you may call me gossip or busybody or anything else.

6 June 1864

I had a letter from Sir John Lawrence by this mail, dated "Simla, 6 May." He is extremely indignant at the non-arrival of our sanitary schemes. After graciously and *contemptuously* accepting (like a great man, as he is) our Mediterranean report, out of which he hopes to "gain some"thing, but not much (you will perhaps remember that in General Pears's letter, enclosing the minute from Mr Strachey, president of the Bengal Sanitary Commission, "Sir C. Wood presumed that" we should use *this* as our scheme for reforming India in sanitary things), Sir John Lawrence goes on to say "but our great want is your standard plans and rules, without which we are quite at sea *and, so far from doing better than formerly,* shall *be in danger of doing worse.* As it is now, the reconstruction of some of our worst barracks is at a standstill, until we get these documents."

It would have been a broad farce, if it had not been so deeply painful, to hear Sir C. Wood's, General Pears's and Sir P. Cautley's reiterations that they could not possibly send out our sanitary plans and schemes "for fear of irritating the government in India," when I was hearing by nearly every mail from the head of that government (personally or by his people) all the permutations and combinations that could be made out of these phrases: that they were "at a standstill" for want of these plans and suggestions, that they were "quite at sea" in consequence of our delay, that they were "in danger of doing worse" and that it was all our fault.

Are all official assurances of the nature of Sir C. Wood's ("Let us by a song conceal our purposes"—vide Canning) and Sir P. Cautley's? Sir John Lawrence goes on to describe his inspections of diverse stations and barracks. He also writes (of the soldiers' libraries) that there is a great improvement, that Sir Hugh Rose has done much *in re* workshops, that he has "issued a G.O. reducing the dram of spirits which a soldier can have, one half." (You know he, Sir J. Lawrence, was very anxious that the sale of spirits in regimental canteens and bazaars should be entirely discontinued. I hope this is a step.)

*Private.* Sir J. Lawrence mentions casually (and as an apology!! for not having inspected two stations) that he has had a "sudden attack of illness." But he writes as if he were well. And I should not have mentioned this, if I did not know you wished to be kept *au fait.* It certainly is not my duty to keep the India Office "au fait"—nor my wish.

I cannot sing for joy loud enough at Sir J. Lawrence's government, for whose appointment we are in a great measure indebted to you.

Source: From a letter to Douglas Galton, Add Mss 45762 ff135-36

14 June 1864

N.B. I have had more letters from India by this last mail reminding me that it is *six months* (this last week) since Sir John Lawrence urged the *immediate* sending out of plans and sanitary suggestions, and that it is *twelve months* (all but three weeks) since the India sanitary report came out. I make no reply.

Source: From a typed copy of a letter to Charles Hathaway, ADD MSS 45782 ff153-55

18 June 1864

*Private.* Your account of the military department reply to the Indian Army sanitary report is much what we thought it would turn out to be. The whole question at issue is simply this: "What *is* a fair formula of mortality?" The Registrar-General's department and the royal commission say that, the longer the term of years you take (within limits), the safer you are. . . . [They] used all the annual tables at their disposal. (It is rather hard to be blamed for not using what they could not get. Although they applied to India for tables subsequent to 1856 and suspended their proceedings for a whole year to wait for these, none were sent subsequent to 1856.) It is no reply to the commission's tables to adduce years subsequent to 1856. They should show that the returns used for Table 10 are either incorrect or improperly used.

I could not help laughing at *your* critics who "exclude" specific diseases, such as "cholera," accidents "proving fatal," etc. (It is very convenient indeed to leave out all deaths that *ought not* to have happened, as *not having* happened. And it is certainly a new way of *preventing preventible* mortality to omit it altogether from any statement of mortality.) Then they would "exclude" "deaths above 60." Their principle, if logically carried out, is simply to throw out all ages and all diseases; and then there would be no mortality whatever. . . .

Mr Strachey's minute on the Calcutta jails exposes a state of horrors altogether inconceivable—and which, if known, would make a great outcry. . . . I have to thank you for the third section of Mr Strachey's cholera report. There is much experience in England about cholera which might be useful to India. . . . I think we could have improved the practical instructions in some important particulars.

Source: From four letters to Lord Stanley, Liverpool Record Office, Derby Collection 920/15/46-49

14 June 1864

*Private.* I had letters, by the last India mail, both from Calcutta and Simla. You will perhaps like to see the printed contents, which you will be so good as to return to me. (I am told that, as this kind of papers is *not* forwarded to the India Office, I am to consider them private. But I expressly stated that I should consider you the exception.)

The Simla letter is (briefly) this: that the papers sent to me, at different times, "will show you that nothing you have ever written or conceived of the horrible state and practices pursued at Calcutta comes up to the reality," that a "counter-blast or reply to the report" (of Lord Stanley) "has been prepared by the military department and submitted." (I do not know whether the India Office has noticed its receipt to you.) "Without actually denying that 6 percent *is* the real mortality when taken on the average of past years, they contend that it is not a fair way of stating the present mortality, or rather that the present mortality (which was as low as 2 percent for 1863) should only have been given" (it is rather hard to withhold "the present mortality" from your commission, which repeatedly wrote for it and delayed its proceedings for a year in consequence, and then to abuse it for *not* giving "the present mortality").

However, the India government seems roused to the truth, for the next sentence is a complaint that the very same absurd objection has been made to their (the government's) own statistics of jail (and other civil) mortality, the "authorities" stipulating that "cholera shall be left out," that such and such years and such and such diseases "shall be left out." (It is very convenient indeed in estimating mortality to say that all the deaths which *ought not* to have happened, shall be "left out," as *not having* happened. And it is certainly a new way of preventing preventible mortality to omit it altogether on a statement of mortality.)

The next sentence states that nearly the whole of the jail mortality *is* "preventible," that, in Bengal, the jail deaths are actually "10 percent" whereas "4 percent" has been (in the Punjab) and can be achieved, that the present condition of the jails "converts a sentence of brief imprisonment into one of capital punishment" "in many cases."

I have a letter from Sir J. Lawrence's private secretary, in which he says that, though Sir J. Lawrence has been ill "from excessive hard work," he has not been ill at all from climate and is very well now. He says, speaking on the subjects above: "It is indeed strange how such revolting, cruel and barbarous practices could have been pursued for years in the metropolis of India *by government officials* (sic) under the very eyes of different viceroys, living on the spot." (But, you will understand, that is not a kind of remark in which Sir J. Lawrence himself at all indulges.) The Calcutta (Bengal Sanitary Commission) letter merely says: they will adopt our "filter system" (in the Mediterranean) for their water, asks for advice on "recording of proceedings," etc. . . .

You will be glad to hear that work *from* India is coming in to the War Office commission. The plan for a Sabathu barrack, to be criticized here, arrived by last mail, "in compliance with the orders in Sir C. Wood's minute of 15 August." . . .

Lastly, I am bitterly reminded that it is six months plus a week since Sir J. Lawrence begged for *immediate* sending out of plans and sanitary works schemes, that it is *twelve months* all but three weeks since your report came out (8 July 1863). I make no reply; since government used the duke of Wellington, as they did in the Peninsula, I think there is no instance like that of a governor general actually *asking* for work from government at home and not getting anything but delays—or rather, we are the Spanish troops and the British government combined (against the duke of Wellington).

7 July 1864

*Private.* As you are engaged in unmaking ministries, I am inopportune. Here is the specification of sanitary work asked for, for India, by Sir John Lawrence this day seven months ago, upon the recommendations of your report, which came out this day *twelve* months ago.

Accompanying this specification are twenty-seven lithographs, of which seven only are original, the remaining twenty having been taken from our other "Local Government Act Office" and "War Office" works. To do seven original plans has therefore taken the W.O. seven months. Up to 20 May, the delay was occasioned principally by the India Office, which persisted in repeating that we should offend the India government by sending out plans, which the head of that government was asking for by every mail till at last he himself sent home a printed minute (at my request).

But the War Office is scarcely less to blame. For in fact, the whole of this work was nearly ready in December last, except the seven plans, which ought to be the seven wonders of the world, but are not. In short, I know that what Sir John Lawrence will say is: Is *that* what I have been kept waiting for these nine months? (which it will be before he receives them). Finally the *Bengal* presidency has not as yet received its copies of your two-folio report, as we hear by last mail.

I have had a passage-at-arms with the Horse Guards, which it is as well to tell you. They volunteered to tell me that they were aware of Sir J. Lawrence's "application and of the War Office delay" but that "it was Sir J.L.'s only interest" (sic) "whereas the W.O. was pressed by a thousand." To which I responded that the greatest living administrator, who rules over one tenth of the human race, who holds in his hand the destinies, territorial, communicational, international, judicial, of 120 millions—in endeavouring to bring health and civilization, for the first time, to his 120 millions—has been foiled by the torpid self-sufficiency of a petty peddling War Office, ruling over at most half a million ("cumbrous torpor" was poor Sidney Herbert's own word for his own office. It suffocated him, it ended by strangling him, like that horrible bronze colossus, in some legend, which throws its brazen arms round the wretched votary and strangles him) and this with the ease with which soldiers are ruled over compared with races—or words to that effect.

There was a great deal more. And I was a little afraid of spoiling Sir John Lawrence's affairs by too much vehemence. But, on the contrary (you must just choke the colossus back again, if you want to breathe), I received an ample apology for Sir J. Lawrence. I am about to send you a copy of the twenty-seven lithographs, also of the enclosed proof corrected, with your leave. I have to write to Sir J. Lawrence by the mail of the 10th.

9 July 1864

Accompanying this is the proof, completed, of which I sent you the uncorrected proof last Thursday. On 3 July the Horse Guards, in the form and countenance of Sir R. Airey, chairman of Barrack Improvement Commission, "pass" this valuable document—a year's growth, seeing that your report has been out just one year. It will then be sent to the India Office with three documents by the General-Register Office to illustrate Section VI on the method of introducing our registration system in India.

Owing to the impassable nature of the roads between Pall Mall and Victoria Street, a considerable delay will necessarily elapse before it can be even forwarded to Sir John Lawrence. But, as I do not live in that direction, I forward all these documents to him by the first India mail after completion. And I shall forward this to him as soon as it has passed the commission next Wednesday, 13. I trust that you will take into consideration the unprecedented haste that we have made, in that we have really completed this document in one year, which is twelve months, which comprises fifty-two weeks.

23 July 1864

*Private.* Here is the first (signed) copy of the first product of your parent commission. I send by book post to Sir John Lawrence direct a number of copies on Tuesday.

It is understood that sometime in the course of the present century the I.O. will send out copies officially. By the document's own showing, it is 7½ months since it was asked for. Of these, about 7½ days were occupied in real work. We understand that the surplus time was occupied by the military members learning to write their names. But, as Sir J. Lawrence and I have profited by your good hint "not to offend the military," we are silent on this fact.

"Occasional papers" have now to be written and sent out, containing explanatory matter. But, if it is expected that this can possibly be accomplished during Sir J. Lawrence's governorship, that expectation must be the offspring of a wild imagination.

The W.O. is utterly demoralized, the I.O. does not speak the truth, the Horse Guards deserve a V.C. [Victoria Cross] for their cool intrepidity in the face of facts.

But I conceal my opinion, as Sir J. Lawrence does his: that the native races are the recipients of civilization, but that the military authorities are a savage tribe whom kindness cannot tame nor suavity conciliate. Please, burn this note.

Source: From a letter to Charles Hathaway, Florence Nightingale Museum, typed copy Add Mss 45782 ff156-57

27 June 1864

Nothing was done, nor would ever have been done, had it not been for a printed minute (Mr Strachey's) from India (5 April) [reminding London of Lawrence's request].

Source: From a letter to John Strachey, Columbia University, Presbyterian Hospital School of Nursing C71

26 July 1864

*Private.* I send by this mail the *Suggestions* for sanitary works for Indian stations, drawn up in obedience to your minute of 24 March, forwarded to me by the Indian Office here on 20 May (dated 5 April). It is rather irregular my sending it to you direct. But you may perhaps like to see the first (signed) copy. And it is about to be forwarded officially in the usual manner to India by the India Office here.

Source: Typed copy of a letter, ADD Mss 45781 f233

32 South St.
London, W.
10 August 1864

*Private*

My dear Sir [James Pattison Walker][36]

I sent to you and to Mr Strachey copies of the *Suggestions* (by book post a fortnight ago) drawn up in compliance with Mr Strachey's minute of 5 April.

These *Suggestions* have now received the sanction of the military committee, of the Council and of the secretary of state of the India Office here. And they are about to be forwarded to you officially by the India Office.

But our people are so slow that, if I were not afraid of being profane, I should say that Sir John Lawrence is always a great deal more ready to hear than we are to pray.[37] Therefore I forward to you (by book post today) four more copies of the *Suggestions*, in case you may wish to apply them at once.

yours very faithfully
Florence Nightingale

## *Suggestions in Regard to Sanitary Works*, 1864

**Editor:** Before leaving for India as viceroy in December 1863, Sir John Lawrence had asked the War and India Offices for guidance in the application of the report of the royal commission. He wanted to be clear about the practical features of the sanitary reforms recommended by the commission, while knowing that such a guide would have to be adapted to Indian circumstances. He repeated his request in a letter dated 6 February 1864 and once more on 6 May from Simla. Because of incomprehensible administrative delays in London, Nightingale resolved in June to draft the *Suggestions* herself in consultation with Drs Sutherland and Farr, and Robert Rawlinson. Her proposals "were submitted to the Barrack and Hospital Improvement

36 James Pattison Walker (1823-1906), secretary of the Bengal Sanitary Commission. See the biographical sketch below in Appendix A.

37 An allusion to the collect for the Twelfth Sunday after Trinity in the Book of Common Prayer.

Commission and, with slight alterations, were adopted by that body" "in accordance with letters from the Secretary-of-State-for-India-in-Council"; in fact, they had been prepared by "Nightingale in accordance with the wishes of Sir John Lawrence."[38] Though mainly her work, Nightingale's name does not appear among the signatures. She herself sent copies to India at her own cost before the official document was mailed. This important document functioned as the charter of sanitary improvements to be implemented at the Indian stations. That it took so many months to reach India greatly embarrassed both Nightingale and Lawrence. Nightingale subsequently sent out these *Suggestions* to many people.

The recommendations are mainly of technical measures required to ensure health at Indian stations and surrounding "native" towns. They include minute details of the sewers and drains needed, the size and shape of pipes, materials used (should not be porous), water supply for toilets and washing facilities, etc., complete with illustrations. There are specifications for the minimum cubic space needed per man in barracks and hospitals, a subject to which Nightingale would often recur for ordinary hospital and workhouse infirmary construction. Comparative material from the U.K. is cited, notably the drains of Windsor Castle.

After all this detail on the material infrastructure come the requirements for administration: inspection, reporting (including a sample death return used in Marylebone) and remediation of defects. These measures, presented as essential to ensure the health of Indian nationals living nearby, are bold indeed. Nightingale and her colleagues were laying out a comprehensive and detailed scheme for a civil Public Health Department. Heading the list of the health officer's varied duties was: "It should be the special duty of the officer of health to keep a constant watch over the health of the population, particularly with regard to the occurrence of epidemic disease" (see pp 364-65 below). No wonder *Suggestions* caused such a storm and had to be repeatedly defended.

38 Cook, *The Life of Florence Nightingale* 2:48.

Source: *Suggestions in Regard to Sanitary Works Required for Improving Indian Stations*, prepared by the Barrack and Hospital Improvement Commission, 15 July 1864, Blue Book (London: Eyre and Spottiswoode 1864; revised edition 1882)

## Introduction

The following suggestions are intended to embody in a practical form those points of home experience in sanitary works and measures which appear to be more or less applicable to conditions brought out in evidence and described in the Report of the Royal Commission on the Sanitary State of the Indian Army. They are in no sense intended to fetter the judgment of local authorities, either military or civil, in India. It would indeed be impossible, without careful local examination, to lay down precise measures and works required for abatement of causes of disease at any given station. Such an examination can be conducted only by persons on the spot, and suitable works can best be designed for India by engineers of Indian experience. The sole advantage which this paper seeks to attain is to bring under the notice of local authorities in India and elsewhere those general principles and forms of procedure which have been found useful at home and which, it is hoped, with the required modifications, may be useful in India and in tropical stations generally.

The reports transmitted to the royal commission from Indian stations show that improvement of those stations includes the following elements:

1. A thorough drainage of ground occupied by stations;
2. An abundant supply of pure water distributed over stations;
3. The adoption of healthy principles of construction in barracks, including suitable provision of means of employment and recreation in the way of gymnasia, workshops, games, soldiers' gardens, reading and day rooms;
4. Improved principles of hospital construction;
5. Improving the sanitary police of stations, bazaars and adjacent native towns.

All these improvements require to be carried out more or less before it can be said of any station that every removable local cause of disease has been removed. It would be a grave error to trust to any one of them for improving the health of the troops. Each has its uses, but all are necessary. No improvement in barrack or hospital accommodation will compensate for a malarious subsoil or for bad water;

and, on the other hand, no improvements in drainage and water supply will neutralize the influence of an ill-ventilated, badly constructed, overcrowded barrack or hospital. And even if these works were carried out, much removable sickness would still exist, unless the men's leisure were profitably occupied and the sanitary police of bazaars and towns efficiently attended to.

When it is contemplated to erect barracks at any station, the question of improved construction should be considered as one only of the elements affecting the health of a station. All the points enumerated above should be carefully provided for at the same time and a consistent scheme drawn up for making the station habitable and healthy. In not a few cases this may possibly involve the question of whether a better site for a station than the one proposed to build upon may not be found within the strategic limits of the position. This point also should receive attention.

The next question of importance in the improvement of stations is the extent to which sanitary methods and appliances suitable for barracks in Europe would answer for barracks in India and in tropical stations generally. It is possible, for example, to subsoil drain any extent of ground in England. And this process is attended not only with increased productiveness but with improved health. Wherever subsoil water comes within a certain distance of the surface of the ground, it interferes with healthy vegetation and generates damp, fogs and malaria, which have been found to diminish or disappear when the water level has been lowered by drainage.

The universal prevalence of malarial disease at Indian stations indicates a malaria-generating condition of the earth. And one of the first improvements required is to diminish or remove this condition. But in order to do so there must be the necessary materials and skill for subsoil draining and an outlet for subsoil water. (At stations over which malaria is carried by winds from a distance, a screen of trees or of bamboos or other quickly growing vegetation will be useful in shielding the station from malaria. But this expedient should be considered as temporary only until the malaria is removed by drainage.)

The question, therefore, occurs whether proper drain tiles can be obtained or manufactured in India, or whether the same result could not be obtained by some equally efficient local expedient. The mere fact of difficulty should not be allowed to overbalance other considerations. Great difficulties were at first experienced in introducing land drainage in England, but they gradually disappeared as improvement advanced.

A similar remark applies to the question of town and barrack drainage. Not many years ago these improvements were as little known in many parts of England as they are at present in India, and much controversy and opposition preceded their introduction. Yet populous districts have been drained in the face of great difficulties, even where they not only had no fall, but were considerably below the level of the drainage outlet.

The introduction of this class of drainage works would of course necessitate the use of closed drainpipes or built drains, with a sufficient fall obtained either naturally or by mechanical methods, such as pumping. A sufficiency of water would be required for flushing these drains, but this could be readily afforded by waste water from baths and ablution rooms, or water might be carried by hand to a small flushing tank, if there be no pipe service. The ablution apparatus, latrines, etc., now extensively used in England, are new to India and other tropical countries, but they could be obtained either from England or manufactured in India. It is understood that excellent earthenware is made in India.

There would be some difficulty at first about fittings on account of the want of skilled labour, but this might be in time overcome by attaching trained workmen to each station or, what would be much better, by selecting from among the soldiers men who had formerly worked at the required trades or who might be trained to such work in the regimental workshops. There is reason to believe that almost every regiment would afford the requisite amount and kinds of skilled labour.

The accompanying barrack and hospital plans have been prepared on the supposition that works of drainage and water supply are to be carried out at stations, and that improved sanitary appliances are to be introduced in both classes of buildings.

We next proceed to give a few general principles, based on experience both in warm climates and in England, on each of the heads of improvement laid down above.

## Section I Drainage of Stations

### 1. Surface Drainage and Paving

(*Recommendation of the royal commission respecting drainage and water supply.* "8. That works of drainage and water supply be carried out at all stations.")

*Roof Gutters.* All rainwater from roofs within the limits of stations should be collected by eaves-gutters and either conducted to tanks for use after being filtered or passed directly into the drains of the station. The immediate surface surrounding buildings should be flagged or paved with closely jointed non-absorbent paving stones, with a sufficient slope to the surface channel to conduct water away from the building by carefully laid surface drains. In large stations, in cases where the surface becomes soft and sloppy, flagged or paved footpaths between the different buildings, properly raised and drained, should be provided for use in wet weather. The whole surface of the station, and also that of its vicinity, should be carefully levelled; all inequalities, pits and holes should be filled up and collections of surface water carefully drained away.

*Trenching.* Deep open trenches dug in the ground, although an excellent means of drainage for temporary camps, are not adapted for surface drainage of permanent stations. They are apt to become irregular and to retain water. They act partly as filters through which water passes into the subsoil, leaving its impurities to ferment in the drain and they are liable to be more or less filled up. Wherever open surface drains are required they should be formed of impervious material; they should be smooth and carefully laid so as to convey away water as speedily as possible.

*Paving.* Paving of towns is one of the first sanitary improvements that will tell on health. The material available for this purpose in India will vary in every district. In Europe almost every geological rock is used for paving. As much of the excellence of the surface depends on the manner of laying the material as on the material itself, hence great care should be bestowed on the workmanship. There is nothing better than flagged footways and roadways paved with close fitting square setts or well-laid macadam. Rubble and boulder paving of every kind should be avoided; these make a bad surface, difficult to cleanse. Small close courts and passages should all be flagged or paved.

A smooth surface, from which water readily runs off, is best suited for purposes of health. There should be carefully formed side drains for receiving and conveying away water. All roof water, if not tanked for use, should be collected by eaves-gutters and turned away from the foundations of houses. All gully-grates should be carefully trapped and all water-traps kept supplied with water.

Paved streets and roads are costly in their first formation and require skilled labour to prepare the stone and to lay it; but they are cheaper in maintenance than other roads when properly made. Paved streets are more easily cleansed than any other; they do not absorb organic matter and the air over them is less impure than over macadamized roads. The most recent and best paving in England is formed with the hardest granite or whinstone, not exceeding nine inches by three inches, and nine or twelve inches in length, set on edge; that is, in courses three inches wide and nine inches deep. The preparation for pavement will be in every respect as for road-making. The foundation should be carefully prepared, firm and well drained. A dry bed of evenly sorted gravel or of broken stone, as for road-making, not less than three inches in thickness, should be spread over the prepared subsoil, upon which the paving stones will be set in sand and then beaten down with a nine lbs. beater.

### 2. Sewerage and Drainage

*Surveys and levels.* As the question of drainage is intimately connected with the question of levels and of outlets, the first step to be taken before beginning the drainage of any station, town or district is to make a detailed survey, on a suitable working scale, of the whole area to be drained in order to settle the levels, with a view of ascertaining the fall and where the outlet should be placed.

*Subsoil drainage.* The great amount of miasmatic disease already mentioned shows that subsoil drainage is necessary as a means of prevention. Miasmatic diseases appear to be most severe at times when surface water, proceeding from heavy rainfall, water-logs the subsoil. It is not at all improbable that the generation of malaria, under such circumstances, is in its effect local rather than general and that, by removing subsoil water to a sufficient depth from the surface, the generation of local malaria may be to a large extent prevented. At many stations it would be in vain to attempt to remove the whole of the rainfall in this way. Well-formed impervious bottomed surface drains would afford the only possible outlet for heavy rains.

But heavy rains are less injurious to health than a wet or damp soil surcharged with organic matter under high temperature. Even in the cooler climate of England it has been found necessary for health to afford a ready means of exit for subsoil water from barrack and hospital grounds. This kind of work is usually carried out, like ordinary agricultural drainage, by means of drain tiles laid in lines 4 or 5 feet below the surface and 15 or 16 feet apart. We would strongly recommend that this improvement be tried at a few of the larger Indian stations and the effects of it upon the soil and upon the health of the men carefully noted.

The chief difficulty in low flat stations, where subsoil drainage is most required, is to find an outlet for water. The question of drainage outfall is, indeed, as important to a station as the question of water sources. In all new stations the outfall for drainage should be a special subject for inquiry and sites which are found to be defective in this respect should be rejected, just as they would be if there were no water. As regards existing stations, absence of outfall should be taken into account in determining whether a station is to be retained. But where a station must be held, an outfall must in some way be provided.

*General suggestions.* The following general suggestions respecting works of sewerage and drainage for stations, towns and districts are intended to embody the chief points of experience obtained in England and may be adopted in India so far as they may be found applicable under local and special peculiarities of surface, of contours, subsoil, rainfall and drought. Drainage sanitary works should aim at producing a dry and wholesome subsoil, a clean surface and a pure atmosphere around and within houses, barracks and hospitals. Defective surface contours may be improved by surface trenching and by providing safe and ready means of escape for surface water, by deepening, straightening and improving natural valley lines and watercourses or nullahs, as also by forming new surface conduits.

*Land drains.* Wet water-logged subsoils, where an available fall can be obtained, may be improved most cheaply by land drains. The depth to which such subsoil can safely be drained will depend on local peculiarities. Not less than six feet vertical depth ought to be attained for main land drains if practicable. Land drainage is applicable to the suburbs of towns and stations, to barrack yards and enclosed lands adjoining, to hospital sites and to lands surrounding hospitals or in their immediate vicinity. Tubular earthenware tiles from one inch to six inches internal diameter make the cheapest and best land drains.

All drain trenches must be set out perfectly true in line and must be bottomed true in gradient. The several lines should be parallel and all the junctions should be carefully made. The tiles should be laid in the trenches truly and evenly, with the joints sound, true and close. Filling in over the tiles should be most carefully performed, so as not to disturb the line of grade, nor break nor injure any tile or tile joint.

Manholes should be brought up to the surface at all main junctions of land drains, so that the working of the drains at these points may be inspected from time to time. The mouth of the outlet drain should be protected with a fine wire grate or by some other efficient means to prevent the drains being choked from without.

If drains are injured during the hot and dry season, on account of drying and cracking in the ground, such drains should be repaired and made good before the rains commence.

Land drains should not be used to convey away surface water other than filters through the soil. There must not be any direct communication from the surface, such as a grate or gully. Sewers and drains must be provided separately for surface and refuse water. Land drains should not be laid near tree roots nor amongst rank vegetation, but should be adopted for cleared and open spaces, where a dry subsoil is essential to health.

Every district, not an absolute swamp or area embanked in from tides or land floods, will have surface fall and natural valley lines. The removal of surface water, in dry and in wet seasons, should be provided for at the surface. Surface water should not be passed into sewers. Valley lines, natural streams and surface contours should in all cases be improved so as to diminish any inconvenience or injury caused by excess of water during wet seasons.

Natural streams should not be arched over to form sewers, as a natural stream may drain an area many times greater than the area to be sewered, and the volume of water to be passed will constantly be varying from a minimum in drought to a maximum in excessive wet. This variation in England is at times from 300 up to 500 to one. Sewers and drains should be made to serve a special purpose and as much as is practicable should be confined to such purpose, namely, to remove all slop and refuse water immediately to some common outlet.

*Sewers.* Main sewers may be constructed with bricks, tiles or stone. In each case hydraulic lime should be used for mortar. All main sewers should be egg-shaped on cross-section, the small end down. The invert in all cases ought to be struck with a short radius and the crown should be a semicircle. Bricks or tiles molded to the radii will make the cheapest and strongest sewers. Stone may be worked to the radii or, if the mortar is good and the stone suitable, rubble masonry may be used.

Plan I gives the forms, sizes, number of bricks, the cost of each section per lineal yard and the prices of the various materials in sewers of different dimensions. The prices are those at which the work was actually executed at Berwick-on-Tweed, Carlisle, Chorley, Lancaster and other places. It will be seen that, in every instance, double courses of bonding bricks were put in at or near the springing to ensure the rings being tied together. Side junctions for branch drains should be provided and fixed in the main sewer as the work proceeds. All such junctions should be properly closed for after use and an accurate record should be kept of their depth, diameter and true position, so that the point of junction can be found when required.

Main sewers should be absolutely true in line and in gradient from point to point. At each change of line or gradient in a main sewer a manhole should be provided, so that the entire system of sewers may be perfectly under command and may be inspected.

At each manhole there should be means for flushing and for permanent ventilation. In providing for ventilation there should be a fixed screen or filter of charcoal, through which the sewer air must pass before escaping into the atmosphere.

The radius of no curve on a main sewer should be less than ten times the cross-sectional diameter of such sewer, excepting that, when a change of line is not greater than 22½ degrees, the curve may be formed in the manhole, an extra fall of three inches being provided.

Sewers of unequal diameters should not join with level inverts, but in all cases tributary sewers should have their inverts at or above the level of the ordinary flow of sewage in the main. The junction should curve in the direction of the main flow and have extra fall so as to deliver freely from the tributary sewer to the main sewer. All main sewers should have full means for permanent ventilation at the upper or higher ends through charcoal air filters, and means for flushing at such points should be provided.

*Flushing of sewers and drains.* Flushing arrangements may be made by a manhole or a surface tank may be adapted to this purpose. A large volume of water is not required so much as a volume of water let off quickly, to act with a cleansing effect. In one instance sewers of rude workmanship were effectually cleansed by flushing from an ordinary wine cask filled by hand with sea water and discharged suddenly into the sewers. Sewers should not enter buildings nor pass beneath buildings, but should terminate outside and have full means for permanent ventilation. A side drain or side drains may be laid from the head of any main or tributary sewer so as to remove the point of outlet for ventilation to any safe distance.

Duplicate systems of sewers are not required, that is, sewers for storm flood waters and sewers for sewage. As previously stated, surface contours and natural valley lines may be improved and main sewers may have overflow communications with such valley lines and natural watercourses, so as to relieve the sewers at all available points during heavy rains. At such times any sewage will be in extreme dilution and the whole district will be in flood, so that any sewage will be washed away without causing injury.

*Causes of obstruction of sewers.* Sewers are liable to choke from several causes:

1. Irregular lines and uneven invert gradients;
2. Defective workmanship and a porous subsoil, allowing fluids to filter away and leaving the solids to accumulate;
3. Sewers too large and having wide, flat and uneven inverts, which the ordinary volume of fluid sewage can neither cover nor scour;
4. Sewers liable to be water-logged either by tides or by rain or river floods.

Where sewers have to be formed on open gravel, sand or rock, a lining of puddle should be placed so as to render the sewer watertight to half its vertical sectional depth. Great care must also be taken to form the invert of any sewer over such subsoil true, sound and watertight.

*Trapping.* All sewer mouths must be protected so as to prevent the wind blowing in and driving sewage gases back. A single flap for small sewers or a compound flap for larger sewers or a fall of canvas, weighted, may be applied. Means must be adopted to protect the mouths of all sewers and drains.

*Ventilation of sewers.* Manholes should have moveable covers at the surface. There should be a side chamber for ventilation, "step-irons" to give access to the invert and a groove to allow of a flushing board being inserted at will for flushing purposes. The side chamber may have a charcoal screen or filter.

Fig. 1 shows a system of ventilation of sewers which has been successfully brought into use in England. The figure shows the usual manhole and shaft with moveable iron cover, made to fit tight and prevent the passage of sewer air. Across the shaft are laid two or more moveable charcoal filtering screens, through which the sewer gas, deprived of its noxious matter by the charcoal, passes into a side ventilating chamber and thence through an open grating into the street. The chamber is intended to receive any solid matter falling in from the street, which can be removed when necessary by a slide at the lower end of the chamber. In a hilly town the system of sewerage should not be so connected as to permit the accumulation of sewer gases in the higher parts of the district. In such cases, the sewer should be divided by steps or falls with a flap valve at the discharging end of the sewer, as shown in fig. 1, to compel the gases to pass through the ventilating shaft.

**FIGURE 1**
**Manhole, Tumbling Bay and Double Ventilating Arrangement**

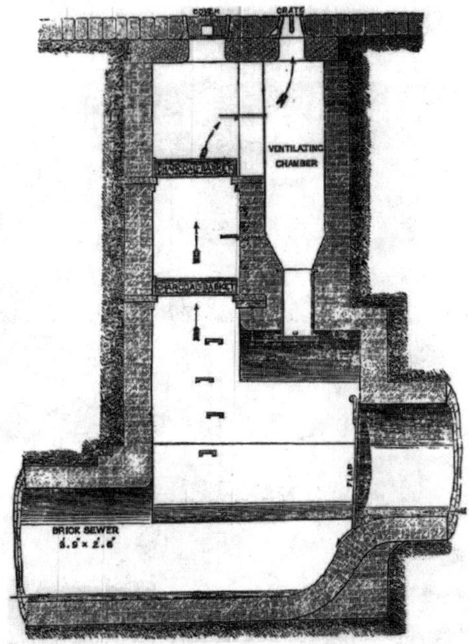


The details of other ventilating arrangements at present in use for brick sewers at their junctions and along their course are shown on Plans II and III.

*Pipe drains.* Earthenware pipes make the best drains up to their sectional capacity, say fifteen inches. Half-socket pipes, laid with the half-socket down, make the best drain, as any pipe can be removed without breaking a pipe. Common circular vitreous earthenware pipes with ordinary junctions are the best.

Drainpipe joints may be made with well-tempered clay in sound ground, but should be made with cement or with hydraulic mortar in open or in sandy ground. Plan IV gives the usual construction, junctions and water-traps adopted in laying down earthenware pipe sewers.

Manholes, as for sewers, should be provided on all drains, with means of flushing and ventilation. On Plan V are shown sections and plans of different forms of manhole and lamphole for examining pipe drains.

The usual method of ventilating pipe drains is shown in fig. 2, where the charcoal screen is placed vertically between the manhole and the ventilating shaft.

**Figure 2**
**Manhole and Ventilating Shaft**

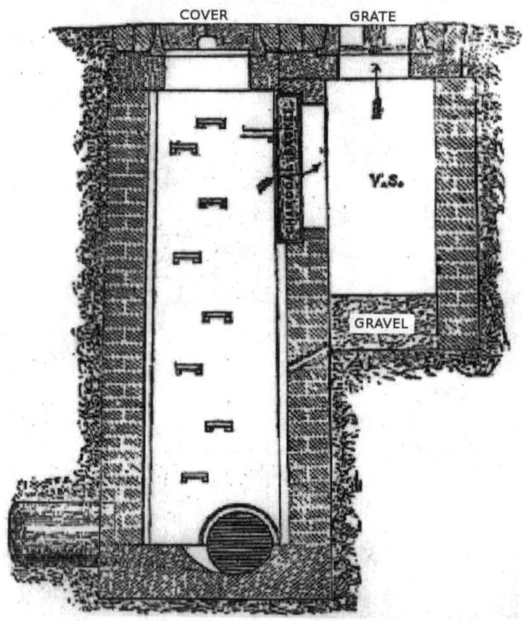


Earthenware pipes of 4 inches in diameter are sufficient for water closets and sinks; these may join drains of 6 inches, the 6 inches joining 9 inches, 12 inches and 15 inches, and these forming a tributary main or passing to a main sewer. (The town of Alnwick, in Northumberland, stands on part of a natural drainage area of 2000 statute acres with steep gradients. The population is about 7000. There is a water supply of 150,000 gallons per day and some 1400 water closets regularly in use. Common privies have been abolished. The outlet sewer is eighteen inches in diameter, upwards of 2000 yards in length, having a fall of one (1) in 400. There are sewers of 15 inches, 12 inches, 9 inches and 6 inches; all house drains are 4 inches. These sewers are entirely of earthenware pipes and have acted perfectly during ten years. There have been falls of rain, tropical in character, causing great destruction at the surface, but the sewers were not injured, nor did anyone complain that they were not larger. It would have required a sewer ten feet in diameter to have removed the flood water; this passed over the surface as such floods had done in all former periods. Alnwick Castle, standing on several acres of ground, is sewered with earthenware pipes of 12 inches to 4 inches diameter. They answer perfectly.)

Large cities and towns are exceptional and will require large constructions where natural streams, such as the Fleet ditch in London, are arched over. But in this instance the Fleet ought not to have been used as a sewer; intercepting sewers should have been formed on both sides, with flood or storm water overflows from the intercepting sewers to the Fleet river.

In India and at all tropical stations where there are heavy rains, any attempt at proportioning main sewers to area and rainfall must break down. Sewers cannot be formed, at any reasonable cost, to remove all the surface water during heavy rains and, if they could be so formed, such sewers would be enormously too large for the ordinary dry-weather flow of sewage, and so far as a sewer is larger in sectional diameter than is requisite to remove the ordinary refuse, soil, roof, yard and waste water, such sewer becomes a cause of nuisance in dry and hot weather. Sewers of small sectional area will answer best even in India.

*Leading principles of drainage and construction of sewers and drains.* The leading principles to be kept in view are:

1. To provide by carefully formed surface drains for the removal of all the rainfall except what sinks into the ground;

2. To provide for the rapid removal of this subsoil water by land or subsoil drainage;

3. To drain away the refuse fluids of all houses, barracks, hospitals, stations and towns by close sewers and drains.

"Sight-rails" should be put up at all convenient points to mark the proposed line and level of the sewer or drain before the ground is opened. The longest lengths of trenching that the ground will allow should be opened, trimmed and bottomed truly before commencing to lay in drainpipes or to construct sewers. To construct drains or sewers in short lengths is to increase the risks of defective workmanship.

Sewer and drain trenching requires skilled labour. Deep trenching may require staying, propping and "polling." Quicksand will require special means, "close timbering" and working in short lengths. Stable litter mixed with ashes placed in the joints of close timbers arrests quicksand better than any other means of filling in. But no general instructions can be given for dealing with quicksand; the engineer must use his practical knowledge. Where quicksand occurs in narrow streets or near buildings, the proposed line of sewer or drain may have to be abandoned for a line at a safer distance.

Heavy clay ground should not be allowed to fall in large masses on the finished sewer or drain. Bricks may be displaced and earthenware pipes may be crushed by allowing large masses of the sides of trenches to fall. If there is danger in removal of timber stays and props from trenches, when filling in over a finished sewer or drain, it will be better and cheaper to leave such timber undisturbed and fill in the trench, burying the timber.

Sewers formed of a single brick in thickness require more care in filling in than where two bricks in thickness are used. The sides and "spandrils" may, is some cases, be filled in with concrete up to the level of the crown of the arch. Ordinary gravel mixed with one seventh by measure of lime will make concrete sufficient for such purpose.

"Fall" or "grade" in any sewer or drain is not absolutely necessary. A proper arrangement of manholes and flushing will preserve sewers clean and sweet having no fall. There must, however, be a free outlet.

As a proof that sewers laid without gradient can keep themselves clear, it may be stated that the main sewer at West Ham, a section of which is shown at fig. 3, is laid level for half a mile at low water of spring tides and then for 2½ miles with a fall of three feet in a mile. This sewer is four feet six inches high and three feet wide. The surface of the ground under which it is laid is from 10 to 12 feet below high water in the Thames. The subsoil was so porous that the water could not be kept, by pumping, below the line shown in the figure. The iron invert had to be so planned that it could be laid underwater by feeling only. Upon this cast-iron invert cement blocks were laid and the sewer built on them in the ordinary manner. About three miles of this sewer have been in use for four years. And although the outlet has been obtained by pumping, the sewer has been kept clean. Means of flushing were provided but the only fall was the surface gradient or water head in the sewer.

It is not advisable to construct sewers and drains without fall, nor will it be necessary to do so excepting on rare and special occasions. A comparatively steep fall will not in all cases serve to preserve sewers and drains clean and sweet in very dry weather and with a limited supply of water passed down in driblets. There must be flushing at regular and short intervals, once a day at least.

**FIGURE 3**
**Main Outlet Sewer: West Ham**

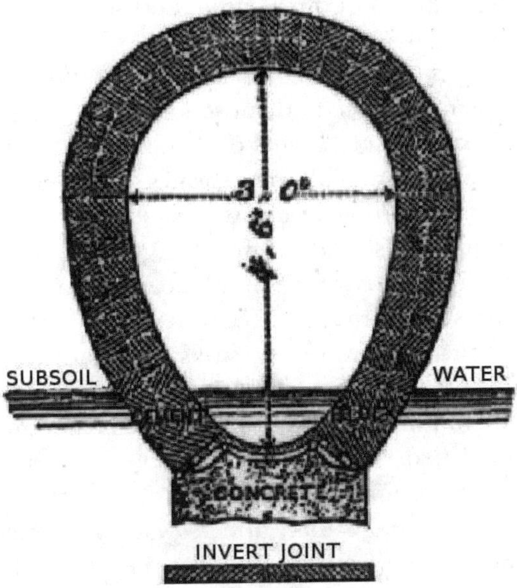


Sewers, drains, sinks, water closets, latrines, lavatories, baths and urinals cannot be so constructed as to act without constant care. The superintendence of these arrangements must be intelligent and unceasingly regular. In a system of sewers and drains, a full provision of manholes, ventilating chambers, described above, and flushing arrangements will enable the engineer to be absolute master of the situation. Inspection can be made of the sewer or drain at any and at every manhole; flushing can be brought into use at all the upper ends of sewers and drains, as also at all intermediate manholes, whilst the ventilating chambers secure an unceasing distribution and dilution of sewage gases at numerous points, settled by the engineer.

No system of sanitary works should be considered satisfactory if the engineer is not absolutely master at every point, without the necessity of excavating one cubic foot of earth or removing one brick or drainpipe.

Sewers "sufficiently large for a man to enter" ought never to be considered necessary for cleansing. Men need not be required to enter any sewer. Flushing or mechanical means, such as a rope or chain passed from manhole to manhole, will serve to remove even heavy road grit sediment, if the invert of every sewer is true, smooth and struck to a radius not greater than 9 inches. No egg-shaped sewer, however large, need have an invert of greater radius than 9 inches. A velocity of one foot per second may be easily obtained through a sewer of the flattest gradient by flushing, and such velocity will remove silt and coarse sand.

*Gullies.* All sewers and drains should have gullies and other inlet connections with the surface and subsoil or other water, so formed as to prevent solids larger than grains of coarse sand being admitted, *see* Plan IV. Silt and sediment of all sorts should, however, be prevented as much as possible from having access to sewers and drains. Gullies should be small and numerous, rather than large and open. Each gully should have a sediment box which may be easily removed and emptied.

For all purposes of drainage of barrack and hospital buildings, for latrines, closets, urinals, lavatories, sinks and baths, glazed earthenware pipe drains, of 9 or 12 inches in diameter, will be found sufficient for 1000 men. Pipes require to be carefully laid on a well-formed and hard rammed bed. The joints should be tight so that no sewage can escape from the drain into the subsoil. It is a cardinal principle in barrack and town drainage that, after sewage has once entered the drain, it shall not escape from it except at the outlet. The water from latrines, urinals, lavatories and baths may be so used and discharged down the drains and sewers as to have a flushing effect. This should be provided for and should also be regularly attended to. The purpose of drainage sanitary works and regulations should be to remove all refuse mixed in water, all surplus, dirty and waste water immediately or before fermentation and decomposition commences.

*Disposal of sewage.* Tanks should never be used in India to store sewage and foul water, but the produce of each day should be expended so as to prevent the commencement of putrefaction, either by discharging it from the outlet or by applying it to the surface of the ground for manuring soldiers' gardens or for similar purposes. Fresh sewage is not injurious, but sewage retained in cesspools, in imperfect drains and sewers, fouls the subsoil and contaminates the wells, and its decomposition produces gases of a most noxious and injurious character.

Sewage and waste water ought, if possible, to be used for purposes of irrigation during dry portions of the year. Fresh sewage properly applied for promoting the growth of suitable vegetation will be found a profitable undertaking. The solids and flocculent matter may be strained out of sewage in any simple and cheap manner. (*See* Appendix No. I.)

No form of filtering, precipitating or treating sewage, either mechanically or chemically, can do more than separate the grosser solids. The effluent water, after any form of treatment, remains essentially sewage water and should only be used for irrigation purposes.

Fresh sewage passed at once over light soils need not have the coarser particles removed, but for many plants it may be advisable to remove the sediment and flocculent matter so as to use the effluent water alone. The solids removed from sewage may be used as ordinary manure.

*Sewage outlets.* Sewage outlet works should ever be simple in design and inexpensive in construction. Brick tanks are not needed. Canal-like tanks, with earth sides, through which there shall be an unceasing flow not greater than three inches per second, answer best. There should be two or more such tanks so arranged that either one or both combined may be used and one may be cleansed whilst the other is in use. It is frequently necessary to carry the outlet of a sewer to a river having a low summer level and a high or flood level. To prevent nuisance arising from the sewage running over the surface at low water, a plan such as that adopted at Windsor Castle and shown in figs. 4 and 5 has been found to answer. An iron pipe was fixed at the bottom of the sewer with a slight dam in front of the junction. This simple arrangement ensured the discharge of all the ordinary sewage below the summer low-water level, while the brick sewer above gave free passage to the storm water. In England a sewer, four feet high and three feet wide, might be required for the removal of storm water, while an iron pipe, 12 inches in diameter, would remove all the ordinary sewage.

Land below high-water level of the sea may be embanked, as in Holland, the fens of England and other places. Such land may be sewered and drained as at West Ham on the Thames, near London, and as is intended on the lowlands at Bombay. Sewers may be laid at the depth of low water, the outlet being protected with self-acting tidal valves, fixed permanent valves being also provided to use at will and as occasion may require.

Where sewers communicate with rivers liable to rise in flood, the area used must be embanked and such sewers must have self-closing valves as also duplicate valves to be closed by hand. The river floods must be banked out. At the city of Carlisle, in England, river floods rise at times 23 feet vertical above the invert of the sewer and some fifteen feet vertical above the land through which the outlet sewer is laid. All manholes are carried above the highest level of floods.

**Figure 4**
**Dry-Weather River Outlet at Windsor Castle**

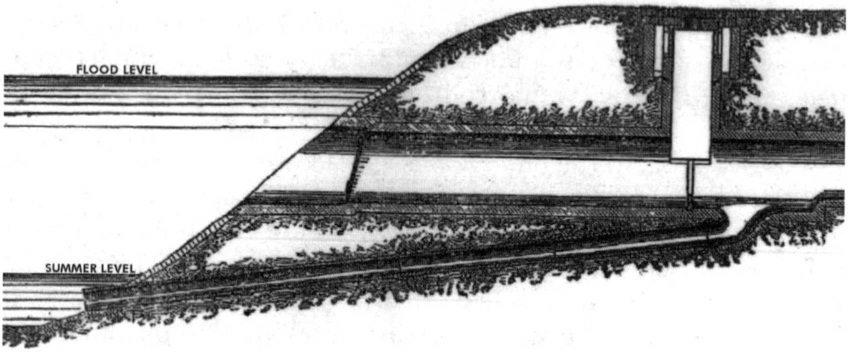


**Figure 5**

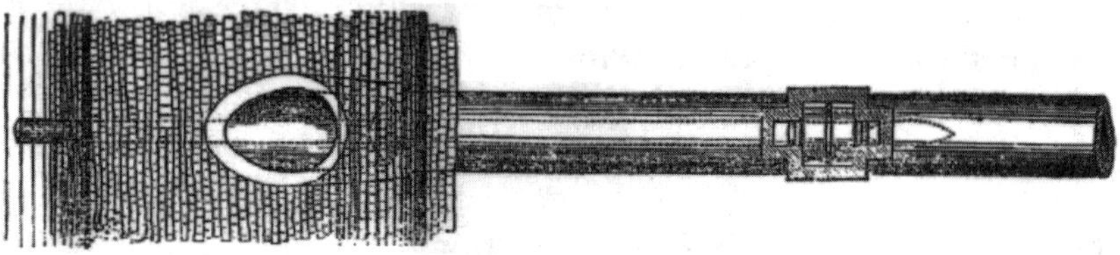

Where lands desirable to be used for building purposes are waterlogged by artificial constructions, it will be a question of removing the cause of obstruction or of artificially draining the site proposed to be used.

Pumping is resorted to for drainage purposes in many places and will pay for purely agricultural uses. Sewage is pumped at West Ham, near London, and at Worthing, in England. The low levels of London will be pumped as also the low levels at Bombay. The sewage pumps at West Ham are so arranged as only to lift to the actual head or level of the tide as each tide rises and falls, and not to a fixed extreme high-water head. Steam is the cheapest pumping power for large volumes of sewage of towns. For small volumes of sewage, proceeding from barracks or military stations, animal power may be made available; windmills cannot be depended upon nor river currents, where weather and rainfall are variable.

*Importance of meteorology to drainage.* In dealing with questions of drainage, it is important that the sanitary engineer should make himself acquainted with meteorology generally, and special attention should be paid to the meteorology of the district he is about to work in. There are many natural signs to be observed in a new country, indicating the meteorological character of the district. If violent rain floods take place, steep ground will be furrowed, rocky ground will be bare and watercourses and valley lines will show the violent effects of flood waters. In Great Britain, rivers rise in flood from low-water level some 20 feet: the river Eden at Carlisle, the river Ouse at York and other rivers of a similar character. In South Africa, rivers rise 60 and 70 feet vertical in floods. In many parts of Europe, Spain, Italy and other places, there is no water visible in dry seasons where roaring torrents come down occasionally. Many parts of India are similarly affected, as is known to Indian engineers. The engineer should ascertain to what extent extreme variations range. "Mediums" and "averages" only mislead, unless the full truth has been mastered and is comprehended.

The seasons and years vary in Great Britain as much as one to two, that is, at any point or place where a long average of years shows a mean rainfall of thirty inches, then, during such period, it will be found that the driest year has been as low as 20 inches and the wettest year as high as forty inches, intermediate years oscillating between these extremes. All embankments, bridges, culverts, viaducts or other waterways must be sufficient for the largest possible flood that can take place. In Great Britain the dry-weather volume in a river is increased by ordinary floods 300 times and occasionally up to 500 times the dry-weather volume. In tropical countries with heavy continued rains the excess will be much greater. In most parts of Great Britain the dry-weather flow from land down streams and rivers is half a cubic foot per second from each 1000 statute acres of land, and of course in ordinary floods this will be 150 cubic feet per second and during extreme floods 250 cubic feet per second. It will be of the utmost importance, in dealing with questions of drainage and water supply, to ascertain and record all meteorological extremes.

## Section II Water Supply

(*Recommendation of the royal commission respecting water supply.* "8. That all existing water sources be subjected to analysis and those rejected which contain matters injurious to health. That the present method of drawing and distributing water be discontinued wherever practicable. That all water used for drinking purposes be filtered or otherwise purified.")

*Examination and selection of water sources.* Every existing water source, supplying a station or town, should be examined as to its available quantity and also analyzed by a competent chemist to ascertain:

a. Its hardness, by Clarke's test.

b. Nature of its constituents, suspended and dissolved.

c. Quantities of each constituent per gallon.

It is a first principle that water, containing suspended matter, should never be distributed in that state for the use of troops. The most important soluble ingredient in water is its organic matter. The amount of this should be very carefully estimated and its nature ascertained whether it be of animal or of vegetable origin. Any appreciable quantity of animal matter subject to putrescence is objectionable in tropical climates and in such climates as those of India. Water containing it should either be purified from its presence or, if this cannot be done, it should be rejected altogether. A grain or two of vegetable matter per gallon is not so objectionable.

Waters containing a large amount of dissolved saline matter, especially of chlorides or sulphates, are not suitable for use on account of their action on the mucous membrane of the bowels. If at any station there be a water source containing two or three grains of saline constituents not of injurious character, no appreciable quantity of animalized matter and only a grain or two of dissolved vegetable matter per gallon, such water may be retained for use. If any existing water source can be made to afford water, after filtration through sand and charcoal, with or without artificial magnetic oxide of iron, of a degree of purity similar to that stated above, it may be used for the supply of troops. Every proposed new water source for supplying troops or for extending the existing supply should be analyzed in the manner recommended and only those sources selected which afford water of the requisite purity.

As the amount of constituents, organic and inorganic, per gallon will vary according to the season, whether it be rainy or dry, the purity of any water source should be judged of from analysis, conducted during the dry season as well as during the season of the rains.

In addition to these preliminary inquiries, all water sources should be examined chemically from time to time to ascertain their state of purity. Such inquiries are just as necessary in a country like India as are periodical inquiries into the amount of water supplied from the source. The purest water is that obtained from the rainfall flowing from primitive rocks. The most impure is in all probability tank water, receiving the surface drainage of a populous district, and water from shallow wells dug in a foul subsoil.

Granite, gneiss, mica slate and clay slate, millstone grit and some other analogous formations produce soft water. Mountain limestone, new red sandstone, the oolites, chalk and some of the tertiaries produce hard water. Water from the chalk is generally from 14 to 16 degrees of hardness. A geologist who has studied the subject will tell with tolerable accuracy the sort and quality of water any of the great geological formations will give, and a chemist who has analyzed many samples of water from the several great geological formations will indicate the formation by an analysis of a sample of the water proceeding from it. As a rule, bright sparkling water is hard water. The lime in the water throws down any vegetable tinge. A brown or brownish water tinged by vegetable matter will most probably be soft water, as the vegetable tinge would not remain if lime were also present in the water. Water may be hardened by containing in solution iron, sulphur and other substances besides lime and in combination with lime.

Iron and sulphur are found in the oolites and lias shales, so that deep-well sinking in these formations is attended with considerable risks. Hard water fit for use is, however, to be obtained in abundance from the oolites.

Salt rock is found in the new red sandstone formation. There is risk in deep sinking from this cause, but good water is frequently found in the new red sandstone. The coal measures rarely produce good water. Lime, iron and sulphur are generally combined with the water obtained from this formation. Chalk and upper green sand produce hard water. Water from the chalk formation is mainly derived from fissures in the chalk. Water springs flowing from sand or débris will be pure or the reverse, according to the chemical constituents in the sand, whether, for example, there be soluble saline matter or soluble organic matter mixed with it. Water from marshes or marshy ground should always be rejected.

The most common source of animal organic impurity in mountain districts is superabundance of decaying vegetable matter from trees and jungle. Waters of this class are unfit for use unless they are purified by filtration. The most common source of animal organic matter in Indian tanks is surface filth. Well water will vary in purity according to the nature and the soluble matters contained in the ground from which the well derives its supply. Shallow wells are always liable to pollution from vegetable matter or even from animal matter in the surface soil. Deep wells only, i.e., wells of a sufficient depth to afford water of the requisite purity, should be sunk and the surface soil water should be cut off from the deep water by casing the well above.

Rainwater from roofs and other impervious surfaces would afford an important source of supply at many Indian stations. Probably nearly every station in India might obtain sufficient rainwater from roofs for all drinking and culinary purposes, reserving all the other water merely for drainage and for cleanliness. In some instances, flagged or cemented surfaces of ground might be used for collecting the rainfall. In hilly districts it may be practicable in some cases to construct storage reservoirs for collecting and keeping water for use during the dry season. Such reservoirs, if above the level of stations, would enable water to be laid on by gravitation. In every case, except there be positive chemical proof that filtration is not required, water for supplying the troops should all be passed through filters of gravel, sand and charcoal, with or without artificial magnetic oxide of iron, to free the water not only from suspended matter but from dissolved organic matter, when water of this character only is obtainable.

*Means of distribution.* The means employed for distributing water should be such as to fulfill the twofold condition of having the water always laid on by pipes for use and delivering the water for use as pure as it is at its source. This principle necessitates the abandonment, at least for stations and towns, of the present system of water drawing and water carrying. In every instance, except where the water source is at a sufficient elevation above the station, water would have to be pumped up for distribution.

Almost every form of water distribution is in use for towns and barracks in Great Britain. In some cases, water is laid on at head-pressure from a public reservoir, at a higher elevation than the barrack. In other instances, the pressure is obtained by steam power employed to throw the water to a sufficient elevation in a standpipe, from which water is conducted for town use and supplied to the barracks. In some towns, water is raised by steam power from deep wells to an iron tank, supported on a water tower of sufficient elevation to distribute water by gravitation. There is one fort in England having a water tower and tank supplied by horse labour. In other instances, raised tanks are filled from deep wells by force pumps, worked by hand. Improved windmills have also been recently introduced for the same purpose.

So far as can be judged of from the Indian stational reports, there is hardly a station that could not be supplied with water all over it, and at all times and in any requisite quantity, by one or other of these methods. The chief difficulty in India will be the question of fuel for steam power, but fuel can be dispensed with wherever animal power can be obtained. The power of running water, where there are rivers, might also be employed, or windmill power, but this, as already stated, is very inconstant and therefore requires great storage capacity.

At most stations probably the best arrangement would be to raise a water tower to a sufficient elevation to distribute water as high as the roof of the barracks. An iron tank should be placed at the top of the tower and protected from the sun's rays. This tank might be supplied either from a deep well, river or surface tank, and it should be large enough to hold a day or two's supply.

The general principles of water supply may be stated briefly as follows:

1. To select the purest available source after careful analysis;

2. To filter the water in order to free it from suspended matter and from dissolved organic matter;

3. To store it in covered tanks and to raise it a sufficient height for distribution by gravitation.

Applying these principles water may be obtained:

from rivers and streams,

from natural springs,

from wells artificially formed,

from impounding reservoirs,

from tanks and cisterns,

from a combination of two or more of the sources named.

And may be conveyed for distribution:

by means of open conduits (before filtration),

by means of covered conduits, always *after filtration*,

by means of pipes under pressure.

Aqueducts of masonry or brickwork are not named, as cast and wrought iron will, even in India, be probably cheaper than such constructions. Water may be brought in by gravity, that is, water obtained at a distance may be found at such an elevation above the station, barrack or hospital requiring to be supplied as to allow of its flowing through conduits or pipes to the tanks or cisterns from which it is to be distributed. Water may be obtained from springs and wells at so low an elevation as to require to be pumped. The mode of pumping, as regards power to be used, will have to be regulated by the volume of water to be raised, the height to which it must be lifted and the most efficient form of power at command.

A gallon of water weighs ten (10) lbs. One horsepower is equivalent to the work of raising 3300 gallons or 33,000 lbs. weight of water one foot high per minute.

Steam is the cheapest form of power for lifting large volumes of water continuously, such as for the supply of a city, large town or large station. Animal power (bullocks) may be used for supplies for barracks or stations where steam-engine power cannot easily be obtained.

A pump for water supply, if the lift is more than thirty feet vertical, must of course be double action—lift and force. Such pumps do not need to be described, as they can be obtained ready-made of the best character from many makers.

*Storage of water.* A spring is the lowest point or lip of an underground reservoir of water in the stratification. A well sunk in such strata will most probably furnish an additional supply of water.

In Appendix No. II are given improved principles of construction of large storage reservoirs in England, together with an improved method of drawing off the water. India contains so many excellent examples of impounding reservoirs that it is hardly necessary to state that amateur engineering should never be admitted in devising and constructing such works. No general rules indeed can be laid down on the subject. Nothing short of competent practical knowledge and experience can obviate the numerous chances of failure. Natural springs may be utilized by storing the water in a reservoir which will contain the flow of one entire day. Such reservoirs should be walled with masonry and may be covered in to protect the water from contamination.

*Water pipes.* Springs of water at a distance may be conducted in channels contouring the intervening distance. The fall for a conduit may vary according to circumstances. The fall should not be less than one in 1000 nor greater than one in 300 unless cast-iron pipe conduits are used.

In forming an earthenware pipe conduit great care must be taken to make the trench watertight and then to lay and joint the pipes so as to secure that the conduit shall be sound and watertight through its whole length to prevent leakage into the subsoil and to obviate the risk of impure water from the subsoil entering the pipe. In forming a conduit the pipes should be laid in straight lines from point to point. There should be means of inspection and of ventilation at all curves. The radius of all curves should be ten times the diameter of the conduit. There should be means of ventilation and of inspection in each quarter mile. There should be means of washing out at all convenient points.

Valley lines may be crossed by means of cast-iron syphon pipes, that is, a pipe may be laid across a valley to conduct the water under pressure. All valley or syphon lines should have double the fall in their length of the ordinary contour conduit. There should be means provided to wash out and cleanse such syphon pipe or pipes. For town and station service cast iron should be used for all pipes above two inches in diameter. Cast-iron pipes should be coated inside and out with black varnish. Turned and bored joints are cheapest. Wrought-iron pipes with screw joints may be used up to 1½ inch diameter. Lead for pipes and cisterns should not be used under any circumstances. Wrought-iron pipes from 3/8 up to 1½ inch may be used for services in houses and buildings and cast-iron pipes from three inches up to three feet diameter for mains in towns. Cast and wrought iron alone should be used for tanks and cisterns, not lead.

*Rainwater tanks.* Tanks to store rainwater may be of masonry. They should either be arched over or be roofed so as to protect the water from the direct action of the sun and from fouling. The ground excavated for the formation of a tank should be made perfectly watertight. The bottom may be covered with clay puddle and the side walls be backed or lined with clay puddle. The thickness of the puddle should not be less than 12 inches. If the site selected for a tank is sand, gravel or open-jointed rock, great care must be taken to give the puddle a full and even bearing over the whole surface area; open joints in rock must be cleaned out and then be filled up with concrete. In gravel large stones must be removed and the entire surface brought to a level, smooth and even plain. Clay puddle will only resist the pressure of water when it rests solidly on an even bed so as to prevent the water forcing holes through it, which will be the case if there is a rough uneven surface and open spaces beneath.

Tanks require to have an inlet pipe, an outlet or supply pipe, a wash-out or cleansing and an overflow pipe. These latter, the cleansing and overflow, may be joined. The main tank or tanks should have valve wells so arranged as to enable the system of supply to be carried on independently of the main tank.

On Plan VI is shown a plan and section of an underground storage tank with valve wells, as at present used in England. By this arrangement the supply of water is passed direct to the inlet-well and may be passed on through this well direct to the main tank; the supply may be obtained from the outlet-well by opening the valve in the main tank and the valve in the supply well. By closing the valves communicating with the main tank in both wells and opening the valve on the end of the connecting pipe in the inlet-well and the valve on the supply pipe in the outlet-well, the supply of water may go on independently of the main tank. The overflow must be formed at the inlet-well to be connected with the wash-out. There must be manhole openings in the covering arches and end windows in each bay, as shown in Plan VI. This is, of course, merely a sketch to show the general arrangements.

Elevated tanks for immediate or daily supply of water should be of cast iron or of wrought iron. Cast iron requires more care and practical skill in construction, but will last longer than wrought iron. In arranging cast-iron tanks of large dimensions care must be taken to support the bottom and stay the sides by wrought-iron tie rods in the best manner. Cast-iron or wrought-iron tanks should be arranged so that the supply of water may be carried on in a small corner compartment (as shown in the sketch of a cast-iron tank with a separate supply cistern, Plan VI) to allow of the main tank being repaired, cleaned and occasionally painted or varnished.

At the junctions of cast and wrought iron, wrought iron will waste more rapidly than cast iron and junctions of bolts and tie rods may give way if not repaired in time. Cleaning and painting should be regularly done once a year.

The sketch is not complicated by showing the details of tank-plates or tie rods, but is intended only to show the proposed mode of arranging a small inner tank within which all the operations of supply may be carried on independently of the larger tank. This will be found to be of the utmost importance in use. The small tank will be connected with the larger tank by means of a pipe having a valve on it.

In arranging a main pipe from pumps, the pipes should have sectional capacity sufficient to allow of the velocity in such main pipe not exceeding two feet per second, as friction increases in proportion to the velocity, as is shown by the law governing the delivery of water from pipes under pressure. Water presses equally in all directions and the pressure is due to the vertical head and not to the volume of water in a long horizontal main.

Where water is to be collected from rainfall, great care is requisite to preserve the surfaces on which it falls perfectly clean, as also the conduits to the reservoirs and tanks. When rainwater is collected from roofs, the first washings of the roofs should not be collected. Where wells are sunk or used, the lining of the well should be made watertight, so as to exclude surface water. The possibility of contamination by sewage should be prevented.

*Watering troughs.* Watering troughs for cavalry horses should be so arranged that each trough may have an independent supply of water. One trough should not be supplied out of any other trough, as the water is rendered unpalatable when breathed in by other horses or cattle. It does not require more water to supply twenty watering troughs independently than it does to arrange them in line, so that the overflow of one trough shall pass into the next below and so on through the whole line. A pipe or trough conveyed the length of the whole may be made to supply each trough independently.

*Water filters.* All water before being stored in tanks from which it is to be pumped direct for use should be passed through filters. Every rainwater storage tank should have its filter. The cheapest and best form of filter may be readily made with gravel, sand and charcoal, to which may be advantageously added artificial magnetic oxide of iron in cases in which the water contains much organic matter. The addition of artificial magnetic oxide of iron increases the oxidizing power of all filters and renders them more effective for destroying organic matter.

The following figs. 6 and 7 show plans and sections of filters, single or double, for stations or barracks; either of which will be found useful, according to the quantity or degree of impurity of the water to be filtered.

When considerable bodies of water have to be filtered, the arrangement of filtering material shown on Plan VII is the one usually adopted in England. But in using such filters in India, it would be necessary to place a layer of charcoal between the layers of gravel, to destroy as much as possible any organic matters which may exist. All possible and practicable means should be taken to collect, store and utilize pure soft water. Springs, wells, conduits, service reservoirs and tanks should be covered or otherwise protected from contamination.

The laws of hydraulics were known in the East ages before civilization sprang up in the West; but the uses of cast and wrought iron for

**Figure 6**
**Detail of Single Filter for Rainwater Tank**

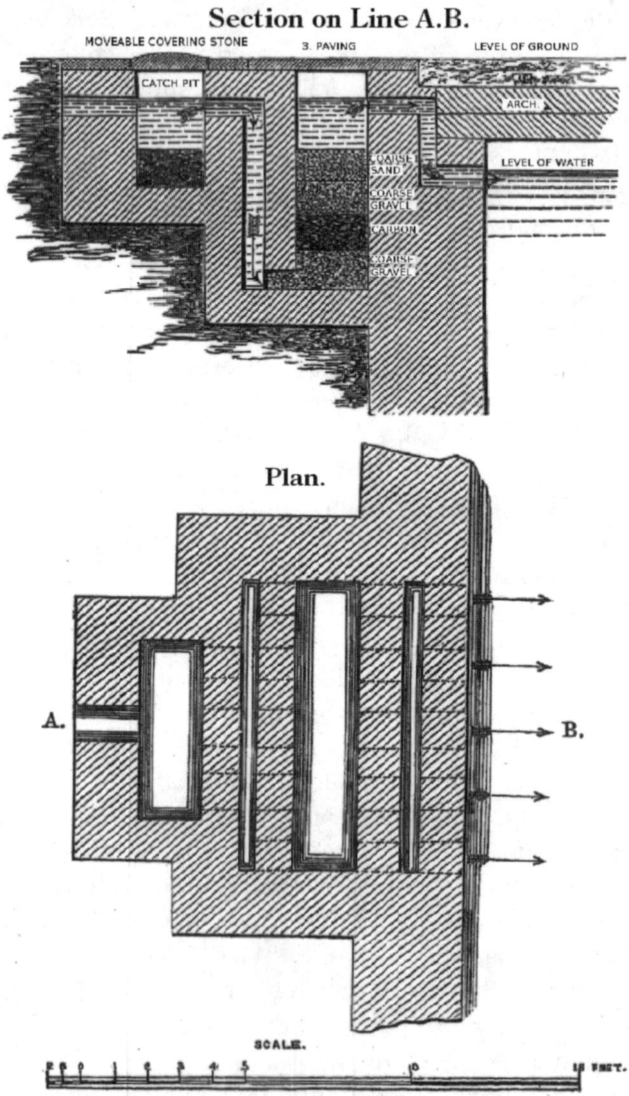


**B 4**

**Figure 7**
**Detail of Double Filter for Rainwater Tank**

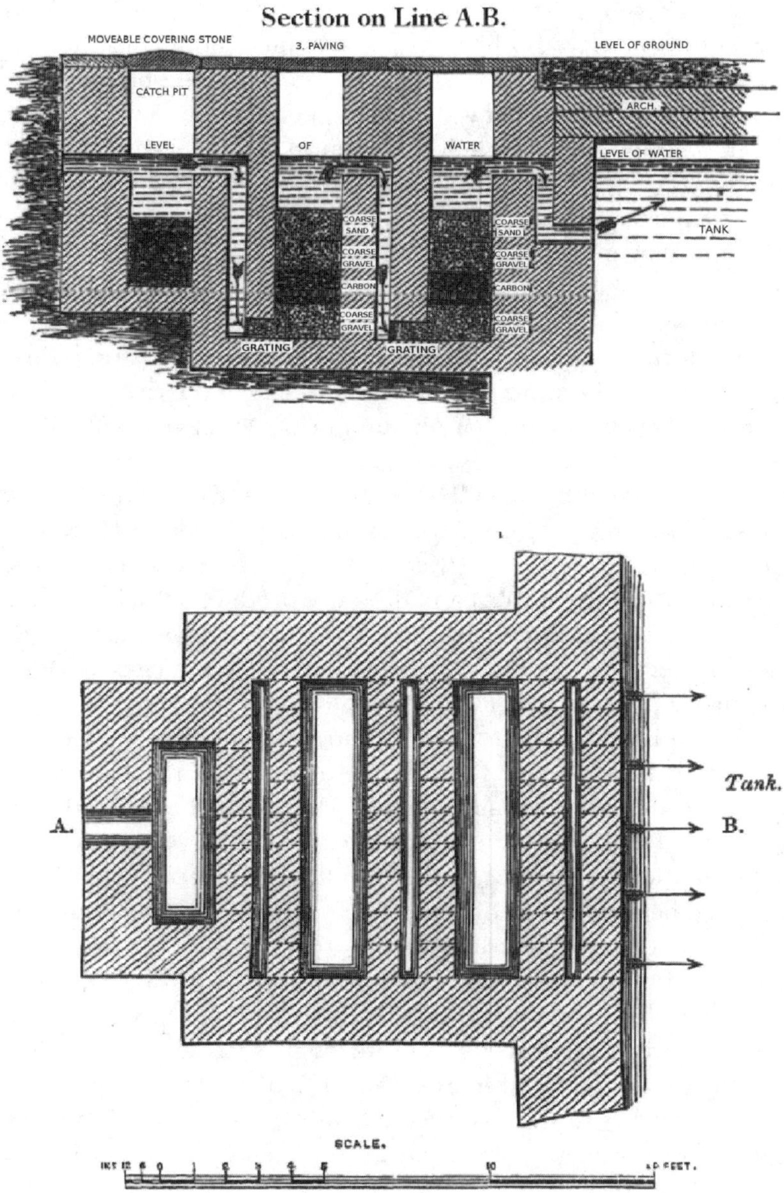

conduits, pipes, reservoirs and tanks have materially simplified the arrangements for waterworks. Masonry aqueducts to span valleys of vast extent are not now required. A syphon pipe of cast iron will convey water across a valley cheaper and better. Elevated tanks of cast or of wrought iron may also be constructed much more cheaply than of brickwork or of masonry. As a rule, if water can be obtained near a station at a low elevation, it will be cheaper to pump than it will be to bring in water by gravity from long distances.

A supply of soft and pure water may cost considerably more to obtain than a supply of harder and more impure water. The soft and pure water may nevertheless be the cheapest to use, though works to bring it in may cost double the sum required to furnish the harder and worse water.

Where a river flows through a valley over porous substrata, sinking a well or wells in the strata within the influence of the river filtration is a cheap and ready method of obtaining river water naturally filtered. The water supplied to Windsor Castle is obtained from wells sunk in the alluvial valley of the river Thames (gravel) and is pumped by water wheels and steam power up to a reservoir above the level of the castle. Wells so situate[d] must be carried above the level of extreme floods.

If a single well on a river bank does not produce sufficient water or if the subsoil is clay impervious to water, then trenches may be excavated parallel to the river or stream, in which trenches perforated earthenware pipes may be laid, leading to a well or wells. The trenches above such pipes should be filled in with fine assorted gravel, charcoal and sand so as to form a filtering medium within reach of the dry-weather flow of such stream or river. These trenches should not be less than six feet deep to the top of the pipes. After water has been filtered it should not again be exposed to the chances of contamination, but should be pumped or flow under cover direct into covered service reservoirs or elevated tanks for use.

Any overflow or waste-water pipe from a service reservoir or tank should deliver the water at an open end into a channel sewer or drain so as to prevent gases rising back through such overflow or waste-water pipe to the water in the reservoir or tank, a result very apt to follow if the pipe is directly connected with the sewer or drain. Water readily absorbs foul gases and may become poisonous by such means. The possibility of such contamination taking place must therefore be prevented. Earthenware conduits should be laid at such depth and be so covered with earth as to prevent the water becoming heated unduly by the rays of the sun. Brick and masonry tanks, if arched, may be covered in with sand or fine earth to the depth of 18 inches, which will preserve the water cool. All covered reservoirs and tanks should be ventilated.

*Service pipes and cisterns.* All service pipes may be of wrought iron from 1½ inches diameter to 3/8 of an inch diameter for single services. All the joints must be screwed. The taps should screw on to the service pipes. A lead or soldered joint should not be required. An ordinary fitter may then fit up and maintain any water service. All supply pipes should be arranged in such manner as to allow of easy inspection and subsequent repairs. Stop-taps should be placed betwixt the main and the building in all cases so as to allow of isolation of any line of service pipe for repairs. All service tanks and service pipes should be fixed in such manner that the rooms shall not be flooded in case of leakage or overflow. Ready means of access to all tanks and cisterns should be provided to allow of inspection, cleansing or repairs.

Up bends should not be formed on lines of main pipes or on service pipes. If up bends are inevitable, air valves should be provided to let out the air at such bends. Bends should not be formed at right angles on pipes, but the pipe should be brought round in a curve.

If a tie rod supports weight at both ends, the strain at either end must not exceed three tons for each square inch of cross-sectional area of the rods.

Iron tanks should not be exposed to the direct action of the sun, but must be enclosed or clothed. An enclosure of boards with felt beneath will form a good protection. Water, especially for drinking, must be kept cool.

*Waterworks.* All mortar used in waterworks should be capable of setting under water. Cement similar to Portland or Roman cement may be used for jointing earthenware conduit pipes. Before deciding to commence waterworks, a most careful examination should be made for several miles around the site to be supplied so as not to leave any reasonable doubt about the best source of supply and the best position for the works having been chosen. Existing means of water supply may be improved by combining with them such portion of the new works proposed as is requisite. If a supply of water is now pumped direct from a river or stream, filtering wells or filter trenches may be formed as suggested.

Open tanks may be cleansed, improved and covered, either by being arched in or by having a roof placed over so as to prevent fouling and the direct action of the heat of the sun, and the surface from which they derive their water should be kept clean and free from filth.

Wells liable to be fouled by surface infiltration may be puddled or lined with brickwork set in cement, or may be cased with iron to a sufficient depth to cut off the water from the alluvial soil, as such water is liable to become tainted from organic matter either on the surface or in the soil itself. Open conduits may be cleansed, deepened and covered, or a line of earthenware pipes may be substituted for the open and exposed channel.

Gathering grounds, catchment areas from which rain is to be impounded, may be formed, cleansed, channelled and paved so as to present a clean surface, and great care should be taken to prevent all gathering surfaces becoming fouled or covered with vegetation.

Deep-well sinking or deep boring necessarily involves special knowledge and appropriate and special tools. A description of such work and such tools is not needed by a practical well-sinker and would not be of use to anyone else.

A steam engine, working with coals at 20*s.* per ton will raise 90,000 gallons of water, 900,000 lbs. or upwards of 400 tons weight, 100 feet high, at a working cost of one shilling. One man making six journeys per hour with two gallons, or 20 lbs. weight and working at this rate eight hours would carry up to an elevation of 100 feet 96 gallons of water or 960 lbs., so that it would require the united labour of upwards of 900 men working eight hours to perform one-shilling's-worth of steam-engine work, such as is daily performed at the large waterworks pumping establishments for London. Small steam engines do not raise water so economically as large engines but the smallest engine, with fuel at a very high rate, will be far cheaper than manual labour if 10,000 gallons of water per day should require to be raised 100 feet.

Private filters of various kinds are purchasable and, where water cannot be filtered at the works, service filters will be useful. A company is about being formed in London to supply filters, not only to remove mechanically suspended impurities, but also to soften and otherwise purify water. Such filters or filtering media may probably in due time be made available for India.

Where waterworks are in use, care will be necessary to preserve the works in effective order. Storage reservoirs must be fenced in. Conduits, open or covered, must be regularly looked to so as to prevent fouling of any kind.

A report as to the state of any local water supply may with advantage be required monthly from each principal medical officer and engineer officer. The engineer officer should give the volume used, the volume in store and the loss or waste, if any. The medical officer should give the quality of an analysis each month. If any men are peculiarly affected by drinking water, the facts should be recorded and the causes should be explained, so that a suitable remedy may be provided. Leaking reservoirs, conduits, tanks, cisterns, pipes or taps should be repaired at once. Every possible means should be used to preserve the water for use in bulk and in the greatest possible purity.

*Amount of water required.* The amount of water required for consumption at home, including washing, is about seven gallons per head per day of the whole population. In hospitals it is 25 gallons per day per head for the whole hospital population (sick, attendants and officers), including baths but *not* washing. At Indian stations, where there is a large preponderance of adults and where the circumstances of the climate and country require so much greater attention to cleanliness, it is probable that about twelve gallons per head per day for healthy people, and 30 to 35 gallons per head for sick in hospitals, would be required for every purpose, including baths, but *not* including laundry work, and allowance must be made for waste. In England waste amounts to about two thirds of the supply to the civil population. In barracks this can be to a great extent avoided.

At stations where the supply of pure water is limited, as, e.g., where the rainfall on the buildings affords the only pure water for cooking and drinking, this part of the supply would require to be filtered, tanked and distributed by itself. Underground tanks for drinking and cooking water possess the advantages of coolness and freedom from vegetation. But wherever such tanks are made, they should be very carefully constructed and lined so as to prevent leakage either from the tank into the subsoil or from the subsoil into the tank. They should be constructed at some distance from the barrack buildings. And they should be carefully arched and covered to prevent the entrance of surface impurities.

*Water distribution for buildings.* As regards barrack water supply, water should be laid on to all barracks and outbuildings for every required purpose. It should always be available by day and night for drinking purposes, ablution rooms, baths, cookhouses, latrines, urinals. Also for stables. Every barrack room should have a pure cool water supply for drinking to be drawn from a tap. Every day room and reading room should have drinking water at hand, laid on in a similar manner. And there should be drinking fountains at convenient points throughout the cantonments, especially in connection with guard rooms, gymnasia, workshops, etc.

Although it is desirable that the whole supply should be laid on from one centre, it is expedient, with a view of watching and, if necessary, of checking waste, in certain cases to provide each separate block of building with its own tank. When this is done, care should be taken not to place any water tank under the same roof as the barrack room. The water tank should be kept separate, closed and ventilated. It is a fundamental principle in the water supply of stations that every drop of water brought into them for use should be conveyed away again by drains; otherwise it will remain, more or less, in the subsoil and become an added source of unhealthiness.

In laying on water for bazaars and towns, the same general principles should be kept in view. All water brought in should be removed by drains. Each house should have its own water supply, wherever practicable, otherwise the supply should be from fountains or hydrants.

## Section III Principles of Barrack Construction

(*Recommendations of the royal commission respecting barrack construction.*

"5. That the means of instruction and recreation be extended to meet the requirements of each station. That covered sheds for exercise and gymnastics be provided. That workshops be established and also soldiers' gardens in connection with the station wherever practicable.

9. That all future barracks be erected on raised basements with the air circulating under the floors. (Report, Vol. I. fol. li: In low, flat and damp districts each barrack should consist of two floors, the upper one only to be used as a sleeping room and the lower floor to be a covered place for exercise and amusement.)

10. That all new barracks be constructed to hold no more than a quarter of a company in each building or at most half a company in one building, in two separate rooms having no direct communication with each other.

11. That barracks be in future constructed with single verandahs only and for no more than two rows of beds between the opposite windows.

12. That the cubic space per man in future barracks be from 1000 to 1500 feet and the superficial area from 80 to 100 square feet, varying according to the airiness of the position.

13. That the beds be so arranged with respect to windows, doors and wall spaces as to ensure the benefit of free ventilation without exposing the men to drafts. That in all future barracks the wall space be made sufficient to keep the beds at the least three feet apart and at the same time out of the door draft.
14. That the ventilation of barracks be sufficiently provided for independently of doors and windows.
15. That in all cavalry barracks saddlery rooms be provided and saddles removed out of the barrack rooms.
16. That all barracks be provided with sufficient glazed window space to light them.
17. That all barracks be provided with sufficient ablution and bath accommodation with a constant water supply. That drinking fountains supplied with filtered water be provided.
18. That barrack cookhouses be improved and better ventilated.
19. That wherever practicable, iron or earthenware water latrines supplied with water and drained to an outlet be introduced instead of the present system; that where this is impracticable, all cesspits be abolished and metal or earthenware vessels to be removed twice a day substituted. That improved urinals supplied with a jet for lavatory purposes, as well as with a free supply of water for the cleansing and drainage of the urinals, be provided.)"

The accompanying plans are intended to illustrate the construction of barracks for accommodating British troops in India and in tropical climates generally. They embody the principles contained in the evidence of witnesses examined before the Royal Commission on the Sanitary State of the Army in India and in reports sent from stations in India and Ceylon.

### 1. BARRACK ROOMS TO BE RAISED ON BASEMENTS

The first improvement suggested by the evidence is that all future barracks and hospitals should be erected on raised basements.

*Height of basements.* In high airy positions, these basements may be 3 or 4 feet in height; they should be arched and the floor of the barrack room should be laid on the top of the arches; means should be taken to prevent water running under the basement; the outer openings should be grated to prevent animals obtaining access or nuisance being deposited under the arches; the basement should be sufficiently lofty to admit of the entrance of work people to keep it clean and its floor should be formed of concrete.

One use to which the basement might be devoted would be as a place of exercise for playing bowls, walking, etc. To answer such purposes the floor of the basement would have to be raised above the ground and paved, and the height of the basement should be sufficient to enable it to be used in the proposed manner.

A damp-proof course should be carried round the entire basement a little above the ground and also in all the piers of the arches to prevent damp rising.

If the basement were used for exercise and were of a sufficient height, say 10 or 12 feet, barrack rooms constructed over basements of this height would be raised sufficiently above the ground to be occupied in most districts with comparative safety to health.

But in low situations, the higher men sleep above the ground, the better. And under unfavourable local circumstances, it would be advisable to interpose between the barrack room and the ground not only an arched basement but an additional floor of rooms. A barrack block so constructed would consist of a basement of, say, three or four feet high, a floor of rooms, fifteen feet or more high, which might be devoted to purposes of recreation, etc., and the sleeping rooms over.

*Uses of lower floors.* There is an apparent waste of space in this form of construction because, in each block, the same amount of floor surface, devoted to the men's sleeping accommodation in the upper floor, has on the lower floor to be occupied by other accommodation. In occupying this space sufficient area might be given for the following purposes:

a. dining, day and recreation rooms;
b. orderly rooms;
c. sergeants' mess;
d. schools and lecture rooms, theatres;
e. guard rooms;
f. certain kinds of workshops;
g. in cavalry barracks, saddlery rooms;
h. stores.

The canteen must be quite separate but all other accommodation could be placed on the ground floors without interfering with the healthiness of the sleeping rooms above.

It is necessary to state distinctly that it is unadvisable to have more than one floor of men's sleeping rooms in any tropical barrack on account of the difficulty of ventilating lower floors sleeping rooms sufficiently for the climate.

## 2. Number of Men per Room and Block

*Size of barracks.* The royal commission recommend that future barracks be built to accommodate not more than a quarter of a company per room and that each block shall consist of one single quarter company room or at the most of two such rooms in line, completely cut off from each other, with separate doors to the open air. This rule precludes the construction of barrack rooms for a greater number than the quarter of a company and also the construction of rooms divided into quarter company sections by arches.

The sanitary principle on which this construction of barracks in quarter company rooms is based is that considerable subdivision *in buildings* is absolutely necessary for health in tropical climates and that, in carrying this principle into effect, it is necessary that the air be allowed to play freely over as large a surface of the buildings as possible. To each quarter company room there should be a non-commissioned officer's room attached. A separate barrack block would thus contain say twenty-four men in one room and one sergeant, or forty-eight men in two rooms and two sergeants.

## 3. Space and Area per Man and Proportions of Rooms

*Space per man.* The royal commission recommend that in future the cubic space per man in barrack sleeping rooms should be between 1000 and 1500 feet, and the superficial area between 80 and 100 square feet, according to the nature of the position. They propose the smaller space to be given in elevated healthy stations, the larger in low and less healthy districts. In disposing of this area the barrack sleeping room should be suitably proportioned in length, width and height.

Assuming 22 feet as the minimum width of the room, the length would be 87 feet 6 inches, and the height 12 feet to the top of the wall, exclusive of the roof space, in cases where 1000 cubic feet are given. But a foot or two of additional height of wall would make a much better room. Where 1500 cubic feet are given, the length would be 100 feet, the width 24 feet and the height 15 feet to the top of the wall, exclusive of the roof space.

*Barrack plans.* These are the proportions which have been used in designing the barrack block shown in Plans VIII, IX and X. At certain very hot stations a greater height of wall is required than could be given with these allotments of space.

## 4. Windows and Doors

*Wall and window space.* There should be a window for every two beds. And the beds should be arranged, two and two, between the windows with their heads to the wall. The wall space between the windows should be sufficiently wide to allow a space of three *feet at least* between the two adjoining beds and to keep the beds free of draught from the doors. Wall spaces of from 9 to 10½ feet, according to the cubic contents allowed, would be sufficient for these purposes.

In the majority of instances, five doors per room, two in each side and one at the end, as shown in Plan VIII, will afford sufficient door space in a room for twenty-four men. But in unhealthy positions it has been customary to have doors only, instead of windows, to barrack rooms. This arrangement has been considered necessary to increase the circulation of air and so to prevent the deposition of moisture within the room. It has the disadvantage of exposing the men to draughts and causing sickness—an evil which may be diminished by introducing screens on each side of the door, as shown on Plan VIII, to shield the men from draughts while in bed. At most of the stations, the advantages of having numerous doors can be obtained by suitable independent means of ventilation.

*Doors.* Each door should have a window on hinges over it, carried up to within a foot or 18 inches of the ceiling. As already stated, it is necessary to shield the beds nearest the doors from air blasts, when the doors are kept open, by thin partitions a few feet in height and three or four feet in width.

*Windows.* The window sills should not exceed two feet or two feet six inches in height. And the head of the window should be carried up to within a foot or 18 inches of the ceiling. Every window should be glazed. Every window should consist of two parts; the upper portion, about two feet in depth, should be hinged on its lower edge to fall inwards to form a species of large louvre for ventilation.

On each side of the hinged portion there should be a triangular cheek to prevent air currents falling upon the men. This louvred portion of the window should admit of being easily closed by a rope and pulley. To whatever extent it is opened, air currents will be directed towards the ceiling of the room. (It may be here mentioned, as a point of experience, that great care is required in warm climates in the fitting of doors, windows and ventilating apparatus; allowance should be made for warping and shrinking. Sometimes, from want of care in this particular, windows are broken or become fixed and immovable, and ventilation is obstructed. Often on such small matters the entire success of improvements may depend.)

The lower portion of the window should be a casement opening inwards in two halves. And each window should be provided with sliding jhilmils [wooden blinds] on the outside, having the blades directed upwards and inwards. The windows should be four feet wide.

Besides the doors along the sides of the room, it will be necessary to have a door at one end of the room opening into the verandah near the entrance to the night urinal, hereafter described.

### 5. VERANDAHS

*Construction of verandahs.* Each barrack block should have verandahs all round. In the plans, these are shown supported on iron columns; but arches or pillars of stone or brick might be used; they should be eight or ten feet wide at the least, to correspond with the breadth of the terrace giving entrance to the rooms. As the terrace for the ground-floor rooms would rest on the arched basement, this basement would have to be longer and broader than the barrack room in proportion to the breadth of the verandah. The roof of the verandah of the upper floor should be a continuation of the slope of the roof of the barrack room. The verandah of the lower floor, where there are two floors, would be the terrace to the rooms above. But as it might hardly project far enough to shelter the lower rooms sufficiently from the sun, a series of louvres should be carried the whole way along between the pillars, sufficiently deep to afford the required amount of shade.

*Roof to double.* It is important that the verandahs should be ventilated to carry off the hot air. In the upper-floor verandah this can be best done by constructing the roof of the verandah double with a continuous free airspace of six inches between the outer covering and the inner lining, both of which should be continuous with the covering and lining of the roof, and the heated air should be discharged at the ridge through the airspace continued up from the verandah. The arrangement is shown in Plan XI. In the lower-floor verandah, the hot air would escape by the louvres between the pillars.

An important incidental advantage derived from this construction of barrack rooms is that each half company block, if on two floors, would have about 1200 linear feet of verandah, half on each floor, for the use of forty-eight men with their N.C. officers.

## 6. VENTILATION AND COOLING OF BARRACK ROOMS

*Arrangement of blocks. Ventilation.* Barrack blocks should be arranged so that prevailing healthy winds should blow against their sides.

In laying down the principles on which tropical barracks should be ventilated, it is necessary to state that probably no one plan will answer for every station. Some stations are much hotter than others. Some are in localities exposed to every breath of wind, while others are in close, sultry, damp positions where there is little movement of the outer air. At some stations the temperature varies little between day and night. At others, cold nights succeed very hot days. At stations in India exposed to hot winds, it is sometimes necessary to close the ventilating openings to windward to prevent the rooms becoming too hot for healthy occupation, or to use artificial means of cooling the air by tatties [grass screens] or thermantidotes on its passage into the room. At stations where dust storms occur, there should be the means of closing all apertures while the storm lasts. It is evident that these and other local conditions require careful consideration on the spot. All we propose to do is to lay down general principles and the mode of application which appears most suitable for the majority of cases.

Every barrack room should be ventilated separately by itself and independently of open doors and windows.

The best way of supplying fresh air is to carry a ventilating course of air brick, nine inches deep, entirely round each room at the eaves, or to leave a similar open space entirely round on all sides of the room and close to the ceiling or eaves. This space would act as the inlet for fresh air and should be introduced into every room in the block. At stations where it is necessary to provide for closing the fresh-air inlets, a succession of louvred inlets with the louvres hinged to admit of their being closed, as shown on Plan XI and on Plan XII, figure 2, will be found a convenient method for excluding hot winds and dust.

Where the ceiling is carried up in the line of the roof, the best outlet for foul air in the upper floor would be a continuous louvre carried along the ridge, but with flat ceilings there should be louvred shafts carried up from the ceiling to above the roof, one shaft for every six men.

The construction of a continuous louvre, and the relation which it bears to the ventilation of the room and of the double roof, are shown on Plan XI. It will be seen that the louvre is so constructed as to prevent rain being blown into the room and at the same time to admit of being closed. To obtain these advantages, the louvred outlet along the ridge is constructed in lengths in the manner shown on Plan XI. It consists of a curved shield to prevent the rain being blown into the room and is provided with a flap valve which can be used either for wholly or for partially closing the louvre. In certain cases at home the means of closing and opening these valves are all connected, so that a non-commissioned officer can regulate the ventilation by simply raising or depressing a lever.

Where shafts carried through flat ceilings are used, their construction should be as follows:

a. The aggregate area of the shafts should be one square inch for from 15 to 20 cubic feet of room space;

b. Each shaft should be louvred on the four sides above the roof; the louvres should be inserted at an acute angle to prevent rain blowing in; and for the same purpose the louvred faces of the shafts should be protected by a board placed in front of each louvre at 12 or 15 inches from its face, as shown in the plans;

c. These shafts should be louvred below within the room to prevent downdraughts. And the closed lower end should be hinged for the purpose of being opened to sweep the shaft;

d. In upper-floor rooms, these shafts should be placed equidistant from each other, along the central line of the ceiling;

e. In lower-floor rooms, the shafts should be built in the walls;

f. The non-commissioned officer's room should be ventilated in the same way, i.e., by a ventilating course carried round at the ceiling and by a single shaft.

The construction and arrangement of these shafts is shown in Plan XII, fig. 2. At stations where there are hot winds or dust storms, ventilating shafts and inlets should admit of being temporarily closed to any required extent.

*Warming.* At lofty hill stations in India and at certain damp stations in the tropics during the rainy season, it may be advantageous to introduce fireplaces for warming and drying the air in barrack rooms and hospital wards. When the fuel is wood, a fireplace shown on Plan XIII, where the fuel heats a fire-clay chamber through which fresh air is introduced warm into the room, may be used. When the fuel is coal, the form of fire grate shown on Plan XII, fig. 1 will be found to answer.

*Cooling.* Much yet remains to be done before a satisfactory method of cooling the air admitted into barrack rooms and hospital wards has been arrived at. Various contrivances have been used and proposed, but none of them fulfill all the conditions of health, facility of application and economy.

Of the three methods now in use, the punkah [fan] merely agitates air already more or less impure. The tattie, at present composed of vegetable material, although it cools fresh air passing through it, is apt to occasion hurtful draughts and, if the material is undergoing decomposition, it may become an incidental cause of disease. If made of a non-decomposable substance and supplied with water otherwise than by hand labour, so that no more water was used than was required for evaporation, the tattie, or at least the principle which it embodies, might admit of better application than at present. The thermantidote is correct in principle, but of all the methods of moving air, that by means of a fan wheel used in the thermantidote is the most costly on account of waste of force. Dr Arnott's ventilating air pump, either in the form of a light metal gasometer or of a large light piston swinging like a punkah in a fresh air chamber, with suitable valves for ingress and egress of air and means of cooling, would be the nearest approach to an economical and effective thermantidote. The expenditure of force required to move large masses of air by Dr Arnott's contrivance is very small indeed.

The cheapest source of cold for cooling air in India is evaporation. And air so cooled should be allowed to enter barrack rooms and wards, not in rapid currents but in large slow moving masses. It should pass over no surface of decomposing or decomposable material in its passage. The cheapest mechanical method for moving large masses of air is Dr Arnott's ventilating air pump. We would suggest this whole subject for consideration in India, where improved methods of cooling air could be tried to an extent for which there are not facilities in this country.

## 7. Ceilings

*Flat ceilings.* Every barrack room should be ceiled. If the ceiling be carried across at the top of the wall, leaving a triangular space above it, this space should be well ventilated at the ridge and by openings in the end walls. If the ceiling be carried up in the line of the sloping roof, it would form in reality the inner layer of a double roof and should be separated from the outer roof by a sufficient depth, say, from six to nine inches, to enable a free current of air to pass upwards between the ceiling and the roof through the ridge to keep the room cool.

*Double roofs.* The roof of the verandah should also be double. The outer layer should be continuous with the outer layer of the roof of the barrack, and its inner layer should be continuous with the inner layer of the roof of the room. The entire space between the two layers should be open from the edge of the verandah to the ridge of the room so that a free current of air may pass upwards between the outer and inner layers.

*Materials.* Tiles laid on felt are suggested for the outer roof and wood for the inner. By using these materials, both the radiating and conducting of sun heat will be diminished to the utmost. The construction of this form of double roof is shown on Plan XI. It consists of an outer layer of boarding, on which the tiles are laid. Under this is a second layer of boarding at the distance of 6 inches, leaving a continuous airspace of that depth, through which the heated air from under the outer layer of the verandah and roof is allowed to escape by the ridge louvres. Under this airspace and 6 inches below it is the boarded ceiling of the room and verandah.

### 8. BARRACK ROOM ABLUTION ACCOMMODATION

*Ablution and bathrooms.* In tropical climates, ablution accommodation for barracks may be provided on one of two principles. (1) The whole ablution and bath arrangements may be separate from the barrack blocks and placed in a building to be reached from the rooms by covered verandahs. Or (2) the ablution basins may be fitted up in a small room attached to each barrack room, but placed on the outer side of the verandah. The first arrangement has the advantage of keeping every source of damp away from the barrack room. The second has the advantage of making each barrack block complete and convenient in itself, at least as regards its ablution arrangements; probably it will be found in practice that in some cases one arrangement, in some another, will be the more advantageous. As a general rule in all low, damp, hot situations, where there is little movement of the external atmosphere, it is safer to keep every additional source of damp and impure air at a distance. But in more dry and airy positions, and at hill stations, there is no reason why ablution accommodation should not be attached to each barrack room.

Plan XIV gives the details of a detached ablution and bath arrangement, which will be found suitable for many tropical stations and also for Indian stations at seasons when plunge baths cannot be used. The building is lighted by windows which, at some stations, might require jhilmils; or the windows might be protected by extending the roof so as to form a verandah. Ventilation is provided for the building at the eaves and by roof louvres.

*Baths.* The slate bath shown on Plan XVI might be found suitable (in England these baths are the cheapest, but sometimes enamelled or painted iron or zinc are used). Wherever a separate ablution and bath-room is provided, water should be laid on and the waste water should be conveyed away by the general sewerage of the station. The ablution building should be connected with the barrack block by a verandah.

In cases where it is considered advisable that a small ablution room should be attached to each barrack room, it should contain only a few basins and footpans. It would be unadvisable to introduce the ordinary ablution table and moveable iron basins on account of the large exposed wet surface which this arrangement entails.

*Ablution basins.* We would suggest for ablution rooms, whether separated from barrack rooms or connected with them, the introduction of fixed earthenware basins sunk in slate slabs, each basin having a water tap over it and a discharging plug at the bottom as in Plan XV. These basins are found to answer perfectly in England and with due care they would be a great improvement on the existing Indian practice. Four basins per room of twenty-four men would be sufficient. And each basin should have about four feet of front to afford plenty of room for the men for washing.

*Footpans.* Three footpans would probably be sufficient. Of course these arrangements are contingent on a proper water supply and drainage being provided for each barrack block. The ablution room, when attached to the barrack room, should always be reached from the barrack room by passing out into the open air under cover of the verandah, but never direct from the barrack room. The best form of this arrangement is that shown on the hospital Plan XXIV, though of course without the bath, which in barracks should always be separate.

### 9. Drinking Fountains

On each floor of the barrack block, at each end, there should be a water tap supplied with pure cool drinking water with drinking cups over a small sink. These fountains could be placed in the same compartment as the ablution room, if the ablution room is attached to the barrack. If there is no such ablution room, the fountains should be outside the barrack rooms. Drinking fountains should also be attached to all recreation rooms, gymnastic sheds, etc., throughout the station.

### 10. Night Urinals

It is proposed to provide a compartment for the night urinal attached to each barrack room to be locked during the day. Also a separate set of day urinals away from the rooms. The most efficient form of night urinal yet made is one constructed for the War Office by Mr Jennings, Plan XVII. (In giving the names of manufacturers of sanitary apparatus, it is not intended to be implied that no others are capable of supplying suitable apparatus. The names given are those of persons who have voluntarily devoted time and capital to contriving sanitary appliances in conformity with the requirements of the War Office.) It consists of a basin, valve and syphon trap, supplied with water, and has an overflow. It is cleansed and filled by raising the handle and dropping it, and it requires a very small quantity of water. For a urinal of this construction a constant water supply from a tank is required and the urinal must be drained. In the absence of water and drainage, or in cases where it might be considered unadvisable to introduce a water urinal, a moveable urinal of wood lined with pitch or of enameled iron or earthenware might be used, in some such manner as is shown on Plan XV.

*Position.* On barrack Plan VIII is shown a small compartment attached to each barrack room to contain the night urinal, which may be either a moveable vessel or a water urinal. A small closet is also shown for containing brushes and cleansing materials for the room.

### 11. Structure of Walls

*Hollow walls.* We propose that the walls should be built hollow so as to substitute an airspace instead of thickness of wall as a means of coolness. This airspace should be ventilated by air bricks, above and below, to ensure a current of air upwards, between the outer and inner walls, to carry off the sun heat. All inner walls should be plastered. Every barrack and outbuilding, and all covered verandahs, should be supplied with eaves-gutters and rainwater pipes to convey the rainwater away from the foundations and walls of the buildings.

### 12. Drainage of a Barrack Block

*Principles.* The following principles are suggested for application in barrack-room drainage.

a. Abolishing cess pits altogether.

b. Conducting all drains outside and free of the walls of the building.

c. A six-inch or nine-inch glazed earthenware pipe is sufficient for the main drain of every barrack block.

d. Into this drain should be led the water from the ablution room, if an ablution room has been attached to the block, and from the night urinal, if a specially constructed night urinal has been provided, as well as all the roof water not tanked for use.

e. The drain should be trapped outside the building and ventilated by a rainwater pipe or by a small pipe carried from between the trap and the wall above the roof of the barrack. Drains from all other buildings should be similarly ventilated.

### 13. Water Supply of Barrack Blocks

Unless every barrack block is supplied with water at pressure from one common centre, a closed iron tank, capable of holding two or three days' supply, should be connected with the barrack block, this cistern to be filled from the central tank of the station. Water will have to be laid on from it to the drinking taps, to the ablution basins and footpans where the ablution accommodation is attached to the block, and to the urinal.

### 14. Barrack Latrines and Urinals

*Latrine buildings.* The present practice in tropical climates of having the latrines and day urinals detached from the barrack blocks and reached under cover is the most suitable arrangement for these conveniences. The question whether or not the construction of latrines and urinals can be improved depends on the possibility of draining the station and providing a water supply.

Whatever form of latrine and urinal is adopted for the future should involve the abolition of cesspits or soak wells. No cesspit should be permitted within the boundary of any cantonment. Cesspits poison the air, earth and water.

If it is impracticable to sewer and drain a station, the best form of latrine consists of moveable metal vessels which should always be emptied twice a day at the least, and the arrangement should be such as to avoid any contamination of the surface of the latrine with filth or fluid, and no washing of the latrine should be required.

Where the surface of a station is so flat as to render it doubtful whether the discharge from the latrine would keep the drain clear, additional fall can always be obtained by raising the latrine and latrine buildings any required height above the level of the ground.

*Jennings' latrine.* The most efficient form of drained water latrine for hot climates is that made for the War Department by Mr Jennings,

Plan XVIII. It requires little water, it exposes a comparatively small surface, it is discharged, cleansed and refilled by raising a handle, it is not liable to get out of order and it has been successfully used for a considerable time. Whether there is smell from it or not depends only on the frequency with which it is discharged and cleansed.

*Macfarlane's.* Cast-iron water latrines, Plan XIX, made by Mr Macfarlane of Glasgow, have been successfully introduced for barracks at home. But it may be doubtful how far they would answer in warm moist climates from the larger water surface they expose.

*Urinal.* Urinals should never be under the same roof as latrines. They are best placed under a simple lean-to roof, with a suitable screen. They should never be drained into the latrine, as this is found to give rise to great additional nuisance. In the absence of drainage the best day urinal is a moveable metal or glazed earthenware vessel.

The best form of drained urinal for India is that one which exposes the smallest surface and has fewest angles. The material should be impervious and have a glazed surface, and water for cleansing it should be readily available. Mr Jennings's white glazed earthenware urinals made by him for the War Department, Plan XVII, are apparently the best hitherto contrived for use in warm climates. They require very little water, they are self-cleansing, they expose a small surface only, they can be discharged and cleansed any number of times a day by simply raising a valve and with ordinary care they are not liable to damage; they have besides been used with entire success in barracks at home. Plan XIX shows a form of slate urinal attached to Macfarlane's latrines. Over every urinal should be placed a water tap for purposes of cleanliness for the men.

Latrine buildings should be placed well to leeward of prevailing winds. They should be simple in construction and thoroughly ventilated at the eaves and along the ridge. There should be divisions between the seats, with partial doors to each seat and there should be sufficient light to admit of doors being used. It would be best to subdivide latrines so as to have one set and one building for not more than a company. In tropical climates latrines and urinals should be connected with the barracks by covered passages in the manner adopted at many Indian stations.

## 15. Cookhouses

*Construction.* The first requisite for cookhouses in warm climates is sufficient ventilation. This can only be secured by having cookhouses detached from other buildings, windows or doors on all sides, together with openings at the eaves and louvres along the roof.

*Drainage and water supply.* Efficient drainage is also required. Surface drains should never be used for the discharge of cookhouse water and cesspits to receive the drainage are inadmissible. The floors should be well raised above the level of the ground outside and well flagged or paved.

If an outlet cannot be obtained for cookhouse drainage, perhaps the best way of disposing of it would be to carry a discharge pipe from the sink to a moveable vessel which could be carried away as often as necessary.

Every cookhouse should have a constant water supply from a water tap placed over a sink; waste water should be drained away from the sink, either to an outlet or to a moveable vessel in the manner stated above.

*Improved kitchens.* It is worthy of consideration whether the introduction of improved cooking apparatus might not lead to more wholesome cooking and to greater economy both in fuel and in food. It is found that steel boilers and steel ovens set in fire-clay lumps, Plan XX, are very economical in fuel and it is suggested that they might be tried in warm climates. Every cookhouse should be provided with suitable tables and racks. The arrangements shown on Plan XXI will be found to be convenient.

## 16. Means of Employment and Recreation

Considerable advances have recently been made in India in providing this class of accommodation. We shall therefore merely suggest generally the points in the accommodation requiring attention as regards health.

*Gymnasia.* The best gymnasium for tropical stations generally is a large covered shed, open on all sides, like a railway station, sufficiently high to contain the apparatus. The floor should be raised two or three feet above the level of the ground. And roof water should be collected by gutters either into a tank or to be removed by the drains. The same shed might very well answer for a variety of outdoor games and exercises.

*Ball courts, etc.* All ball courts and skittle alleys should be covered to enable them to be used in hot weather and in rains, and roof water should be carefully disposed of.

*Workshops.* Workshops for lighter kinds of labour, tailoring, shoemaking, printing, harness and saddle making, watch making, certain kinds of woodworking, might be placed in the ground floor of new barracks. For other heavier trades shed buildings would be required.

*Reading and day rooms.* All library, reading room, day and lecture room and schoolroom accommodation could very well be placed in ground floors of new barrack blocks. But where day rooms, lecture rooms, reading and game rooms have to be provided separately, they should all be placed in a single block at a distance from the canteen, and this "institute" should have the means of supplying tea, coffee and other non-intoxicating refreshments to the men. It is not improbable that accommodation of this nature would be required in India for two thirds of the men. N.C. officers' rooms should be attached to day rooms and libraries for the sake of discipline. In barrack blocks of two floors, two such rooms would form part of the construction under the N.C. officers' rooms of the floor above.

The general sanitary principles as to ventilation, doors, windows, etc., already laid down, will be found applicable to this class of accommodation. It need scarcely be pointed out that reading and recreation rooms should be made comfortable and attractive, and of sufficient dimensions and height to prevent closeness and crowding. Broad verandahs should be provided on all sides and each block should have latrine and urinal accommodation. Also a sufficient supply of pure cool drinking water laid on.

*Soldiers' gardens.* If soldiers' gardens, properly laid out, were permanently attached to stations, all waste water and sewage of stations might be used for watering and manuring the ground. If this were carefully done these gardens might be placed, say, 600 or 700 yards to leeward of the nearest barrack room. The irrigation might take place at times when the men are not employed in the gardens.

## 17. QUARTERS FOR OFFICERS, NON-COMMISSIONED OFFICERS AND MARRIED SOLDIERS

*Government should provide quarters.* The most suitable arrangement of officers', non-commissioned officers' and married soldiers' quarters for tropical climates is probably that of separate bungalows at present in use in India. But it would be very advisable that all quarters should in future be constructed by government and form part of the barrack or station establishment, an arrangement which would enable quarters to be built on some uniform plan with due regard to health and to the execution of repairs.

All separate quarters should be erected on raised basements constructed on the principles already suggested and with ventilation beneath. The height of the basement should vary with the sanitary condition of the district. The higher sleeping rooms can be raised above the ground the more healthy will they be.

There should of course be a suitable allowance of rooms for officers of different ranks. We would propose for tropical climates to fix the minimum space at two rooms for a married soldier and to add on additional rooms to suit the requirements of each rank.

*Construction of quarters.* The general principles of construction for health should be similar to those already suggested for barracks, viz., windows or doors on all sides, glazed, made to open and with sliding jhilmils, verandahs, a sufficiency of ridge and eaves ventilation, means of ablution and of bathing.

Drainage should be carefully attended to as far as it may be required for detached dwellings of this class. The roof water should be removed and collected for use, the subsoil should be drained, the surface paved and guttered. It might not be practicable in many cases to improve the present latrine arrangements in detached quarters by using water closets and drainage, but where married soldiers' quarters are grouped together, water latrines, one set for men and another for women, as shown on Plan XXII, may be introduced. Ablution water and all refuse water should be very carefully drained away from all detached quarters and should not be allowed to sink into the ground in the immediate vicinity.

One general cookhouse provided with a sink, water laid on, with drainage and ventilation and means of cooking separately for each family, will probably be sufficient for each group of married soldiers' quarters.

### 18. Washhouse and Laundry

Although all washing in India is performed by washermen, there are certain climates and seasons when it is very difficult to dry and get up linen, especially for hospital use. In the moist climate of England, the washing and drying arrangements shown on Plan XXIII have been introduced with complete success. And it is possible that there may be stations at which similar apparatus might be advantageously introduced.

## Section IV Principles of Hospital Construction

(*Recommendations of the royal commission respecting hospital construction.*
"9. That all future hospitals be erected on raised basements with the air circulating under the floors. Report, Vol. I, fol. lxviii. The only way to prevent malaria from the ground entering the sick wards is 'to construct hospitals always of two floors, placing the sick only on the upper floor.'
10. That hospitals be constructed in detached buildings containing no more than from 20 to 24 beds.
11. That hospitals be in future constructed with single verandahs only and for no more than two rows of beds between the opposite windows.
14. That the ventilation of hospitals be sufficiently provided for independently of doors and windows.
16. That all hospitals be provided with sufficient glazed window space to light them.
22. That the cubic space in hospitals be fixed at 1500 feet and upwards, and the superficial area at from 100 to 120 and 130 square feet according to the healthiness of the position, and that the wall space per bed be never less than eight feet.
23. That every hospital be provided with a constant supply of pure filtered water and with drainage.
24. That every hospital be provided with ablution accommodation, with fixed basins and with baths, having hot and cold water laid on, conveniently accessible from the wards.
25. That wherever practicable, water closets with drainage and water supply be introduced for hospital wards and privies converted into water latrines.")

*Proportion of sick and convalescents.* For tropical stations generally, 10 percent hospital accommodation will be sufficient. But making allowance for epidemic seasons, hospital accommodation should be provided at Indian stations for from 10 to about 15 percent of the strength, according to the healthiness or otherwise of the station. Considering the local peculiarities of the climate and the nature of the prevailing diseases, every Indian hospital, except perhaps at convalescent stations, should consist of two divisions: (a) for sick, (b) for convalescents. The convalescent division should be sufficient to accommodate about 25 percent of the total hospital inmates.

Every Indian hospital, and every hospital at the more unhealthy tropical stations, should consist of detached wards in separate blocks, one ward to each block. Each ward or block should hold no more than from 20 to 24 beds.

*Space per bed.* The space per bed in the more healthy districts should be 1500 cubic feet at the least and the superficial area 100 square feet per bed. In the less healthy districts, the space per bed should exceed 1500 cubic feet up to 2000 cubic feet, and the superficial area should be 120 to 130 square feet per bed according to the locality.

*Sick to be always in upper floors.* Each hospital block should consist of two floors over an arched basement at least four feet high. In India and at all tropical stations sick and convalescents should sleep on upper floors only. The lower floors might be used for day rooms, dining rooms, book room, waiting room, surgery, pack store, clean linen and bedding store, utensil store, without detriment to the sick. (In damp climates it will be necessary to provide a drying closet, possibly in the room under the ward scullery, for airing linen before issuing it to the sick.) Accommodation might also be found, at healthy stations, on the ground floor for European regimental orderlies and sergeants. If the surgery is placed under a ward, it should be at one end of the block, on account of the large class of native patients, servants and others who resort to it. The surgeon's room should be next the surgery. In very unhealthy localities, the attendants should all be lodged on upper floors.

*Ward doors and windows.* A ward for twenty-four beds should have eleven windows and doors, placed at equal distances along each of its sides. And the beds should be arranged, one bed to each pier between two windows and one bed placed about 18 inches or 2 feet from each corner. A large door at each end of the ward would be sufficient at all healthy or comparatively healthy stations. But in very close positions it may be deemed advisable to place a door or two on each side of the ward. As these doors, where introduced, will open close to the beds it may be advantageous to place a thin partition a few feet high between the nearest beds and the door to shield the patients from blasts of air.

*Hospital plan.* Plans XXIV, XXV and XXVI show a plan, section and elevation of a hospital block for twenty-four sick, embodying the principles laid down by the royal commission. The ward is 111 feet long, 26 feet wide and 15 feet high to the top of the wall, and 21½ feet to the ridge. These dimensions allow upwards of 120 square feet and 1800 cubic feet per bed, counting the space to the top of the wall only.

As the upper floor of a hospital block will always be occupied by the sick through the day, it is of the greatest importance that the radiating and heat-conducting power of the roof should be diminished to the greatest possible extent. This may be done either by making the roof of the verandah and ward double throughout, with a ventilated airspace between as already recommended for barracks; or a transverse plastered ceiling, having a space between it and the roof well ventilated, may be carried across the ward at the top of the wall. The double roof has the advantage of giving additional height and additional cubic space to the ward. The construction of double roof we propose for hospital wards is the same as that shown on Plan XI and already described.

Each ward block requires a hospital sergeant's room, a scullery, an ablution and bathroom, water closets, a sink for ward slops and a urinal. We propose to arrange these offices in the manner shown on Plan XXIV.

A place for a slipper bath is also required, with the means of filling it with hot and cold water, and also for running the water off. There should be for each ward a water tap supplying pure cold water for drinking.

All the ward offices must be arranged in such manner as to leave the air to play freely on each of the four sides of the block. Among sick, after the convalescents have been removed, about ten out of every twenty-four sick would be greatly benefited by being moved from the ward into a separate dining room, if under the care of a hospital sergeant.

*Dining room.* Each sick block should therefore have dining and dayroom accommodation for this number on the ground floor, as sketched on Plan XXIV and shown in section on Plan XXV.

*Operation room.* To each general hospital for a large station there should be an operating theatre attached to one of the wards, to be used as a surgical ward. The operating theatre should be lighted from the north and means should be provided for moderating the light, as the operating surgeon may require. For operation cases, not less than 2000 to 2500 cubic feet per bed should be given, according to locality. We propose to attach the operation ward to a surgical block of such dimensions as to allow of these amounts of space being given, in the manner shown by the dotted lines on Plan XXIV. In regimental hospitals the sergeant's room would afford all the accommodation required for operations, which are very few in number in such hospitals.

*Construction of hospital.* Every hospital block should be surrounded by single open verandahs and terraces, 10 or 12 feet wide, supported on pillars or arches. The upper verandah should be continuous with the roof. Its roof should be double and ventilated, as already mentioned and shown on Plan XI; the amount of shade may be increased to suit local position by carrying louvres along between the columns.

The construction of windows should be the same as that recommended for barrack blocks, i.e., each window should consist of an upper part made to fall inwards and capable of being closed by a rope and pulley, and the lower part should open in two halves like a casement. There should be a similar glass window to open inwards over each door. Each window should have sliding jhilmils. And all windows should be glazed. The windows and doors of the floor below the sick ward should be constructed on the same principles, but their arrangement will of course differ in different blocks to suit the purposes to which the lower floors are devoted.

*Ventilation.* The ventilating arrangements for sick wards should be generally the same and subject to the same local variations to suit circumstances, as already mentioned with regard to barracks. The great principle to be kept in view is that the ventilating arrangements should be independent of doors and windows; continuous-ridge ventilation where the ceiling is carried up in the line of the roof, with inlets for fresh air along the eaves, as shown on Plan XI or shafts carried above the roof for removing foul air where a transverse plaster ceiling has been adopted, together with inlets for fresh air round the outer walls close to the ceiling, like those on Plan XII, figure 2, are suitable alike for hospitals and barracks.

*Ablution and bathroom.* Every sick and convalescent ward for twenty-four beds requires for lavatory purposes three sunk earthenware basins, with water laid on, as on Plan XV and one bath also with water laid on, as on Plan XVI. Rufford and Finch's bath is best for hospitals.

Each sick and convalescent ward requires three syphon water closets of the best construction, and one glazed earthenware sink for ward slops, all with water laid on. The compartments, where these ward conveniences are situated, require thorough ventilation. They should be quite detached from the ward block and reached under cover of the verandah, as shown on Plan XXIV.

*Scullery.* Each ward scullery requires a glazed earthenware sink, with water over it for washing up and means for warming drinks, etc., required for patients. There should be a small glazed window from the scullery, looking into the ward.

*Sergeant's room.* The hospital sergeant's room should be large enough to hold a bed and bedroom furniture with coolness and airiness. It should also have a small inspection window into the ward. The hospital sergeant must be in charge of his wards by night as well as by day, as every efficient head nurse is. Both hospital sergeant's room and scullery should be ventilated on the same principle as the ward.

*Convalescent wards.* Each convalescent block should consist of the sleeping room above, with a dining and day and game room, and reading room below. This day accommodation should be overlooked by the hospital sergeant from a room at the end of the block corresponding to his sleeping room above.

*Hospital drainage and water supply.* All that has been said regarding drainage and water supply of barracks applies with even greater force to hospitals. Special care should be bestowed on the formation of the surface and on the surface and subsoil drainage of every hospital enclosure. Roof water should be carefully collected by eaves-gutters and rainwater pipes, and tanked or conveyed away from the ground. The space immediately round each hospital block should be sloped and paved or cemented to allow of the water running freely away from the building to the surface drains. Any surface drains should be smoothly laid with impervious bottoms to remove the rainwater as rapidly as possible. There should be no cesspits, and the hospital drainage should be part of the general drainage system of the station.

Detached ablution rooms, baths, latrines and urinals for hospitals in addition to those connected with wards should be constructed on the principles already suggested for barracks and exhibited in Plans XIV, XV, XVI and XVII, XVIII or XIX.

*Kitchen.* Improved kitchens and cooking apparatus on general principles similar to those recommended for barracks and shown on Plan XXI are required for hospitals. These should also be in detached buildings.

*Arrangment of buildings.* Buildings allotted to sick or convalescents should be arranged so as to receive all healthy winds on their sides. Crowding of buildings should be avoided. Care should be taken that nothing interferes with the free outer ventilation of the blocks and all such buildings should be connected by verandahs for facility of administration in wet and hot weather. Where it is considered necessary to provide a ward for a small number of beds, in order to admit of the segregation of special cases, the ward may be placed in the position of the operating room in Plan XXIV shown by dotted lines; or, if in a separate block, the general construction of such wards as regards doors, windows, ventilation, etc., should be the same as that described above. But for such cases, the cubic space per bed should never be less than 2500 cubic feet.

*Enclosure.* Enclosures of all hospitals in tropical climates should be formed of railings on dwarf walls, never of high walls.

## Section V Sanitary Police of Barracks, Hospitals and Stations

The following points relating to the prevention of disease and the current efficiency of sanitary works at stations have been raised in the report and evidence of the royal commission, and require to be embodied in an improved sanitary code for India.

### 1. Sanitary Duties of Regimental Medical Officers and of Military Sanitary Officers of Stations

The royal commission has made recommendation (No. 32) that the sanitary duties of regimental, garrison and inspecting medical officers, described in the new medical regulations of 7 October 1859, be applied or adapted to all stations in India.

(*Recommendations of the royal commission regarding a new sanitary code and sanitary regulations for India.*
32. That the sanitary duties of regimental, garrison and inspecting medical officers, prescribed in the new medical regulations of 7 October 1859, be applied or adapted to all stations in India, and that properly trained army medical officers of health be appointed to this service at the larger stations.
37. That a code of regulations embodying the duties and adapted to the specialities of the Indian sanitary service be drawn up and issued under authority.
These sanitary duties, extracted from the army medical regulations with alterations in italics to render them suitable for Indian service, are given in Appendix No. IV.)

*Duties of medical officers.* These regulations are to the following effect: By Section XX, Nos. 5 to 21, the surgeon is charged with the duty of examining and reporting on the condition of barracks, hospitals, canteens, quarters, places of amusement and recreation, lavatories and baths, ventilation, lighting, limewashing, urinals, latrines, drainage, water supply.

By regulations 22 to 25 the principal medical officer or sanitary officer, if such has been appointed, is required to do the same duties for garrisons, camps and stations.

By Section II, Nos. 1 to 36, the inspector general or deputy inspector general of hospitals of the district is charged with inspectorial functions in all of these matters, and each class of officers is required to report to their commanding officers on all defects they may discover.

*Duties of commanding officer.* The commanding officer is bound by the regulation to take steps for remedying the defects so represented to him, unless he have sufficient reasons for not doing so, in which case he is bound to transmit his reasons to the superior military authority. Some subjects of complaint the commanding officer could deal with himself, but for all matters beyond his own immediate jurisdiction, such as repairs of works, etc., he would have to apply to other departments.

*Duties of executive authority.* Any code of sanitary regulations, intended for Indian stations, should therefore lay down in a manner not admitting of mistake the relation which is to exist between the commanding officer and the executive authorities, whoever they may be, in order that the requirements for health made on the commanding officer by the medical or sanitary officer may be complied with, and that works of repair, cleansing, draining, etc., may be carried out. It will be observed that by Section XX, Clause 23, the duty of reporting on the health of troops by the sanitary or medical officer includes not only reporting on causes of disease within a station but causes in "its vicinity" which will include all nuisance or cause of unhealthiness, beyond the boundaries of such station, likely to influence its health.

*Causes of disease to be removed.* Provision would therefore have to be made in the code for the immediate abatement, removal or prevention of all causes of disease connected with stations, bazaars, native towns on receipt of complaints or representations from commanding officers. The code should state clearly the necessary course of proceeding, the local authorities or other persons to whom representations are to be made and the steps to be taken for abating the nuisance.

The chief causes likely to give rise to complaints to commanding officers on the part of regimental surgeons or medical sanitary officers at stations, as brought out in evidence before the royal commission, are as follow:

1. Surface filth. Defects in cleansing;
2. Excavated and broken ground;
3. Marshy or wet ground. Unwholesome collections of water;
4. Dung heaps and stables;
5. Unwholesome latrines and urinals. Cesspits;

6. Nuisance committed by natives;
7. Nuisance from animals and slaughtering places;
8. Impure or deficient water. Fouling of water supplies;
9. Want of drainage or bad drainage of surface or subsoil. Foul gutters and drains;
10. Growth of jungle and underwood. Old walls or useless buildings interfering with the ventilation of the station;
11. Repairs of buildings necessary for health, including windows, doors, floors, ventilators, etc.; lighting, cleansing, limewashing of barracks and hospitals; lavatories, baths, etc.;
12. Unwholesome means of disposing of dead;
13. Other removable causes of unhealthiness.

It will be seen that among the matters which the medical officer will have to represent are certain causes of disease for the removal of which permanent works will be required. It is necessary, therefore, to provide for the execution of these works. When all the stations are properly regulated and their sanitary defects removed, representations on such points would probably be unnecessary, but until this is done provision would have to be made for attending to any such representations as speedily as possible.

*Army sanitary officers.* With regard to the appointment of military medical sanitary officers for the larger stations, as directed by the new medical regulations, it is apprehended that such appointments will be made in India. The medical officer so appointed should be specially conversant with sanitary duties. He should perform the inspectorial duties required of such officers by the new army medical regulations; he should make representations to the officer commanding at the station who, in his turn, should represent defects requiring remedy to the local executive authority, which authority should be directed to execute the necessary improvements with as little delay as possible.

## 2. Duties of Sanitary Inspectors at Stations, Bazaars and Native Towns

*Appointment of inspectors.* It is of the greatest importance that the sanitary administration should be special and that the local authority should make it someone's special duty at each station to remove, abate or prevent all nuisances, either by bringing cases before the magistrate or by himself and his agents taking whatever steps may be necessary to keep the station and its vicinity in a good sanitary condition.

It is found to be indispensable for this purpose in home practice for every local board of health to appoint inspectors to see to the execution of various sanitary works and measures ordered by the local authority; one of these officers is called inspector of nuisances, whose duty it is (in larger districts) to report nuisances for removal by other officers or to combine in his own person the inspectorial and executive functions. It is suggested that perhaps an officer of this latter class would best suit the case of Indian stations and smaller towns. Wherever there are municipal councils, commissioners or other executive sanitary authorities, the inspector of nuisances should be an officer acting under that authority. He should be an efficient and well-paid officer and should have a sufficient staff for all cleansing purposes placed under him. In larger towns and cities it would be advantageous to divide the town into manageable districts, each with its sanitary staff.

*Duties of inspector.* If such an officer is appointed, it would be necessary to lay down:

a. The limit within which he is to perform his duty. This limit should be extensive enough to prevent any nuisances or causes of disease, beyond the limit, being injurious to the health of troops.

b. The inspector to see that the whole area within the prescribed limit is kept free of nuisance or removable causes of disease.

To prevent any deposit of filth on the surface and to provide suitable means for collecting all house and other refuse matter.

To see to filling up of broken ground and to levelling the surface.

To draining away of foul water from the surface of the ground.

To removal of all refuse matters from the station and its vicinity.

To prevention of dung heaps and other accumulations of foul matter.

To see that animals kept within his district are so kept as not to be a nuisance or injurious to health.

To see to cleansing, filling up and abolishing of all cesspits.

To see that all gutters and surface drains are kept clean and in proper level, so that no water may accumulate in them.

To see that all latrines and urinals are duly cleansed.

That slaughterhouses are properly kept and offal disposed of immediately.

To prevent ground within his district being fouled by the native population.

To see that sources of water supply are kept from contamination.

To see that old walls and useless buildings are removed and that the growth of underwood likely to be injurious to the health of the station is prevented.

To do all other matters and things required for the cleansing, keeping clean and preventing a recurrence of nuisance within his district.

If these inspectorial and executive functions are properly carried out by the inspector of nuisances, the regimental or medical sanitary officers of stations will have fewer complaints or representations to make. If they did complain, it would be rather a proof that the inspector of nuisances had failed in his duty and there would hence be an efficient check over him.

There is another duty placed on sanitary inspectors in England which it would be very desirable to extend to India, if practicable, and that is the inspection of meat sold in bazaars. Bazaar-fed pork is unfit for human food and the sale of it should be prevented, at all events inasfar as concerns the soldier. In the comparatively small area of the city of London many tons of meat are seized by the inspector every week, of which it may be said that it is much more wholesome than bazaar pork.

*Markets to be constructed.* With reference to the question of bazaars generally, it would be very desirable to consider whether properly constructed markets for the sale of all articles of human food might not be erected by government or by the local authority and placed under suitable regulations as to drainage, water supply, cleanliness, inspection of food, etc.

*By-laws.* It would be almost impossible in any general regulations as to duties to provide for every case likely to happen over such an immense extent of country, and it would be necessary to provide for making by-laws to meet special cases. Under sanitary acts in England these by-laws are drawn by the local authorities and sanctioned by the home office.

### 3. Regulation of Bazaars and Native Dwellings

A common cause of unhealthiness of stations is the want of some regulation respecting native dwellings and bazaars. Bazaars and native population are apt to increase almost imperceptibly in cantonments. The people encourage their relatives to live with them. These bring others and eventually there is little real limit to their numbers. It sometimes happens that the native population encroaches on cantonments in every direction so that, except to the initiated, there is apparently no cantonment boundary. With such a state of matters, sanitary regulation is hardly possible. At present there appear to be doubts as to the legality of interfering with these encroachments. And it is necessary in any sanitary code to provide for the difficulty.

*Heads of regulation.* There appear to be many bazaars which ought to be removed entirely from their present position. Powers to effect this removal are required. The simplest way of meeting the difficulty in new stations, or in cases when bazaars or native dwellings can be removed or where they have become ruinous and require to be rebuilt, would be for some authority to provide:

That bazaars and native dwellings shall in future be erected to the leeward of stations, at a safe distance from the nearest point of the station to the nearest point of the bazaar.

That a plan be prepared by the local authority, showing the position of the houses and the general arrangement of the bazaar.

That streets be so arranged and of such width as to ensure freedom of ventilation.

That streets be drained in such manner as to remove readily all rainfall and other water.

That provision be made for a water supply and for cleansing and preventing nuisances, in the manner already pointed out.

That public latrines be provided and nuisance at the outskirts of the bazaar prevented.

That excavations in the ground be prohibited.

That provision be made for the sanitary inspection and cleansing of the bazaar by the inspector of nuisances.

That the local authority draw up by-laws, subject to approval, for the regulation of the bazaar.

And that infringement be punished.

Beyond this there should be powers for removing nuisances, draining, water supply, laying out streets, cleansing, etc., of native houses near stations, similar to those required for bazaars.

### 4. SANITARY POLICE OF NATIVE LINES

*Causes of disease.* A defective sanitary condition of native lines is not only a cause of disease among native troops, but is likely to react on the health of European troops in the vicinity. The sanitary defects in these lines, as described in evidence are:

Crowding of surfaces;

Irregularity of arrangement;

Absence of suitable drainage and water supply;
Bad water;
Excavations and broken ground among the huts;
Foul drains or ditches;
A filthy state of the surface;
Want of latrines.

To obviate this state of matters, it is suggested that before native lines are constructed plans should be prepared, showing a healthy arrangement and suitable distance between the huts, also roads, pathways, drainage, latrines and water supply. With regard to existing lines, provision should be made in the code in order that nuisances be prevented, the ground properly drained, levelled and kept clean, and suitable arrangements made for supplying latrines and water.

## 5. Officers of Health Appointed for Civil Duties in Towns

A very important recommendation in the report of the royal commission (No. 35: That trained medical officers of health be appointed to act in peace as in war in connection with these presidency sanitary commissions) is the appointment of officers of health for civil purposes to act for towns and districts in the same way as military sanitary officers are to act for stations. We have considered that it may be useful to give the following general suggestions as to the duties to be fulfilled by this class of officers.

*Duties.* The special object of the inspectorial duties of the civil officer of health appointed for cities and towns is, in the first place, to keep himself thoroughly acquainted with the movement of disease and mortality among the population over which he is placed; secondly, to ascertain as far as practicable what are the causes, local, personal and climatic, which influence the prevailing amount of sickness and mortality, especially when epidemics prevail or threaten to do so; thirdly, to report on the whole subject to the local authority charged with executive duties for protecting the public health in order that the local authority may take steps necessary for removing local causes of disease or for mitigating attacks of epidemics.

*To ascertain amount of disease.* In fulfilling these duties the officer of health of any city, town or district should keep himself acquainted with the nature and amount of disease, especially of epidemic or endemic disease prevailing among the civil population, also of the mortality, with the diseases from which it has arisen.

*To report to authorities.* He should be prepared at all times to make such reports or representations on the subject of prevailing diseases and mortality to the executive authorities under whom he is acting as he may consider necessary to bring before them. He should make a careful examination into the sanitary state of the city, town or district for which he is acting in regard to the following points:

1. *Water supply:* With reference to the amount and chemical constitution of the water, especially to the amount of organic matter, animal and vegetable, which it contains, together with his opinion as to the influence of the water supply on health; state of the tanks and other water sources, with special reference to the condition of the water they contain and to the cleanliness of the ground around them, the risk of filth being washed into the water, the use of water from the same sources for drinking, washing or bathing, the manner of storing water for use among the population, the manner in which refuse water is disposed of and into all other points regarding water supply in which the health of the population is involved.

*On drainage.* 2. State of the *drainage* of the district and of the bazaars, streets, compounds, villages, houses, etc., whether the drains are built or merely covered or open, with the condition in which they are kept, whether they convey away or retain filth or water near the houses, the condition of any ravines or nullahs likely to affect the health of the population, the existence of broken ground, waterpits, cesspools and their influence on health, the state of the subsoil drainage, whether it is sufficient to keep the subsoil dry and prevent malaria, the extent of damp, wet or marshy ground and the extent of wet cultivation, the extent of tank surface or of muddy ground on the banks of rivers or creeks sufficiently near to affect the health of the people.

*On surface cleansing.* 3. The condition of the *surface drainage,* paving and cleansing in public streets, bazaars and other public places, whether the streets are paved, with the nature of the paving, as to its material, its surface equality or inequality, its power of turning off or absorbing moisture and impurities and its adaptation for facilitating surface cleansing, similar particulars as regards the state of the surface of private streets, passages and courts, including compounds, the condition of open spaces of ground, ruinous buildings, river and sea margins in the vicinity of the town, as regards their cleanliness, the growth of underwood, prickly pear or other rank vegetation, dung heaps, nuisances, obstructions to ventilation.

*On sanitary works and measures.* 4. The provision of latrines, urinals, etc., for the population, arrangements as to their cleansing, the condition in which they are kept and their probable effect on public health.

5. The general state and efficiency of the sanitary or conservancy police.

6. The influence of the general structure and arrangement in streets, courts, etc., on the external ventilation of the town, especially as regards the effect of ruinous or useless walls and buildings which it might be desirable to remove or of closed courts or alleys requiring to be opened up.

7. The effect of the construction of houses on ventilation and on the health of their inmates.

8. The existence of overcrowding in houses or on town areas, setting forth the proportion of inhabitants in different districts to a square mile.

9. The condition of stables and other places where animals are kept, of slaughterhouses, skinning ghats, etc., offensive or unwholesome trades, such as tanners, curriers, cowhide stores, soap manufacturers, etc., and nuisances proceeding from any such causes.

*On food and drink.* 10. Much disease is engendered in India by unwholesome food; the officer of health should therefore, as far as practicable, ascertain and report on the condition of articles of food exposed for sale.

11. Unwholesome or poisonous drinks are frequently sold in Indian bazaars. This subject should also be from time to time carefully reported on by the officer of health.

*On disposal of dead.* 12. The officer of health should further examine into the state of burial grounds, burning ghats and generally into the manner of disposing of the dead and into the effect of this on public health. He should also recommend to the local authority such precautionary measures on the subject as he may deem necessary at all ordinary times, but especially when epidemics prevail.

*Times of reporting.* 13. He should report at least once a week at ordinary times and oftener during epidemics. And he should prepare an annual report, entering minutely into the whole subject for the preceding year.

## 6. PRECAUTIONS AGAINST EPIDEMIC DISEASES

*Sanitary inspectors.* It should be a special duty of the officer of health to keep a constant watch over the health of the population, particularly with regard to the occurrence of epidemic disease. He should take means to ascertain this point; also the nature and extent of the disease, the localities where it has appeared, especially as regards the first cases; the sanitary condition of affected houses and districts in regard to the points already mentioned, viz., water supply, drainage, state of the surface and subsoil, cleansing, nuisances, ventilation, proximity of rank vegetation, ruinous buildings, old walls, overcrowding of houses; also as regards any other circumstances connected with food, habits, etc., of the population, which may have tended to predispose them to the disease. In his reports to the executive authority the officer of health should enter with sufficient fullness into these particulars and should indicate any causes of disease which in his opinion require to be removed by the executive authority.

*Measures during epidemics.* Some general regulations appear to be required as to the sanitary measures to be adopted when epidemic diseases are imminent either among troops or among the civil population of the station. These measures will of course receive the best attention from the presidency medical authorities. But in order to ensure unity of action, it might be advisable to lay down some general enactments and to give the authorities power to issue special regulations and to see to their execution. The following points are suggested by the evidence and reports obtained by the royal commission.

a. Promptitude of action on the first suspicion of epidemic disease among the native population;

b. Taking every necessary measure for protecting the public health in districts threatened by the disease;

c. Spreading the population and removing part of them into the open air;

d. Thinning the troops out of barracks and the sick out of hospitals;

e. Cleansing and removing nuisances;

f. Limewashing;

g. Examination of the water supply;

h. Providing dispensaries, medicines, medical relief, including inspection of the troops for the discovery of diarrhea, when cholera or dysentery prevail. And as far as possible, similar measures for the native population;

i. Devising measures for safely disposing of the dead.

During the prevalence of epidemics, the civil officer of health might be entrusted with certain executive duties of a medical kind, such as keeping an oversight of the measures of medical relief provided for the population, especially as regards the treatment of the premonitory symptoms of cholera and other epidemics, the removal of people from infected houses and districts and seeing to the satisfactory carrying out of temporary measures of cleansing, limewashing, etc., in the houses.

## Section VI Registration of Deaths, etc.

The concluding recommendation of the report of the royal commission is that a system of registering deaths and causes of death should be established in the large cities of India with a view to publication as in England.

("No. 39. That a system of registering deaths and the causes of death be established in the large cities of India and be gradually extended so as to determine the effects of local causes on the mortality of the native as well as of the European population, the results to be tabulated and published annually by the presidency sanitary commissions.")

We have communicated with the Registrar-General of England on the subject, who has been kind enough to forward to us copies of the forms in use in his office, the heads of which we append. He has further suggested that for Calcutta at least a method of dealing with the mortality statistics similar to that adopted in London should be introduced, viz., that a weekly mortality table should be prepared and published, showing the deaths and diseases of the preceding week. We beg to recommend that the Registrar-General's suggestion be carried into effect, as one specially adapted not only to Calcutta but to Madras, Bombay and indeed to all the larger groups of population throughout India.

The occurrence of epidemic diseases among the native population always indicates more or less of danger to troops in the vicinity and it is highly desirable that the earliest possible information as to the movement of epidemic diseases among the natives should be available for the purpose of prevention, both among them and among the troops.

*Weekly return of deaths.* A weekly publication of the mortality statistics in London, and even a daily summary during epidemic seasons, has been found of the greatest public service, and it is presumed this will be still more the case in India.

*How obtained in London.* 1. The method of obtaining the facts in London is as follows:

London is divided into districts and sub-districts; to each of the former is appointed a superintending registrar, to each of the latter a registrar, who is supplied with a register book, divided into columns as follows:

**1836—Deaths in the *District of Marylebone North* in the County of *Middlesex***

| No. | When and where died | Name and surname | Sex | Age | Rank or profession | Cause of death | Signature, description and residence of informant | When registered | Signature of Registrar |
|---|---|---|---|---|---|---|---|---|---|
| *17* | *4 February* | *William Green* | *Male* | *48* | *Carpenter* | | *Rebecca Green, widow 17, North Street Marylebone* | *5 February* | *John Cox, Registrar* |

(The words and figures in *italics* in this schedule to be filled in according as the case may be.)

In this book each death is registered from information supplied by some person present at the death, who is required to produce a medical certificate on the following form:

**FIGURE 16**

*To the Registrar of the Sub–District in which the Death took place*

*Name* ________
*Age* ________
*Last seen* ________
*Died on* ________
*At* ________
*Cause of Death* ________
*(a)* ________
*(b)* ________
*Signed* ________
*Date* ________

***Certificate of Cause of Death.***

*I hereby certify that I attended* ________ *aged* ________ *last Birthday; that I last saw h* ___ *on* ______ *186*__ *that he died on* ________ *at* ________ *and that the cause of h* ___ *death was*

| | *Cause of Death.* | *Time from attack till Death.* |
|---|---|---|
| *(a) First* | | * |
| *(b) Second* | | * |

*Signed* ________
*Profl Title* ________
*Address* ________
*Date* ________

* Each form of disease, or symptom, is reckoned from the commencement *till death.*

When the death is registered by the officer, he gives a burial certificate, which is produced and placed in the hands of the clergyman by the undertaker at the cemetery, thus authorizing the funeral. Without this certificate the burial cannot take place, except in rare cases of urgency, when the clergyman himself is bound under a penalty to give the registrar notice. The registrar's books are examined by the superintending registrar, who keeps the books, when filled up, in safe custody for future use. He is bound to give certificates of deaths to anyone who asks for them and who pays the stipulated fees.

The registrars in London supply copies of the entries of all deaths occurring in the week ending on Saturday in the form No. 1, which reaches the central office by post on Monday morning and in the course of that day the forms are analyzed on the abstract sheet form No. 2, according to the nomenclature and classification given on form No. 3. The total deaths in form No. 2 are then classified on a precisely similar form, except that the sums of each order and class of diseases are given instead of the deaths from individual diseases, and both are published. A very important summary is made on form No. 4 which is intended to show the number of deaths during the week in each registrar's sub-district in London from zymotic diseases. This summary if adopted for Indian cities would enable the state of health of the native population to be readily ascertained. A further summary of deaths in public institutions is made on form No. 5 which is intended to show the total weekly mortality in each class of establishments and also in each separate workhouse, prison, hospital, etc. The abstracts of the registrars' returns are sent to the printer on Monday evening, with a meteorological table supplied by the astronomer royal and a short commentary. This constitutes the weekly return for London of the Registrar-General. It is sent to the newspapers on Tuesday and published for public information on Wednesday morning. After the facts are abstracted from the registrars' returns, these returns are sent to the officers of health of the different London parishes on Wednesday and, as they contain not only the causes of death but the residences of each fatal case, the officers of health are enabled to ascertain the movement of disease and mortality in every part of their districts.

2. *Quarterly returns.* Besides the weekly return of London, the births and deaths for every registration district in the kingdom are published once a quarter in the "Quarterly Tables" and also annually. The registration of deaths is conducted on the same principles all over England. But the facts are supplied to the Registrar-General in a somewhat different manner, as follows:

*How obtained.* Every registrar in England and Wales is required to fill up the form No. 6 at the end of each quarter and to transmit it to the Registrar-General. In this form he enters the total births and deaths for the quarter, with notes on the movement of births and deaths and of the causes of mortality, in compliance with the requirement printed on the form. At the Registrar-General's office the sum total of births and deaths contained in these quarterly returns are entered on form No. 7. Copies of the same form answer for both purposes, *i.e.*, one copy of the form is used for abstracting the births, another for abstracting the deaths. The facts so tabulated for the registration division, counties and districts in England are published in the Registrar-General's quarterly report. This report contains also the meteorology of the quarter, the state of the crops, the prices of provisions, together with any points of interest regarding the movement of the rate of births, deaths, marriages, diseases, etc., contained in the notes appended to the registrar's return.

Certified copies of the marriage registers are collected by the registrars and transmitted to the central office in London once a quarter but, on account of unavoidable delay in their collection, the quarterly publication of marriages does not take place for three months later than the publication of births and deaths.

3. *Annual reports.* Duplicate copies of all registers in England certified by the superintending registrars are sent every quarter to the central office, at which indexes are made.

*How made up.* The Registrar-General's annual report is made up at the central office by abstracting the facts, not from the registrars' quarterly returns, but from the original certified copies of their books, which have been sent as already mentioned by the registrars to the Registrar-General. The quarterly and annual totals for the annual report are abstracted from these books on form No. 7. The same form No. 7 is also used for abstracting the births and in doing so, legitimate, illegitimate and multiple births are distinguished. From the same sources, but by a separate examination, the causes of death, with the sexes and ages for the whole year, are abstracted on form No. 8.

The marriages for the year are abstracted from the certified copies of the registrars' books in the Registrar-General's office on form No. 9 for the annual report.

The annual report, besides the statistical tables, contains much useful information on various subjects connected with the public health, occasional papers and occasional tables illustrative of special points in vital statistics.

The weekly report is published within three days of the time when the data are received, the quarterly report within 30 days and the annual report within 15 months from the end of the year.

In every country in Europe, not excepting the remotest provinces of Russia, the births, deaths and marriages are now registered. And there appears to be no reason why this should not ultimately be done in India, with such machinery as is suitable to that country.

The circumstances of the population in Indian cities differ so materially from those of the people of England that it may not be practicable to introduce so complete a system of collecting facts. It is necessary, of course, that the methods employed should be fixed by the India government. The results in the first instance may be by no means satisfactory, but we should consider it of great importance, nevertheless, that they should be obtained to the utmost practicable extent and in the best practicable way, in the expectation that in time this important branch of the public service will become sufficient for all necessary purposes.

[signed by]

RICHARD AIREY, quartermaster general and president
DOUGLAS GALTON, assistant under secretary of state for war
JOHN SUTHERLAND
T.G. LOGAN, inspector general of hospitals
EDWARD BELFIED, deputy director of works, War Office
PROBY T. CAUTLEY, member of the Council of India
J. RANALD MARTIN, inspector general of hospitals
ROBERT RAWLINSON, Local Government Act Office
J.J. FREDERICK, secretary, Barrack and Hospital Improvement Commission
War Office, 15 July 1864

**Editor:** Agitation for the implementation of the royal commission recommendations continued, now often with the specifics of the *Suggestions* used in argument.

Source: From an undated memorandum sent by Nightingale to Lord Stanley, Liverpool Record Office, Derby Collection 920/15/59

[1864]

[report of the Indian commission] *Of your recommendations: to be done by War Office and Horse Guards.* [13 items]
*Of your recommendations: to be carried out by government in India.* [7 items]

Source: From a letter to William Farr, Wellcome (Claydon copy) Ms 5474/73

Hampstead
5 August 1864

*Private.* I will attend to what you wish (about the Bath Meeting) and in the meantime I send you a copy of the first fruits of your Royal India Army Sanitary Commission, with your section on registration in it. (Probably you have received a copy already.) Sir J. Lawrence has been writing home most impatiently for it. And I have sent him copies direct by H.M.'s book post. (It is understood that some time in the course of the present century he will receive them officially from the India Office. It took the members of the commission 7½ months to sign their names to this document.)

You are aware of the fruits of your India royal commission in the creation by Sir John Lawrence of the three presidency commissions (of which the Bengal one is working actively. He sometimes sends me its minutes) and in his willingness to carry out any suggestion sent him by the home commission—indeed he is more willing to hear than they to pray.

I am sorry to hear of your griefs. I do not find that mine close my hear to those of others and I should be more than anxious to hear of yours—you who have been our faithful friend for so many years. I had heard of your father's death, but not of any other loss. Sidney Herbert has been dead three years on the 2nd. And these three years have been nothing but a slow undermining of all he has done (at the W.O.). This is the bitterest grief. The mere personal craving after a beloved presence I feel as nothing. A few years at most and that will be over. But the other is never over. For me, I look forward to pursuing God's work soon in another of his worlds. I do not look forward with any craving to seeing again those I have lost (in the *very* next world), sure that that will all come in His own good time and sure of my willingness to work in whichever of His worlds I am most wanted, with or without those dear fellow workers, as He pleases. But this does not at all soothe the pain of seeing men wantonly deface the work *here* of some of His best workers. But I shall bear your faith in mind, that good works never really die. Alas! Good Tulloch. But I think his work was done. Pray, if you speak of him, remember, had it not been for him, where would our two army sanitary inquiries have been? . . . I am very sorry.

ever yours sincerely, overflowingly

F.N.

I sent Sir J. Lawrence your registration papers by book post with copies of the "Suggestions." Depend upon it, he will register all India.

The thunder of the India military authorities has been heard. It was nothing but an echo of Colonel Baker's paper—the complaining of our not having incorporated the years since the Mutiny (which they did not send us) in the statistics, of our not having taken into account the diminution in mortality of late years. Sir J. Lawrence sent me word of this. The India Office were to receive this remonstrance. But they have subsided and make no sign. Though it must have been at least two months before the end of the session that they received it, and Sir C. Wood promised and threatened to lay it before the House of Commons, he wisely held his tongue. And no soul has heard of the receipt by the I.O.

F.N.

Source: From a letter to Lord Stanley, Liverpool Record Office, Derby Collection 920/15/51

Hampstead, N.W.
16 August 1864

*Private.* I think you may like to see the accompanying letter from Sir Hugh Rose. I must sing an ode to *him* now for *he* has carried out the recommendations of your sanitary commission [regimental workshops and soldiers' gardens] (of his own accord *he* says of course—not for anyone else—so they are done, we do not care). We know very well that the questions sent out by your commission prompted the four first, and Sir John Lawrence forced upon him the last. However, he has behaved *a great deal* better to us than our War Office at home has, or our Horse Guards. And this is the greatest real step made yet. You will perhaps have forgotten that in conjunction with Sir John Lawrence I drew up a kind of list by which the recommendations, which *he* was to carry out himself, the recommendations the War Office was to carry out and those, viz., five, which were regimental reform and which only the military authorities could carry out, were specified.

After the usual amount of delay, the W.O. wrote to the Horse Guards and the Horse Guards wrote to Sir Hugh Rose. And this is his answer to the five points. It is a private document. And I must ask you to return me this, which is my copy. Would it be desirable to move for it in the House of Commons?

You will be glad to hear that the authorities of an invaliding establishment at Netley themselves attribute the decrease of Indian invalids to the measures carried out in India according to your recommendations—they wrote this of their own accord (in a letter I had from the governor today). I am rather sorry that, at Bombay, the Presidency Sanitary Commission, only lately appointed, has not been filled up according to your intentions exactly. There is no civilian on it at all. A medical officer is the president (Dr Leith, a very able man); there are only two members and a secretary. And all, except the president, may be ordered anywhere any day, when they give up their duties on the commission.

Source: From a letter to Sir Harry Verney, Wellcome (Claydon copy) Ms 9001/50

Hampstead, N.W.
16 August 1864

We have a letter from Sir Hugh Rose who has carried out all *his* part of the recommendations of the royal sanitary commission (of course *he* says, of his own accord, *not* of theirs—so they are done, we do not mind). I have sent it to Lord Stanley—when it comes back, I will lend it you. It is a private document—more creditable to Sir H. Rose. We mean to have it called for, somehow or other, and printed. Perhaps you would like to do it. Sir H. Rose will be delighted to have his great deeds sung in public. But they really are (five) great deeds and the workshops one of the five. We are truly indebted to him. It would have taken *our* commander-in-chief a long time to do likewise.

Source: From two letters to Robert Rawlinson, Boston University 1/3/44 and 45a (both written from Hampstead, N.W.)

19 August 1864

*Private.* Since I wrote to you yesterday, Mr Delane,[39] of the *Times,* has offered in the kindest way to "do all and more than" I "ask if' I "will but give" him "the materials." This being the case, I think it would be better, if you would kindly send me what it would be well to have said on the Indian *Suggestions,* leaving me to negotiate the putting it in the *Times.* I hope this will reach you in time.

[20 August 1864]

*Private.* For fear of mistakes, my second letter to you was to say that I have had a letter of Mr Delane, saying in the kindest manner that he will do and say "all and more" than I want done or said about the Indian suggestions.

To appear to distrust that tremendous potentate is the worst policy. I therefore think that it would be better if you will send me anything

39 John Thadeus Delane (1817-79), editor of the *Times* 1841-77.

you are kind enough to put down, and not set in motion Mr Taylor this time. To husband our resources, so as to have said at any time what we want said, in the *Times,* is wise. Please, burn.

Source: From a letter to Douglas Galton, Add Mss 45762 ff208-9

Hampstead, N.W.
19 September 1864

*Private.* I have been asked to reprint and publish my pamphlet on "How People May Live and Not Die in India." I shall put a preface to it, showing how much has been done.[40] May I quote from Sir Hugh Rose's letter to the Horse Guards? There is an account of how the Rifles said "we *won't* have cholera" and gardened so hard they did not have cholera, which I should like to put in verbatim. The letter *has* been quoted in the *Times.* By the way, *I* did not send it to the *Times.* I sent the "Abstract" and *Suggestions* to Mr Delane through Count [Paul Edmond de] Strzelecki and told them of the existence of Sir Hugh Rose's letter, and got those articles written [on the sanitary needs of India]. But I did not give them Sir H. Rose. Probably they came to you for it.

Source: From a letter to Lord Stanley, Liverpool Record Office, Derby Collection 920/15/54

Hampstead, N.W.
22 October 1864

*Private.* I had a whole batch of papers from Simla by last mail. I enclose one to you—the *Gazette of India.*

This is the first governmental result of your royal commission. It is a very startling one. It will revolutionize the whole of India, either for good or for bad, by creating a number of little separate governments and lots of separate officers. My own feeling is that it is a very glorious revolution[41] and entirely due to your commission which, while aiming at one thing, has done (not only that but) a great municipal work, of which it is impossible to see the end, but of which you have certainly laid the beginning.

If you will read at page 12 (the blue marks are Sir C. Trevelyan's) and then turn back to the first page, you will see a great deal better

---

40 In the preface "she gave 'Three Cheers for Sir John Lawrence'" (Cook, *The Life of Florence Nightingale* 2:53).

41 An allusion to the "Glorious Revolution" of 1688-89, during which King James II was deposed and William and Mary of Orange were invited to assume the throne. It is also called the "Bloodless Revolution."

than I do what I mean. It seems to me that you have hastened the political growth of India by half a century in self-government.

Source: From a letter to Sir Charles Trevelyan, Newcastle University Library 35/42-43 and 45-47

26 October 1864

*Private.* I cannot tell you how I thank you for sending me the *Gazette of India* of 14 September (about the municipalities). One copy I sent to Lord Stanley, one I have most carefully read through.

You have begun an immense work, which will revolutionize India for good or for bad by creating a number of local self-governments, of different sets of officers. My own feeling is that it is a glorious revolution. All honour to the men who have done it. This is the critical time for India. Now she must go on. She cannot stop. And may God grant that she may keep the wise hands who are guiding her!

For of course we only see the rough cast (in this *Gazette*), the perfect thing has to be worked out. But, fanatical as is my enthusiasm for what poor Sidney Herbert used to call my "child," the royal (sanitary) commission, do you know I should hail as its most blessed result that it has been doing not only its own proper sanitary work, but helping in another far greater one, viz., the showing that all these things must be done by municipalities, by local self-governments? . . .

We have been waiting with much interest to see how you in India would provide for the execution of sanitary works, and this proposal to act through new local authorities will in time alter the whole face of India. . . .

As soon as the municipalities begin to act, they are quite certain to commit enormous blunders. This danger must be met and warded off. But why will you not stay in India and finish your own work? It sounds most unfriendly to say so. And probably I should not say it, if I did not know it would be of not the slightest use. Everybody I know of the least authority says the same thing. The greatest work in the whole of God's world is to be done in India now. And there is no one but you and Sir John Lawrence to do it.

(If I were a statesman in India, I would do *everything* to preserve my health, but in order to stay there, not to come away.) . . .

Note on relation which should exist between the powers of raising and spending taxes, proposed to be granted to local authorities throughout India, and the proper execution of sanitary works and measures:

Taking for granted that the measures proposed in the *Gazette of India* of 14 September 1864 for the future police administration of towns and districts are the best adapted to meet local circumstances, it is most desirable that every precaution be taken that the money raised for conservancy purposes is spent in such manner as not only to do no harm to health but to benefit health. These two principles flow from ascertained experience at home. Much of the work of sanitary improvement in England has consisted in undoing, tearing up, destroying and reconstructing works already existing, which had been planned and constructed by local authorities and paid for out of the rates.

Again, it has happened, even under the Public Health Act, that works have been so imperfectly planned and executed by local authorities, from want of sufficient power of control by some better informed authority, that such works have had to be reconstructed. It is obviously of the greatest importance to derive all possible benefit from this experience in India and to provide for the following successive steps in the procedure:

1. Some competent sanitary and engineering authority must determine the drainage area and general limits, within which sanitary works and improvements are to be carried out by every local authority. The reason of this is obvious. It relates to questions of outfall for drainage, the application of sewage to agricultural purposes, the deposit and utilizing of solid refuse matters, the draining and reclaiming of unhealthy ground near towns and the prevention or removal of distant sources of nuisance.

2. The same authority should either prepare or sanction a general survey and map of the whole district, laying down the contours, levels, outfall, course of sewers and drains, streets, roads, houses, properties.

3. The same authority should prepare or sanction a general scheme of sanitary improvement, including works of drainage, water supply, paving, cleansing, opening up of streets, laying out new streets and other sanitary measures, which are to be carried out in detail and for the execution of which the local authority is to raise the required sums of money.

4. The same authority or some similar authority should inspect works in course of execution, to see that they will fulfill the required object.

5. The same authority or some similar authority would have to see that the works were kept in proper and efficient repair and working order.

The royal commission proposed the appointment of the existing presidency sanitary commissions for the express purpose of giving a beneficial direction to all expenditure for sanitary purposes, whether civil or military. And the question has now arrived at this point that it will be necessary to arrange the order in which the various authorities should act. The following questions arise:

1. Should not the sanitary commissions take the initiative and inspect by themselves or by officers acting under them?

2. When it is judged to be necessary to improve a city or town, should not the commissions either directly or through the government, have the necessary surveys and schemes of works prepared by the Public Works Department?

3. Should not the commissions sanction the scheme before it is sent to government?

4. Should not the scheme, when finally sanctioned by government, be executed by the Public Works Department from money provided by the local authorities?

5. Should not the certificate and sanction of the commissions of health be given as to the completeness and efficiency of all work executed?

6. Would it be practicable for the local authorities to borrow money, repayable (principal and interest) in thirty years, as is done in England?

These points have been suggested by what will apparently be the probable result of entrusting uncontrolled execution of works to such local authorities as India is likely to supply. They are not put forward as affording a solution of the difficulty, but solely to show what the difficulty is and how apparently it might be met, in conformity with the inference drawn by the royal commission from past practice in India, viz., that constructive works should be executed under the Public Works Department.

But you have illustrations of another method of procedure in the cases of Calcutta and Bombay, in both of which places the municipal authority has employed its own engineer as is done in England. Such a course would be most in conformity with the extended introduction of municipal authorities throughout India. But again it would be very difficult to find enough of competent sanitary engineers even to make a beginning. The way would be wonderfully smoothed, if the capitals were once put into a good sanitary state. A number of engineers would be trained in the process, who might be drafted to other cities. And possibly the chief engineers of the presidency capitals might act as consulting engineers to other municipalities.

There are difficulties anyway and the whole case has been stated above (only so much as our knowledge here extends) in order that you may have an opportunity of considering in what manner the works (described in the *Suggestions* prepared by the War Office commission) may be carried out inasfar as these works are applicable to Indian cities and towns.

Source: From two letters to William Farr, Wellcome Ms 5474/75 and 76, copies ADD Mss 43399 ff226 and 229-30

6 December 1864

I send the method proposed by the president of the sanitary commission of Madras presidency[42] for collecting births and deaths. It is proposed that the forms shall be filled up by native village officers and native police, that the filled-up forms be sent by them to the public health officer of district or city (this officer is a purely inspecting officer to see that the health machinery is kept in operation).

This officer is to tabulate the returns under the general supervision of the district magistrates, in the same way as the criminal statistics are now tabulated.

The president of the Madras presidency sanitary commission (our commission) to be registrar-general of births and deaths in the presidency and to keep up direct inspection of the civil and military registration, by means of his health inspectors (officers having large districts similar to military circles). Returns to be made *monthly* by the public health officers to the president of the sanitary commission for his annual registration report, to be published with his health report, for the military and civil population of the whole presidency.

I fancy you would like to know how they propose to carry out your *Suggestions*. And, if you would send me any observations, I would gladly forward them.

9 December 1864

I am very glad to find that you think the (Madras) general plan for registration will answer: it has no reference to the details which I have no doubt will be carried out in conformity with the *Suggestions* as far as practicable. I now send you the Madras proposal for registering the deaths and births *in cantonments.*

---

42 Robert Staunton Ellis (1825-77), president of the Madras Sanitary Commission and sanitary commissioner 1864-67.

1. The cantonment sanitary committee (to be appointed under the act) to keep the registers in their office.

2. The public health officer of the cantonment to be registrar without fees.

3. Father or mother to report birth of child within fifteen days. Neglect entails fine up to 50 rupees.

4. Some person present at death to report to registrar within eight days, under penalties up to 50 rupees.

5. Persons giving information of births or deaths shall sign their names in register book. Registration incomplete without this.

6. Police officers of cantonments to inform themselves of all births and deaths and to send certified lists at the end of each week to public health officer.

7. Census of cantonment to be taken.

Pray let us have any observations of yours upon this.

Sir John Lawrence started for India a twelvemonth this very day. And how much he has already done for us. I believe he would receive and adopt with eagerness any proposal of the nature you mention. I should not feel the least scruple in forwarding it to *him directly* and privately. We never get anything *done* in any other way.

Source: From three letters to Lord Stanley, Liverpool Record Office, Derby Collection 920/15/58, 60 and 63

Christmas Eve
[24 December 1864]

*Private.* I said that I would not trouble you with Indian papers. But I must, for we are in a great difficulty. Among those which have recently been sent me is the enclosed. (It is by our former enemy, Colonel Crommelin, but who is adopting all our principles.) It is just one of those papers which are of consequence, as involving sanitary principles of permanent importance. And it should certainly be brought under revisal before being issued for the guidance of officers.

A good paper of this kind is extraordinarily useful, but all depends, of course, on the principles laid down. If these papers are sent to me privately, as they now are, I can do some good, but in a roundabout way. If they were sent officially to the (W.O. and I.O.) "Barrack and Hospital Improvement Commission," I should be able to give the same amount of criticism (for they send their papers to me) but in a much more direct and official manner, under their name. (About a year ago, Sir C. Trevelyan sent me a similar paper of Colonel Crommelin's on the construction of *barracks*—an uncorrected proof, which

I think you saw. They have never sent the finished paper, as they should have done, for the official revisal of the home commission.)

Would you think well to ask Sir C. Wood to refer this (the enclosed) and similar papers to the W.O. commission? If he answers "that he already does so," what he has referred (besides Dr Leith's report) have been sanctioned plans, which the W.O. commission have been obliged to pronounce very bad. But as they were already "sanctioned," it was rather too late. If he says that what he receives from the Government of India are not papers at all, but plans only, then we have still a recourse, for I might write direct to Sir J. Lawrence. Or I might write even (privately) to Colonel Crommelin, whom however I do not know, but who knows me, through Sirs Lawrence and Trevelyan, enough not to take amiss.

We should be glad of your advice in any and every case. And we should be very glad to find that you thought well to induce Sir C. Wood to do the thing officially. (I must invoke your discretion to judge what is best to say as to how this paper reached you. I do not know if these papers are sent to the India Office at all from India.)

Mr J. Strachey, the president of the Bengal Sanitary Commission, is at home on three months' leave (for his health, I am sorry to say). The next best thing to having a viceroy at home and in one's hand is to have a president of sanitary commission at home and in one's hand. He brought a good many papers for me. He has asked for help. And we might be able to put him in the way of many things. He does not need to be taught. He has shown immense energy and ability in the Bengal matter.

[January 1865]

*Confidential.* We are getting on very well with the business which Sir John Lawrence wanted done, to be sent out to India. Nearly all is gone to press, including the section for having a registration and weekly table of deaths at Calcutta, Madras and Bombay, the same as we have in London. Mr Rawlinson, C.E., who has been placed on the (home) joint I.O. and W.O. commission by Lord de Grey, is writing the drainage section. The commission met for the first time on Tuesday week and passed a good deal of the work, including barrack plans. Sir Richard Airey, who is its chairman since Sidney Herbert, has come out in the light of a great sanitary reformer (new). By Sir John Lawrence's desire, I have seen Lord de Grey to settle with him under whose respective jurisdictions the different recommendations of your report came. And I made out a list in order that the W.O. might draft a letter to the I.O. But this has hung fire. For the respective jurisdictions of governor general, Horse Guards, commander-in-chief in India, War Office, India Office are as much chaos (in this kind of thing) as if India were the Sandwich Islands. And it appears to have occurred to these persons for the first time that it would be better if their respective powers and duties were defined. Sir John Lawrence would act and not wait.

But these persons wait and don't act. However, the thing is being inquired into.

19 January 1865

*Private.* I see that you are good enough to say that, when you come to London, we might discuss the Indian sanitary matter verbally. I think good might come of our doing so, if before you become pressed with House of Commons business, you would be so kind as to make an appointment. I think Sir John Lawrence might be enabled to make the first step, which has not been made yet—which no governor general but he ever will make—and, after that, all will go of itself. And Indians will wonder how they could have lived so long as they are.

As to how far diminution in mortality is due to invaliding . . . as regards India, the invaliding effect was of such a kind that, after the Mutiny, there was a clearing out of all the bad constitutions (indeed of all, it seems, who had not a "good life" up to 100 years of age). And the death rate has been much lowered in consequence. But it is not safe to take their figures any way. Their "strength" [Stanley: apparently] does not tally with the muster rolls, their "deaths" do not [Stanley: apparently] tally with the adjutant general's "casualties," nor do they appear to include all the deaths in the Mutiny. They are now wading and wandering through all the discrepancies of ill-kept statistics, in which we were for two years (1856-58) up to our chins. And they must struggle out of these as we did and establish reliable statistics as we have done.

Source: From a typed copy of a letter to Thomas Graham Balfour, ADD MSS 45772 f266

20 January 1865

*Private.* Your report stood me in good service lately, when "the military," my esteemed patrons, made a private attack, which came to me from Lord Stanley, saying that all the improvements in the health of the British Army not [now] in India, was due to invaliding only. It shows how wise you were to put the deaths of invalids in your columns, and I was able to show what the improvement was, even including these.

I assure you I have not neglected in spirit your letter of 18 November. I mean to make another attack. But I thought it best to wait awhile. We have not a secretary of state now [Lord de Grey and Ripon] who will impose his will for good on the Horse Guards. We expected better things of him. But there are many worse.

Source: From a letter to Sir Harry Verney, Wellcome (Claydon copy) Ms 9001/107

2 February 1865

I feel so used up and I know nothing about Indian finance. It seems like putting myself forward to ask to see Mr Massey, unless there is something positive to say. I have no power to teach a man sanitary things in an hour. It was different with Sir John Lawrence and Sir C. Trevelyan. But should Mr Massey,[43] *par extraordinaire*, think he has something to say to me after glancing at these books, then I should feel I was failing in my duty not to see him.

Source: From a letter to Lord Stanley, Liverpool Record Office, Derby Collection 920/14/67

19 February 1865

*Private.* Colonel Sykes has given notice of a question to Sir C. Wood, on Monday, as to the disinfectant for Bombay. (About these abominable disinfectants, references have been continually made from the Bombay government, through the I.O., to the "Barrack Improvement Commission".) The question is one, as I need not tell you, of primary importance. Is India to be laid down in disinfectants? or is she to be drained and water supplied, like other civilized countries? Are we to have sanitary works or disinfectants to cure India? Colonel Sykes's question refers to Macdougall's powder.[44]

Sir C. Wood's best reply would simply be to lay the report of the "Barrack and Hospital Improvement Commission" (on this subject) on the table of the House. In that report, they enter into the question of disinfectants for India, in its length and breadth. They show to what

43 William Nathaniel Massey (1809-81), finance minister of India under Lawrence and Mayo.

44 Colonel Sykes asked whether a requisition from the Bombay government for a large supply of disinfecting powder had been received and whether it was being complied with. Sir Charles Wood replied that it had been received, referred to the War Office for a report, and from the report did not feel justified in complying (Hansard, *Parliamentary Debates*, 3rd series [1830-91] 20 February 1865:450).

extent disinfectants can be used. These can never be used as a *substitute* for works or for cleanliness. They point out that lime or charcoal answer the purpose of destroying smell temporarily, though not so completely as the powder, and they recommend that lime or charcoal be used, before the more expensive article is obtained from England. The disinfectors have, from the first, attempted to substitute their *charlatanerie* for your (royal commission) report. I wonder that Colonel Sykes should allow himself to be their agent.

If you thought well to see Sir C. Wood and induce him to lay the said answer on disinfectants before the House of Commons, it might be the most advantageous course for the progress of our works.

Source: From a letter to Benjamin Jowett,[45] Add Mss 45783 f25

5 March 1865

I do assure you that, if I had not made myself "intolerable" to the "kings" of the India Council, I never should have got my 7 millions. One of the "kings" told a friend of mine that, since I had put him on the royal commission and he had had to stand by its principles, he had not had a moment's peace of his life. Next time I want 7 millions, I shall give notice, as Lord Panmure does in the House of Lords, that I mean to make myself "intolerable" to "kings," "even pious ones," till I get it. I thank thee, Jew, for teaching me that word. (Lord Panmure's motion tomorrow night is against Sidney Herbert's measures. And he told a man privately, who told me, that he means "*not* to spare S. Herbert's memory." And we have no one but Lord de Grey to answer him!)

Source: From a letter to William Farr, Wellcome Ms 5474/85, copy Add Mss 43400 f30

4 April 1865

I have received the enclosed table from Calcutta this very morning. Dr Sutherland thinks it will be in your line. Pray return it to me when not wanted. The table is by Dr Bryden[46] of the medical department.

---

45 Benjamin Jowett (1817-93), master of Balliol College, biographical sketch in *Theology* (3:645-47).

46 James Lumsden Bryden (1833-80), assistant surgeon at the Bengal Medical Department 1856, author of vital statistics of the Bengal presidency, author of a report on epidemic cholera in India in 1870; he believed that cholera could be spread by airborne means.

(There was no time, the covering letter says, to calculate the percentages before mail.) . . .

You see, Lord Stanley has moved for your returns. We hope to see soon your reply. Probably, in the course of ten years, the returns may come in.

Source: From a letter to Lord Stanley, Liverpool Record Office, Derby Collection 920/15/74

17 May 1865

*Confidential.* I hope you will not think me profane if I say that, God and Lord Stanley and Sir John Lawrence being on our side, we have nothing to fear. And indeed your very kind note encouraged me more than I can say. But Sir John Lawrence is in very low spirits.

My immediate reason for troubling you again (in consequence of the kind encouragement you have given) is the enclosed extract from one of the Calcutta papers, sent me by Sir J. Lawrence, which shows the backward state of opinion, and also of practical engineering ability in Calcutta. I forwarded the article to Mr Rawlinson, C.E. (Local Government Act Office) for his opinion. And he has sent me the accompanying paper. I intend writing to Sir J. Lawrence and shall enclose the Rawlinson reply. (Tomorrow is next Indian mail, by Bombay. But it is of less consequence for me to catch that mail than to communicate with you.)

The whole matter shows the need of giving them the benefit of home experience and pointing out to them how to meet difficulties which were at one time the same here. It was partly to meet these civil cases that we wished the W.O. commission to be put in communication with India, and Mr Rawlinson to be put upon it, which you brought about. So far as the troops are concerned, you have well said (in your report) that the sanitary state of the civil population is so intimately connected with that of the troops that they cannot be separated. So long, e.g., as the smell of Calcutta reaches Fort William—and it will cease to do so (and thank God that it does do so) only when the city is improved—so long will the troops suffer in health. The same principle holds good in all large groups of population where there are troops stationed. They may build barracks and spend their seven and their ten millions—as Mr Massey told me just before he went out, they should—but till they improve the water supply and drainage of the stations, they will not save their men.

2. As to Sir J. Lawrence: his letter is dated Calcutta 7 April. Of course he touches sadly upon the finance question. But, as I know nothing about Indian finance, and you know everything, it is no use

my troubling you. (I hope that the discredit of this will not recoil upon Sir J. Lawrence's administration. We feel rather as if India were holding down his head, and we cannot be too thankful for your powerful words in time of trouble.) Sir J. Lawrence says: "Our difficulties are very great—very much beyond your conception." (Yes, I can conceive. But you can conceive better.) Also: "Everybody (English) is a bird of passage; none look to India as a home; all are anxious to get away as soon as may be practicable. This evil tendency has greatly increased of late years. The general idea is that 'sufficient for the day is the evil thereof'[47] in the worst sense. Few take any real interest in improvements. The natives themselves are ignorant, apathetic or even opposed to sanitary improvements. They will not expend money on such matters. We have no easy job in raising the necessary income to meet the public demands. Then the very reforms in themselves are difficult of execution and are very expensive."

He then goes into some details about Calcutta water supply and says: "Though Calcutta is the richest place in India, the inhabitants grudge the expense, and I doubt much if they will consent to incur it. The city is under municipal management, which is defective and feeble in its character, but, if one abolished it and put in a dictator, ten to one but we put everybody against the government. Then would commence vituperation and lamentations *which re-echo in England.*" However, Sir J. Lawrence does not succumb. On the contrary, he goes on to say that he is going to "see what can be done." I need hardly say that I do not communicate Sir J. Lawrence's letters to anyone but yourself.

With regard to sanitary and statistical matters, you know Sir J. Lawrence is no statistician and only an amateur sanitarian. It would be very odd if he were otherwise. He does not see, either, the defects of the enclosed newspaper article. But he is always willing to do *more,* instead of less, *than he says.* And of all men he should have help. Would you please return me the newspaper article and Mr Rawlinson's paper with your remarks, if you will be so good as to make any.

3. We have seen the copy of Dr Farr's reply, with your alterations inserted. It is very greatly improved, if I may say so. Dr Sutherland will be glad to sign it, and Dr Farr agrees to this. In haste.

your very faithful servant
Florence Nightingale

---

47 Matt 6:34.

Sir J. Lawrence says he shall be at Simla "before long," where he has had to "send" his Bengal Sanitary Commission, "they were so ill," and where he will set to work with them upon our sanitary matters.

## Defence of the Report

**Editor:** Attacks on the report came from many quarters, the bluntest of which came from "Indians," that is, British officials in India, who were offended by a report that seemed to ignore their own efforts at improving sanitary conditions. Nightingale referred to "the thunder of the India military authorities" (see p 372 above) in their response. Some criticisms were due to the inevitable differences in standpoint and time, for by the time the report reached India some of the evils mentioned in it had already been remedied—the data for the report had been collected mainly in 1859-60, but the report itself was not issued until 1863, and did not reach India until 1864. The competence of the authors was questioned by some, but the bulk of the criticism was aimed at two aspects of the report: that it was exaggerated, and its statistics flawed. Nightingale complained to Harriet Martineau that "they charged us with exaggeration. . . . So little is understood of the whole subject of statistics that . . . it was stated that the report of the royal commission was false and had been demolished by the India government."[48]

The most serious attack on the report was made by the president of the Bombay Sanitary Commission, Dr A.H. Leith, whose *Report on the General Condition of the Bombay Army*, 1864, was first published in the *Times of India.* He questioned the statistics used and was incensed at the lack of recognition recent, completed, sanitary work had received. John Lawrence himself seemed to agree with Leith's frustration at the London commission's failure to recognize that officials in India had acted to put their house in order.

A firm reply, however, was imperative. Nightingale thought that all the points raised by Leith could be answered, but he was a respected professional and she wanted his co-operation. She wrote a conciliatory letter to him directly and received a cordial reply. As she explained to Lord Stanley, "It is most important not to alienate the president of the Bombay Sanitary Commission from reform. It is really a matter of

48 Letter 13 August 1865, in *Women* (8:628-29).

very delicate management" (see p 389 below). A careful process had to be devised for an effective reply. On this, E.T. Cook comments:

> Lord Stanley thought that Dr Leith ought to be answered at once, and wrote to Nightingale (25 October) for her advice on the subject. She suggested that the answer should be sent in the form of a report on Dr Leith's letter by the Barrack and Hospital Improvement Commission—an ingenious plan, as it gave opportunity to that expert body for giving further advice to one of the presidency commissions. Miss Nightingale and Dr Sutherland drafted the report, which was adopted by the commission on 6 January 1865. "I have pleasure," wrote Lord Stanley to her (26 December), "in sending back the draft reply to Dr Leith with only one or two verbal amendments suggested. It seems to me well done, moderate in tone and conclusive in argument."[49]

Nightingale did not take criticism lightly and she was inclined to find any hesitation on the part of officials discouraging or irritating. Replies and rejoinders scattered in these *Remarks* sometimes betray bad-humoured authors. "The suggestion that, to reduce the mortality of the army, the sole course is to avoid war in future, requires no discussion" (see p 416 below). Of the soldiers' deaths at the time of the Mutiny the reply repeats that "It was disease and not the enemy that killed" them (see p 418 below). "It was not the uncontrollable 'climate' that killed them" (see p 421 below). Lord Stanley was eager to reassure Nightingale, saying that "the Indian authorities only want time to set things a little in order—that they are willing to mend, but not inclined to give us the credit of having first put them in the right way" (Cook, *The Life of Florence Nightingale* 2:55). Improvements already achieved in India were a promise of a brighter future. "The Indian authorities did mend; and so successfully has the work been carried out by a long line of commanders, administrators and engineers that the death rate from preventible disease among the British Army in India has fallen far below the figure which the royal commission named as a counsel of perfection" (Cook, *The Life of Florence Nightingale* 2:55).

It is obvious that much care went into the formulation of the reply, which was officially adopted by the Barrack and Hospital Improvement Commission in January 1865, and published as a Parliamentary

---

49 Cook, *The Life of Florence Nightingale* 2:54.

paper. It appears below as *Remarks on Dr Leith's Report.* In the end it turned out that Dr Leith's attack had been a welcome gesture in that "it has enabled the War Office commission to state more fully than it otherwise could have done (without, possibly, giving offence) the principles on which surveys of stations should be carried out" (see p 394 below). It showed that the report's statistics were under the mark when soldiers, invalided and returned to die at home, were added to the deaths that took place in India. It also led to Nightingale's proposal, made to Lord Stanley, of "an annual report to be laid before Parliament, including mortality statistics, civil and military, sanitary reports on stations, proposed works sanctioned and executed works" (see p 395 below).

David Arnold offers the following account of the controversy in retrospect:

> Ironically, historians have tended to ignore the views of writers like Ewart[50] and to accept uncritically the uniformly gloomy view presented by the royal commission and by Florence Nightingale. . . . In consequence, credit for improvements in the army's sickness and mortality rates after the 1850s has gone to the royal commission and not to the medical establishment in India, seen, in contrast, as obstructive, obscurantist and woefully out-of-touch. Certainly, many medical and military officers in India did not take kindly to what they saw as outside meddling in their domestic affairs. The commission was strongly criticized in India at the time by doctors indignant at its apparent failure to acknowledge their own (albeit limited) achievements in military health and hygiene since the 1830s. The significance of the statistical and sanitary inquiries of the 1850s and 1860s was that . . . they gave medical officers and advisors, such as Ewart in Bengal or J.R. Martin (now in London), the opportunity and the confidence to press their professional claims on a previously indifferent administration and . . . to stress the urgent necessity and practical value of sanitary reform and preventive medicine.[51]

---

50 Joseph Ewart, *A Digest of the Vital Statistics of the European and Native Armies in India,* 1859.

51 David Arnold, *Colonizing the Body: State Medicine and Epidemic Disease in Nineteenth-Century India* 71-72.

Source: From two letters to Lord Stanley, Liverpool Record Office, Derby Collection 920/15/54 and 55

Hampstead, N.W.
22 October 1864

*Private.* I also send you Dr Leith's report on and objections to your report (Dr Leith is president of the Bombay Presidency Sanitary Commission). (You will find it on the first sheet of the Bombay *Times*). *Every paragraph of it can be answered.* And, if you see fit to have it answered, we could send the answer for your inspection. It really is a matter of statesmanship to decide what is to be done. And I have no opinion.

The logical result of Dr Leith's conclusions would be: to do nothing for Bombay presidency. *This* must not be left unanswered. At the same time, I have had a most kind and cordial letter from Dr Leith (whom I do not know) by the very same mail. And it is most important not to alienate the president of the Bombay Sanitary Commission from reform. It is really a matter of very delicate management.

(I should add that yesterday, before a meeting of your War Office and the India Office commission, was brought a proposal from Bombay presidency that, instead of draining, it was to be laid down in Macdougall's disinfecting fluid—one of those notable expedients by which people who like to keep their dirt, instead of removing it, try to blind themselves into thinking it safe.)

If, as is most probable, you have all these documents sent to you, pray return these to me. If with your own remarks, we shall deeply value them. But should you not have the *Gazette* and newspaper, they will be of more value in your hands than mine. . . . I need hardly say that I shall (basely) take advantage of the opportunity of Dr Leith writing to me to answer (to him and his objections).

26 October 1864

As you are so good as to ask my opinion as to the best form of answer to Dr Leith (Bombay Presidency Sanitary Commission), I cannot but say that I think he wants an official answer and that I believe the best way would be, if you would be so very good as to induce Sir Charles Wood (Pilate) to refer the report of Dr Leith to your own (W.O. and I.O.) "Barrack and Hospital Improvement Commission" to answer, my reason being that several important points, indeed the really important points, are engineering in character. We would ourselves get an answer (to the statistical matters) appended separately by Dr Farr. The real evil of Dr Leith's report is that Dr Leith had meddled with practical points which he is not acquainted with, and that he contradicts the engineering and architectural *Suggestions* drawn up by the "Barrack and Hospital Improvement Commission," apparently before having seen them.

Since receiving your note of yesterday, I have gone over Dr Leith's report with Dr Sutherland, and he and I have jotted down some answers, which will be submitted to you and which, if you think well to refer the matter to the "barrack commission," might be incorporated into its answer. But Dr Sutherland concurs with me in thinking that, as these answers are chiefly engineering, they ought to receive the authority of the said commission, upon which are an Indian, an English Army and a civil engineer. With regard to the other matter, the municipalities (in the *Gazette of India*), I take the liberty of sending you the notes I made for my answer, which is gone today, relatively to the application of municipal powers to our sanitary question. And, as I have no other notes of my correspondence with Sir J. Lawrence, I should take it as a great favour if you would, at your convenience, return me these.

Source: From a letter to Douglas Galton, Add Mss 45762 ff243-44

10 November 1864

*Dr Leith's Report on the Sanitary State of the Bombay Army.* I dare say you know that Lord Stanley and I have been in eager correspondence about this and that he and Sir C. Wood, in conference, agreed to refer it to your Barrack Improvers. I have a copy of Dr Leith's report. And Dr Sutherland and I have already written the heads of an answer, in accordance with Lord Stanley's desire, and have already solicited *and received* an answer from Dr Farr to Dr Leith's statistical objections.

Please, what you have to do is to get (in a meeting of the Barrack Improvers) the thing remitted to Dr Sutherland to write a reply, as having been the person who knew all about it on the *royal* commission. And the reply *must then be printed* together with Dr Farr's. For it must be distributed in India as Dr Leith's (which is also printed) has been. And I shall myself send copies to Sir John Lawrence and to the Bengal sanitary commission.

The reply will, of course, be practical and may be made the vehicle of information as important to India as that conveyed in the "Suggestions."

N.B. The reply will be short, occupying but a few folio pages of print. Of course the proof will be circulated amongst the members before being adopted.

Source: From two letters to Lord Stanley, Liverpool Record Office, Derby Collection 920/15/56 and 57

11 November 1864

Sir C. Wood has sent Dr Leith's report to the "Barrack Improvers" at the War Office, with a very proper (!) letter of "submission." We (Dr Sutherland and I) have already written our reply. I have already received, from Dr Farr, his. I understand the W.O. is to print it. And of course a proof will be submitted to you before it goes any farther. But a meeting of the W.O. "Barrack Improvers," who are by no means so rapid as Yankee "improvers," has to be held first (who can tell when?)

We are getting on steadily in India. I received a whole batch of papers by last mail, which perhaps I may trouble you with. Had we but known that such skill and energy and wisdom were to be found in Bengal, it would have been well to subordinate the other presidency commissions (sanitary) to theirs. Not one out of 100 bodies in England could show the experienced zeal they have. I wish we showed the same at home. I wish, e.g., Mr Gladstone could be brought to look upon an army otherwise than as the old schoolmaster looked upon women: as "only the evils, that belong to this state o'probation, which it's lawful for a man to keep as clear of as he can in this life, hoping to get quit of 'em forever in another."[52]

The beginning that has been made in India is entirely due to your royal commission and to the hero whom I am proud to call my "noble friend," and whom you have had so great a share in elevating, Sir John Lawrence.

13 November 1864

*Private.* With our usual dispatch, we have succeeded in producing the first rough proof of a reply to Dr Leith's report this very day. Sir C. Wood, as you are aware, and in consequence of your recommendation, referred Dr Leith's report to the "Barrack and Hospital Improvement Commission." After the necessary delay, these met and referred it to a sub-committee consisting of Dr Sutherland, Sir P. Cautley and Sir Ranald Martin. The two last have not yet seen this proof, which is only just arrived. It incorporates, as you will see, Dr Farr's remarks, which we applied to him for, as a reply to Dr Leith's *statistical* objections. Would you be so very good as to look over this first rough

52 George Eliot, *Adam Bede* chap 21.

proof with Dr Leith's report (of which Sir C. Wood sent you a copy—a thin green folio) and return it to me here with any remarks and criticisms, which you would be kind enough to make to help us?

I would farther ask you a question, but this is only from myself. Scarcely a mail passes that Sir John Lawrence, Sir C. Trevelyan (poor Sir C. Trevelyan: he has been so ill; though returned to Calcutta, he is in constant danger of a relapse and in absolute certainty of one if he does not return home before the next hot season), Mr Strachey, president of Bengal Sanitary Commission, Mr Ellis, of the Madras one, do not send me copies of sanitary codes and those kinds of things emanating from your presidency commissions. Mr Ellis shows great administrative ability. He is the only one who has apprehended the position you intended the chairmen of these commissions to hold, viz., the executive of the consultatives. Mr Strachey shows immense energy, practical ability and determination to proceed at once. But all these papers fail in the initiative. Nothing has really been done. No plan has yet been framed embracing how the thing is to begin. I am afraid of sending you even a selection of these papers—they are so voluminous. Otherwise you would see at once what I mean. What I thought was that, if we could (in this compulsory reply to Dr Leith) introduce something more specific than we ventured to do in the *Suggestions* as to modes of initiative, of procedure, of administration—it would then come with official authority—I would send copies privately to Sir John Lawrence, Mr Strachey, Mr Ellis, who are not only willing but eager to receive help. Do you think this possible or desirable?

yours very faithfully
Florence Nightingale

P.S. I have received a very kind note from Sir C. Wood, but which is extremely aggravating. He, evidently quoting from Dr Leith, alleges the last year's mortality (12) of Bombay as a proof that nothing more of progress is wanting. Now the fact is, Bombay has done nothing, less than Bengal or Madras, less than nothing, in truth. And if they think that nothing wants doing, next epidemic year they will have a cholera or something which will sweep half of them off the face of the earth.

Source: From a draft letter to Dr A.H. Leith in Dr Sutherland's hand, ADD MSS 45799 f71

[ca. 1 December 1864]

Some time ago I received your letter written in consequence of my having requested a friend to introduce me to you. My object was to discuss with you the general principles of sanitary improvement for the Bombay stations and towns and to render any assistance I could in carrying out the work. Very shortly after receiving your note I also received a copy of the *Times of India* containing a report of yours in reply to the report of the royal commission and I subsequently got copy of the report itself from Sir R. Martin. I need scarcely say that all the friends of the cause who read the report did so with much regret, and Sir C. Wood sent a copy of it to the War Office commission for their remarks. They have drawn up a paper on the subject, of which no doubt a copy will be sent you. I am personally sorry that such a difference should have arisen, especially as I feel certain that it would not have arisen if you had had an opportunity of following similar controversies which have taken place in this country many years ago. However it is to be hoped that good will come of it and that the interests of the army and of the civil population will not in the end suffer.

Source: From a letter and a note to Douglas Galton, ADD MSS 45762 ff279 and 281

5 December 1864

We send you the draft of the reply to Dr Leith's report. It is absolutely necessary, they tell me to say, that it be set up in type. Will you be so good as to give the necessary directions, and desire six proofs to be sent here as soon as possible?

[December 1864]

Certainly I think it's perfect luck for us that Leith has put out that mess of blunders.

Source: From a letter to James Pattison Walker, Florence Nightingale Museum (LMA) H1/ST/NC1/64/23

19 December 1864

Sir C. Wood (but this is STRICTLY IN CONFIDENCE) referred the report of Dr Leith on the sanitary condition of the Bombay Army to our Barrack and Hospital Improvement Commission for reply. We have replied to it. I shall send you a copy of the reply (you have of course seen Dr Leith's report) as soon as it is through the press.

Source: From a letter to William Farr, Wellcome Ms 5474/78, typed copy ADD Mss 43400 f3

4 January 1865

I send you back a revise (with your proof) of the answer to Dr Leith's report. In looking over Mr Strachey's tables, you may possibly find some illustrative matter which you would like to add to the revise. If you add anything, please return the revise as soon as you can.

It would be very curious, if the mortality and invaliding, in Mr Strachey's tables, could be compared with the mortality and invaliding, separately, of the years preceding 1858. Do these figures not lead to a suspicion that the Indian mortality was augmented in former years by the low rate of invaliding, if there were such, compared to the high rate since the Mutiny? If so, it is to be feared that sanitary improvement has had little to do with [here the letter is cut] . . . expiry of time have lowered the rate.

The War Office commission meets on Friday to sign Dr Leith's doom (answer, I mean). If possible, it would be a great advantage to us to have your opinion by that time.

Source: From a letter to Lord Stanley, Liverpool Record Office, Derby Collection 920/15/62

18 January 1865

*Private.* You will see by the thin Blue Book [*Remarks*], herewith sent, that the "Barrack [and Hospital] Improvement Commission" has adopted the reply to Dr Leith's report. And I have this day sent copies by book post to Sir John Lawrence. The great thing now is to have its recommendations put to practical use in India. We are lucky perhaps in that Dr Leith made the attack on your royal commission, because it has enabled the War Office commission to state more fully than it otherwise could have done (without, possibly, giving offence) the principles on which surveys of stations should be carried out (v. para 2, p 12). At Calcutta and Madras (as for Bombay, she appears to be doing nothing) the sanitary commissions have been engaged in drawing up draft sanitary codes. But these codes have dealt only with questions of police and cleansing. There is not a word about sanitary works in them; and perhaps there could not be.

What is now required is that the presidency governments should each direct surveys of stations to be made in the way pointed out in the *Remarks.* One or two selected stations in each presidency would be enough to begin with. If we only had a few of the larger stations fully improved, the work would go on of itself afterwards; for all would see the benefits of the new system. It was in this that we were so very anxious to have your help in pressing for a few such surveys, although we do not know whether the India Office can order such. I have been told by the highest authority in India, and since this year began, that there are not men in India (sanitary *engineers*; we could send them such from England) competent to undertake the work. All that is wanted is a good surveyor, generally acquainted with sanitary requirements (and we have sent them a perfect library of books on the subject) together with a sanitary medical officer. The sanitary medical member of each commission might, in the meantime, do the work. (He of Bengal is quite equal to it.) What we want is a beginning.

Would it be possible, and if possible would it be desirable, in the present state of the question, to call for an annual report to be laid before Parliament, including mortality statistics, civil and military, sanitary reports on stations, proposed works sanctioned and executed works, etc.? If the House would order these reports from each presidency, it appears to us that a great deal of good would be done. . . .

I am afraid I must have made some misunderstanding as to our meaning about the kind of communication we want between the War Office commission and the presidency commissions. We never intended that the communication should be *direct.* At present Sir C. Wood sends what papers he does send to the secretary of the commission and the secretary of the commission writes direct to General Pears. The papers do not pass through the War Office *in transitu.* This answers quite well. All we want is that *all* sanitary papers should be sent to the W.O. commission by the India Office for opinion.

Source: From a letter to John Strachey, Columbia University, Presbyterian Hospital School of Nursing C78

19 January 1865

*Private.* I send you one of the earliest copies of the "Remarks" on Dr Leith's report. They are, in fact, a sequel to the *Suggestions.*

The first thing now to be done is that the presidency governments should have surveys made. The steps would be these:

1. the sanitary commissions to advise the government as to the stations most requiring improvement;

2. government to appoint a committee to survey the station or town, as laid down in the *Suggestions* and "Remarks." There is no objection to the sanitary member of the commission acting as sanitary member of the survey commission;

3. *survey* commission to report, as advised in *Suggestions* and "Remarks";

4. *sanitary* commission to examine reports and plans, and make their recommendations;

5. reports and plans, etc., then to be sent home to the India Office for sanction (when they would be submitted to the War Office Commission). If you have no sanitary engineers capable of making the survey, I have reason to believe that we could find you men who would gladly go to India to do this work.

I hold it as a fortunate thing that Dr Leith's ignorance has enabled the War Office Commission distinctly to recommend a course of proceeding to be followed at all Indian stations.

I trust your health is improving.

Source: From a letter to Lord Stanley, Liverpool Record Office, Derby Collection 920/15/64

20 January 1865

*Private.* I heard last night from a man, not in the India Office but in connection with it, that "the answer of the Government of India to Lord Stanley's sanitary report has now arrived" and that "a competent judge has pronounced it admirable." Pray have it referred to the (W.O. and I.O.) "Barrack Improvement Commission." I really can hardly keep from swearing, not because I do not believe that the very worst state for action is when everybody pronounces you right, but because, when we had only just finished the reply to Dr Leith (*we are so slow*), there now is another reply to do. It is too bad.

yours very faithfully

Florence Nightingale

I feel so violent that, if I were to say what I think, I should be put into Dr Pusey's "Small Debts Court" where he put Mr Jowett.[53] I feel like the Fury in Orestes,[54] who wakes her sister Fury with a gripe on the back of her neck and worries her, as a terrier does a rat, crying: Awake! arouse! rouse her as I rouse thee!

53 E.B. Pusey (1800-82), high church leader and a critic of Benjamin Jowett's liberal theology.

54 Aeschylus, *The Libation Pourers* 957-64. Fury (a curse) pursued Orestes after he had killed his mother.

Source: From a letter to Douglas Galton, Add Mss 45763 ff15-19

26 January 1865

*Private.* I understand from Dr Sutherland that there has been a tempest in a pint-pot, about Sir C. Wood receiving from me a copy of your *Remarks* upon Dr Leith's report. That report was publicly circulated *in extenso* in the newspapers of India as far back as August last. It was widely quoted from, in such terms as these, viz., that it showed the royal commission's report to be all nonsense. I first received it in a newspaper from India from a private hand. I wrote to Lord Stanley to ask Sir C. Wood to submit the report, which was doing such extensive mischief to your commission. And then (and not till then, I believe) it was sent you from the India Office. Another 2½ months elapsed before the reply was ready. In the meantime I received (on 18 November) a note from Sir C. Wood, who had taken the trouble to find out my direction—a very kind note—but quoting Dr Leith's mortality of 12 per 1000 as a kind of triumph. After your *Remarks* came out I waited for several days, not only till after I knew they had been officially distributed, but till after I was informed that the covering letter had been written and sent to Sir C. Wood. I then replied to his note, already two months old, and sent him a copy to his own house.

All that *I* regret is my *excessive* discretion (which indeed is my besetting sin), which prevented me from forestalling the reply to Dr Leith, and answering Sir C. Wood, instead of waiting for some days till after it had come out. Since it would be far better if the temporary 12 per 1000 had remained at 69 per 1000, if people are to be deluded by it into the belief that any material improvements securing a *permanent* improvement in health have been made at Indian stations.

As we are going to have exactly the same game to play in replying to Colonel Norman's answer (to the royal commission's report) which has arrived at the India Office, and may arrive in the course of years at your office, I have submitted to your honour my sentiments on the occasion. As for Sir John Lawrence, *of course* I send him all this class of papers. The extreme celerity with which the *Suggestions* were prepared, which he begged (and prayed for on 1 December 1863 when he was appointed governor general), and for which he wrote repeatedly in these terms, "we are standing still for want of them," "we are in danger of doing worse," etc., emboldens me to hope that, as it is desirable such papers should reach him during his lifetime, my master will condone the sin I have committed and shall commit, in sending them him by book post direct. . . .

To sum up: it will be fully seven months and a half since the public circulation of Dr Leith's report by newspapers in India, before the reply, sent by me direct to Sir John Lawrence, will reach him. (It may be seven *years* and a half, for aught I know, before the copies sent by the India Office will reach him.)

O'Connell said it was worthwhile to make a lie to last twenty-four hours. How very much worthwhile, then, for Indians to make a lie which lasts 7½ months, at shortest! I hope, then, that the overhaste and indiscretion, with which this lie will have been treated, so as to receive its reply in less than eight months, will be pardoned!!

Source: From two letters to Lord Stanley, Liverpool Record Office, Derby Collection 920/14/69 and 70

23 March 1865

*Indian Sanitary.* We appear to be "in for" another reply. But so far as can be judged of from the *Times* article of today, it will be mainly statistical. We should not like to do anything except under your advice. If you would kindly say what ought to be done by us? Unless there is some sanitary heterodoxy, perhaps the home ("Barrack and Hospital") Commission cannot interfere. But we have not seen the paper and are in the darkness which Lord Panmure thinks so conducive to health. The difference in the statistical estimates we fear to be mainly due to invaliding, i.e., in the earlier periods taken by Dr Farr for estimating the mortality, the men were kept till they died, while, of late years, since the Mutiny, sickly men have been sent home either to die or recover. It may turn out that Dr Farr's part of the "reply to Dr Leith" will cover most of the ground. As we whistled, cried and shouted to them for their statistics after 1856 and could get no answer, as we tried alternately threatening, intriguing, "soaping" and going on all fours, and they were as silent as if they were dead, it is truly hard upon us to make an accusation against us that we have not put in the statistics which they had not, or pretended they had not.

25 March 1865

I have not seen the Parliamentary paper containing the Indian government's reply (sanitary), and should be very glad if you will be kind enough to send it me. I am afraid it has annoyed Sir J. Lawrence very much.

Dr Farr has asked Colonel Sykes, I understand, to move for the "remarks on *Dr Leith.*" And he has also sent a copy to Mr Delane (*Times*). If you decide on a reply, another point for you to say will be, by whom the reply is to be signed? . . . Dr Farr says the statistical points raised are the same as those raised by Dr Leith.

Source: From a letter to William Farr, Wellcome Ms 5474/89, copy ADD Mss 43400 ff44-46

10 May 1865

Both Dr Sutherland and I have gone over your very able reply, and compared it with the despatch. Your reasoning on the facts is conclusive. Would it not be advisable, *also,* to bring out (at the end) tersely the points at issue? The great body of the public do not understand a word of the controversy—no more, in fact, does the Government of India—and the *Pall Mall Gazette* shows that all that this class of people want is to get something to say which they do understand.

It is easy to lay hold of the general impression that the royal commission told a falsehood. It is not so easy for the same people to understand how it was that the royal commission did *not* tell a falsehood. A few roundly true assertions, prominently put forward, either at the beginning or the end, would meet the case. Would something as follows (proposed for your consideration) do?

1. To point out and establish briefly what the death rate was, up to the time of the conclusion of the inquiry of the commissioners? Quite terse: the fewer words, the better.

2. To point out that the jubilation of the Government of India is based on returns obtained since the close of the inquiry of the commission *and for too short a period to be reliable,* as yet.

(3. To point out that the royal commission actually sent forms to India to be filled up for the years following those for which they were able to find returns at home, and that no reply was ever sent, although the publication of the report was delayed for nearly two years in waiting for them.)

4. To point out that the sanitary state of stations is not to be estimated solely by mortality, but by the diseases attacking persons there, and that, viewed from this point, it cannot be said that any of the stations, put forward by the India government as well chosen, *are* healthy—as, at all of them, fever, dysentery, cholera have prevailed.

5. That, whatever sanitary improvements may, in the estimation of the Government of India, have been carried out, it is quite certain that the stational reports, published in Vol. 2 of the royal commission report, show that all the stations were, at that date, suffering from diseases, the result of bad sanitary condition, and that the condition of a great many of them was bad indeed.

(6. That, wherever the royal commissioners had any evidence in proof of improvements having been carried out, they noticed it and were only sorry they had so little to notice of this kind.)

7. That the new evidence brought forward by the India government in this despatch is confirmatory of the conclusion of the royal commission as to the possibility of lowering the death rate to the ratio estimated by the royal commission; and that, after this despatch, the public will have every reason to be indignant, if the high death rate of the British Army in India is not swept away.

Lord Stanley should sign alone or with you. We agree that it would be better to have the two replies to the Government of India and to Dr Leith separate but called for together. But this is a matter for Lord Stanley to decide.

Source: From a letter to Lord Stanley, Liverpool Record Office, Derby Collection 920/15/75

20 May 1865

Drs Farr and Sutherland signed the reply to the Government of India yesterday, and you probably received it last night, with a request (which nevertheless I take the liberty of seconding) that, if you saw no objection, you might think well to move for it on Monday. Also, that, as the reply to Dr Leith is referred to in the reply to the Government of India, and as it completes the case, we should be very glad if you thought well that both documents should be moved for together—on two separate notice papers—so that each might be separately printed. (Colonel Sykes promised Dr Farr some time ago to move for the reply to Dr Leith, but has not done so.) The titles are: (1) Copy of letter addressed to Sir C. Wood in reply to despatch of Government of India on Report of the Royal Sanitary Commission for India, and (2) Copy of remarks of Barrack and Hospital Improvement Commission on a report by Dr Leith on the general sanitary condition of the Bombay Army.

I am extremely grateful to you for your kind letter about Sir J. Lawrence.

Source: From a draft letter to William Farr, ADD MSS 43400 f56

[26 May 1865]

The reply [to the despatch of the Government of India on the report of the royal commission] will now do. It has been much improved. Dr S[utherland] will be glad to sign after Lord Stanley and you if you will transcribe it, sign and send it here. As soon as it is sent to Sir C. Wood, Lord Stanley might move it in the House.

Source: From two letters to Lord Stanley, Liverpool Record Office, Derby Collection 920/15/82 and 87

19 June 1865

In case Dr Farr has not sent you your Parliamentary return, with the *rates* calculated by himself, I send you my copy. But, if he has, I think I will trouble you to return me mine. You will see how, alas! the rates of Invaliding increase with the diminution of the rates of mortality. (Still there is an improvement during the last five years. This is the first return we have had of the years '57, '58, '59.)

your faithful servant

Florence Nightingale

The return for the E.I.C.'s troops, which you called for, is not yet come. Probably it will, in five or six months.

4 October 1865

*Private.* I have received in the most "Confidential" manner from the I.O. (and I am to swear that I have never seen it) the enclosed reply of Dr Leith, president of Bombay Sanitary Commission, to the *Remarks* of our home commission. The reason of the "Confidential" is that the government means to smuggle Dr Leith's reply and to close the controversy. I must say I think Dr Leith has written this in a very nice spirit (he was obliged to say something) and that the gist of it is that he had no business to make any answer to your report before, and that the time is come now to make practical progress and not to quarrel. (He and I have had, in a most "coming-on disposition," a private correspondence.)

Please return me this document by return of post and, whether they have the grace to send you a copy or not, please to say that you have never had one from me. (I am completely callous about telling lies—the I.O. tell so many. So do we.)

## *Remarks on Dr Leith's Report*, 1865

**Editor:** As explained above, the following "official" report is included here because its original and quasi-final draft was the joint work of Dr Sutherland and Nightingale. It entirely conforms with the position expounded in *Observations.*

Source: Parliamentary Papers No 29: 467-81, [Lord] Hartington [secretary of state for war], *Remarks of the Barrack and Hospital Improvement Commission on a Report by Dr Leith on the General Sanitary Condition of the Bombay Army*, copy [originally adopted by the Commission on 6 January 1865]

26 May 1865

As this report has been submitted to us by the secretary of state for India, we deem it necessary to make a few remarks on certain portions of it:

1. Dr Leith's report appears to have been drawn up in consequence of an instruction from the Bombay government, the object of which, as stated in paragraph 4, is, that the report might point out "how far the improvements of late years, and the elimination of exceptional data, modify the conclusions of the royal commission as to the general sanitary condition of the Bombay Army."

2. In directing such an inquiry, there has been apparently some misunderstanding regarding the nature of the report of the royal commission and the objects it was intended to fulfill.

That report does not deal specially with the sanitary condition of Bombay presidency. It discusses, generally, the sanitary question as regards the whole of India. And the conclusions arrived at are those following on a very general inquiry as to the sanitary condition of stations occupied by British and native troops, and of groups of population in their vicinity. The conclusions were founded on the evidence of witnesses and on answers to questions sent to all the leading stations. But neither the evidence nor the replies can be said to give a complete account of the sanitary condition of any one station.

The object of the inquiry was simply to enable the commission to obtain a knowledge of the great leading facts of the case, so as to recommend general principles for future guidance, leaving their conclusions, together with the evidence on which they are founded, to be used by the authorities in India as a basis on which to rest a searching investigation on the spot, to be conducted by competent sanitary and engineering officers, in order that the real sanitary condition of every station might be reported on in detail, and suitable works devised for removing causes injurious to health which might be discovered.

This having been the object of the report of the royal commission, it will be seen that the course directed by the Bombay government could not have resulted in supplying the information required, either for enabling a correct judgment to be arrived at as to the real condition of any station, or for enabling sanitary works and proceedings to be devised and recommended for sanction.

3. Dr Leith, in complying with his instruction, appears to have called for replies to questions sent by him to the stations, and he has compared the information so received with the conclusions of the royal commission, which, as already stated, were not specially applicable to Bombay, and with the reports from the stations contained in the second volume of the commissioners' report. And the result is that, although Dr Leith shows that certain improvements have been carried out since the commissioners began their inquiry, and although there are a few discrepancies between the two sets of replies, Dr Leith's report leaves the question of the sanitary condition of the Bombay stations very much in the same position it was left in by the royal commissioners, so that a thorough searching inquiry, followed by well-digested proposals for improving the stations, has yet to be carried out.

4. We might have concluded our remarks at this point, had it not been for certain statements which Dr Leith has made, involving the accuracy of a few points in the report, and in the estimates of mortality contained in it; as also, for certain views advanced by him on sanitary and engineering questions, which are of so much importance to the improvement of Indian stations generally as to require notice.

5. In paragraph 10 of Dr Leith's report, he directs attention to an apparent discrepancy between a statement in the royal commissioners' report, that "some means of passing the time are provided for the soldiers at all stations. The usual games are long bullets, quoits, fives and cricket, and almost every station has its ball court and skittle alley" (which, he says, is the case in the Bombay Army) and the summing up in the recapitulation that "the means of recreation are few, of exercise none."

The discrepancy is, however, only apparent, and only such as is incidental to a general conclusion, one object of which was to lead to a provision being made for exercise on such a scale as did not exist at any Indian station. Even with regard to the Bombay stations, the reports published by the commissioners show the following results: At the town barracks, Bombay, and at Malligaum, there were no means of recreation whatever. At Sattara there were no ball courts, skittle grounds, library, nor reading rooms, no gardens, workshops, nor gymnasia. At Surat there was no ball court, library, reading room, no gardens, workshops, nor gymnasia. With the exception of a small library and a reading room, not lighted at night, the deficiencies were the same at Baroda. At Ahmedabad and Neemuch there were no ball courts, workshops, nor gymnasia, nor any means of exercise except skittle grounds. At several of the larger stations which had ball courts, the provision was insufficient. At several the ball courts were uncovered and useless during the heat of the day. As a general rule, the men were confined to barracks from eight o'clock in the morning to four or five in the afternoon, eating all their heavy meals during the heat of the day, in eight or nine hours of inaction. There were no gymnasia, no covered places for exercise; although there were generally skittle grounds, these could certainly not be considered as sufficient. And from almost all the stations there were demands for increased means of exercise and occupation.

The next sentence in the recapitulation, not quoted by Dr Leith, viz., "the soldier's habits are sedentary where they ought to be active," explains what the commissioners meant.

6. In the same paragraph 10, Dr Leith takes exception to the statement made by the commissioners, that "the men's amusements, such as they are, are always connected more or less with drink." The statement was made on authority of Dr Colvin Smith, one of the witnesses examined, in answer to a pointed question put by Colonel Greathed, who is one of our best authorities on such subjects. And another witness, of excellent authority, Brigadier General Russell, stated in evidence, that in endeavouring to improve the habits of the men, by providing day rooms, etc., it was necessary to keep the canteen as far as possible from the place of amusement, "the very smell of the liquor being a temptation." Besides, Dr Leith himself confirms the statement in the report that the cost of the means of recreation (Dr Leith says "implements of play") is paid for out of the profits of what men drink at the canteen.

7. In sections 12 and 13, Dr Leith touches upon a far more important subject, and one which the royal commissioners state to be an "indispensable sanitary improvement," for all Indian stations, viz., what is included in England under the general term of "house drainage." Dr Leith states that this recommendation was made "from imperfect data, derived probably from observations made on the banks of the great rivers of the Bengal presidency and Burma." The recommenda-

tion was certainly not based on such data. He states that such drainage requires a very copious water supply. But in reality no more water is required for house drainage than is required for household purposes. He is mistaken also in supposing that, for house drainage, an outfall is required into "an abundant ever-flowing current."

The question of drainage is one of ordinary sanitary engineering, not to be settled by general assertions as to its possibility or impossibility. The only way to arrive at sound conclusions on the subject in India is to do what is required everywhere else, viz., to make an inquiry at the station which it is proposed to drain. Such an inquiry would include the levels and outfall, besides a survey and scheme of works. There may be exceptional cases, but so far as can be judged of from the Bombay stational reports, there is no station in this presidency in which works of house drainage could not be executed and an outlet found. Dr Leith very properly objects to fouling streams by sewage. There is no difference of opinion on this point. But the fact that streams in England have been so fouled is no objection against drainage works, either in England or in India. The evil has been in selecting streams for outfalls and thereby sacrificing a large amount of valuable manure, besides polluting the stream.

The evil and loss were all foreseen in England before the Public Health Act was passed. But although public opinion is slow in forming itself in England, it is satisfactory to know that at length attention has been awakened to the subject, and that the evils adduced by Dr Leith, as affording an argument against draining Indian stations will, it is hoped, be grappled with and removed by the application of sewage to agriculture. Dr Leith is mistaken in saying that "in England there are as yet but comparatively few of even the larger provincial towns that have house drainage such as is considered indispensable for our military stations." Not to speak of the immense population of the metropolitan districts, amounting to nearly three millions, which has house drainage, and the large provincial cities and towns executing works under private acts, there are between 400 and 500 towns and places in England which have been placed under the provisions of the Public Health Act and the Local Government Act, and at most of these places works have been completed.

It must not be forgotten that whether Indian stations are provided with "house drainage" or not, a water supply of from 20 to 30 gallons per head per day for every station must be brought into it for household purposes, and that it must be removed out of the station either by drains or by hand labour. The same drains which remove the ordinary refuse water would remove the latrine drainage, whilst the latrines might so be placed as to act as flushing tanks (which tanks must in any case be provided) for the main lines of sewer, so as to increase the general efficiency of the whole system. In any case an outlet must be found for the water supply, and the safest, as well as the most profitable outlet for it, would be on land under cultivation. There is not only no reason why the latrine drainage should not be disposed of in the same manner, but there is every reason to believe that it would be a very profitable use to make of it. It is highly probable that, in the vicinity of every station in India, a few acres of wasteland could be found on which to dispose of the whole sewage, or it might be used for gardens at a safe distance from barracks. The exceptional cases, both as regards barracks and towns, would probably be those in which the sea or a large river would form a more convenient outlet.

8. It may here be stated that in the 32nd paragraph of Dr Leith's report, he considers that the impracticability of providing a proper outlet precludes the possibility of adopting the recommendation of the royal commission, that iron or earthenware latrines supplied with water be introduced instead of the present system. This, it will be seen, is the same question as that dealt with above, and if an outlet can be found for the drainage of any station, the difficulty of course vanishes.

As a point of experience we may mention that the camp at Aldershot was for a number of years provided with latrines consisting of moveable vessels. But after sufficient experience of this system it was deemed desirable to abandon it, to drain the camp, introduce water latrines and to find an outlet. This great improvement has already been carried out for three fourths of the troops, occupying an area of 500 acres. Water latrines, quite inodorous, have been introduced over this large area, and 150 acres of sandy soil have been let on lease to a gentleman who will apply the whole of the sewage for agricultural purposes, chiefly the cultivation of vegetables for the troops, and of fodder for cows, from which milk and butter will be derived for the camp. In a few months the works will be in complete operation. This case in point shows what in all probability might be done at many stations in India.

9. The next matter of importance is the question of water supply, which is discussed in paragraphs 14 to 23 of Dr Leith's report.

In paragraph 21, Dr Leith alludes to the classification of water sources, contained in the evidence given by the late Dr R.D. Thomson before the commission. And as there has apparently been some misunderstanding as to the nature of the classification of sources, it may be well to restate the points of importance in regard to it.

Three sources of water are recognized for sanitary purposes:

(a) Water proceeding from mountain drainage. As mountain districts at home are generally used for pasture, this water is called "pastoral water." It comprehends springs, heads of streams or rivers, mountain lakes or artificial impounding reservoirs for collecting and storing the rainfall in upland districts. This water is the purest of all for sanitary purposes, especially when derived from primitive and igneous rocks. It contains very little solid matter, perhaps not more than two or three grains per gallon, and only a trace of organic matter of vegetable origin.

(b) The next most pure water source, but one much less pure than mountain drainage, consists of rivers. As rivers at home flow through agricultural districts, this water is usually called "agricultural water." It contains a considerable quantity, very often from 15 to 20 grains per gallon, of dissolved inorganic matter and a sensible proportion of organic matter, often amounting to several grains per gallon, derived from soluble substances in the land through which the river passes.

(c) The third sources are wells, which differ in many important points from either of the others.

Dr Leith states that, from information collected by him, the wells in use throughout the Bombay presidency belong to the two first sources, viz., mountain drainage and agricultural drainage, mentioned above. It is of importance to state that well water can never belong either to the one source or to the other. It is true that by driving a tunnel through primitive rocks a supply of water might be obtained. But this water would be essentially well water, and would either have or want certain soluble constituents which would distinguish it from the mountain drainage of the district. The great characteristic of wells, that in which they differ essentially from the other water sources, consists in their being dug through the superficial strata, and it is these strata which confer upon the waters any peculiarities they may possess. Thus, if wells are dug through ground long occupied by population, such as the area of the metropolis, the well drainage will contain in solution whatever soluble matter it has been able to take up in its course in filtering from the surface to the bottom of the well. The matters held in solution are usually inorganic compounds of various kinds, organic matter, animal and vegetable, or compounds of nitrogen, resulting from the decomposition of organic matter of animal origin. None of the London well waters are fit for use from this circumstance. But Dr Leith is mistaken in supposing that these waters are "assumed" (by the royal commissioners in their report) "as illustrative of what the wells of Indian cantonments are" (paragraph 19). The London experience is merely used to show what the water in shallow wells may become, under certain conditions of surface and population. Wherever in India these conditions are reproduced, we may feel satisfied that shallow well waters will exhibit similar impurities. Where wells are dug through rich vegetable soil, the dissolved organic matter will, of course, be of vegetable origin. These conditions, derived from the surface soil, are quite independent of the rock in which the well is dug. The rock may be of the most insoluble character, and yet the water may be polluted by impurities in the surface soil. Notwithstanding this danger, wells may be made perfectly safe as water sources, provided they be dug to a sufficient depth to obtain water of the requisite purity, and provided the surface water be cut off by casing the well above, as recommended in our *Suggestions.*

10. It is impossible to state whether the water from any source is sufficiently pure for use in such climates as those of India, without a careful qualitative and quantitative analysis. And so far as this indispensable information is concerned, Dr Leith's report affords no additional information to that previously in our possession.

There are, it is true, the analyses of four well water sources at Pune, given at pp 18 and 19 of the report. They are stated as follows:

| | Per Imperial Gallon | |
|---|---|---|
| | Organic Matter, Grains | Saline Matter, Grains |
| Of one well | 0.635 | 32.80 |
| Other well | 0.726 | 40.00 |
| First well | 1.68 | 14.40 |
| Second well | 2.24 | 37.60 |

For sanitary purposes, analyses of this class are of little or no use. With one exception, they show the waters to be very impure, as a whole, but before their probable effect on health could be stated, it would be necessary to give both the organic and inorganic constituents in minute detail.

We have given in our *Suggestions* the chief points requiring attention in the analysis of water, but we may add that, as impure drinking water is the most fruitful source of water diseases, it is necessary that the water in the condition in which it is drunk by the men should be analyzed, both as regards its suspended and dissolved impurities, in addition to the analysis of water taken from the source of supply.

11. Dr Leith states that "the physiological test," viz., the effect of water on the health of troops, may be presumed to supply in some degree the absence of a chemical test. In reports from the stations appended to Dr Leith's report, the writers state their opinion that the waters are not injurious to health, notwithstanding the prevalence of cholera, dysentery and other bowel diseases, and fevers at the stations. The point at issue is to determine to what extent the existing water supply contributes to this diseased predisposition. And the first step towards an answer is to ascertain accurately what is the composition of the waters. With our improved knowledge on such subjects at home, the occurrence of any extent of bowel disease, especially of dysentery or cholera, would necessarily lead to an analysis of the water. And our experience has certainly shown that not a few preconceptions as to the physiological effects of impure water have been erroneous, and that it is a far more frequent and important cause of disease than was formerly believed. In such cases no medical opinion taken by itself can settle the question.

12. There is one other point regarding the analysis of water which may be noticed, viz., the precautions required in using the microscope for ascertaining the extent of animalcular life in water. At paragraph 18, Dr Leith takes notice of an apparent error on the part of a medical officer at Hyderabad, who writes, in regard to a certain water mentioned in the stational report, "Although I have never examined it microscopically, I have no doubt it swarms with animal life." In the abstract of the stational reports, the first member of this sentence was omitted in abstracting, as being apparently unnecessary, seeing that a medical officer was not likely to be mistaken in such an opinion. Dr Leith says of it, that it was a "surmise," which "has been found to be groundless." We notice this, in order to call attention to the conditions absolutely necessary for ascertaining the amount of living organisms in water. And unless the method has been adopted in this case, it may be found, after all, that the water does contain them.

The following is the proceeding usually followed in examining water by the microscope:

(a) Half a gallon of the water to be examined should be allowed to remain at rest in a scrupulously clean glass vessel for six or eight hours, and the sediment carefully collected and examined under the microscope.

(b) If the sediment be small in quantity, the lower portion of the water should be transferred to a clean conical glass vessel, and allowed to stand for three or four hours. The sediment should then be submitted to the microscope.

13. There are one or two other points in regard to the water supply which require notice. Appended to the report of the royal commission is a report from Asseerghur, giving an account of the water supply of the station. Dr Leith, in paragraph 16 of his own report, states that the commissioners, misled by the want of precision in the Asseerghur report, mislead others by the way in which they quote it. The statement in the stational report bearing on the question is as follows: "The water supply is derived from tanks and rainfall, these tanks being open and generally well filled. The tank surface is 163,000 square feet in the fort, and about 7000 square feet in the lower fort and village." "One tank is used for drinking and bathing; for the former, the natives slightly clear away the surface. The water supply is sufficient for 3500 inhabitants inclusive of the water in the fort. The water in the sweet well reserved for Europeans is good. But that in the tanks very bad, though not considered so by the natives when filtered; and the tanks are preserved for the use of the garrison, and used only for drinking."

Now, at this station the report states that there were present of Her Majesty's 95th Regiment (a detachment merely) ninety-three men and nine pendalls (native barracks) for fifty native soldiers each, 450 in all. The water supply is intended for both, and it is such as is described above. It is surely not an inaccurate representation of the text quoted above to state, in the abstracts Dr Leith represents as misleading, "water derived from tanks, same tank used for drinking and bathing, for the former natives clear away surface. Water in the sweet well for Europeans is good, that in the tanks very bad."

But, besides, it must never be forgotten that the object is not only to provide a proper water supply at Asseerghur for a small European detachment, but for half a native regiment and a civil population, among which no epidemic disease (often arising from bad water) can occur without endangering the health of the troops.

It is a very limited view of such questions, to include in one's vision only the requirements of ninety-three men, and even these we should in this country consider were very imperfectly provided for by simply having a well from which they could draw water.

We are glad to find that Dr Leith sees no valid reason why the recommendation of the royal commission for a constant water supply, laid on by pipes, over stations should not be adopted.

14. Dr Leith deals with the question of the superficial area and cubic space allowed for men in barracks and sick in hospitals, in paragraphs 24, 25, 26 and 34. In these paragraphs and in the reports from the stations given by Dr Leith, there is some discrepancy between the amounts of space and area per man and the amounts given in the Appendix report of the royal commission. Dr Leith's report gives the cubic space and superficial area available at the time he received the information, and both elements are calculated, after deducting guards, prisoners and sick from the occupants of the rooms. The information asked for by the royal commissioners, in the barrack and hospital returns, was the *Regulation* space, *i.e.*, the number of men which could be placed by regulation in every barrack room and sick ward, together with the dimensions of the rooms and wards, and the superficial area and cubic space each man had a right to. The stational reports show this for most of the stations.

This element, namely, the "regulation space," is quite different from the accidental occupation. The cubic space and superficial area, recommended by the commissioners for future adoption, was so recommended, with the intention of its being made matter of regulation.

15. In the same paragraphs, attention is directed to certain important discrepancies between the measurements of some barracks and hospitals, given in the Appendix to the report of the royal commission, and measurements of the same barracks and hospitals obtained by Dr Leith. The mistakes were made in India, and though of no very great moment as regards the general result of the inquiry into the question of cubic space, still it would have been as easy for the committees at the stations to have been accurate in the measurements as not.

16. We are glad to find, from paragraph 29, that increased glazed window space has been introduced into both barracks and hospitals in the Bombay presidency, although Dr Leith informs us that there is still often a great deficiency of daylight both in barracks and hospitals.

We would call attention also to his statement that there is nothing, except the cost, to prevent barracks and hospitals from being lighted with gas. There are several excellent forms of portable gas apparatus, such as are used at home for lighting country railway stations, which might be tried for lighting military stations in India.

17. In paragraphs 35 and 36, Dr Leith deals with the recommendation of the royal commission as to the introduction of iron bedsteads and horsehair mattresses into hospitals. He states that there is not at present a hospital in the Bombay presidency in which the sick have any but iron bedsteads. As it might be inferred from this that the recommendation of the commissioners was unnecessary, it may be as well to state that the reports from the stations show that, at the date they were sent in, the hospital bedsteads at Malligaum, Kolhapur, Neemuch and Hyderabad were of wood. At Nusserabad they were chiefly wood; at Karachi partly wood; at Aden planks on iron trestles; at Surat the hospital bedsteads were the same as those in barracks. It is satisfactory to know that the great improvement of substituting iron bedsteads has been completed.

18. As regards the introduction of hair mattresses for hospitals, the commendation bestowed on this kind of bedding by the commissioners was the result of experience both in civil and military hospitals. In the Bombay presidency, Dr Leith states that straw is the usual stuffing for hospital beds, but that cotton or coir are substituted in special cases. Both straw and cotton are inadmissible materials. The choice at present lies between coir and hair. After due consideration and experience the introduction of hair mattresses was made matter of regulation in the hospitals of Her Majesty's regiments, and in conformity with the regulation they should be introduced throughout India. This is, indeed, the object of the recommendation.

19. In paragraphs 39 to 42, Dr Leith calls in question the representations made by the royal commissioners as to the sick rate and death rate of the Indian Army. He adduces certain statistical tables to show that the Bombay Army is much more healthy than could be gathered from the data referring to the whole of India given in the report. As the analysis of the Indian returns was made under the directions of Dr Farr, he has been so good as to place at our disposal the following remarks on the subject:

20. Dr Leith says in his report,

> *The data on which the conclusions of the royal commission regarding the sickness and mortality of the Indian Army were founded are returns that extend to periods far back, during many years of which the troops were exposed in the field to the inclemencies of weather, and privations in food and shelter, as well as to losses in battle, and to periods during which much new territory was occupied with, as usual, increase of sickness and loss of life, from the now acknowledged rules of sanitary science having then been as little attended to in India as elsewhere. The heavy sickness and mortality*

> *of India have thus been made* TO APPEAR IN BLACKER RELIEF THAN THEY WOULD OTHERWISE HAVE DONE. (Report of Dr Leith 11.) (The italics and capitals are not Dr Leith's.)

Dr Leith charitably adds: "It is to be hoped that good will flow from attention having been thus directed, more forcibly than might have been expected, to the existing evils, which it is desirable should without delay be removed or at least lessened by all practicable means."

In the next paragraph, Dr Leith intimates that the ratio of 84 men constantly sick in a battalion of 1000 is too high; the royal commission has applied, he says, "a heavy ratio of sickness which existed in one presidency" (Bengal) to the whole of India.

The royal commission writes, in the recapitulation, "the annual death rate for the whole of India has hitherto been 69 per thousand, and Dr Leith proceeds to controvert this statement by showing from returns "that for fifteen years back there has been progressive improvement in the health of the troops (in Bombay)" (page 11).

The fifteen years ended in 1863 and his returns relate only to the troops in Bombay, and, after 1856, are based on the strength and mortality in regiments, neither including non-effectives nor deaths that happened among invalids after their embarkation. Dr Leith gives no information about the numbers of invalids.

The commission has been charged in other quarters, and on the same grounds, with having exaggerated the mortality of the army of India. Now, this charge is unfounded, and the commission cannot accept the equivocal compliment that good may possibly flow from the overcolouring of their report.

The dates are of some importance. The commission was no sooner appointed (31 May 1859) than the members who were specially entrusted with the statistical part of the inquiry proceeded to the India House, and were supplied with all the documents available in the department. They were anxious to obtain information down to the latest date, but found nothing later than 1856. The Mutiny and consequent campaigns had produced great disturbances in the returns, and some of the records of regiments which had suffered most severely were, it appears, entirely lost.

All the commission could then gather was that the mortality of the battalions of the East India Company in the Mutiny had been excessively high. (The director general of the Army Medical Department could give no information in 1861 about India in 1859 in his report. *See* Dr Balfour's letter attached to the report, dated March 1861. The

Annual Returns of Bengal for 1860 were not received by the director general in the early part of 1862. *See* second report, dated May 1862. He gave the mortality from Quarterly Returns, including neither the European nor Asiatic troops of the late East India Company.) This was confirmed by the subsequent information, and to avoid uncertainty on the one hand, and any overstatement on the other, the investigation was closed at the end of the 1856, thus not including the excessively high rate of mortality in the Mutiny, which began in May 1857 and ended early in 1859.

The deaths of the whole of the European troops in India during the years 1857, 1858 and 1859 have never yet been published, and the director general's second report begins with the Indian returns of 1860.

The report of the royal commission was written earlier than, but it was dated 19 May 1863, in order to include the latest information which the director general could supply. That information related to 1860 (The returns of India are necessarily, and perhaps unnecessarily, slow in reaching England. Dr Balfour, in all his Indian reports, has to say, "The Annual Reports from the Bengal presidency being still in arrear, etc." *Report for 1861*, p 108) and was used to show the rates of mortality in particular stations down to recent [ti]mes. (*See* pp 38-39 of 8vo report of royal commission. To prevent confusion, it may here be stated that there are three editions of this report, viz., (1) the *folio* edition of 1863, with Précis and Minutes of Evidence and Addenda (two volumes folio); (2) the 8vo edition of 1863, with Précis of Evidence only; and (3) the 8vo edition of 1864, with abstract of Evidence and of reports received from Indian military stations. The (1) folio edition and (3) 8vo edition of 1864 are quoted in these remarks.) But the collective information available respecting the four years 1857, 1858, 1859 and 1860 confirmed the commissioners in the opinion they expressed in their report of the average losses of the armies in India exposed to the evils which continued to exist down to the date of its appointment. Their statement is to the following effect, and it has often been misquoted:

> Sir Alexander Tulloch gave, in his evidence, a series of War Office Returns of the strength, deaths and mortality of the Royal Army in India during thirty-nine years, 1817-55, from which it appears that the mean strength in the three presidencies was 20,332, and the deaths 55,584, so that the annual rate of mortality was 70 per thousand. The Maratha, Pindari, Burmese, Afghan, Sind, Satlej, Punjab and Chinese campaigns, account, according to his estimate, for 10 of the 70 annual deaths. (*See* p 319 of Evidence, folio edition, and

p 283, 8vo edition, 1864; also, pp 178-86 of Evidence before commission of inquiry into the organization of the Indian Army, 1859.) Those who are conversant with military statistics are well aware of the difficulty of obtaining results at once exact and precise. This difficulty is increased in India, and the necessary calculations are further complicated by the distribution of European officers among the Native corps, by the mixing up of officers and men, or of the Royal Army with that of the late Company, or of men at home in depot with men in India, and by the confusion of invaliding from disease with the discharge of soldiers whose terms of service have expired. The medical returns for some time appear to have included only the deaths in hospitals.

After carefully examining all the documents at our disposal, we selected for analysis the nominal rolls of strength and casualties at the India House relating to the late Company's European troops. The collection of annual casualty rolls at the India House was "compiled upon the principle of accounting for every man becoming ineffective in the year." Verified by the signatures of the commanding officers and adjutants of corps, the rolls are perfectly intelligible and substantially correct; they have been, therefore, analyzed elaborately for the purposes of this inquiry. The troops of the Company, unlike the Royal Army, served only in India, where they remained until death, or until they returned home. The deaths in the fifty-seven years, 1800-56, among all the Company's non-commissioned officers and men, including invalids in India, amounted to 40,420 out of an aggregate of 588,820 years of life, obtained by adding up the average annual strength in those years; so the annual rate of mortality has been 69 in 1000 during the present century. The mortality rate was as high as 134 in 1804, in the first Maratha war, and it was as low as 41 in 1852. It was high again in the years of Mutiny, and it has been subsequently lower than the Indian standard. From the rate of 55 in 1700-99, the rate rose to 85 in the thirty years, 1800-29; and the mortality fell to 58 in the twenty-seven years, 1830-56; so that the death rate of the British soldier, since the first occupation of the country down to the present day, has oscillated round 69 per 1000. If the mortality is set down at 69 in 1000, it follows that, besides deaths by natural causes, 61, or taking the English standard, 60 per 1000 of our troops perish in India annually. It is at that expense that we have held dominion there for a century; a company out of every regiment has been sacrificed every twenty months. These companies fade away in the prime of life, leave few children, and have to be replaced at great cost by successive shiploads of recruits. (Report, 8vo Edition of 1864:9 and 10).

It will be observed, that the mortality, deduced from the latest War Office returns which Sir Alexander Tulloch could give in, closely agreed with the mortality deduced by the commission from still better materials, the nominal returns of the Company's European troops. By the one, the mortality of our European troops was 70, by the other 69, in 1000.

The soldiers who were invalided from the Royal Army and from the Company's force included many who laboured under slow fatal diseases, such as chronic dysentery or consumption, which were contracted in the service. The commission did not bring them into account, yet the returns showed that, while in a strength of 1000 the annual deaths during fifty-seven years were at the average rate of 69 in 1000, the other casualties were 82 in 1000, making the total "casualties" from all causes, including invaliding and discharges, 151 in 1000. (*See* Report, vol. 1 *folio* p 531. This is clearly set forth in the report and in the tables, yet Dr Bird, in a paper which appears in the *Journal of the Statistical Society* Vol. 26, 1863:401, says: "The above-mentioned high rate, 69 per 1000, is not simply the mortality, but includes other rates of *decrement* from the effective strength, as those of *invaliding*, and of extraordinary war service in climates not Indian.") The commissioners only brought 69 per 1000 into account.

The commission discussed the effects of war in a special chapter (*See* Report, vol. 1 (*folio*) p xvi; and pp 19, 20 of 8vo Report) and showed that the years of war were those in which the mortality was generally highest, but that the greater part of this mortality was the direct effect of cholera and other diseases, leaving a small proportion from deaths in battle and wounds.

Sir Alexander Tulloch, who estimated the mortality of the Royal Army at 70 deaths in 1000, referred 10 of the 70 casualties in the field, and the commission was of opinion that more than 10 of the 82 men discharged for other casualties, including chronic maladies, would die of diseases induced in India.

It is evident that the mortality of an army in war cannot be omitted in any investigation of the general mortality to which armies are liable, and it is in war chiefly that the deficiency of their sanitary organization is seen. Thus, as it would not be right to leave out the years of the Crimean War in investigating the aggregate mortality of the British Army, neither could the commission exclude the years of war in India from their survey. The suggestion that, to reduce the mortality of the army, the sole course is to avoid war in future, requires no discussion.

For the reasons stated, the commission did not include the years of the Persian War and of the Mutiny, for, imperfect as the returns in their possession were, the returns by the commanding officers of regiments, published in detail (at pp 757-79 of vol. I, folio Report), convinced the commission that, had the returns been brought down to the latest period, the rate of mortality would not have been lowered by that operation.

This is evident in the Table A appended to these remarks, by which it appears that in the military year April 1857, the 64th Regiment engaged in Persia lost in deaths 237 men; the 70th, 117 men; the 1st battalion of the 60th, 194 men; the 81st, 170 men, and other regiments also great numbers. In the year following, twelve regiments or battalions lost 105, 384, 223, 280, 128, 175, 107, 106, 228, 284, 140 and 121 men out of strengths often below 1000 at the beginning of the year. In the military year 1859, 17 regiments lost 116, 187, 107, 104, 120, 123, 118, 113, 141, 176, 123, 139, 112, 112, 165, 141 and 148 men in India; and of other regiments the losses were heavy. After the war, the invalids and disabled, many of whom died, were sent home in large numbers, and thus reduced the deaths in India during the following years.

The following table, not including all the deaths in India, shows that the mortality during the excluded years must have been higher than the average of the previous years of Indian experience:

| Military years, ending 1 April | Estimated mean strength | Deaths | Mortality per 1000 |
|---|---|---|---|
| 1857 | 21,260 | 1504 | 70.74 |
| 1858 | 22,057 | 2956 | 134.02 |
| 1859 | 42,194 | 4355 | 103.21 |
| 1860 | 62,110 | 2329 | 37.50 |
| 3 years 1857-59 | 85,511 | 8815 | 103.09 |
| 4 years 1857-60 | 147,721 | 11,144 | 77.51 |

*Note:* The facts from which this table is derived will be found in Vol. 1 of folio Report, pp 757-79, "Statistics of regiments which have served in India," an analysis of which is given in the Table A annexed to this paper and referred to above. The estimated mean strength in each of the years is obtained by taking the mean of the strength at the beginning and end of the year, excepting in 1857, which is the number given as the actual strength on the 1 April of that year.

These regimental returns will be of use to the future historian of the war of the Mutiny, but the commission, desiring to avoid anything like overstatement of the case, did not bring the mortality of any regiment during the years 1857-58-59 into account; they only paid a just tribute to the men whose military virtues were so loudly proclaimed by their deaths:

> It is impossible to read the losses of particular regiments in the war of the Mutiny without being struck by the inextinguishable valour of the British soldier, but it was disease and not the enemy that killed him, for out of 9467 men dying among regiments in India prior to the Mutiny, or sent out in 1857-8, only 586 were killed in action or died of wounds (8vo Report 1864:19).

The reform in the army statistics of India, which Lord Herbert's commission suggested, had not come into operation in 1859, and the Indian returns gave very little information respecting the proportional numbers constantly in hospital for sickness, and no information about the diseases by which that constant sickness was caused.

Dr Leith says, "The existing returns of the daily sick in the hospitals of the Bombay Army extend only four years back, from 1863 to 1860; they show 73 sick in every 1000 of strength" (p 11). The estimate of the commission for all India was 84 in 1000, a "heavy ratio of sickness," which Dr Leith thinks inapplicable to the Bombay presidency.

No returns exist, but it is found that there is a certain relation between the "sick" and the dying, and Dr Leith shows, that while in the four years (1860-63) the mortality was at the rate of 21, the sick were 73 in 1000. Now, following out this proportion and taking his figures, if 21 deaths gave 73 constantly sick, 29 deaths annually, his rate of mortality from 1849 to 1863 would imply that the sick were 101 per 1000 of the strength. This is Annesley's proportion (8vo Report 1864:20) and it is higher than the low rate (84) which the commission intentionally adopted.

It was a current opinion among Indian writers, the able author [J. Ewart] of "Vital Statistics of the Anglo-Indian Armies," for instance, that the "European Army in India has hitherto disappeared in about 13½ years." This result, deduced from the facts by a mathematical oversight, and some unintentional exaggerations of other writers, the commission corrected (8vo Report 1864 pp 12-14); and to calculate the prevailing loss of men by death, invaliding and other causes, the life table for the English soldier in India, and the greater part of the deductions, were based upon the facts observed in the last available ten years, 1847-56, when the current annual rate of mortality was 51.2 per 1000 in India; namely, 67 in Bengal, 39 in Madras and 38 in Bombay (8vo Report 1864 pp 133-35).

Public attention has been directed to the health of the army; the measures which Lord Herbert and Miss Nightingale originated began to bear fruit; the appointment and the inquiries of the royal commission gave an impulse to sanitary affairs in India; and finally, the new stations in Oudh and the Punjab opened to the Bengal Army some of the advantages of a healthier country, which had before been realized by the European forces of Madras and Bombay. Thus it happened, as subsequent returns prove, that the mortality was reduced in the year 1860 to 35 per 1000, in the year 1861 to 37 per 1000, and in the year 1862 to 26 per 1000 (*See* Dr Balfour's report to the director general of Army Medical Department on returns for 1860, 1861 and 1862). During the latter year, 28 per 1000 were invalided from India for discharge or for change of climate.

The mortality per 1000 of Bengal was at the rate of 28, of Bombay 25, and of Madras 21. This most happy occurrence, which has come to light since the inquiry of the commission commenced, is cited by a certain class of writers to prove that the commission, in their report, overstated the deplorable mortality which prevailed during the present century down to the year of the Mutiny. Other critics, by excluding years of war, as well as even the deaths from cholera, and selecting years after war had cleared the army of invalids, contrived to exhibit low rates of mortality, but none have impeached the accuracy of the calculations of the commissioners. They have only reasoned in this inconclusive form: "The mortality in the years since the commission was appointed has been lower than 69 in 1000; therefore that rate could not have accurately represented the mortality of soldiers in India up to the date of the last returns." The answer is that the mortality which the commission cites is an incontestable fact.

With regard to recent lower death rates, it is necessary to bear in mind that numerical records made for short periods (still more for a single year) are usually either in excess or in deficiency. And no general law, either as regards sickness or mortality, can be deduced from them. By selecting particular years, all the stations even on the west coast of Africa might be shown to be among the healthiest places in our foreign possessions.

It is always possible, by selecting years and localities skillfully, to prove that the mortality of the troops in a great country is either high or low. The commission was well aware of this, and to avoid all such misleading fallacies, based their estimate on returns during long series of years, displaying, however, the facts for each year, and for each presidency. The commission not only described the mortality of each presidency separately, but, as far as was practicable, of each station, each regiment and each arm of the service.

Dr Leith is apparently able to show that in 1863 the mortality was so low as 12 in the 1000 in Bombay (p 12). This result may require some correction for deaths not included by Dr Leith, as he makes the mortality of Bombay in 1862, the previous year, 20.8, while Dr Balfour shows that the mortality was 24.6 per 1000 in that year (Dr Balfour states the strength of the troops in Bombay to be 11,870, and the deaths among them in India to be 274, while 18 of the invalids died. Dr Leith makes the strength 11,971 and the deaths in India 249 (*Report of Army Medical Department,* 1862 p 123).

But allowing for any necessary correction, the reduction of the mortality of the Bombay Army, which for fifty-six years had been 66 per 1000 (68 in the ten years 1840-50 and 31 in 1850-56), to (say) 15 per 1000 is a most gratifying fact, particularly as Dr Leith is able to say that "the progressive decrease of mortality may reasonably be attributed to the increasing attention that has been paid to the welfare of the soldiers in barracks and in hospital" (p 12).

So far as the commission could discern, there was less disposition among Indian authorities to believe that the mortality of European troops had been high, particularly during active service, than to admit that the mortality could possibly be reduced below the past standard; it was all the fault of the burning implacable sun, according to popular belief. The commission addressed itself, therefore, especially to this branch of the inquiry, and they proved (1) that in several of the hottest stations of India the mortality had been as low as 30 and 20 in 1000 during a series of years; (2) that the mortality was mainly due to certain diseases which are the result of various excremental organic compounds and marsh malaria, producing the same class of diseases in Europe; (3) that the mortality of the population from the same class of diseases was formerly higher in London than it is now in Calcutta; (4) that the dietary, regimen, barracks, sanitary arrangements, particularly in the field, had been inconceivably defective during a long series of years; (5) that the native cities and bazaars of India were in a deplorable sanitary condition, that they were centres of disease, but that the native troops of the East India Company lost less than 20 per 1000 by death; (6) that the military officers of the Company died at the rate of 31 in 1000, while the civil servants exposed to the climate died at the rate of 20 in 1000.

All this seemed to show that if British soldiers died at the rate of 69, or even 50 per 1000 annually, it was not the uncontrollable "climate" that killed them.

From these and other elaborate inquiries, the commission concluded that the "climate" of India includes various elements, and that the mortality of our army in India and of the European race is due chiefly to those elements which are to a large extent under control. The diet of the men could be improved; the excessive doses of poisonous spirits under a burning sun could be commuted into other drinks; the mind of the soldier could be occupied; troops could be transferred from stations irreclaimably bad to stations proved by experience to be comparatively salubrious, and susceptible of being rendered more salubrious still; the same sanitary measures, too, as had driven plague from Europe, and mitigated malarious fevers, must, it was inferred, produce the same salutary effects in Bombay, Madras, Calcutta and the other cities of India.

Upon all these grounds the commission saw a brighter prospect before the English Army in India. It is thus described:

> We have, in the course of our inquiries, endeavoured to ascertain the probable excess of mortality in the Indian Army, occasioned by the sanitary defects we have described, as well as the reduction of mortality which would follow on the adoption of improvements in existing stations, combined with the use of hill stations, and the abandonment of as many unhealthy localities as may be practicable. The statistical evidence shows that the mortality varies from 11½ percent in the most unhealthy to about 2 percent in the most healthy places, even in their present unimproved state. It has been estimated that the lowest of these rates, or 2 percent (double the rate at home stations since the introduction of sanitary improvements) may be taken as the possible mortality under improved sanitary conditions (8vo Report 1864 pp 124-25).

Nay, they go further, and hypothetically predict a still better state of things:

> A careful examination of the causes of disease and of the character of diseases prevalent at the more healthy stations would lead us to hope eventually for a greater saving of life than we have here estimated. Causes of disease such as exist at these stations, would even at home be sufficient to account for one half of the 20 per 1000; and if

> the time should ever arrive when, under the influence of improved culture, drainage and sanitary works, India should be freed from the local malaria which exists everywhere there now, as it once did in some form or other over Europe, we may cherish the hope of realizing what statistical inquiries appear to point to, namely, that the natural death rate in times of peace of men of the soldiers' ages in India will be no more than 10 per 1000 per annum.

Now, although Dr Leith and other writers have not proved that the mortality of the British Army in India, down to the date of the inquiry, was less than the calculations of the commission indicate, they have shown that the somewhat sanguine prediction of the commission, that a future low rate of mortality is to be obtained in India, may be realized, and Dr Leith tells the government that the mortality in Bombay is at the rate of 12 in 1000. He ascribes it to an unusual degree of freedom from cholera, and to "increasing attention to the welfare of the soldier." But very much remains to be done before such a rate can become permanent.

21. After a careful consideration of Dr Leith's report, although we are glad to find that there has been a lower death rate since the royal commission began its work, and although there have been some improvements in a few matters of detail regarding barracks and hospitals, we are of opinion that the report contains no satisfactory evidence that any material improvement has yet been effected in the sanitary condition of the Bombay presidency. In comparing its statements with the recommendations of the royal commission, we find:

(1) That the sale of spirits in canteens, at the date of the report, was pretty much in the same condition as represented by the commissioners. But we are somewhat surprised to find that at Colaba Sanitarium, where men are sent for the recovery of their health, "a quart of malt liquor and two drams of spirits are allowed to be bought by each of the invalids in the barracks at the canteen," and that, at Ahmadnagar, the quantity of spirits which the men can purchase at the cavalry canteen appears to have been doubled since the date of the report made to the royal commissioners. Surely this requires reform.

(2) That the means of instruction, exercise and recreation are still very deficient.

(3) That invalids are not yet embarked for home with the necessary speed.

(4) That works of drainage and water supply have still to be carried out at all the stations, that the existing water sources still require

to be analyzed, and that means of filtration, combined with improved distribution of water, have still to be provided.

(5) That plans for improving the existing barracks and hospitals, as nearly as practicable in conformity with the principles laid down by the royal commission for building new barracks and hospitals, have yet to be prepared and carried out.

(6) That the ventilation of barracks and hospitals has still to be completed on sound principles.

(7) That a sufficient amount of glazed window space has still to be provided for lighting barracks and hospitals, and that gas has still to be introduced.

(8) That the ablution and bath accommodation for barracks and hospitals is still very deficient, and the supply of water for cleanliness quite inadequate. (Dr Leith shows that at Hyderabad, on the banks of the Indus, the allowance of water is only five gallons per head per day, and even shower baths cannot be used.)

(9) That drinking fountains, supplied with pure, cool, filtered water, have still to be provided.

(10) That barracks cookhouses are pretty much in the state they were.

(11) That in consequence of the want of drainage and water supply improved latrines, water closets and urinals cannot be provided for barracks or hospitals.

22. With the view of supplying these deficiencies, we would recommend as follows:

(1) That each station be carefully examined by competent sanitary and engineering officers, and that a careful survey be made and a well-digested scheme for improving the station be prepared and submitted for sanction. This scheme to include:

(2) Levelling, filling up, paving and otherwise improving the surface drainage of the station.

(3) Drainage and water supply, including subsoil drainage, house drainage, filtration and distribution of water over the station.

(4) Improving existing barracks and hospitals, including raised floors, with ventilation beneath, or providing upper floors for sleeping rooms, in localities where it may be necessary to do so.

(5) Ventilation of barrack rooms and hospital wards, on the principles laid down in our *Suggestions.* Improvements in lighting barracks and hospitals.

(6) Fixing, *by regulation,* the superficial and cubic feet to be allotted per bed in barracks and hospitals, the amount being regulated accord-

ing to the healthiness or otherwise of the locality, on the principles laid down by the royal commission. In doing this, rooms or wards unfit or doubtful for occupation should be excluded, and the amount of additional barrack and hospital accommodation necessary to admit of the regulation being complied with should be stated.

(7) Subdividing long barrack rooms and sick wards, so as to have no more than from twenty to twenty-four beds per room, and providing that each room is completely cut off from the others and ventilated separately.

(8) Improved latrines, water closets and urinals for barracks and hospitals.

(9) Improved and extended ablution and bath accommodation for barracks and hospitals.

(10) Improvements in cookhouses, hospital kitchens and cooking apparatus.

(11) The provision of sufficient accommodation for exercise, recreation and instruction in the way of gymnasia, workshops, reading and day rooms, soldiers' gardens, covered ball courts, etc.

23. It is impossible for us to do more than indicate generally the more important points of such an inquiry. Nothing short of actual examination on the spot, by persons competent to conduct such an examination, is of any real use in determining the nature of the influences affecting the health of troops at any given station, and the nature of the works required for improving its sanitary condition. Such an inquiry, followed by a carefully drawn up report on each station, accompanied with the necessary maps, plans and surveys, affords the only basis on which a practical opinion could be arrived at as to the extent and class of improvements required.

[signed by]

Richard Airey, quartermaster general and president
Douglas Galton, assistant under secretary of state for war
John Sutherland
T.G. Logan, inspector general of hospitals
Edward Belfield, deputy director of works, War Office
Proby T. Cautley, member of the Council of India
J. Ranald Martin, inspector general of hospitals
Robert Rawlinson, Local Government Act Office
J.J. Frederick, secretary
Barrack and Hospital Improvement Commission
War Office, 6 January 1865

## Table A. Statistics of Regiments

Statistics of Regiments which have served in *India* during the years which the commissioners did not include in their estimate of the mortality.

| Regiment or Corps | 1857 | | 1858 | | 1859 | | 1860 | | 1861 | |
|---|---|---|---|---|---|---|---|---|---|---|
| | Strenth on 1 April | Deaths in Prev. Year | Str. On 1 April | Deaths In Prev. Year, 1857-58 | Strgth. | Death | Strgth. | Death | Strgth | Death |
| 14th Hussars | 656 | 7 | 706 | 18 | 630 | 62 | — | — | — | — |
| 24th Reg. (1st Btlion) | 952 | 79 | 954 | 105 | 1141 | 27 | 1058 | 16 | 633 | 11 |
| 29th Reg. | 949 | 69 | 913 | 37 | — | | — | — | — | — |
| 32d Reg. | 742 | 82 | 510 | 384 | — | — | — | — | — | — |
| 78th Highlanders (Persian Ex. 1856-57) | — | — | 756 | 223 | 540 | 48 | — | — | — | — |
| 83rd Reg. | 940 | 18 | 1006 | 45 | 1101 | 54 | 1048 | 30 | 965 | 18 |
| 84th Reg. | 918 | 29 | 803 | 280 | — | — | — | — | — | — |
| 64th Reg. (Persian Ex. 1856-57) | 1088 | 237 | 852 | 39 | 1228 | 24 | 993 | 12 | — | — |
| 10th Reg. (1st Btlion) | 898 | 30 | 796 | 128 | — | — | — | — | — | — |
| 8th Reg. (1st Btlion) | 891 | 40 | 845 | 175 | 870 | 56 | — | — | — | — |
| 86th Reg. | 937 | 40 | 977 | 90 | — | — | — | — | — | — |
| 70th Reg. (1st Btlion | 745 | 117 | 963 | 82 | 975 | 59 | 915 | 18 | — | — |
| 9th Lancers | 611 | 13 | 547 | 107 | 399 | 41 | — | — | — | — |
| 87th Reg. | 890 | 58 | 889 | 58 | 943 | 58 | 1036 | 27 | — | — |
| 53rd Reg. | 1093 | 35 | 961 | 106 | 863 | 13 | 807 | 64 | — | — |
| 75th Reg. | 937 | 22 | 816 | 228 | 1091 | 39 | 1039 | 27 | 951 | 57 |
| 60th Reg. (1st Btlion) | 882 | 194 | 789 | 43 | 900 | 61 | — | — | — | — |
| 52d Reg. | 871 | 63 | 888 | 25 | 1204 | 12 | 1131 | 13 | — | — |
| 61st Reg. | 945 | 27 | 787 | 284 | 885 | 44 | — | — | — | — |
| 81st Reg. | 1047 | 170 | 1044 | 32 | 1074 | 41 | — | — | — | — |
| 43d Reg. | 1094 | 50 | 1,041 | 31 | 979 | 116 | 950 | 26 | 969 | 11 |
| 74th Highlanders | 978 | 22 | 972 | 18 | 1065 | 40 | 911 | 27 | 932 | 13 |
| 27th Reg. | 930 | 33 | 988 | 140 | 935 | 34 | 1040 | 12 | 1042 | 22 |
| 35th Reg. | 656 | 66 | 933 | 66 | 934 | 187* | 959 | 38 | 1102 | 19 |
| 6th Dragoon Guards | — | — | 632 | 71 | 661 | 28 | 659 | 13 | — | — |
| 12th Lancers | 610 | 3 | 644 | 20 | 608 | 52 | 404 | 34 | — | — |
| 37th Reg. | — | — | 841 | 121 | 705 | 36 | 862 | 37 | 998 | 84 |
| 5th Reg. (1st Btlion) | — | — | — | — | 663 | 88 | 828 | 104 | 805 | 38 |
| 90th Reg. | — | — | — | — | — | — | 858 | 32 | 929 | 25 |
| 33d Reg. | — | — | — | — | 1233 | 12 | 1168 | 41 | 991 | 64 |
| 89th Reg. | — | — | — | — | 979 | 38 | 1058 | 81 | — | — |
| 23d Reg. (1st Btlion) | — | — | — | — | 1191 | 107 | 1046 | 53 | 1166 | 23 |

| Regiment or Corps | 1857 Strenth on 1 April | 1857 Deaths in Prev. Year | 1858 Str. On 1 April | 1858 Deaths In Prev. Year, 1857-58 | 1859 Strgth. | 1859 Death | 1860 Strgth. | 1860 Death | 1861 Strgth | 1861 Death |
|---|---|---|---|---|---|---|---|---|---|---|
| 13th Reg. (1st Btlion) | — | — | — | — | 1058 | 98 | 917 | 61 | 989 | 36 |
| 82d Reg. | — | — | — | — | 1112 | 104 | 1039 | 31 | 1153 | 27 |
| 34th Reg. | — | — | — | — | 730 | 83 | 1175 | 58 | — | — |
| 1st Reg. (1st Btlion) | — | — | — | — | 1079 | 120 | 1279 | 43 | 1013 | 18 |
| 42d Highlanders | — | — | — | — | 961 | 123 | 1009 | 20 | 990 | 23 |
| 95th Reg. | — | — | — | — | 1047 | 50 | 1037 | 32 | 985 | 38 |
| 88th Reg. | — | — | — | — | 916 | 118 | 961 | 43 | 1000 | 25 |
| 2d Btlion Rifle Brigade | — | — | — | — | 1043 | 113 | 1106 | 48 | 1133 | 18 |
| 3d Btlion Rifle Brigade | — | — | — | — | 1069 | 141 | 1156 | 29 | 1047 | 79 |
| 3d Dragoon Guards | — | — | — | — | 701 | 16 | 663 | 30 | 657 | 14 |
| 1st Dragoon Guards | — | — | — | — | 605 | 9 | 704 | 11 | 699 | 25 |
| 38th Reg. | — | — | — | — | 982 | 176 | 1059 | 40 | 1014 | 22 |
| 19th Reg. (1st Btlion) | — | — | — | — | 1108 | 87 | 965 | 65 | 905 | 40 |
| 20th Reg. (1st Btlion) | — | — | — | — | 1015 | 123 | 964 | 56 | 975 | 17 |
| 97th Reg. | — | — | — | — | 799 | 139 | 1 013 | 93 | 986 | 35 |
| 7th Reg. (1st Btlion) | — | — | — | — | 1 222 | 68 | 1182 | 30 | 1254 | 19 |
| 93d Highlanders | — | — | — | — | 911 | 42 | 1 069 | 41 | 1098 | 1** |
| 2d Dragoon Guards | — | — | — | — | 604 | 112 | 605 | 22 | 585 | 29 |
| 44th Reg. | — | — | — | — | 1139 | 33 | 1176 | 18 | — | — |
| 7th Hussars | — | — | — | — | 546 | 112 | 723 | 19 | 737 | 19 |
| 79th Reg. | — | — | — | — | 949 | 165 | 967 | 25 | 1016 | 12 |
| 60th Rifles (3d Btlion) | — | — | — | — | 1 178 | 24 | 1 176 | 13 | 934 | 23 |
| 72d Highlanders | — | — | — | — | 1061 | 48 | 892 | 23 | 968 | 15 |
| 66th Reg. | — | — | — | — | 1270 | 18 | 1,204 | 25 | 1036 | 9 |
| 8th Hussars | — | — | — | — | 559 | 41 | 711 | 24 | 704 | 19 |
| 69th Reg. | — | — | — | — | 969 | 29 | 974 | 38 | 1010 | 9 |
| 51st Reg. | — | — | — | — | 1 188 | 33 | 1 148 | 46 | 1070 | 19 |
| 7th Dragoon Guards | — | — | — | — | 568 | 39 | 601 | 9 | 645 | 15 |
| 94th Reg. | — | — | — | — | 1081 | 46 | 1125 | 31 | 1023 | 15 |
| 98th Reg. | — | — | — | — | 991 | 17 | 1 046 | 17 | — | — |
| 80th Reg. | — | — | — | — | 858 | 67 | 838 | 22 | — | — |
| 56th Reg. | — | — | — | — | 792 | 21 | 976 | 51 | 924 | 36 |
| 54th Reg. | — | — | — | — | 1 057 | 141 | 1004 | 47 | 1011 | 52 |
| 17th Lancers | — | — | — | — | 568 | 21 | 599 | 74 | 632 | 28 |
| 71st Light Infantry | — | — | — | — | 967 | 65 | 907 | 40 | 868 | 106 |
| 18th Reg. (1st Btlion) | — | — | — | — | 1 179 | 61 | 1031 | 18 | 992 | 4 |

| Regiment or Corps | 1857 | | 1858 | | 1859 | | 1860 | | 1861 | |
|---|---|---|---|---|---|---|---|---|---|---|
| | Strenth on 1 April | Deaths in Prev. Year | Str. On 1 April | Deaths In Prev. Year, 1857-58 | Strgth. | Death | Strgth. | Death | Strgth | Death |
| 6th Reg. (1st Btlion) | — | — | — | — | 679 | 148 | 798 | 43 | 951 | 32 |
| 92d Highlanders | — | — | — | — | 1150 | 65 | 991 | 22 | — | — |
| 68th Reg. | — | — | — | — | 1261 | 13 | 1202 | 25 | 1112 | 9 |
| 77th Reg. | — | — | — | — | — | — | 934 | 51 | 877 | 116 |
| 46th Reg. | — | — | — | — | — | — | 875 | 18 | 1085 | 14 |
| 6th Dragoon | — | — | — | — | — | — | 686 | 13 | 702 | 5 |
| 91st Reg. | — | — | — | — | — | — | 893 | 27 | 1090 | 30 |
| 48th Reg. | — | — | — | — | — | — | 787 | 71 | 979 | 40 |
| 4th Reg. (1st Btlion) | — | — | — | — | — | — | 991 | 37 | 933 | 50 |
| 73d Reg. | — | — | — | — | 765 | 49 | 765 | 34 | 704 | 4 |
| TOTAL | 21260 | 1504 | 22853 | 2956 | 61534 | 4355 | 62687 | 2329 | 50029 | 1526 |

*Notes:* It is not clear whether deaths in this return always refer to the military year ending 1 April. No satisfactory information on that head could be procured from the Adjutant General's Office, to which application was made.

*Of the 187 deaths in the 35th regiment in 1859, 101 were killed in action.

The returns of deaths for 1861 are imperfect; the regiments not having remained in India during the whole of the military year, their deaths during a portion only of the year were returned. Thus the 93rd Highlanders, 1098 strong, return 1 death, that is, in a week or so.

(The returns are by the commanding officers of regiments, and are given in detail in the report of the "Royal Commission on Sanitary State of Army in India," Vol. I, pp 757-79).

## Home and Presidencies' Sanitary Commissions

**Editor:** The first task to be tackled in the implementation of the recommendations of the royal commission's report was to create the proper machinery to carry out those recommendations. To that end a double instrument was devised. First a home commission (also called "joint commission," sometimes "War Office commission") with advisory power was formed. It was incorporated into the existing War Office's Barrack and Hospital Improvement Commission, itself formed in 1858 and now expanded to include members of the India Office; from 1865 on this commission was called the Army Sanitary Commission (A.S.C.). Second, presidency commissions were constituted in Calcutta, Bombay and Madras, with consultative and, through their presidents, administrative powers: "the germs of local self-government" (see p 442 below). Close co-operation with the viceroy, John Lawrence, aided the introduction of the presidency commissions, since the Bengal commission, based in the capital, Calcutta, operated as a "model" (see p 497 below) for the other presidency commissions.

The urgency of the creation of those two instruments is emphasized in the material below. The commissions should be "immediately appointed. Without them, we shall be ruined," Nightingale said (see p 437 below). Their importance could also be gauged by the amount of material devoted to the formation and operation of those commissions. Attention was thereby directed, as has appeared in the *Suggestions,* to the improvement of the sanitary conditions of both the Indian stations and the surrounding population. Some of the necessary army reforms dealt with the right diet to be followed by soldiers during the passage to India and after arrival. Neglect of diet meant deplorable consequences. Then the stations had to be examined and rebuilt if necessary in order to protect the soldiers' health, and the "native lines" around the stations brought to a level of salubrity that would no longer contaminate the stations.

Many more organizational initiatives were imperative in both England and India if sanitary measures were to be effectively introduced, but these two instruments were crucial. The need for home and presidency sanitary commissions was anticipated at the time the report was written and well before it was officially issued, as the correspondence above and below shows. The aforementioned Army Sanitary Commission, as it was called from 1865, operated till the late 1880s, when the need for its reconstitution was felt and a reorganization took place. The presidency commissions were established as early as 1864; they were initially made of five members each but were reduced in 1866 to two members, a commissioner and a secretary, thereby enhancing their executive power as well as their efficient functioning. In 1888 the presidency commissions were replaced by sanitary boards, which operated in close co-operation with municipal councils and local boards, thus giving more profile to local instances. At home, in 1867, an India Office Sanitary Commission/Committee was added to those two main instruments in order to monitor the sanitary work done in India more closely; it functioned only to the end of 1874, by which time the local commissions had become more experienced and could "walk alone." All those "commissions" contributed their share to the improvement of soldiers' health and in the birth of a public health system in India. Summarizing her views, Nightingale wrote to Sir Charles Trevelyan in 1863: "The India administrative arrangements are . . . the main thing. And these can only be settled by you there. It concerns nothing less than the creation of a Public Health Department for India" (see p 439 below).

Source: From four letters to Douglas Galton, ADD MSS 45760 ff249-53, 256-57, 267 and 273

14 February 1863

Lord de Grey's letter has touched our great difficulty with India. Perhaps the best way would be to wait a little for the Indian report, which is now in proof, and you will see what we have said on the subject. Of course all we can do is to lay down general principles. You know but too well that general principles, like regulations, won't act by themselves. They only lead the way to practical results.

Our difficulty will be to obtain these. Lord Herbert wisely recommended the appointment of your Barrack and Hospital Improvement Commission to apply general principles; without that commission they never would have been applied in this country. Some such commission is absolutely necessary for India.

I have written this to Lord Stanley some time ago and talked about it to Dr Sutherland always. But the question of stations is so intimately connected with that of barracks that, unless you improve the stations, it is of little use putting up (or pulling down) new barracks. A commission is wanted to bring our English sanitary knowledge (painfully acquired) to bear on Indian questions as a whole. It is quite certain that there is no hope of this in India, for the very last barrack they built is the very worst.

No: there is no "Indian Sutherland." Nothing is more striking (in the reams of manuscript replies which we have now waded through) than the clearness of sight with which they see the evils and the vast gap between this and their knowledge of any remedies.

If the India government would appoint some commission at home to guide the local health commissions in India, this is the only hope. Your Barrack and Hospital Commission (with Indian additions, well selected qua India) would do very well. I would add Rawlinson, who is the first water engineer now, is he not? India is not so much farther off than the West Indies but that plans could come over here. And Dr Sutherland might make a run out there to a few of the stations reached by railway. The fact is, I see in Lord de Grey's letter an opening to all we had hoped for India.

At all events, the members of the Barrack and Hospital Commission, if not selected as members, might be selected by the India government as individuals. And we would find the very best India men to add. The principle is a *home commission* to apply our home experience to India, and to inform and, so far, guide the first movements of the local authorities in India.

*Private.* If you should talk this over with Lord de Grey, I would gladly help with the heads of a memo [see next letter].

18 February 1863

I send you the memo asked for, also a letter from Sir John McNeill, which please return to me. If you like to show it to Lord de Grey, pray do.

Sir John McNeill being an old Indian officer, I sent him my abstracts, paper, etc. (for the Indian sanitary commission). You see how strongly he thinks of the necessity for an organization to initiate sanitary works in India. . . .

If anything comes of this, I should be very glad to write the instructions for the commission, as I used to do for Lord Herbert.

19 February 1863

If Sir G. Lewis, instead of writing a "Dialogue on the best form of government," would write (or rather silently act) a *Mono*logue on the dual form being the worst "form of government," the War Office would be much the gainer.

19 March 1863

I have just received your Indian (Strachey) paper and am looking at it as fast as I can. It is a very important paper. And I am afraid I shall not be able to send it back till tomorrow or Saturday, will that signify? You must really put it to Lord de Grey on the score of health. The India Office is by no means so prompt itself as to justify it in complaining of us. The reason of my delay is I have been very ill, like you. Dr Sutherland I never see. For he says that he is "so ill" he can only do just *what he likes.* And I am doing work for Lord Stanley.

Source: From a letter to Douglas Galton, ADD Mss 45760 ff276-77

20 March 1863

I sent this morning to the War Office your India (Strachey) paper with my observations. I was so appalled by it (is that all the India authorities know about the remedies to be applied to their gigantic evils?) that I compelled Dr Sutherland to come. He backs *with horror* my observations. It is only another proof of what I so much dread being dreadable, viz., the establishment of a controlling authority in sanitary things at Calcutta (and this is also recommended in Strachey). I think

I convinced Lord de Grey of the undesirableness of this. And since that I have seen Lord Stanley. And he actually (a most unusual zeal) went off to Sir C. Wood and persuaded him to sanction the establishment of a (consultative) Barrack and Hospital Commission at the I.O. here, with some modifications. I hope to see you when you come back, as I have much to tell you about this. In the meanwhile, it is all in (the recommendations of) the report, which I received back (complete) from press yesterday. I have not yet sent Lord de Grey a copy.

Source: From a letter to Lord de Grey, ADD Mss 43546 ff27-28

21 March 1863

*Confidential.* I saw Lord Stanley about that matter of the commission *at home* for the purpose of advising the (home) India government on sanitary matters. He so far consented to it that he allowed it to be put into the report (together with the three presidency consultative commissions). And he even went to Sir Charles Wood to convince him of the utility and necessity of the (home) commission. Probably you have heard of this from the latter.

I shall have to consult you farther some day, according to your kind permission, about the constitution of this said commission.

Source: From a letter to Douglas Galton, ADD Mss 45760 f287

27 March 1863

I send you our Indian report, confound it! at last. It is *confidential* and unrevised. A sorry performance, in my opinion, so different from the masterly touch of our first report. But at least it is complete and exhausts the subject.

Please return it to me in a few days. I think I told you that I had carried the home commission (Barrack and Hospital) with Lord Stanley and he with Sir C. Wood.

**Editor:** Sir George Lewis died suddenly on 13 April 1863 and had to be replaced as secretary of state for war. Nightingale was quick to realize the opportunity for having an effective secretary to see to the introduction of the sanitary commissions and to support her India work in general. She asked Harriet Martineau to use the press to create a movement in favour of Lord de Grey, urging her in a telegram to "Agitate, agitate for Lord de Grey to succeed Sir George Lewis."[55] In

55 Letter 16 April 1863, ADD Mss 45788 f174.

the end Lord de Grey was chosen and Nightingale welcomed him as a solid collaborator. We will see him play an even greater role later as Lord Ripon, governor general of India 1880-84.

Source: From a draft letter in Dr Sutherland's hand to Lord Stanley, Add Mss 45781 ff80-81

18 May 1863

I am afraid from what I have heard of the Saturday's discussion on the report that there is great danger of the Indian inquiry arriving at no practical result. . . . It is absolutely necessary that there should be local commissions in India to carry out the works there, but it is as certain as experience can make it that those commissions, constituted as they must be out of the best available material, will not of themselves arrive at a good practical solution of the multifarious questions they will have to deal with. Were it practicable to pick out a sufficient number of able men in England and send them out to form these commissions, there would be a fair hope of success, but I think I know well what the probabilities are of this being practicable and I feel assured you would hardly be able to get men for money to undertake the work, that is, men thoroughly up to the sanitary question in all its bearings. . . .

All the real practical work which has led to the great reduction of army mortality [after the first royal commission] has been done by persons determined to carry out the principles which were laid down in it, who would not be turned aside by any obstacles and who from long previous experience were competent for the work.

Source: Letter, Liverpool Record Office, Derby Collection 920/15/13

4 Cleveland Row, S.W.
18 May 1863

*Private*

Dear Lord Stanley

I was much distressed to hear the unpractical views, taken by some of the members of the India sanitary commission on Saturday (at the meeting). And I trust you will excuse my rewriting to you on this score.

I am afraid there is great danger of the Indian inquiry arriving at no practical result. I urged the necessity of using home experience in dealing with India sanitary questions, because, from the evidence and from the reports (from Indian stations), it was obvious that there was no hope of any practical reform springing up from India. It is quite necessary that there should be local commissions in India to carry out the works there. But it is as certain as experience can make it that those commissions, constituted, as they must be, out of the best available material, will not, *of themselves*, arrive at a good practical solution of the multifarious questions they will have to deal with. Were it practicable to pick out a sufficient number of able men in England and send them out to form these commissions, there would be a fair hope of success. But we know well what the probabilities are of this being practicable. You would hardly be able to get men for money to undertake the work, i.e., men thoroughly up to the sanitary question in all its bearings.

If then you stop with the recommendation of "India presidency commissions," your report will amount to this: "This is how bad the things are in India. They have grown up into their present state under the guidance of such amount of practical ability and intelligence as was obtainable in that country. We recommend you to form commissions out of the same material and to go on as before. It is true that great practical advances have been made in sanitary works at home, and the result has been a reduction of the army death rate to one half. But it is not necessary to make use of this practical experience in India."

Yet we are interfering in Ceylon at this moment. For instance, on what principle can be justified the introduction of home experience in Ceylon and keeping it out of India? Their diseases are the same, the causes the same, the troops the same and the measures required would be the same.

The formation of a home commission was urged, because you thought (when you were so good as to see me on this subject) that the I.O. would not like to have to do with the W.O. But if the I.O. does not object, there is no other reason why the W.O. should not help with its own commission. Unless some such arrangement can be come to, it really matters very little practically whether the report is issued or not. It will only be a nine days' wonder, as the first army report was. That report did nothing of itself. All the real practical work which has led to the great reduction of army mortality has been done by persons determined to carry out the principles laid down in it, who would not be turned aside by any obstacles and who from long previous experience were competent for the work.

Nothing can show more the *imminent* importance of the work that has to be done in India than the fact that plague is gradually surrounding Calcutta. Cholera came out of the Sunderbuns (epidemically) and spread over the world. Plague did the same in the Nile delta and thence spread over Europe in the Middle Ages. Egyptian plague is now coming up from the Sunderbuns and drawing slowly round to hem in Calcutta. It requires no great length of vision to see what is likely to follow from this Sunderbuns plague in the present state of Indian cities. Believe me,

yours apologetically
Florence Nightingale

PRIVATE. N.B. I was quite appalled to hear what is the advice that the I.O. do take on these matters, according to Sir Proby Cautley. They apply to Dr Mapleton,[56] member of the Director General's Office at the Army Medical Department. When Dr Mapleton was appointed, under General Peel's term of office, Sidney Herbert lay awake all night, thinking of the mischief this man's gross ignorance would do, and went the first thing the next morning to General Peel, before he was up, to try to have the appointment cancelled. And it was only on assurance that Dr Mapleton should have nothing to do with sanitary matters that he remitted his efforts. This is the man whom the India Office, when "taking home experience," apply to.

Source: From a letter to Harriet Martineau, ADD Mss 45788 ff184-85

19 May 1863

*Private.* I cannot help telling you, in the joy of my heart, that the final meeting of the India sanitary commission was held today—that the report was signed—and that after a very tough battle, lasting over three days, to convince these people that a report was not self-executive, our working commission was carried, not quite in the original form proposed, but in what may prove a better working form, because grafted on what exists [on the Barrack and Hospital Improvement Commission]. This is the dawn of a new day for India in sanitary things, not only as regards our army, but as regards the native population.

The present form of the working commission proposed is to add for India work Sir Proby Cautley, Sir Ranald Martin, as two members of the India government, and Mr Rawlinson on to the standing War Office commission (for these purposes) and to let them hold their meetings at the India Office, when desirable. The two Indians themselves proposed to be called in at all the War Office meetings for War Office work in order to learn their mode of working. Sir Charles Wood and Lord de Grey will thus be our heads, instead of our having a special chairman, Lord Stanley.

---

56 Dr Henry Mapleton, proponent of the unsanitary site and design of the Netley Hosptial.

Source: From a letter to Lord de Grey, Add Mss 43546 ff47-48

2 June 1863

*Private.* I send, as I promised, the Indian sanitary report, as determined upon in the final sitting of that commission. Of course you will have a copy as soon as it is signed. But it is not even gone in to Sir C. Wood yet. It goes to Lord Stanley this week for him to affix his signature.

We carried the two things we had at heart (but after a closer run than Epsom), viz., (1) the "working" commission *at home*, in connection with the three "presidency" commissions recommended (how odd it is the tendency of men to think a report self-executive instead of seeing that, when the report is ended, the work begins!); (2) the *not* recommending any (French) medical police regulation system, in connection with lock hospitals.[57]

**Editor:** With the issue of the royal commission's report on 8 July 1863, the need for the formation of the home and presidency sanitary commissions, recommended in the report, became more urgent if practical results were to be obtained. Nightingale knew how important the new commissions were, and vigorously spurred every responsible person to action. Her main allies in this matter were John Lawrence and Lord de Grey.

Source: From an incomplete letter to Sir Charles Trevelyan, Newcastle University Library 35/14

18 June 1863

Colonel Booth's notes, for which I thank you heartily, are very satisfactory. On certain points he differs, on others he writes remarks stronger than any I should have dared to write. But in the cases wherein he differs, his reasons are rather against his conclusions. And as a whole his remarks not only strongly corroborate the evidence laid before the commission (I wish we could have had him as a witness or as a commissioner) but there are certain test points Colonel Booth mentions which show the statements I have made to be understatements. The case is more than proved. And we now have to seek the administrative remedies.

The royal commission has recommended committees of health at each presidency seat of government. But as these committees are as

57 The French were practising a system of registration and regulation of prostitutes with the expectation of better controlling venereal disease; the English saw that system as encouraging prostitution, as the debate on the Contagious Diseases Acts demonstrated. See *Women* (8:411-515).

likely to blunder as not, until they learn, and as your £300,000 (for which God be praised and *you* most cordially thanked) are as likely to be misspent on small new barracks as larger sums have been misspent on large old barracks, the royal commission has advised the India Office either to constitute an advising commission at the I.O. in England, to help the presidency commissions with advice, experience and the recent improvements introduced in Europe (even at Malta and Gibraltar), or else to add an Indian engineer and medical officer (Sir Proby Cautley and Sir Ranald Martin) to the existing War Office "Barrack and Hospital Improvement Commission" which has done such good work here.

Source: Letter, Add Mss 43546 ff60-63

4 Cleveland Row, S.W.
8 July 1863

Dear Lord de Grey

By dint of sending three times a day to Spottiswoode's, and every half hour to the lithographers, I have got for you the very first copy of the India Army sanitary report, *before* it is ready for issue.

The next point is to have the three presidency commissions appointed, and also to make some arrangement about the home commission. It is certain that, without home influence, Indian improvement in the sanitary line is hopeless. But, if home assistance were given for a time, until the presidency commissions were able to walk alone, the improvements would go on. This is the most urgent point now in hand. And, after you have given your consideration to the whole matter, you will choose the best way to bring about the required co-operation between the home and Indian sanitary service, I know. If your own Barrack and Hospital Improvement Commission is to be adopted as the basis, then Sir Proby Cautley and Sir Ranald Martin will have to be added onto it when Indian questions come before it. And Mr Rawlinson, C.E., when the great water supply and drainage questions in India come on, will have to act upon it. If an I.O. commission were appointed, its members should be: Sir Proby Cautley, Sir Ranald Martin, Dr Sutherland, Captain Galton, Mr Rawlinson, C.E.

I will not trouble you with a long letter as the subject is so fully before you. Sir C. Trevelyan writes me word that he has provided £300,000 in his budget for our barrack purposes, which, he thinks, is as much as can be expended in the *first* year. But, he says, if more is wanted, it shall be forthcoming.

Might I add that, for sanitary members of the *presidency* commissions, the documents point out none but Inspector General Dr

MacPherson, Madras; Dr Norman Chevers, Calcutta; Dr Joseph Ewart who was at Kherwarrah; and also Dr Dempster and Dr MacClellan. If you bid me look out for engineers, I will do so (from the documents).

I will send the very next copy I can extract from the printers to Sir C. Wood's own house. But as I have not the honour of knowing him, I shall do so without a name. Believe me, dear Lord de Grey,

ever yours gratefully and *beseechingly*

Florence Nightingale

"La reconnaissance n'est qu'un vif sentiment des bienfaits futurs" [Gratitude is but the keen anticipation of future benefits].

Source: From a letter to Harriet Martineau, Add Mss 45788 f189

8 July 1863

To me it is inexpressibly sad bringing out this report, begun as it was with Sidney Herbert, and now two years after he is gone.

But enough of this. The main point is to get the three presidency commissions appointed, and also to have some arrangement about the home commission at once. It is certain that, without home experience, Indian improvement is hopeless. But, if home assistance were given for a time, until the Indian (presidency) commissions could walk alone, the improvements would *go on. This is the most urgent point now.*

Source: Letter to Douglas Galton, Add Mss 45761 ff39-42

4 Cleveland Row S.W.

9 July 1863

With the bayonet I have obtained some copies of the India sanitary report *before* it is issued. But I shan't give you one because I am furious with you and Hilary. Hilary goes and tells you about Sir C. Trevelyan's £300,000. And you go and tell her that it had better all be locked up, instead of saying we must none of us rest day or night till we get the working organization settled.

I sent a copy of this report to Lord de Grey yesterday, and also one to Sir John Lawrence, and to each of them I wrote, urging and pressing the immediate appointment of the presidency commissions (giving some names therefore) and the immediate arrangement of the joint India Office and War Office commission at home, in whatever way may prove most convenient, the names being yourself, Dr Sutherland, Sir P. Cautley, Sir J.R. Martin, Mr Rawlinson. And now, from your knowledge of Lord de Grey, you must tell me any way in which I could further these commissions being immediately appointed. Without them, we shall be ruined. And all this reporting had better not have been. . . .

I am obliged to give up this house on the 21st, owing to my abominable proprietor. But I can take rooms at No. 2.

Swear that you will, if you see the least thing that I can do, tell me in time. For to miss doing the slightest thing by being away at Hampstead would be misery.

I send you Sir C.T.'s note which please return at once.

ever yours

F.N.

Lord Stanley does not do the least thing for us. He is sulky. We must fight the more. When does the House of Commons break up? Shall we have questions asked in the House for our report? I could get several men to do so. When does Lord de Grey go away? When do you? I have just heard from Sir John Lawrence: *he* thinks the having an India Office commission with you, Dr Sutherland and Mr Rawlinson on it will work the best. But he is completely besotted with his Dr Hathaway, the author of that idiotic sanitary Punjab report, and wants to have him on a presidency commission.

Source: From an undated draft letter to Sir John Lawrence in Dr Sutherland's hand, Add Mss 45777 f20

[1863]

As regards the home commission, either plan proposed in the report would do. The commission could only deal with questions positively laid before it by the Indian government, and it could give no more than its opinion. . . .

In my last letter I ventured to give a few names of medical officers who might serve advantageously on the Indian presidency health commission. The names were all those of Indian officers whose reports and other works show them to possess the species of practical advising talent suitable for the purpose.

Source: From a letter to Robert Rawlinson, Boston University 1/2/33

13 July 1863

*Private.* Lord de Grey and Lord Stanley are arranging with Sir C. Wood the home commission, consisting of yourself, Dr Sutherland, Captain Galton, Sir P. Cautley, Sir R. Martin. I only hope and pray that it may be done this month, before London disperses. As to the India administrative arrangements, we are putting what pressure we can upon authorities out there to have them carried out. The question is nothing less than the creation of a Public Health Department for India.

The report proposes commissioners of health, one for each presidency; probably a fourth will be necessary for the Punjab, and a consultative commission, with a responsible administrative head, would appear to be the best. And the whole might possibly be raised into a department of government.

Source: From a letter to Sir Charles Trevelyan, Newcastle University Library 35/20, incomplete copy ADD Mss 45798 f137

13 July 1863

The big sanitary report is on its way out to you. One comfort is that you will not do what a War Office official proposed to do here, viz., take six months' leave to read it. The chief thing now is to have its recommendations carried out as fast as possible. Every day's delay is a loss.

Lord Stanley and Lord de Grey are already arranging with Sir Charles Wood about the consultative (home) commission here.... Sir John Lawrence interests himself very much for us, and gives me valuable hints as to how to proceed. But he is, after all, like a great fish out of water here—or like a great Roman proconsul—returned for Marylebone to serve as an MP.

The *India administrative arrangements are however the main thing. And these can only be settled by you there.* It concerns nothing less than the creation of a Public Health Department for India. The royal commission's report proposes presidency commissions of health. A consultative commission, with a responsible administrative head, would appear to be the best arrangement. And the whole might possibly be raised into a department of government. What a noble work for an India government! We can help in all matters of detail and experience from this end. Before anything is decided, should you think well to send us a sketch of what you propose, we will obtain the advice of all our sanitary administrators about it.

Source: From two letters to Lord de Grey, ADD Mss 43546 ff66-67 and 68-69

13 July 1863

*Confidential.* Lord Stanley would like to be "asked by Sir C. Wood" for his "assistance in giving effect to the sanitary projects" (India Army sanitary report), but does not like to "offer such help." (How unlike Sidney Herbert, who "offered his help" to the man who displaced him—the difference to my mind between a great man and a little one. But as I did not make Lord Stanley, the reflection is out of place!)

I leave it to your judgment entirely to make use of this hint or not. I have none—no judgment, I mean. But, although Lord Stanley in no way claims my secrecy, I think whatever you do had better be entirely as from yourself, without in any way quoting me or him. I need hardly say that he is perfectly unaware of my writing to you.

Lord Stanley further wishes to know "what the War and India departments will do"—he means, as to attaching the home commission to the War or to the India Office—as "the first step."

Please destroy this note.

20 July 1863

*Private.* Our Indian work looks bad. The home commission is objected to on the ground that there is no direct communication on sanitary matters between the home India government and the governments in India. What is wanted is to bring about such an arrangement as will enable all plans and improvements of barracks, etc., to be sent home and to be considered by a home commission. This point is essential and, unless arranged, I cannot see what result can follow the work of the royal commission. All will depend upon bringing about this arrangement. So far as I can ascertain, the procedure which you have at the W.O. is doubly requisite at the I.O., viz., to have plans and proposals for spending money on works remitted home for sanction. And, on this, to raise the question of the adaptation of such plans to their objects (just as is done by your Barrack and Hospital Commission). And such alterations and improvements to be suggested as appear necessary, and in this way gradually to be introduced.

Please could you do anything with the I.O.? It is urgent.

Source: From three letters to Sir Charles Trevelyan, Newcastle University Library 35/21-23, copy of first letter Add Mss 45798 f143 and 24-25, copy of third letter Add Mss 45798 f170

22 July 1863

*Private.* I am afraid we are in a bad way here as regards our home commission which, if at all, is, they say, to be attached to the India Office, to which we have no objection. But if it is to be at all is the question. Lord Stanley is very lukewarm in helping us. And Sir C. Wood does not understand the subject. We miss our Sidney Herbert so much *who never wanted anything but a reason for doing anything.* He would have gone straight to Sir C. Wood himself and settled it all and been chairman of it himself. The next help must come from you in India. I will tell you how matters stand.

Practical difficulties have arisen in giving effect to the administrative proposals of the royal commission, which you in India must remove. Our object is to bring European experience to bear on the

Indian health question without in any way interfering with freedom of action. And the point at issue is how is this to be done. All the sanitary work must be done in India. It cannot be done in England. All we can do (or propose to do) is to give to the commissions in India, if appointed, the benefit of English experience and to prevent the mishaps and failures quite certain to ensue if the Indian commissions of health are left to gain their own experience. The report of the royal commission only states the most general principles. But the question really lies in the application of these principles to suit specific cases.

At present there is no direct reference of plans from India to England, and such a reference as regards sanitary works is what is required. It would work as follows. Suppose that the Madras presidency commission of health (if appointed) were to draw up at the request of the Madras government a plan for the sanitary improvement of Secunderabad or of Madras itself. They would do this without any practical experience of how such cases had been dealt with elsewhere. If such a plan were carried out, without consulting this experience, it would be mere matter of chance whether the whole did not prove a failure. The only way to prevent this as far as practicable would be to refer the plan home without loss of time to the India Office here. It would then come before its special commission, the details of the plan would be minutely canvassed by experienced men and, after the best practicable decision had been arrived at, the plan would be sent back with all needful information as to matters of detail in water supply, drainage, latrines, construction and improvement of buildings, etc. And then, after the Madras commission had profited as much as possible by the criticisms and information, the plan would be put forwards for sanction in the usual way.

It has been proposed here to send out ready-formed commissions of practical men to deal with the India question. But it is quite certain that for some time the men will not be forthcoming. There are as yet very few men practically conversant with this class of works, and all we have are occupied on duties here. To send out inferior men would be to misspend money. The Army Medical School at Netley is now training young men in sanitary knowledge. But it will be some years before any number will be available. Cadets of engineers for Indian service will, it is hoped, before long be trained in this branch of knowledge. But as yet nothing has been done.

As regards India, your latest barrack at Fort William is one of your worst and you are now draining Calcutta apparently without a water supply. There is then no reasonable hope of progress, unless some arrangement be made whereby the I.O. here may by good advice prevent such mistakes. All plans or proposals for sanitary improvements should be sent voluntarily from India, direct and without circumlocution, to the I.O. here. There is no need of any jealousy. For all wish to help you. The interests, though by no means the sole interests at stake, are those of our queen's regiments. And we cannot understand, after the War Office has had a commission of practical men at work to improve our home barracks and hospitals, thereby reducing the former death rate to one half, why the troops which have had such care bestowed on them here should go to India and be there decimated and deteriorated, because there is no authority sufficiently informed to deal with these health questions.

The plan proposed is similar to the W.O. method. At present all sanitary works are sent from every station (from the West Indies to China) to the W.O. The plans are carefully examined and corrected by Sidney Herbert's special commission and then returned to the station. This is what is wanted for India and there is no reason, is there? why it should not work as well. If not strictly in accordance with existing system, surely the system should bend to the greater necessity, not the necessity to the system.

2. The report has created a great impression here and is continuing to do so. Not a day should be lost in taking the matter up in India. For the report has passed into the administrative stage. Could you consider at once about your presidency commissions? They ought in reality to be Public Health Departments of the government of each presidency. Much good would not be done by making them deliberative bodies. Such bodies waste time and breath, create jealousies and do nothing. Should you not have an executive head responsible for carrying out the requisite reforms? And in this case the commissions would be consultative. Large powers will be required and promptitude of action. In the infancy of the question it is probable that you will have to work through inspectors and officers of health, waiting the time for granting local powers where at present they could not be exercised with advantage. Immense changes will grow out of this report in India, for it really contains the germs of local self-government under central supervision, a kind of transition period between military rule and municipal action. (I know your darling project is local self-government.) The only other way would be for government to do all, if the military system is to be retained, and to pay everything out of revenue. One way

or other the thing must be done. Our moral title to hold India has been called in question, on the ground of what we have left undone there. Now is the time to make our title good.

3. I have been desired to ask you, if you reprint for India, to make up a readable book, containing say in two 8vos (1) the report, (2) the evidence, (3) my *Observation*, (4) abstract of stational returns (all in Vol. I of the big books). All these papers have a direct bearing on the reforms to be carried out.

The stational reports, given *in extenso* (in Vol. II of the big books), are all important for the work at each station and each station should have copies. But for the general reader Vol. II would have little interest. The statistics in Vol. I are important for reference. But the results are all given in the report.

4. We are making inquiries about the best men for the presidency commissions. And I shall, if you will allow me, suggest some names by next mail.

[continued] 24 July [1863]

I have just heard from Lord de Grey that Sir C. Wood consents to the home commission but proposes to form it by adding two India members to the W.O. Barrack and Hospital Commission. As however nothing official has been done, I still send my letter, as we want all the help we can get from you. I was sorry to see Sir C. Wood's entire ignorance of sanitary statistics in his speech last night in the House of Commons.[58]

25 July 1863

*Private.* Lord Stanley tells me that Sir C. Wood has finally decided to adopt one at least of the recommendations of the royal commission as to the home sanitary commission, viz., to make use of the W.O. Barrack and Hospital Improvement Commission, with two additional India members, to form the home centre for Indian sanitary improvement.

The next thing is to have your Indian Health Departments organized with men of the best available knowledge and experience. At first there will be difficulty. Lord Stanley says: "It is probable that difficul-

---

58 Wood's speech minimized the mortality in the Indian Army by saying that the facts were so out-of-date that they did not afford "a good index of the sanitary state" of the army at present; he also claimed that intemperance of the soldiers was worse in "former years than now" (Hansard, *Parliamentary Debates*, 3rd series [1830-91] 23 July 1863:1299).

ties will arise out of the conflicting claims of the Indian and home authorities, but these we must be prepared for and deal with as they come up. So far, all has gone well."

If you thought well to send me home a plan which would enable the Indian commissions to act in concert with the home commission, we could try here and, by your help, we could come to an agreement. The functions of both Indian and home commissions are sufficiently sketched in the report to enable you to judge how their powers should be arranged.

Next in importance is the finding of good men for India commissioners and officers of health. I have been able as yet to obtain the names of medical officers only, herewith sent [appended]. They are proposed partly from the kind of knowledge shown in the reports they sent to the royal commission and partly from independent inquiries. We want in addition Indian civilians, military officers and also engineers, to act both as commissioners and the engineers as inspectors. I will write again about these, if you will allow me.

Your present practice is, I suppose, to send all plans of military buildings up to the Government of India. Should these plans be sent to England before or after they are sent to the Government of India? How would it do to send everything from the presidency commissions direct to the Government of India, thence home, from home back to the Government of India and thence to the presidencies for execution? If this would work, it should include military buildings and all civil sanitary works. Or should there be direct communication between the presidency commissions and the home commission (of course through the secretary of state for India)?

For your consideration we put these points to bring out what would be the best administrative arrangements.

[list of possible members of presidencies' sanitary commissions]

*Bengal* – Medical commissioners: *Dr Norman Chevers, *Dr Joseph Ewart, *Dr E.I. Mouatt, *Dr T.E. Dempster

– Officers of health: Dr A. Grant, *H.M. McPherson, *I.F. Beatson, C. Hathaway, I.R. Playfair, A. Christison, G.S. Sutherland, *A. Maclean, assistant surgeon 42nd Highlanders

*Madras* – Commissioners: *Dr Duncan Macpherson, I.G., E.G. Balfour

– Officers of health: S.A. Reynolds, D. Macfarlane

– Officers of health: M. Rogers, S.W. Mudge, W.S. Leslie, C.M. Duff, G. Mackay, I. Donaldson, W.N. Chipperfield

*Bombay* – Commissioner: *Dr D. Grierson, surgeon-major

– Officers of health: J. Vaughan, G.G. Maitland, J. Peet, W.C. Coles, J.G. Fraser, G.R. Ballingall, J. Miller

I have put * to the names of those whose own returns recommend them. But possibly you have better information as to men. This is only as a help.

Source: From two letters to Douglas Galton with a comment by Galton, ADD Mss 45761 ff46-51 and 54

27 July 1863

You bid us "think over instructions." Before drawing them up, it must be determined what should be the plan of working. The simplest and I believe the best plan would be to constitute the conjoint commission and then to put into its hands the royal commission report and its recommendations, with a simple instruction to take the whole matter as regards the sanitary condition of Indian stations, bazaars and native towns and of the troops generally into its hands, and to advise the secretary of state for India as to what he should do. The executive work would of course have to be done in India, the advising work in England.

I send two other schemes, I and II, either of which if adopted would become a basis for instructions; I is the best and the most direct; II presupposes a certain amount of knowledge in India which does not exist. Could you have them both considered and us told which is most likely to answer the purpose, with any remarks or suggestions, that we may proceed with the instructions. . . .

[Scheme] I

1. Conjoint commission when constituted to proceed at once with the framing of proposals for the sanitary improvement of existing stations, bazaars, towns, barracks and hospitals (including officers' and married quarters), taking for their guidance the stational reports and evidence laid before the commission and such other evidence as can be obtained from documents in the possession of the India Office and War Office, that they also obtain additional information from Indian officers who may be in England. [DG: Sir C. Wood would not entertain this plan because it appears more roundabout than the other, although it would really be shorter.]

2. That having selected a station for improvement, the joint commission prepare a report setting forth the sanitary condition of the station, etc., together with the proposals for improvement.

3. That this report be sent to the secretary of state for India and be transmitted to the government in India with the view [DG: The committee might draw up a scheme.] of obtaining such additional information or observations as the local commissions may be able to afford.

4. The local commissions to report on the scheme proposed after inquiry on the spot.

5. This report to be sent to the secretary of state for India and to be referred to the home commission.

6. The home commission to reconsider the case with the additional information thus obtained and to report their final recommendations to the secretary of state for India with the view of their being communicated to the local commission and to the public works department for execution.

7. All plans of officers' quarters, barracks, married quarters, hospitals, to be prepared by the works department in India in consultation with the local commissions and to be sent direct to the secretary of state for India for reference to the home commission on points of sanitary details.

The advantage of this plan of working would be that the initiative would begin at home. There is an apparent interference with the functions of the authorities in India. But it is more apparent than real, and it may very well be argued that these authorities, who have allowed things to get into their present state, are not the most likely to move in a right direction out of it.

[Scheme] II

1. The presidency commissions to proceed at once to the selection of stations, etc., to be improved.

2. That in doing this they take for their guidance the evidence contained in the stational reports and given by witnesses before the royal commission, with such other evidence obtained by inspection or otherwise as they may think necessary.

3. That they report on the sanitary condition of each station together with the improvements required.

4. That this report be sent to the secretary of state for India to be referred to the conjoint commission.

5. That the conjoint commission take the proposed scheme of improvement into consideration and report on the same with any suggestions they may have to make to the secretary of state for India.

6. That this report be sent to the Government of India and its recommendations adopted as the basis of the sanitary improvement of the station.

7. That all plans of barracks, hospitals, etc., be prepared in India and sent to the secretary of state for India for examination by the conjoint commission before being sanctioned.

By this scheme of working the initiative would be in India and nothing could be done at home until the Indian authorities had moved. Apparently it would interfere less with their freedom of action; but really it would interfere more than if the initiative were at home, because they would be quite sure to send stupid schemes and plans, which the conjoint commission at home would have to criticize.

29 July 1863

According to your note, we work upon [Scheme] No. II. But before drawing up the instructions, it is necessary that the India Office do concur, because any change would involve a new code of instructions being drawn up.

The enclosed proposal contains the suggestion in your note. It is a preliminary proposal for the India Office and perhaps might now be put forward, if Lord de Grey agrees.

Source: From a letter to Sir Charles Trevelyan, Newcastle University Library 35/26

9 August 1863

I hear that Sir H. Rose has "drawn up a bill" to form divisional boards of health. This is against the recommendation of the commission ("royal sanitary") and would result in failure from want of unity of action. The presidency commissions must be the centre of action. And you in India must arrange how to work the stations from this centre, either by responsible *local* boards or by inspectors sent from the centre, or by both. To set any number of men of any kind to do work in any number of districts, without any community of principles or of action, is to introduce bad and costly sanitary works instead of none. And all that Sir Hugh Rose wants done can be done through the regimental and stational medical officers under the "Army Medical Regulations," at present. Sir H. Rose's proposition would virtually supersede these regulations by something not by any means so good, while it is one of the recommendations of the royal commission that these "regulations" be adopted at all stations in India. They are of course purely regimental and stational, and while you preserve the responsibilities under them intact, you must find some way of combining these under one general system of sanitary reform and administration for each presidency. If *you* would sketch an act which would answer for India, you are the only man who could do it. We would look it over for you.

Source: From two letters to Douglas Galton, Add Mss 45761 ff75-78 and 79-97

Hampstead, N.W.
20 August 1863

We will prepare a draft of instructions for the conjoint India and War Office commission. But, in the meantime, as they have agreed to the conjunction, *pray, pray,* do you, at the War Office, before you accede to it, consider well what the work and the responsibility will be.

We wished for a *special commission,* whose special work it should be to direct this, the greatest movement of our time, *as it may be.* THEY wish to connect it with your Barrack and Hospital Commission. So be it. Amen. But let it be done thoroughly and well, as well as it can be. *It cannot be tacked onto the ordinary work.* Somebody must be responsible. And you must make such provision for the work as will enable it to be *continuously* carried out.

Dr Sutherland says there will be difficulty as to office room. But office room *must* be found, if not in the War Office, at least in some convenient building at hand, as it would be inconvenient for you to go to the India Office.

Everything depends on starting well and on arranging well preliminaries. You will find that in reality the commission will be an India commission with a vast work in its hands, and the War Office barrack work will take a secondary place in it. An India mail may at any time bring you fifty reports and as many plans, all these to be studied in detail. It will be hard work and work of a different kind from what you have been dealing with heretofore.

Out of thirty-nine (39) recommendations in the report of the royal commission, twenty (20) or thereabouts come under the conjoint commission.

Don't let us start without consideration of what is wanted for success. If you begin without laying the ground so well as to prevent a breakdown, a breakdown there will be. The India Office must of course bear its share of expense. Pray consult Lord de Grey.

The royal commission has done its work and done it well. It very much depends upon the first steps the War Office takes to make this a serious commission, whether any good is to be done to India or *none.* The vast advantage we had before (of having Sidney Herbert at the head of all the working commissions) we have not now.

[21 August 1863]

These are the things that have to be done. And whatever the form of instruction may be, the things must be done. The instructions are not sent as final. They are only to inform as to the work which the joint commission has to make itself responsible for to show that adequate preparation must be made for carrying it out.

After you have read it, please return it with any remarks, before it is put into shape for Lord de Grey. . . .

It may be as well to explain that the commission has two sets of duties (under the report) regarding barracks, hospitals, stations, etc.:

1. To report generally and in such a manner as to be useful in India, the principles applicable to the improvement of existing buildings.

2. Checking plans sent from India to see that the principles have been properly applied. This will explain the prominence given to general reporting given in the instructions. But this is nothing new. It is only what you have been doing all along.

Query: Might not the sanitary conditions of the stations be attended to by the following administrative arrangements?

1. The presidency commissions to act as the advising authority of the India government on all matters connected with the health of stations, bazaars, native towns.

2. At each station or town there be constituted a local executive authority with power to employ and pay officers, such as inspector of nuisances and his staff, these local authorities reporting to the presidency commissions and referring to them for all questions in which advice is required, the presidency commissions having power to send sanitary and engineering inspectors to see that all works are properly executed and causes of disease removed. The object of this procedure ought to be that every station in India shall be kept in a proper sanitary condition, whatever be the number of troops in occupation, however frequently the troops are changed and when the station is temporarily unoccupied. It would seem desirable that the Indian stations should be, at all times, kept in a good sanitary condition, quite independently of the troops.

And the next question is, what would be the duty of the commanding and medical officers in occupation? In reply, would it not be advisable to add the commanding and medical officer for the time being to the local authority? If this is not done, the proceeding laid down in the new army medical regulations (Section XX, 77) would come into operation, by which the medical officer represents to the commanding officer whatever requires improvement. And the commanding officer would in his turn represent to the local authority.

At large stations, the officer commanding and the principal medical officer would be sufficient additions to the local authority, but the medical and commanding officers of *regiments* would still represent to the local authorities in terms of the new medical regulations. The necessities of the case will be better understood by the following enumeration of things requiring to be done:

1. Permanent works such as water supply, drainage, levelling ground, improving existing barracks, hospitals and other buildings, building improved barracks and hospitals.

2. Current improvements, such as cleansing and removal of nuisances, repairs seeing to the efficiency of all sanitary arrangements, limewashing.

3. Selecting and laying out stations, including bazaars and neighbouring native dwellings.

Lastly, the whole question of the water supply, drainage and general sanitary supervision of native towns. Judging from this distance, it would appear that the most efficient and economical procedure would be to connect the whole sanitary administration of each presidency with the central commission, the executive head of which should be the minister of health for the presidency. It is proposed to place on these commissions representatives of every interest likely to be affected, viz., a civilian, a military officer, an engineering officer, a medical officer, a sanitary officer, so that there may be no jealousy between the stational authorities and the commissions.

Suppose, by way of illustration, that it is proposed by the Government of India to improve, say, the station of Allahabad, there would be, of course, first, a careful local inquiry and survey, including levels, natural means of drainage, water sources and their analysis, state of the ground within the station and of the river banks adjoining, contouring state of the barrack and hospital buildings, which of them might be improved and whether better sites could not be selected for these barrack and hospital plans, position, distance, laying out, water supply and drainage of bazaars, improvements in barracks and hospitals to be retained. It is evident that such an inquiry would raise questions which could only be settled by the presidency commission. It is apprehended that all the works enumerated above would be *executed* by the Public Works Department, which would benefit immensely by the advice of the presidency commission.

If all these works were satisfactorily carried out, it is evident that the local authority at Allahabad would have its attention chiefly occupied with questions of cleansing and preventions of nuisance, and with a general oversight of the state of the station, its buildings and sanitary arrangements. All improvements and repairs of the buildings it might recommend would be executed by the local officer of the Public Works Department. And all questions of cleansing and prevention of nuisances would be carried out by the officers of the local authority.

As regards native cities and towns, the work would have to be carried out by municipalities where there are such, or by any other local authority that may exist or be constituted. In these cases, the presidency commission should have a power of inspection by officers of health and engineers.

One of the most important functions of the presidency commissions and local authorities must henceforth be the mitigation or prevention of epidemic disease among the native population. And for this purpose they should have the power of inspection and recommending measures. Or they might be vested temporarily with absolute executive functions.

Some doubts have been expressed as to the extent to which sanitary improvements can be introduced among the natives without shocking their prejudices. But hitherto there has been no opposition to improvements forming the basis of all sanitary progress. E.g., Bombay has received a water supply and is about to be drained. Calcutta is being drained and will shortly be supplied with water. Sir C. Trevelyan states that the question of drainage and water supply was a very popular one amongst the natives at Madras. There has hitherto been no opposition to carrying out these fundamental principles of improvement. Again, no native can raise any objection against paving the surface of a street. (There has been no plague in Paris since this simple improvement was carried out.) Again, if the Indian government chose to run new streets through densely peopled, unhealthy native districts, there would be nothing in caste prejudices to prevent this, provided suitable compensation were given. (Is the Muhammadan law of property like that of Naboth's vineyard?[59]) These things can, no doubt, be done. And after they are done, the only remaining points refer to the internal economy of dwellings, which might very well be left to improving civilization. Or at least until the other improvements were completed.

The question of houses might stand till then, because in all probability it will be found quite a secondary one to the others. Of course it is taken for granted in this that native houses are cleansed at present

59 An allusion to 1 Kings 21:1-19.

by mehters [sweepers]. With regard to improvements, the royal commission has recommended that the three presidency cities, and some of the more important stations, be selected and put in a complete state of sanitary improvement, the latter as regards buildings as well as sanitary works. And in this way much valuable experience will be obtained for future progress. But this course should not prevent the more urgent sanitary works being carried out at all the stations.

As to "representations" under Section XX of "Regulations," the Indian sanitary service, if duly organized, should render such "representations" unnecessary. And if they require to be made, they should be considered as proof of neglect in some quarter.

The government supply the spirit on the requirement of the regiment. A tea-total regiment or a temperance regiment would not be obliged to take any spirit. What can be done in India at present is to suppress the sale of spirit in bazaars under the control of the magistrate. We will try here to get the Horse Guards to discontinue the sale of spirit in the canteens.

The apparent reason why Dr Linton would not sign the Cholera Commission report and why it has created so much ill feeling in the Army Medical Department is that one Indian medical officer, Dr McClelland, and one civilian, Mr Strachey, have *not only* exposed fearlessly the sanitary defects of the stations, for on this all parties may be agreed, but because they have criticized rather severely the measures and treatment adopted for the *sick* by the royal army medical officers. They feel that, on this point, Mr Strachey was not competent, while they do not admit that Dr McClelland was any more competent than the men whose practice was criticized.

The following can only be done by the War Office and Horse Guards [see letter of 26 December 1863 below]:

1. Sending none but fully drilled recruits to India.

2. Suppressing issue of spirits on board ship, except on the recommendation of the medical officer; introducing a gradual change in solders' diet during passage, e.g., introducing a larger proportion of vegetables.

3. Regulation of regimental canteens in India, with special reference to the disappearance of spirits from these, and extended use of malt liquor, tea, coffee, etc.

4. Greater stringency in the regulation of regimental and all bazaars over which the military authority has control, with a view to suppress the sale of spirits in them.

5. Flannel underclothing, better boots, improvements in clothing generally, where required.

6. Providing regimental and hospital cooks, properly trained.

7. Introduction of gymnastics, whenever gymnasia are provided.

8. Encouraging trades, wherever workshops have been provided, and also soldiers' gardens.

9. Fixing the period of service in India for the present at ten years.

10. Applying the army medical regulations of 7 October 1859 to all garrisons, stations and regiments in India (including, of course, the statistical records and forms).

11. Provision to be made for passing invalids at the port of embarcation without delay, and for their immediate shipment home.

12. Each regiment proceeding to India to be accompanied by its hospital sergeant and quota of trained orderlies.

13. That all cadets of engineers receive a course of instruction in sanitary principles at Brompton.

The Horse Guards through their regimental authorities could direct compliance with Nos. 3, 4, 7, 8. The W.O. could arrange with Admiralty about Nos. 2, 11. The W.O. direct could do Nos. 5, 10, 13 and in concurrence with Horse Guards could arrange for carrying out Nos. 1, 6, 9, 12.

The following will have to be done by the government in India:

1. Sanitary improvement of stations and native towns.

2. Construction of healthy barracks and hospitals.

3. Water supply and drainage.

4. Improvement of existing barracks.

5. Erection of gymnasia, reading, day and coffee rooms, workshops; providing soldiers' gardens.

6. Question of hill stations.

7. Providing, through the India commissariat, sufficient means, such as vegetables, etc., for varying the soldiers' diet according to season.

[From the Queen's Regulations]

1. Improving entire management of army, e.g., commanding officers seeing to better general employment of men, soldier's institutes, gymnastics. Government [providing] means of occupation, covered sheds, workshops, gardens, tools, apparatus, buildings, better regulation of canteens as to spirits, better police of bazaars to prevent sale.

Question of increased marriages, better provision for wives and children. Improvement in ration, vegetables.

2. Points to be held in India. What unhealthy stations to be given up. Which best hill stations and best way of using them.

3. Sanitary improvements in stations: drainage, water supply, laying out, better construction. We would gladly help with our experience.

4. Habits of the people: improving native towns and dwellings, better water supply imperative, cannot be had without drainage.

5. Must be somebody's duty (presidency commissions'?). Should be appointed at once.

Christian education cannot proceed with bad sanitary conditions. Government in India [does] everything as regards physical progress. It can also educate. It should do both.

[More from the Queen's Regulations]

1. War Office to despatch troops to India at proper seasons.

2. War Office to alter regulations as to issue of spirits to troops on board ship going to India [Queen's regulations], pp 338-60 as follows: no spirits are in future to be issued to troops on board ship except on the recommendation of the medical officer in charge.

3. War Office to urge on the Indian government that the sale of spirits in canteens in India be discontinued and that the sale of spirits in military bazaars be made illegal and suppressed.

4. War Office to come to an arrangement with the India government as to a modification of the ration to suit the season with special reference to a better provision of vegetables. War Office to provide soldiers with flannel underclothing and better boots.

5. For conjoint commission.

6. India government to reduce the period of service in India to ten years.

7. India government to embark invalids immediately for England.

8-19. For conjoint commission.

20. Government in India.

21-25. For conjoint commission.

26. War Office to represent to India government.

27. Ditto. War Office and India government.

28. War Office itself (to provide hospital orderlies for sick).

29. Conjoint commission.

30. Government in India.

31. Ditto.

32. War Office and India government.

33. Conjoint commission and War Office.

34. Ditto.

35, 36. Duties to be arranged between conjoint commission and presidency.

37. Conjoint Commission.
38. War Office and Indian government.
39. India government aided by conjoint and presidency commissions.

*Instructions* for the guidance of the conjoint commission appointed by the secretary of state for India and the secretary of state for war to advise on the sanitary improvement of stations, bazaars and native towns, barracks and hospitals in India.

1. You will take generally for your guidance the principles laid down in the report of the royal commission appointed to inquire into the sanitary state of the Indian Army together with the recommendations appended to that report.

2. In furtherance of these objects, you will advise the secretary of state for India as to the best methods of improving the sanitary condition of individual stations, beginning with those of most importance and in which the evidence collected by the royal commission has shown the sanitary conditions to be most defective and the mortality of the troops greatest.

[in Dr Sutherland's hand] You will examine the evidence regarding the condition of stations contained in the report (and appendix) of the royal commission and you will prepare a general scheme of improvement of the stations, setting forth the pre-eminent levels of sanitary defects which exercise the greatest influence as to water analysis, health of the troops and the order in which these should be dealt with. This scheme should also contain the general principles of procedure applicable to all stations, so framed as to assist the local commissions of health in the practical steps they may take. You will take for your guidance in this matter the recommendations made by the royal commission and make such practical proposals in regard to the carrying out of these recommendations as you may consider necessary.

You will prepare for the consideration of the secretary of state a code of instructions for the duties of officers of health appointed to stations and towns setting forth the duties of these officers as regards the examination of the causes of disease and the steps to be taken for their abatement. All sanitary reports on stations, barracks, hospitals and towns in India and its dependencies will be referred to you with the view to your giving your advice and opinion on the improvements recommended in these reports with special reference to the introduction of the most recent improvements.

All plans of barracks, hospitals, stations, bazaars and other buildings will be referred to you for consideration insofar as regards their sanitary details, and you will report your opinion on the same, with any alterations you think desirable should be made, in their details, to make them more healthy.

[FN resumes]

Hospital construction:

1. The royal commission has recommended that the cubic space for hospital beds in India should be 1500 ft. as a minimum and upwards to 2000 in less healthy situations. Also that the superficial area per bed should be from 100 to 120 and 130 sq. ft. according to the position.

2. They have laid it down as a principle that a hospital should consist of separate detached wards for from twenty to twenty-four beds per ward.

3. It is proposed that these hospital blocks should resemble, as far as is suitable, quarter company barrack blocks, i.e., that each hospital block shall consist of a raised basement with two floors over it, the upper floor only to be used for sick and the whole surrounded by verandahs, 10 ft. in width.

4. Each block ought thus to be exposed on all its sides freely to the wind.

Source: From a letter to Douglas Galton, Add Mss 45761 ff120-21

Hampstead, N.W.
18 September 1863

Sir Proby Cautley has been appointed by Sir C. Wood on your conjoint India Office and War Office (sanitary) commission. This I dare say you know. But he [P. Cautley] wrote above ten days ago to say that they wished to proceed at once, to take the initiative, and to *send out* building plans to India. He even named the days on which he could attend at the War Office.

He was answered that, as the commission was to proceed under special instructions, and as these were not yet issued, nothing could be done until they were. I was in hopes to have heard from you. But as I have not, I now remind you that not a day should have been lost in framing these special instructions. Pray urge Lord de Grey. The India Office is actually ahead of us now.

I only mention what Sir P. Cautley says as to initiative and as to plans being "sent out" from home because it may modify Lord de Grey's opinion as to the instructions—who, you will remember, thought the initiative had better (or rather must) come from India.

Source: From a letter to Sir Harry Verney, Wellcome (Claydon copy) Ms 9000/128

Hampstead, N.W.
19 September 1863

In answer to your kind letter:

1. For carrying out the recommendations of the India Army Sanitary Commission, all depends upon the promptitude of government in forming the four *working* commissions of health—one for each presidency in India, and one at home, to be attached to the India and War Offices.

You yourself know how Sidney Herbert halved the death rate of the army at home by his Barrack and Hospital Improvement Commission (among other measures), which still exists. To this the India Office has already appointed Sir Proby Cautley and is about to appoint two other members. This is to be the advising body of the India Office in all matters relating to the sanitary improvement of stations, etc.

But this commission is of course for nothing more than to give its advice when asked for. It can execute nothing. All practical work must be done in India. And not a day should be lost in appointing the three presidency commissions, or rather "departments of public health," as recommended by the royal commission, to take official charge of the great work to be carried out in India.

2. You know what an impression the report has made in England, even deeper than that of Sidney Herbert's first army sanitary report. People ask if the state of things revealed "is to last another day." MPs are burning to take it up. It is *out of*, rather than *in*, the India Office that the outcry is loudest. It is amazing how easily officials are satisfied of the truth of anything it is held desirable to assert. And therefore it is a simple conformity with the tradition of a government office to denounce as extravagant and exaggerated the lamentable exposures made by this inquiry. Would that our facts could vanish before their denunciations! . . .

The Government *of* India *in* India must take steps itself, and not wait for pressure from England. It must take the initiative well and willingly. It will never sit down quietly under such a weight of responsibility, nor rest till these deplorable evils are removed.

3. The object is to have a department of health under a responsible head for each presidency, to be constituted out of the required elements: civil, military, engineering, sanitary, medical; to place this department in the relation of receiving aid and advice from the India and War Office commission at home; and in the position of advising the Public Works Department and local authorities in each presidency

on all matters connected with barracks, hospitals, stations, bazaars, native towns, etc.; at home we would gladly help with a plan for working out the details. But first let India find the best men and constitute the commissions.

There are some good men to begin with, such as Dr T.E. Dempster; Inspector General MacPherson of Madras; Dr Norman Chevers and Dr Joseph Ewart of Bengal; Dr MacClelland, etc., who would be efficient on these commissions as sanitary or medical members (of course officers of health there must be to act under the commissions. Good names could be given for these too).

4. Unless the death rate and invaliding rate of the Indian Army can be reduced, to hold India by British troops will become impossible.

Already this next year 1864 we want 25,000 recruits. And I have just seen a letter from the Horse Guards who wish to extend re-enlistment by an increase of pay, because they do not know where to turn to keep up the army. But a better method than this would be to improve the sanitary condition of India. And this is the key to holding India by British troops. And on the India government now depends the possibility of doing so.

5. There is the native population too. It is surely something to stir us all, to know that Indian pestilences are of Indian manufacture, that the causes which give rise to them are removeable, now that Indians are as much our own fellow subjects as Londoners. What is wanted is to drain India, to water supply India, to cleanse India by something more than surface cleansing.

What is wanted is that it should not be said now of us as Burke said (?) years ago—that if we were to leave India tomorrow, we should leave behind us no more traces of our civilization than if India had been in the possession of the hyena or the tiger.[60]

6. The question is, in short, nothing less than to create a Public Health Department for India. What a glorious work for an India government! The difficulties are great. But see what Sidney Herbert's confidence in a good cause enabled him to do. He halved the death rate of the army at home. Lord Elgin can do much more than this—the India death rate can be reduced to much less than half. For *everything* is there to be done, as everything had to be done in the Crimea. And this makes it the more, *not* the less hopeful.

---

60 A paraphrase from Burke, *The Works of the Rt Hon Edmund Burke* 2:354.

The discovery, so to speak, of the royal commission is that the cause of ill health in India lies *not* in the climate, but in the absence of all works of sanitary civilization. This produced the very same diseases in Europe, when there was no water supply, no drainage, no sewerage here, and the results are intensified in India by climate. Let this not go on.

Source: From two letters to Douglas Galton, ADD Mss 45761 ff124-25 and 133-34

Hampstead, N.W.
24 September 1863

With regard to the India and War Offices joint commission, as the *Instructions* are the turning point of the whole, pray don't forget to let us see them before they are issued. Also, the India Office do not seem to have appointed an Indian medical officer (Martin) [to the joint commission]. This is necessary. Also, Rawlinson, for the water and drainage.

Also, pray don't forget the room. If men are to work, they must sit down. I have all the manuscript stational reports, and whole fortresses of other Indian papers, which I have kept in my own room for four years. And worlds shall not compel me to give them up, except to a conjoint commission established in a good room at the War Office.

Otherwise, I shall bury them with *me.* Confound me if I don't! We are busy in abstracting the evidence and preparing the 8vo (of the Indian report).... Of course you will let us see the *Instructions* again, before they are decided upon.

30 September 1863

The proposed *Instructions* will do, subject to one or two verbal alterations which I have made, to make them include advice as to the kind of improvements required in existing buildings. If the Indian representatives are added for all purposes to your commission, the heading will have to be as altered.

A good room *must* be. Make haste or I shall bury all my papers and plans, as proposed, with me. The India plans are, I should say, about 60 miles square. The commission will want these. And I shall sing aloud when they can't get them, as they certainly shall not, till I am duly certified of good lodgings and accommodation for them. I want to get rid of them, for I have had two vans, price £4, to move them every time I have moved myself for four years.

We *must* have Rawlinson on the [joint] commission.

Source: From unsigned notes for Lord Stanley, Add Mss 45836 ff15-20

[ca. October 1863]

The course of proceeding recommended by the royal commission for carrying out the sanitary improvement of Indian stations and towns was as follows:

1. To vest the executive in a local authority or commission of health for each presidency;

2. To give to these Indian authorities the advantage of home experience in the details of sanitary improvement, leaving to the Indian authorities the sole responsibility of accepting or rejecting any information or advice which might be sent to them;

3. As a commission already existed at the War Office, which was discharging the function of advising not only at home but at all foreign stations, including Ceylon, on the confines of India itself, it was considered by the royal commission that, unless the secretary of state for India thought it advisable to appoint a special commission, he should add to the War Office commission officers of Indian experience, and that the joint commission should discharge the function of advising and transmitting information to the India authorities. The latter course was followed. And the joint commission is now ready for action.

Some may think that this advising function of a home commission was unnecessary. But, in the first place, it is found to be absolutely necessary for Ceylon, in which the defects of stations are precisely the same as those in India.

And, in the second place, it is perfectly well known to foreign governments that nearly all existing practical experience of sanitary works is to be found in England. It frequently happens that commissions are sent to this country to obtain information, both as regards civil and military improvements. There is surely no reason why India should not also benefit in this way.

There is of course a certain amount of jealousy between the Indian authorities in India and those at home. But surely this jealousy should disappear, as neither interference nor control is proposed in this case, but simply to offer to the India commissions our own accumulated experience. . . .

According to present understanding, the connection between the presidency commissions and the War Office [home] commission would be as follows:

1. The home commission has been already requested to prepare model plans of barracks and hospitals, which are now considerably

advanced. These plans, when completed, will be sent to the India Office. And, if sanctioned there, will be transmitted to India.

2. The presidency commissions are, I believe, to send home to the secretary of state for India any plans or proposals of their own which, before being sanctioned, will be sent to the War Office commission for advice and information. Besides this, however, which is good, so far as it goes, we have been most desirous to help the presidency commissions by a direct statement and description of the kind of sanitary works, improvements and appliances applicable to Indian stations to meet the requirements described in the stational reports. If the home commission were authorized to draw up such a statement, it would clear away at once most of the presumed difficulty in applying improved sanitary methods to the case of India. I have already seen documents printed at Calcutta, since they received the royal commission report, in which difficulties have been raised which could never have occurred to the writers, if they had known what is being done at home. It would be very advisable to prevent a repetition of similar objections.

Source: From five letters to Douglas Galton, Add Mss 45761 ff147-149, 150-53, 154, 163-65 and 166-67 (all written from Hampstead, N.W.)

10 October 1863

*Private.* I very much wish that the War Office would bestir itself about the *Instructions* and room for the India and War Office joint commission. I hear from Sir John Lawrence that "instructions have" already "gone out to India to form local committees," i.e., the presidency commissions, "and for these committees to draw up rules." I would have given a great deal that this had not happened. I mean that you had been beforehand with them.

Lord de Grey had the game in his own hands, by its being their own desire that the commission should be a War Office one. He need not have been so delicate about not "irritating" them.

I also hear from Colonel Strachey (in India) that they are setting their faces against "boards" which they are entirely mistaken in supposing the royal commission to recommend, and that they want an officer of health with responsible powers. *We* want a civilian with administrative powers at the head of a consultative commission. And it is a great pity that the War Office joint commission did not take the lead in explaining what it did want.

Sir J. Lawrence says that Sir P. Cautley and Sir R. Martin were appointed "some weeks ago." He says that "unofficial" only means that the members receive no pay, but that in "all other respects they are just as if they were official members."

Colonel Strachey writes at great length about workshops, but requiring some regulation, which we don't know the Horse Guards will grant. I would gladly submit all these letters to you. But indeed I fear that everyone has been more ready than the War Office, although the War Office itself *very justly* said that "Sir C. Trevelyan had better lock up his money" unless this home commission were got out quickly, for that Colonel Strachey and company were quite incapable of using it well.

13 October 1863

*Private.* If the India Office members of the joint commission are to "prescribe" what that commission is to do, we are lost.

Sir P. Cautley's note alarms me more than I can tell you. "He thinks delay in anything beyond plans desirable." It is true the plans are one essential, but another essential, I had almost said a greater essential, is the "code." The very first thing the commission was to have done was to prepare a working scheme for the practical carrying out of the recommendations of the royal commission, to be submitted to the India Office.

Now you may expect a year to elapse before the "code" comes home—this Lord Stanley told me—and then the best thing that can happen is that you will be able to alter it all.

Do they really think that Sidney Herbert's royal commission was worked this way? Why, the whole working scheme was on paper and carried by himself to Lord Panmure (and afterwards to General Peel) before those four sub-commissions, which carried out all his recommendations, were issued at all.

How do you think it would have been, if the *Horse Guards* had written the "Army Medical Regulations," which is our "code"? Yet the India Office is showing the most undue activity in doing what it knows nothing at all about, and the War Office is showing the most undue inactivity, not to say sloth, in not doing what it knows perfectly well how to do.

I wish you had sent us a copy of Sir P. Cautley's letter of 30 September, if you could not send us the original. Surely it is to those who worked the royal commission that this information is due. I promise that, if you will send me such letters in future, I will take a copy and return them to you in two hours.

I am quite dismayed at our prospects. Indeed they know little of how Sidney Herbert's commissions were worked. Of course the *admin-*

*istrative rules* for the India presidency commissions would have to be drawn up in India. But indeed, indeed, the instructions ought to have gone out from us.

Sir J. Lawrence "advises" me just in the same sense as Sir P. Cautley and I have written to him much what I write now. But I fear it is too late. All that is to be done now is *to hurry on the Instructions of the home commission* as fast as possible. Some danger may still be saved. (To my mind, sending out plans is only a secondary object, though, of course, the India Office thinks it is all.) And I remember you said this too.

I may as well tell you that Colonel Strachey says "he will not move a finger" in constructing workshops, as recommended by the commission, unless the Horse Guards make them a parade. He also says that he will oppose the organization of "boards," whatever orders the India Office sends out, mistaking what we recommend.

14 October 1863

I return Sir P. Cautley['s letter]. I have taken a copy of it for Dr Sutherland, to whom he desired it to be sent and whom I have not seen for some days.

I return to London (32 South St.) on 2 November. I wish I had never left it, for I could have prevented the orders being sent out to India to form the "code" without us, if I had known of them. I feel very uneasy. And you must forgive me.

16 October 1863

*Private.* I was in hopes to have heard from you today, both as to the *Instructions* and as to whether there is a possibility of the home commission still doing the heads of the code.

I cannot tell you how strongly I feel about it. The royal commission, with its four years' labour and expense, had better not have been if India is to do its own commissions and its own sanitary code. For there is an amazing difference, e.g., between the Horse Guards framing its own code and getting it approved by the War Office, and the War Office framing the code and getting it accepted by the Horse Guards. Besides, I see no *certainty* now even that the code, when it does come back from India, will be submitted to your commission. Exactly the same trick may be played again. I shall never forgive myself that I did not keep up such a daily correspondence with the India Office, either through Sir J. Lawrence or by making Dr Sutherland call upon Sir P. Cautley, as would have enabled us to know exactly what the India Office was doing.

For I believe there has been no mystery at all about it. I believe Sir J. Lawrence or Sir P. Cautley would have told us exactly what was doing, if they had known we wished to know it, and would instantly have acquiesced in your commission framing the heads of the code, if they had known we wished it. . . . I would have written to Lord de Grey about the *Instructions*. But Dr Sutherland told me you preferred that it should be left to you.

17 October 1863

I have had your two letters of the 15th and 16th about the India joint commission, for which a very great many thanks. (I did not have either till after I had written my reminder of the 16th.)

I am overjoyed with the result of your exertions. We will do the "heads of a code" as soon as possible. I trust the *Instructions* will soon be out and that, as you have got a room, the commission will soon begin its sittings. I have not seen Dr Sutherland for some time. He has been ill. But I have no doubt he will be "out" as soon as the *Instructions*, and able to attend the first meetings.

Source: From a draft letter to an unnamed recipient in Dr Sutherland's hand, Add Mss 45798 ff171-72

[ca. 17 October 1863]

As I know you take a deep interest in the Indian Army I do not scruple to tell you that no time should now be lost in giving practical effect to the recommendations of the royal commission. The India Office here has appointed members to add to the War Office Barrack and Hospital Improvement Commission, which you may remember was recommended by the royal commission as the advising body of the India Office in all matters relating to the sanitary improvement of stations. But the commission can do nothing more than give its advice when asked for. It can execute nothing. All practical work must be done in India, and there is an urgent necessity for the appointment of the presidency commissions, or rather "departments of public health," recommended by the royal commission to take official charge of the great work to be carried out in India.

The report has made a deeper impression than the report of the first army sanitary commission did, and people are beginning to ask whether the state of things the report reveals is to last a day longer. . . . I have already myself written more than once urging that the presidency commissions should be appointed without delay. It would be much better that the Government of India in India should take steps itself than that pressure should be exercised from this side. . . .

Could you in any way help by writing or otherwise in urging on the work in India? What we want there is a department of health under a responsible head, for each presidency to be constituted out of the required elements: civil, military, engineering, sanitary and medical to place this department in the relation of receiving aid and advice from the War Office commission at home, and in the position of advising the Public Works Department and local authorities in each presidency on all matters connected with barracks, hospitals, stations, bazaars, native towns, etc. On this side we would gladly help with a plan of working out the details. But what is now wanted is that the best men should be found and the commissions constituted. We know some good men to begin with such as - -, who would render efficient aid.

Unless we can reduce the death and invaliding rate of the Indian army we must give up the idea of holding India by British troops. Even now I happen to know that the Horse Guards wish to extend re-enlistment by an increase of pay because they do not know where to turn for recruits next year. The sanitary condition of India is the key to the holding of India by British troops, and on the Indian government now depends the responsibility of doing so.

I have said nothing about the native population, but I must here add that it is an obvious duty to care for their interests also. It is surely something to stir us all up, to know that Indian pestilences are of Indian manufacture, but the causes which give rise to them are removable; that Indians are as much our own fellow subjects as the people of London; that if we profess to govern India we must in the eye of humanity and of public opinion govern it for the good of the people.

Source: From a letter to Douglas Galton, ADD Mss 45761 f175

Hampstead, N.W.
21 October 1863

*Private.* The fact is, your Lord de Grey and your Sir C. Wood understand nothing about it. I enclose a paper, in which, in case you should wish to show it to Lord de Grey, the controversy is put as with Sir C. Wood. *Would it be wise to get from the India Office what their own view is?*

Source: From a letter to Lord de Grey, ADD Mss 43546 ff74-75

23 October 1863

*Private.* It seems odd to me to be writing to you without mentioning what is so desperately near my heart. I mean the India (home) commission *Instructions.* Captain Galton wrote to me about it. And I answered him at some length, i.e., about the *Instructions.* You will know what best to do and what best to settle with Sir C. Wood. . . .

Excuse me for referring to the subject (you know Lord Panmure said I was a "turbulent fellow"). But having gone through step by step with the India sanitary royal commission, both before and after Sidney Herbert's death, for four years, I seem to be the only survivor who can offer viva voce explanations about its gist and intentions.

Source: From two letters to Sir Charles Trevelyan, Newcastle University Library 35/27-28 and 29

26 October 1863

I write now rather to report progress than to make a definite request. Sir C. Wood's despatch to India on the sanitary commissions (1) sent out a summary of the royal commission's recommendations, (2) authorized the formation of presidency commissions, (3) pointed out that all plans for sanitary improvements should, before being carried into execution, be sent to him for reference to the sanitary commission *here*. . . . (4) Sir C. Wood directs that the Calcutta, in communication with the Madras and Bombay commissions, be charged with the preparation of a draft code of sanitary regulations such as is referred to in [the] 37th clause of the royal commission's recommendations, that this draft code is to be transmitted to him for revision in this country and the completed code will then be sent to India for promulgation. Pray take care that the presidency commissions have one responsible administrative head (as we have all along agreed), but a civilian, not an officer of health, as Colonel Strachey advises (*that* would not do).

Pray take care, as Sir C. Wood has left the forms of procedure to be drawn up by the presidency commissions, to get a reference at once to the home India government to ask our Barrack and Hospital Improvement Commission (now constituted with its India members) here to report on the best sanitary arrangements applicable to India, merely to save time and to keep the presidency commissions in the right path.

I remonstrated at the I.O. about leaving "the code" to them and Sir C. Wood has now sent us privately orders to draw up a "memorandum of the heads of a code which he might send to India for the advantage of the presidency commissions." Of course we must be very careful not to set the India authorities against us as, if it is begun by treating them as ignorant and incompetent, must infallibly be the case. The instructions of our home commission are not yet out. Sir

C. Wood did not approve them, though Sir P. Cautley did. And Lord de Grey proposed to compromise the matter by letting the commission act for India upon its home instructions. I remonstrated (having written the Instructions at Lord de Grey's desire) and showed that it was impossible to do so, the circumstances being totally different. For example, sanitary administration *outside*, by local and general acts, has been in progress for years in England and every local administrative body at home has its sanitary powers. It was upon this state of things that our Barrack and Hospital Improvement Commission began its work at home. But there is no such thing in India. There is not a bit of use in beginning the work (in India) *inside*, if nothing is to be done *outside*. Disappointment and deception would alone result. The worst buildings in England were in a better state (from their outside surroundings being in a civilized condition when we began) than the best buildings are in India.

With this knowledge, to begin our commission's work as if we had nothing else to do than at home and merely to send out building plans, as was proposed to us, was simply ensuring failure in effecting any improvement in health.

And here we stand now. I may hear from Lord de Grey tomorrow that Sir C. Wood has acceded to our (new) "Instructions." I have a great deal to say in answer to Colonel Strachey's important letter. But I will only today say, (1) he will see, by the report and evidence, how many barracks there are in India with numbers varying from 100 to 600 men in a single room, (2) the report shows that it would not be "visionary" to employ the men in workshops, even though the H.G. should not make it a "parade" which, of course, would be much better. But of this more at length next mail.

I was pained by the somewhat melancholy tone of your letter, as if you felt your health rather failing. I trust in God that it is not so. But, for God's sake, take all possible precautions. I trust it is *not only* Lady Trevelyan and your children who can get out occasionally quite away from Calcutta. Yours is a health so invaluable. God bless you and keep you safe.

ever yours gratefully and hopefully
Florence Nightingale

26 October 1863

*In re Colonel Strachey's letter.* As regards his proposal to commit the administration to sanitary officers. You will see that this is impracticable, because engineering works and healthy architectural arrangements are the remedies for unhealthy stations. There is no man at present alive, whom one would designate as "officer of health," who would be competent to do this work. Officers of health are indispensable for India. But they should do no more than they do at home, viz., report causes of disease to the executive authority, which should then deal with them, order and see to the execution of works, when necessary. We agree here that deliberative boards do not work. What you want in India is a consultative commission, representing the various scientific elements which enter into health questions, who would advise their executive head, who should be the chief of the Public Health Department and who should be held responsible for directing the execution. A good administrative civilian would perhaps make the best head. The commissions would require to be furnished with officers of health and engineers to make the necessary inspections and inquiries, and the commissions would have to frame the best method of administrative procedure applicable to stations.

Source: From five letters to Douglas Galton, ADD MSS 45761 ff172-74, 189, 190, 195-200 and 206-07

29 October 1863

*India Office joint commission.* You must ascertain very carefully what position Sir P. Cautley and [J.R.] Martin are to occupy. They must represent the India Office in the same sense that the other members represent the War Office. And any decision must be taken as the decision of the commission.

You must avoid any such decision being subsequently reconsidered at the India Office by the Indian representatives. We must guard against any such possibility by the *Instructions.* You must not take anything that Sir C. Wood offers, but what will ensure efficiency. It will not do to take responsibility without the means of discharging it. Everything depends on the *Instructions.* And the sooner we get them out, the better.

Sir C. Wood must not be able to say, Now there are my two men, and I wash my hands of it.

29 October 1863

*No* tidings about the *Instructions*! "Hope deferred," etc. I have never missed Sidney Herbert so much as now. As a *reminder.*

2 November 1863

*Burn.* What could Lord de Grey be about, in declining to press our *Instructions* upon the India Office, "for fear of irritating them," *at the very time* they were sending *their Instructions* to India, and in not knowing even what they were doing till *two months* after it was done!!! The India Office has much the advantage of the War Office now. Well, it can't be helped now. I'm "a gone coon."[61] You see I am "coming down."

2 November 1863

The misfortune is that, while we were proposing a code of instructions, one part of which required the Barrack and Hospital Commission to draw up a scheme for carrying out the recommendations of the royal commission in India, the India Office had actually sent out such a scheme, drawn up in their own way on 15 August. It is clear that they cannot stultify themselves by sending another. But there is nothing to prevent the commission being asked to prepare plans and descriptions of new barracks and hospitals and methods for improving existing barracks and hospitals.

What you want now is an instruction to this effect and also one to give your advice and opinion on all plans and proposals of a sanitary nature sent from India.

In drawing up the "heads of a code," we might introduce such explanatory matters, by way of note, as would cover a good deal of the ground, which your commission can't touch, in the absence of the specific instruction which Sir C. Wood declines giving.

Further: such is the state of things in Calcutta that the Esplanade, which was the only refuge for health of the people, has now become a dangerous source of malaria. Calcutta has a municipal council and they do not know how to begin. They have therefore sent their engineer [Mr Clarke[62]] to England to learn. Now, of whom is he to learn? Would not the wisest thing be to put him into relation with your commission? The *very case* has arisen. And yet you have no power whatever to deal with it. (The above I learn from "Public Works Department" minutes sent me by the last mail by Sir C. Trevelyan and which I have sent to Lord Stanley. But as soon as he returns them, I will send them to Lord de Grey.)

---

61 According to E.C. Brewer, *Dictionary of Phrase and Fable,* "The coon (racoon) being hunted for its fur is a 'gone coon' when it has no escape from its pursuers."

62 Sir Andrew Clarke (1824-1902), engineer, soldier, politician and civil servant; governor of the Straits Settlements 1873-75, where he negotiated the treaty that brought British political control to the peninsular Malay states; minister of public works in India 1875-80.

I enclose a "short instruction," as you desire. But two of the points in the original draft, viz., those relating to the training of officers of health and to the training of cadets of engineers in sanitary principles, are omitted. But, if you think you can carry them, do pray put them into the draft. . . .

*Heads of Instructions.* You will prepare draft plans of barracks, hospitals, married quarters, and other buildings for the accommodation of troops, having special reference, in their sanitary arrangements, to the climates of India.

You will further state generally the principles you would recommend to be kept in view in improving existing barracks and hospitals, in conformity with the sanitary experience obtained in this country, but also having reference to the necessities of Indian climates. You will take into consideration all plans and proposals which may be referred to you for examination, relative to sanitary improvements in India, including the improvement of existing and the construction of new barracks, hospitals and other buildings to be occupied by troops, with a view to the introduction of the most efficient recent improvements. [not in FN's hand] And you will report generally upon any sanitary questions concerning India which the secretary of state for India may refer to you.

7 November 1863

*Private.* I enclose a letter of Sir C. Trevelyan's, which please return to me. It was the enclosure of a great many papers, which Lord Stanley has not yet thought fit to return to me. But the main point of them was the question of the Calcutta municipality, which exists, which is helpless, which is in agonies about its "maidan," which has sent its "Mr Clarke" for information to England. And you are powerless to treat with the question, although the very case has arisen. Has this "Mr Clarke" made any reference to you?

Lord Stanley is coming to me this week, in order to have an interview with Sir C. Wood afterwards about our *Instructions.* Are they out? Please put me *au fait.* As I have urged and baited Lord Stanley to come up to London, I want to know exactly how we stand. I have a vast quantity of other papers from Sir C. Trevelyan about our commission (to the amount of eight- and two-pence per mail). But I am almost afraid of sending them to you, without my answers, at least.

Source: From two letters to Sir Charles Trevelyan, Newcastle University Library 35/31-32 and 34

2 November 1863

*Private.* Since I wrote to you last, matters have somewhat altered their aspect here. Sir C. Wood has definitely declined to grant the instructions to the home (India sanitary) commission which we asked for. And when I see his despatch of 15 August, which he did not communicate to Lord de Grey till more than two months afterwards, I cannot wonder that he does so. In fact, it would be stultifying himself to do so. I have already told you how the home (India sanitary) commission is constituted, viz., by adding two India members on to the W.O. Barrack and Hospital Improvement Commission.

Now, from this despatch, it appears that the only use which the home India government proposes to make of the experience collected by this commission is to ask them to criticize plans of barracks prepared in India. But this is by no means the only duty (and there are others of far more importance than this) of the home commission. The very papers which you were so good as to send me show this. Calcutta has a municipal council. But, in the case of the maidan (a stronger case than anything we have put in our report) they don't know how to begin. They are sending their officer home to learn. Of whom is he to learn? Would not the wisest thing be to put him into relation with the home commission? *The very case has arisen.* And yet the people at home have no power whatever to deal with it. First among the home commission's duties should be to draw up a scheme for carrying out the recommendations of the royal commission, i.e., the laying down of principles in regard to details of sanitary works for India, of which, vide Calcutta municipality, nothing is known in India at present. The home commission has all the experience necessary to draw up such a statement as would keep such authorities in the right groove and prevent their beginning on wrong principles, which they may afterwards decline to change.

Besides this, sketch plans of barracks and hospitals should be prepared here to bring before the Indian engineers the most recent improvements in construction which would not be otherwise arrived at, except by wasting the time and correspondence required for criticizing plans sent home from India.

At present, according to the despatch of 15 August, everything must begin in India. What we proposed was that, before they begin in India, they should have the home experience in black and white, with plans, drawings, etc., before them, then that they should apply them and send their proposals home for examination. If you could (and would) induce the authorities with you to apply for information as to the best methods of conducting sanitary works and building barracks and hospitals, the thing would be done. And if it were done from India, it is probable that Sir C. Wood would apply to the (joint) home commission to give the requisite information.

9 November 1863

*Private.* It may be useful if I repeat the principles of the royal commission as regards the administration:

1. That each presidency shall have its own independent administrative commission, not interfered with in any way by the home commission. This is absolutely necessary for freedom of action in India and also for direct responsibility there.

2. If you in India prefer Dr McClelland's plan of constituting your commissions of *ex officio* members and you can have really efficient men, that is your affair. And we at home can only rejoice.

3. *You* will know whether deliberative boards work in India. We understood *not,* and considered that the president of the board should be the responsible executive authority (or minister of health) and the other members consultative. We considered that inspecting officers, sanitary and engineering, might be placed under each presidency commission to do the inspecting work in each presidency.

4. Further than this, we could not go. For the whole stational administration must, of course, be organized in India, with reference to local circumstances and local knowledge.

5. It would be very important, however, to bear the following points in mind as regards stations. You have two classes of defects to deal with: (a) conservancy defects (what in England are called "nuisances") capable of removal without the execution of works, (b) local causes of unhealthiness, such as bad drainage, bad water, bad construction, bad barracks to be improved, bad bazaars or native towns to be improved or eventually rebuilt, new barracks and hospitals to be constructed. In arranging your central and stational administrative authorities, you will have to provide for all these things. But you in India can alone do it. You will make a fatal mistake, however, if you think to lower the death rate in the army solely by improved conservancy. The reports clearly show what the removal of nuisances can do and can*not* do.

6. Next, as regards the home commission. It never was intended, as Dr McClelland appears to consider, that the home commission should come out to India. The home commission has one function only and

that is to put at the disposal of the presidency commissions the experience in sanitary works and methods which they have accumulated from every station of the British Army, simply with a view of aiding, by their advice and experience, the presidency commissions until they are able to pursue their own course. If this were not done, these would have all their experience to gain and that too at the expense of the soldier's health.

The home commission will send out information, sketches of improvements in sanitary appliances of various kinds. They will look at and give their best advice on any plans and proposals that may be submitted to them from India. But this is all. The responsibility of accepting or rejecting must rest with India and all communications should take place through the India government.

As you state, the great difficulty will be with ignorance and apathy. We shall cure the ignorance, in time, by our present education and examination in sanitary science and hygiene at the Army Medical School. Every officer that enters the service and every medical officer, civil and military, intended for Indian service, must pass through this course. It would be a good addition to teach hygiene in India, as proposed by McClelland. Whether you constitute your local commissions of *ex officio* members or not, it is matter of paramount importance that the sanitary improvement of Indian stations or towns shall be their special work, not entered upon as a *pis aller* [last resort] or as an addition to other employments, but as an office hardly second to any in India. The difficulty of combining *ex officio* employments with this absolute necessity is very great, but possibly might be overcome by having most of the work *not sanitary* done by the members at present, carried out by assistants, as soon as the *ex officio* men are appointed on the commissions. This might not be possible, in which case the *ex officio* membership will have to be given up. In any case the president (the responsible health minister of the presidency) must have no other duty. To show the importance of this, the War Office commission at home had, during the first years of its existence, to confine its work to barrack improvement.

Source: From notes for Lord Stanley, Add Mss 45781 ff101-04

[November 1863]

Course of proceeding recommended by your royal commission for carrying out the sanitary improvement of Indian stations and towns:

1. To vest the executive in a local authority, or commission of health, for each presidency;

2. To give to these Indian authorities the advantage of home experience in the details of sanitary improvement, leaving to the Indian authorities the sole responsibility of accepting or rejecting any information or advice sent to them;

3. As a commission already existed at the War Office, *advising* not only at home but at all foreign stations, e.g., Ceylon, close to India itself, the royal commission proposed, if the secretary of state for India did not appoint a special commission, that Indian members should be added to the War Office commission, and that the joint commission should advise and transmit information to the India authorities. This was done. . . .

According to present understanding, the connection between the presidency commissions and the home commission would be:

1. The War Office had been already asked to prepare model plans of barracks and hospitals—these are now considerably advanced. (These plans, when completed, will be sent to the India Office and, if sanctioned, transmitted to India.)

2. The presidency commissions are to send home to the secretary of state for India any plans or proposals of their own which, before being sanctioned, will be sent to the home commission for advice and information.

Besides this, however, which is good so far as it goes, the home commission should help the presidency commissions by a direct statement and description of the kind of sanitary works, improvements, etc., applicable to Indian stations, as described in the stational reports. If the home commission were authorized to draw up such a statement, it would clear away at once most of the presumed difficulty in applying improved sanitary methods to India.

**Editor:** The Barrack and Hospital Improvement Commission's function was to look after the state of the military stations, their barracks and hospitals. Even before being renamed the Army Sanitary Commission in 1865, the commission became increasingly concerned with Indian nationals, above all those living in the vicinity of military stations. Eventually the A.S.C. worked in concert with the presidencies' sanitary commissions, promoting military well-being and public health in India, and ascertaining that sanitary reforms were in fact taking place. Most proposals mentioned in the following correspondence ended up being included in the *Suggestions* of 1864 (above) when their final version was completed and sent to India.

Source: From six letters to Douglas Galton, Add Mss 45761 ff245, 246-55, 260-69

21 December 1863

I was rather in hopes that the India barrack and hospital plans [requested by John Lawrence] would have been sent up here on Saturday. It is of great importance that these should be transmitted to India as soon as possible.

We have written as much as we can without the plans to write from. And we cannot now proceed, until we have the plans.

24 December 1863

We send back the barrack plans with a criticism. Pray go on with them. We have kept the bungalows and also the hospital plan, which shall be returned with a criticism in a day or two. We will send you a list of the outbuildings for stations. . . .

We want, first, a good hospital ward for twenty-four beds, or rather two wards, showing 1500 cub. ft. and 2000 cub. ft. per bed respectively.

1. One plan to show 100 sq. ft., the other 120 or 130 sq. ft. per bed.

2. Instead of a window for every two beds, there should be a window for every bed, and a bed in each corner.

3. In arranging the ward offices, the ends of the wards as well as the sides must be left quite free, except that the sergeant's room must overlap the ward just sufficiently to have a window into the ward.

4. The scullery must correspond with the sergeant's room on the opposite side of the ward door.

5. The water closet is to be placed in a detached pavilion at the opposite end of the ward.

6. Ablution and bath accommodation to correspond with W.C. Space will be required for a slipper bath.

7. Hospital block to be on two floors, with a basement 4 ft. high below.

8. Verandahs 10 ft. wide.

9. Ventilating arrangements the same; window and door construction the same as for barrack blocks, except that the windows and doors may be modified in width to suit the arrangement of the beds.

*Indian Barracks*

1. The plans are very good and meet the requirements of the royal commission. Small louvred dormers about 12 ft. apart will effect this, similar to Kowloon barracks. But the upper verandahs must be ventilated. Otherwise there will be intensely hot air passing into the barrack rooms. There is a very important question regarding these lower floors which has reference to the general arrangement of the station

[rather] than to the construction of the barrack room. For example, under two barrack rooms to hold forty-eight men at 1500 cub. ft. per man, there are two spacious rooms, each 100 ft. long by 24 ft. wide. It is evident that forty-eight men would never require, even in India, such an amount of day accommodation as this.

Four such rooms would possibly be sufficient for the wants of the entire station. But at the very stations where these two floor blocks are required, the men not only in these blocks but in all the blocks should sleep at least ten or twelve feet above the level of the ground. How would it answer to provide for an entire regiment two blocks with the day rooms and coffee rooms on the ground floor? and to raise all the rest of the blocks on arches? Could some of these arches be fitted up as workshops, the floors being a little raised above the ground? Or they might be used for stores. But on the other hand this would leave all these blocks without day accommodation. And one of our principles is certainly that men should not live and sleep in the same room in India.

The India "standard plans" provide for this thus: they have what they call inner verandahs, extending alongside the barrack rooms and these verandahs are used for day and dining rooms, an arrangement which the royal commission has condemned by abolishing the inner verandah altogether. A day room, half the length of the barrack room, would be enough for sitting and dining in.

Could use be found for all the rest of the first-floor accommodation for stores and workshops?

2. In healthy situations, it would not be necessary to have an under floor. A basement from four to six feet high would be amply sufficient for health. In this case, the day room might be added on at the end of the barrack room.

3. It is said that every barrack room in the Punjab has a reading room and workshops at the ends. In our plans, these might be placed below, as already stated. The amount of room is more than required, which is the only objection.

The plans as a whole are VERY good. There are only a few points in which we think a little more consideration might be well—from information we have received.

1. In the War Office plan the ablution rooms are placed in a detached block at the end of the barrack room. This construction is entirely new in the Indian barracks. All the plans show arrangements of one or two classes: (a) these rooms are either made to fill up two corners

of the verandah . . . leaving the end of the room exposed to the air; or (b) the rooms are made to overlap. . . . Any of the arrangements, either W.O. or Indian, would answer. But the Indian ones have the advantage of leaving the end of the barrack room free from obstruction. Were either A or B adopted, a different arrangement of the staircases would be necessary. The question is more one of construction than of health. And we could quite well suggest the Indian arrangements in the description, leaving the War Office plans unaltered, as an alternative.

2. The allowance of basins and foot pans is too small for India. A daily foot washing is necessary. Let them have four basins with the same linear frontage as at present, and three foot pans at the least. The three might be put along the side wall.

3. We propose two methods of supplying water to the ablution rooms: either directly from a central raised water tank, or from a tank placed over the ablution room. Would it be necessary to show this tank in a section?

4. India is a long way ahead of *plank* barrack doors. She has long ago introduced paneling. Show the doors paneled.

5. Three doors are shown at the end of one of the rooms in elevation and only one door in plan. There should be only one door.

6. Ventilate the upper verandah to allow the hot air to escape. The verandah should be in two layers; the space between the layers is what should be ventilated thus.

Two objects will be served: (1) the solar radiation will be cut off; (2) conducted heat will be diminished by the air current.

7. In the double plan, put a window in the recess in front of the two N.C. officers' rooms, to admit light and air to the end of each barrack room.

8. It must be kept in view that the chief thing now required consists of intelligible plans and sections of the sanitary details. It will not be necessary to proceed farther with the twelve-men room plan. . . . Plans and sections are required to show rooms with 1000 and with 1500 cub. ft. both on the single barrack room model and on the double barrack room model. A double barrack room model with 1000 cub. ft. per man, raised on an arched basement, say 4 ft. high, should be prepared, as an illustration of what is wanted for hill stations. Such a barrack room should show a fireplace.

P.S. to Indian barrack plans. Two Indian medical officers of great experience were consulted on a question of a night W.C. for each barrack room, to provide against sudden illness. One advised it strongly. But today the other considers that, with "a covered way to the latrines," the W.C. would be unnecessary. We therefore decide *against* the W.C. because the necessity is not satisfactorily proved, and because it is advisable, unless there be necessity, to restrict this class of appliances as much as possible.

26 December 1863

Before a letter can be drafted for India Office, some points will have to be cleared up. Following the numbers in the paper [see letter of 21 August 1863 above]:

2. Suppressing issue of spirits on board ship. You will find in the Queen's Regulations, 1859, pp 338, 360, that it is taken for granted that spirits are to be issued with the ration. The regulation concluded thus: "The officer of the day is invariably to attend to see the spirit mixed (with water) in the proportion above specified and issued to the troops." Spirit is thus provided with the ration by the transport service (?). And the queen's officer superintends the issue. Now the report of the royal commission states that recently an issue of malt liquor has been made. And what we require is that malt liquor be issued with the ration instead of spirit, and *that the Queen's Regulation be altered* to permit the issue of spirit *only on the recommendation of the medical officer.*

Next, as to issuing vegetables on the passage out: it is one of the duties of every medical officer in charge of troops to represent what changes are required in the diet. On board ship this power is at present useless, because the means of effecting the required alterations do not exist. The transport service (?) should be requested to supply vegetables and farinaceous substances. And the director general should instruct the medical officer in charge of ships to attend to this. Here again there are two concurrent authorities.

3. Sale of spirits in canteens. The question involved in this is whether the Queen's Regulations are binding on commanding officers in India. The preliminary letter of the commander-in-chief (1 July 1857) states that they are to be obeyed strictly throughout the army and that every officer is responsible for their being observed.

Now the canteen regulations take it for granted that spirits are to be sold in canteens. And you will find in Vol. 2 of the royal commission sanitary report for India specimens of regimental regulations. We know that some regiments permit an issue of two drams spirits per day, others of only one dram. What we want is that the Queen's Regulations should enable commanding officers so to regulate canteens in India that spirits shall be issued to men *only on the recommendation of the medical officer.*

But, to enable this to be done, the India government must provide more beer. And the regimental regulation should state that spirits are to be issued *only on such special recommendation.* Here again there are two collateral jurisdictions.

4. Preventing sale of spirits in regimental bazaars. Here again the Queen's Regulations positively prohibit the introduction of spirits within the barrack boundary except in canteens. In India the station boundary corresponds to the barrack boundary. And, unless the Queen's Regulations are a dead letter there, the commanding officer could suppress the sale in bazaars.

5. Flannel underclothing and better boots—reform in this matter will depend upon whom it is who supplies the boots (?).

6. Trained hospital cooks. Doubtless the India hospital cooks, *such as they are,* are provided at present by the India government. You at home are training hospital cooks for the purveyor. The question is, where these cooks should be trained for the India Army (?). The India government will never train trained cooks.

7. Introducing gymnastics as a parade. Is not this part of the internal work of a regiment and, as such, under the officer commanding? Or must he be ordered to do it by the commander-in-chief in India? That is the whole point at issue.

8. Trades, gardens, etc. The same remarks apply. (When her majesty issues regulations, one would think they were binding upon her army, wherever it is. Or do not Queen's Regulations find in India?)

10. Applying new medical regulations to India you say (on the margin) "India government." I understood Lord de Grey to say that the non-amalgamation, having been carried, paved the way to the War Office applying those new medical regulations.

11. Passing invalids immediately for England. So far as this may depend on the India government, it should be represented to them. But delay has been *most* frequently caused by medical boards at Calcutta, Madras and Bombay; if these boards are in future to belong to the queen's service, the question is, who can either abolish them as unnecessary, or expedite their proceedings? Query, the director general? (The first would be the best.)

12. Surely it does not "depend" on "*India government*" that each regiment shall take its hospital sergeant and orderlies. This is a purely

regimental matter, is it not? But it may be necessary that the India government shall make the requisite changes in their hospital system to admit of this (?).

14. More vegetables in the ration. The matériel for this must of course be provided by India government through India commissariat. But the proportions and general arrangements of ration will depend upon queen's medical officer.

26 December 1863

*Confidential.* I understood Lord de Grey [to say] that the draft (of the proposed letter) was to come to us for our revisal. We are so ignorant of the technical method of dealing (of the W.O.) with the I.O. and I am quite sure Sir John Lawrence is so too, and I believe that H.R.H. the commander-in-chief (though what I know of it I must not divulge) is so too, that it appears to me much better that *we* should revise *your* draft, as Lord de Grey said, than that *we* should write the draft. (What the commander-in-chief said to Sir John Lawrence is widely different from what Lord de Grey said to me. But this is *really* confidential.)

Anyhow you will see that, till the enclosed questions are answered, we cannot write your draft, because we do not know your technical matters.

28 December 1863

We agree with you in thinking that the hospital draft is not good. There is a difficulty in deciding at once on an Indian hospital construction. The hospital should consist of detached wards, arranged for the greatest convenience of administration, which is hard to arrive at. We propose, first, to get a good ward. And the enclosed notes show the points required. Afterwards, let us arrange the block plan.

With regard to barrack ablution accommodation, we think your plan of detached towers at corners unexceptionable. But, for barracks, *any* way that you could arrange to keep the ends open would answer. For hospitals, your plan is by far the best. There is no objection to placing cisterns over ablution rooms. They can always be covered. For urinals, perhaps the best way would be to provide a compartment for a vessel. And we could point out in the description the different forms of improved water urinals, if they choose to adopt them.

2. The lower floors of barrack rooms may be safely used for dining, day and reading rooms, orderly rooms, sergeants' quarters, stores, offices of various kinds, sergeants' mess, schoolrooms, schoolmaster's quarters. These will occupy, it is supposed, two thirds of the whole

space under barrack rooms. And the remaining third must be left to take care of itself. It is what must be paid for the advantage of upper floors. The disposal of all this first-floor space might be left to Indian officials.

In hospitals, the first floors would be used as day and dining rooms, surgery, waiting room, surgeon's room, orderlies' quarters, stores, sergeants' (?) quarters, etc.

[December 1863]

My letters to you are much too improper to be "opened" at the W.O., specially my views about the non-conjugal duties of superintendents and about "Dick" being an ass. But I have never once sent a letter to the W.O. for you without being marked "Private" on the cover, nor (except two big ones which went the same day) without "to be forwarded" or "immediate" on the cover. Do they strip off the covers naked in sending them to you? a process I very particularly object to.

Source: From an unsigned draft letter to unnamed recipient [Lord de Grey?] in Dr Sutherland's hand, Add Mss 45798 ff210-11

[c1863]

1. Has not the time arrived for improving the entire management of the army in India, and bringing it into conformity with advancing intelligence everywhere? So far as concerns the military part this change would involve improved means of occupation, that is, commanding officers seeing more to better general employment of the men; soldiers, institutes, gymnastics, government providing the means such as covered sheds, workshops, gardens, tools, apparatus, buildings; better regulation of canteens as regards issue of spirits and better police of bazaars to prevent sale of spirits.

Next the question of increased marriages and better provisions for soldiers' wives and children.

2. Should not the question be finally settled as to the points to be held in India? Which unhealthy stations could be given up, which are the best hill stations and the best way of using them.

3. Improvements in the ration with reference to vegetable food.

4. Better management of drills. Then as regards general sanitary improvements in stations, drainage, water supply, better barracks and hospitals. On all these points we at home will gladly help with our experience.

But, allied to this, the great thing in India is to improve the social condition of the people. The stational returns show a lamentable state of matters. Can this not be dealt with? Surely under British rule we should try to improve the habits of the people and to raise them in the scale of civilization by laying a basis for this in improving their towns and dwellings. Better water supply is everywhere imperative, and this cannot be got without drainage. Everything must go hand in hand.

5. It is absolutely necessary to make this great work somebody's duty. The presidency commissions should do this. Should not these be appointed at once and instituted to proceed with this work? India has to be educated and Christianized, but we know in this country that education and bad sanitary conditions are antagonistic.

The whole secret of progress is in improving physically, intellectually, morally and Christianly at the same time. This lesson is the last to be learned. We shall succeed in civilizing just in proportion as we recognize the unity of the whole process. Government in India is everything as regards physical progress. It can also educate. It should do both.

Source: From a letter to Robert Rawlinson, Boston University 1/3/38

9 January 1864

I think it better to answer your note at once. What you contemplate doing and what we are authorized to do for India are two, alas! totally different things. The Barrack and Hospital Improvement Commission have no authority whatever to enter into minute details of drainage works in any suggestions to be sent to India. I believe that, even if they were asked, they would refuse to do so. The work required of them by their Instructions is of two kinds:

1. To send general suggestions, merely to prevent the local authorities from going into a wrong groove at first. This is the only object of the paper sent to you.

2. To take into consideration and report on all plans for sanitary improvements, including sewerage, which may be sent to the commission by the India Office. For these plans, minute information, such as you contemplate, will be required. And if it does not accompany the plans, of course the commission will ask for it.

We have information so minute as to the most important stations that we could almost do without any farther information. But still such farther information, if you are not satisfied, can of course be asked for. All that is required of us now therefore is just to state the general principles of the subject.

The woodcuts and general descriptive matter applicable to all kinds of sewers and drains, such as that contained in the pamphlet you have been so good as to send me, will be very useful; and to the extent to which you approve, should be introduced. They are the very things wanted.

Pray let me thank you very much for your Bombay sewerage correspondence and for Messrs Fulton and Williams.

Source: From nine letters to Douglas Galton, ADD Mss 45762 ff3, 8-9, 10-11, 12, 15-18, 19-20, 21-23, 33-35 and 36-38

10 January 1864

As I have not heard from your holiness about the letter to be drafted for the India Office, with regard to the recommendations of the royal commission (vide Sir J. Lawrence and Lord de Grey), can your infallibility tell me what is to be done, in order that it may be drafted into a bull? I have got a copy of the Bombay drainage correspondence from the India Office, so that I need not trouble you to get me one. Dr Sutherland says you do not think it good. It is six months on last Friday since the India Army sanitary report came out. The progress made has not been alarming in carrying out its recommendations. Indeed, had it not been for Sir J. Lawrence, it might have been described as *nil.*

23 January 1864

I have had the reading of a correspondence about victualling troops on board ship going to the East, which you should take up and deal with. It is a War Office paper. . . . It contains a proposal for a new diet scale by Surgeon Major Docker. This paper shows that the old scale (still in use) is abominable. Docker's plan is much better. But if you will send me a copy of the paper I will write upon it more in detail. The whole of the correspondence is curious, not the least so because the India Office think the bad system in use the best possible.

Where is our draft to the India Office on the recommendations of the royal commission (sanitary)?

[January 1864]

*Confidential. Burn. In re letter to India Office.* As soon as you have seen your way as to the best course to pursue, I need not say that we will help in any way you think fit. I never had so strong an impression in all my life as that "borne in" upon me (in evangelical parlance) during my conversation with Lord de Grey on Sunday, viz., that *he* had never considered the subject as to the respective jurisdictions (although having administered in both offices), that *they* had never considered the subject of the respective jurisdictions, that the sooner the subject was considered the better—and settled the better—that at present the jurisdictions of India Office, War Office, Horse Guards, commander-in-chief in India, governor general, are as much chaos as if India were the Sandwich Islands.

But I have communicated with at least three administrators in the last three weeks to whom the idea appeared to have occurred for the first time, viz., that these respective jurisdictions ought to be settled, and were *not* settled.

But pray believe that you are the only person to whom I have made this mutinous reflection. Pray burn.

26 January 1864

I conclude that you have not been able to lay your hands yet on the War Office paper containing Surgeon Docker's correspondence on the victualling of troops on board ship. This is a necessary item of information—could you send it us before the letter to the India Office can be drafted?

28 January 1864

*As to the victualling papers.* These ration papers show that the time is almost past to do any great good (since August 1861) unless through the secretary of state himself.

Surgeon Docker's plans are certainly much better than those proposed by the committee. But even his plans of diet can be improved. The committee's plans are all based on the old naval *possibilities*, i.e., with a certain amount of storage and a certain time at sea, how to keep the largest number of men from absolute starvation. But since the British Admiralty propounded and answered this question in their own rough way, and a number of sailors died not of starvation but of scurvy (confound the Admiralty!), the whole question of diet and possibilities has undergone a great change.

The physiological side of it is shown by Surgeon Docker, not by the committee. The committee's plan would do for a voyage to Canada, Surgeon Docker's for voyages within the tropics. The whole principle of dieting is very simple in either case. For Canada heat-generating materials are wanted, for the tropics not. All that is wanted with soldiers is to supply daily wear and tear, exclusive of work. Sailors work hard and can live on a diet in the tropics injurious to idle soldiers or sailors. The point to be kept in view in the Indian troop ships is to have your men (comparatively idle) in the best state of health to encounter the climate and service of India. This is a very plain problem in physiology. We cannot pasture sheep or grow vegetables at sea, but we can preserve meat and vegetables sufficient. Roughly speaking, a POSSIBLE sea diet should consist of fresh preserved meat every alternate day with salt beef, except one salt pork day, compressed vegetables or potatoes every day, the former on all the salt meat days, a proportion of fresh bread, a proportion of biscuit, tea, coffee, sugar, rice (an exceedingly valuable article), flour for puddings, etc., porter or bitter ale (no spirit on any account except under medical advice: the India commission distinctly recommend this contrary to your committee's opinion). Lime juice should never be required nowadays. It is an old expedient to neutralize an alkaline state of the blood arising from defect of acid-generating elements in the food. And in advising it your committee has condemned its own scheme.

We will help in any way we can. But in the meantime, between two proposed plans, we go for Surgeon Docker's, with the addition of some fresh bread.

To give you trouble in preparing a minute for Lord de Grey, we enclose a draft. It is a matter of extreme importance and, if Lord de Grey would take it up and put it forward, might be settled for centuries to come.

29 January 1864

As to your having "written to General Pears," "given Lord de Grey his reply which came to little": this was done to ascertain how the various administrative questions coming out of the royal commission Indian report were to be raised and who were the persons responsible. As you have an answer, although it comes "to little," we should like very much to see it, before steps are taken upon it.

As to victualling of troops on board ship, one of the highest Indian authorities says that, if the diet scheme of your committee is carried out, one half of the troops will be landed in India with the scorbutic taint, which will declare itself afterwards (inexperienced medical officers not recognizing it as scurvy, as also they did not in the Crimea) in dysentery.

29 January 1864

I cannot tell you how I was shocked by your victualling troops papers. That a committee chosen by those two great bodies, the Admiralty and the War Office, should advocate such practices is monstrous. Monstrous for the ignorance it shows. A book is coming out immediately by a great authority, in which it is said that if "spirits out of pandemonium had set to work to devise a scheme which would destroy *most* men, they could not have succeeded better than the Admiralty did." As to your committee's scheme, I wrote to you (at the War Office) that the most enlightened Indians, not Docker, say that half the men will be landed in India with the scorbutic taint by its means, although it, the scurvy, will not be recognized by the doctors. To this last fact I can add my own personal testimony, that the doctors in the Crimean War left the fact of the scorbutic taint to be discovered by—me!! And this, after half the army were dead of it. It shows itself in dysentery. I deeply regret that we did not bring this question prominently before the India sanitary commission. Had I but seen these papers then, I would. *You must* look to this.

9 February 1864

With reference to the diet on board ship, Lord de Grey's proposal to ask the opinion of the Barrack and Hospital Improvement Commission is perhaps on the whole the best course:

1. Because they have a number of cognate questions before them, such, e.g., as the supply of drinking water (and there are manuscripts in both), cooking apparatus and cooking of ration materials. There is besides a large amount of evidence on the question of ration in the India sanitary report. And as the whole proceedings of the committee on rationing are anterior to the report of said royal commission (except some of the latest correspondence) it will be quite competent to ask the opinion of Barrack and Hospital Improvement Commission on the general principles on which troops should be rationed on board ship, so as to land them in India well and not sick.

All you will have to do will be to address a letter to the chairman of the Barrack and Hospital Improvement Commission to ask them whether they would be so good as "state for the information of the secretary of state for war what, in their opinion, ought to be the general principles on which troops should be rationed at sea during the voyage to India so as to land them in the best health."

2. Another reason for this is that it is stated in a report from Karachi that 10 percent of the troops landed there are ill with the evident disease scurvy, irrespective of those, probably six times the number, in whom the scorbutic taint is latent and only shows itself afterwards under Indian disadvantages.

13 February 1864

It would be infinitely better to fix a ration for the troops at Hong Kong—at least to lay down the principles on which they should be rationed—than to trust to the varying opinion of medical men and commanding officers. The Indian scale is a more healthy one than Dr Home's. And the only objection raised against it by the director general is that it contains ¼ lb. too little meat. But if the soldier wants more, he might be allowed to purchase and so to dispose of part of his surplus pay. For these climates a lb. fresh meat and a lb. vegetables should be your basis. Also, a lb. of bread. And then build on it due proportions of rice, sugar, tea, coffee, etc. Beer (but no spirit except on medical certificate) should be issued at the canteen. I fear your draft letter, without some addition, will lead to constant changes in the ration to suit the views of successive officers, although the principle on which the men should be dieted is really not susceptible of change. It is a fixed one. You might add to your letter either [of] the fundamental points mentioned. Or you might refer the Indian scale to the "board" (as well as Dr Home's) and ask whether it, the Indian scale, could not be adopted.

But I suppose you must make this a separate communication, as you have shut the stable door after the steed has been stolen. I hope you will not refer the dieting of troops on board ship going to India to the Barrack and Hospital Improvement Commission, *after* a decision has been come to.

Source: From a letter to James Pattison Walker, Boston University 2/2/3

10 March 1864

*Private.* I rejoice to hear of your appointment as secretary to the first board of health [Bengal Sanitary Commission] India has ever had. It shows the governor general's wisdom. You may now do more good than falls to the lot of any medical officer, otherwise employed. We will send you out all the reports and books, which we think may be useful to your board. . . .

The Barrack and Hospital Improvement Commission, to which are now added two India members, are engaged with model barrack plans for India, now nearly completed, also a paper of *Suggestions* on the whole Indian subject, which will be useful. All these will be sent out as soon as possible. . . .

If at any time I can send you out any sanitary papers from here, pray command me. I consider the sanitary "mission" in India at this moment perhaps the greatest "mission" in the world. And I envy you.

Source: From a letter to Charles Hathaway, Florence Nightingale Museum, typed copy Add Mss 45782 ff135-38

10 March 1864

*Private.* The appointments [on the Bengal sanitary commission] are excellent and show the governor general's wisdom—at least to three of them I can speak from my knowledge of the men's works.

There is no manual in existence such as you desire. But the moment I received your welcome letter, I wrote to the Local Government Act Office and to the War Office to send out (for your commissions) copies of all their sanitary reports.

The barrack and hospital plans we are preparing for you are nearly complete, and also a printed paper of "Suggestions" on all the subjects which have arisen out of the Indian inquiry and which I hope will meet what Sir John Lawrence wants. This is in the press, and as soon as a complete copy is printed, it will be laid before the Barrack and Hospital Improvement Commission, which has been reconstituted here with two India members, as you are aware. . . .

I am very sorry that our part of the work was not ready as soon as your presidency commission was ready. But the fact is, we should never have got a start at all if Sir John Lawrence had not given us one before he left England. Even since that we have been hopelessly floundering between the vague and confused jurisdictions of War Office, India Office, Horse Guards at home, commander-in-chief in India. Now about such a matter as this, the victualling of troops on board ship going out to India, it seems for the first time to have struck them that it might be better if each office knew what it had to do. Sir John Lawrence acts and does not wait. But these people wait and do not act.

But as I can say, Sir John Lawrence himself can hardly tell what an impulse his appointment has given us—the first we have had since my dear master, Sidney Herbert, died. And I could not explain it without a much longer letter than I can write or you would read.

Of course you will consider this, and any letter I may in future trouble you with, as strictly between yourself and me, and him, if you choose it. You cannot tell what his appointment, his work, his and your news are to me. This is worth living for. I envy you your work.

Source: From two letters to James Pattison Walker, Florence Nightingale Museum (LMA) H1/ST/NC1/64/7 and 8 (copy of first letter ADD Mss 45781 ff219-21) (complete first letter in *Society and Politics* 5:318-20)

3 June 1864

I thank you much for your kind letter of 23 April and its most interesting account of the proceedings of the [Bengal] commission. It is doing its work vigorously and will be a blessing to India. . . .

With regard to the very important question of disposing of the dead, would not the best plan be to confer with the different castes and ascertain what really constitutes religious burial. (This is what even the old Indians [former British administrators in India, now in London] at the India Office here seem not exactly to know.) Then the whole question would resolve itself into the best practicable and most wholesome method of doing the work.

If cremation were adopted, suppose your commission were to send a minute home, desiring that the War and India Office commission here (Barrack and Hospital Improvement Commission) should send them out the best plans of apparatus from this country, where the process has been applied to almost every purpose, except burning dead bodies (and even that has been considered).

I was delighted to see Mr Strachey's minute (5 April), which was sent by the India Office to the Barrack and Hospital Commission in a letter of 20 May, desiring them to send out plans, etc., of sanitary construction to you—because we are so slow (they talk of Hindus being slow, but War Office and India Office in England are slower). These plans are however nearly ready [the famous *Suggestions*]. And they will be sent out almost immediately with general suggestions.

I wish you Godspeed with all my heart. You will have much opposition to encounter. But great works do not prosper without opposition. (Do you remember what, by a curious coincidence, Pope Paul III[63] said to a predecessor of yours in the missionary work in India, St Francis Xavier,[64] viz., that God would always find means to carry out a work which was really God's; that indeed he, Xavier, would find much to suffer, but that the "affairs of God" succeed only by the way of crosses and difficulties. I did not think Pope Paul could have said so good a thing. And I suppose Xavier was half a madman. But, for all

63 Pope Paul III (1468-1549), pope from 1534, was in favour of the creation of new religious orders such as the Jesuits.

64 Francis Xavier (1506-52), Jesuit, apostle to India and Japan.

that, I think it is true, is it not? for *every* work engaged in for the good of men.)

18 June 1864

*Private.* What occurred to me, with regard to your proceedings, is that it would be advisable to make them very short, unless for special reasons. If everything is put in at length, errors in principle, backed by high names, may have to be recorded. There is an example of this in your present minutes, where barrack rooms for large numbers are recommended by a general officer and medical officer, contrary to all sound principle. This is a very great mistake, and even the record of it might lead to mischief. All forget that these overgrown barrack rooms are very obvious causes of disease in India. (Dr McClelland's theory of barrack building shows throughout great lack of sanitary knowledge on such subjects.) It would be better to limit the record of matter of instruction either to the enunciation of sound principles and sound practice by the commission itself or to such principles as it adopted (stated in other's words).

Source: From a letter to Henry Staunton Ellis[65] [president of the Madras Sanitary Commission], Columbia University, Presbyterian Hospital School of Nursing C70

26 July 1864

Mr John Clark (the son of my old friend Sir James Clark) encouraged me to venture to communicate with you direct on the subject of the sanitary commission of which you are president. Otherwise I should be afraid you would wonder who your correspondent was.

I send you, by this mail, the first (signed) copy of *Suggestions* for sanitary works for Indian stations, drawn up in obedience to certain minutes, as you will see by the title page. It will be forwarded to you officially by the Indian Office here in the usual manner. But the roads are difficult and almost impassable, as perhaps you know, between Pall Mall and Victoria St. Her Majesty is much the quickest postman, although it is somewhat irregular of me to use the quick, instead of the slow, method.

65 This ought to be Robert S. Ellis.

Source: From a letter to Sir John McNeill, Florence Nightingale Museum (LMA) H1/ST/NC1/64/SU155, typed copy ADD Mss 45768 ff188-89

Hampstead, N.W.
4 August 1864

*Private.* I send you by this day's book post one of the first (signed) copies of the first offspring of the joint War Office and India Office commission, appointed to carry out the recommendations of the royal Indian Army sanitary commission. (7½ months it has taken them to sign it, while Sir J. Lawrence has been constantly writing home for it with his own hand.) It is expected that, in the course of the present century, the India Office will send it out to Sir John Lawrence officially. But in the meantime copies are speeding out to him direct from me by Her Majesty's book post.

Source: From three letters to Douglas Galton, ADD Mss 45762 ff168-69, 170-72 and 206 (all written from Hampstead, N.W.)

8 August 1864

*Medical Regulations for India.* We thought it better, i.e., safer, to keep these [regulations] and to ask you to ask the question (of director general) upon my note, which gave the requisite detail.

We are quite sure director general is perfectly unfit to write the general or regimental hospital regulations himself and therefore we thought, if he would report to you what are the alterations necessary for India (which why he can't do in this case, as in others, we don't know), *we* would make the alterations upon the existing ones.

I beg to inform you that I sent off by Her Majesty's book post (at an enormous!! expense, I have a good mind to charge it to you!!) to Sir John Lawrence direct no end of copies of *Suggestions*—also to the presidency commissions—by the first mail after signature. And that, as he is always more ready to hear than you are to pray, you sinners, I have not the least doubt that they will have been *put in execution* long before the India Office has even begun to send them him officially.

8 August 1864

*Private.* 1. The original proposal for supplying Indian regiments and civil stations with medical officers was that all candidates should enter by one door, be instructed at Netley and commissioned through the War Office, and then a power was required to enable men so commissioned to volunteer into the Indian staff [at] any period within the first five years. We agreed to this. But, in the meantime, that "precious" squabble with the Horse Guards cut off the supply of candidates. And Sir C. Wood, very properly considering that among them they were not fit to be trusted with the key of the door, asked for power to keep it himself. This was not granted, and now he proposes to act independently of the W.O. It is a very decided slap in the face.

2. He would no doubt get the power he requires to accept volunteers, if he gave up the key. But he does not see his way to getting them without. And now he proposes the only course open to him.

3. The present proposal is that Sir C. Wood shall issue an advertisement asking for candidates and that the preliminary examination shall be conducted—under whose supervision? The director general's? (Has he been at Sir C. Wood's about this?)

4. Your course is clear:

a. let Sir C. Wood advertise;

b. let the amended schedule for the Army Medical Service be the one issued (the schedule making the natural history examination voluntary);

c. let the candidates be examined by the same examining board which examines for the army, and state pointedly to Sir C. Wood that it has not been considered advisable on public grounds to give the director general any control over the examinations;

d. let the men selected by competitive examination be sent to Netley for a session like the others;

e. let their position on the list be decided at the conclusion of the session by the same examination which decides the position of the candidates for army medical commissions;

f. let promotion to the rank of surgeon take place after examination in the same manner as in the queen's service. . . .

This change is very much to be regretted because it introduces elements which will in time bring forth unwholesome fruit. But the emergency is urgent. And you are so long in getting out the amended warrant that it is difficult to see what else can be done. As a proof of the mischief that has been done, nearly the whole of the candidates for the next examination have applied to undergo *voluntarily* the natural history examination, which, as you are aware, was compulsory until the issue of the last schedule. This simple fact is enough to show the absurdity and untruthfulness of the D. and Horse Guards in stating that men are kept back by the examinations. You have lowered the standard *in consequence of a lie.* The result is sufficient to justify you in returning to the former schedule at the next examination.

17 September 1864

At the time the troops are to be sent out again, you must see to this: Inform the India Office that you agree to the *delay* as inevitable, but that Lord de Grey will look upon it only as a *delay* and looks forward to the change being introduced at the time stated, according to Sir C. Wood's letter. . . . Sir C. Wood *is* Pilate, you know, and would let anybody be crucified. Sir John Lawrence—he is leaving to be crucified every day.

Source: From a letter to Lord Stanley, Liverpool Record Office, Derby Collection 920/15/52

8 [18] August 1864

*Private.* In reply to your query, I knew Dr Duncan MacPherson, of the Madras Army, well in the Crimea. He was principal medical officer of our Turkish contingent there. He is one of the best (sanitary) officers in our service. He has large Indian experience. His was one of the best, if not *the* best, sanitary reports received by your (royal) commission, viz., one on the sanitary condition of Madras presidency generally—see 2nd Volume folio edition of your report.

Of course I do not know what his "grievance" is to you. He has made a "grievance" in not getting one of the presidency sanitary commission appointments—to us. The matter is after this wise: some of the members of your (royal) commission told him that he might "make his own terms" in getting one of these appointments. Now Sir John Lawrence did exactly what your royal commission told him to do: he made a civilian the head, the executive, the responsible member, well-paid and having nothing else to do; he constituted the sanitary engineering, medical and military elements as consultative members, and in order to give the sanitary member a position and an office, he made him secretary with a salary and nothing else to do. This last, of course, viz., who was to be the secretary and what was to be the salary, I did not presume to determine when Sir John Lawrence was good enough to talk the matter over with me, as I limited myself strictly to the recommendations of your royal commission.

(I mentioned more than once, to Sir John Lawrence and other members of his government, Dr D. MacPherson's name as an able sanitary man, in obedience to their request to name names.) Dr MacPherson is bitterly offended, because he has been offered the place of sanitary member and secretary (of the Madras Sanitary Commission) at the salary, he says, of an assistant surgeon, it having now been given "to an assistant surgeon who may be ordered away any day" because he was not offered the place of president, which has been given to Mr R.S. Ellis, "who knows nothing about it," "a civilian"! and some of the members of your royal commission, he says, promised it him. (It is really rather hard that any member of a commission should abuse poor Sir John Lawrence for doing exactly what the commission recommended.)

Dr MacPherson is one of the most active, energetic men I ever knew. He has practical means and practical knowledge to carry out his sanitary views, such as not one man in a hundred in the army medical profession has. He would be an immense loss to us. (Long after he had left Kertch, where our Turkish contingent was, the fruits of his sanitary work were evident and he found time, after putting all his camps and hospitals in the best possible—sanitary—order, to dig up antiquities and write a book about them.[66])

The Madras government have behaved very ill to him. And I am afraid we shall lose one of our best tools. If the "assistant surgeon" could be "ordered away" on duty and Dr MacPherson given the sanitary member's and secretary's post at a salary *according to his rank*, he would make the best sanitary advisor in India. And there is not a man who knows the Madras presidency so well.

If, as is said, the India Office at home mean to have an officer like Sir Ranald Martin, but to give them his whole time (Sir R. Martin, who has a large practice, to resign), Dr MacPherson would be the man for the place. But undoubtedly Madras presidency wants him most. . . .

Dr MacPherson being a man of high medical rank, it does not appear as if it would be invidious to give him a higher salary as secretary than the other "presidency sanitary commission" secretaries. N.B. He went out by the same mail with Sir John Lawrence. And I mentioned him to Sir John, who asked him to write a program for the presidency sanitary commissions—his rather differing from that of your royal commission report perhaps rather set Sir J. Lawrence against him. But this would not affect his *sanitary* work. I don't think he is a good administrator. But he has not his equal at the other.

66 *Antiquities of Kertch and Researches in the Cimmerian Bosphorus: With Remarks on the Ethnological and Physical History of the Crimea*, 1857.

Source: Memorandum to Douglas Galton, Add Mss 45762 ff212-13

20 September 1864

*Application of the Army Medical Regulations to India.* We have, as you know, been in communication with the Army Medical Department on the subject and an entire copy of the regulations, altered according to their views, was sent us by you. But, before returning it in order to be forwarded to the India Office, we have tried it ourselves as far as we could and have obtained the most experienced *Indian* advice to be had. The result is that there are many administrative points in Indian practice which differ so materially from the ordinary course of army medical administration in England that we feel we could not venture to ask the War Office to put forward the amended regulations in their present form. We now wish to know what you would advise to be done. It has occurred to us that possibly a good course would be to send a copy of the new medical regulations with a copy of the recommendation of the royal commission, to the India Office, requesting them to adapt the regulations to Indian Medical Service, and to send the result for Lord de Grey's consideration. They would have to send to India to have this done. (They would not do it in the present state of relations between Sir C. Wood and Sir J. Lawrence: Editor's note.) If you chose me to write to Sir John Lawrence and do the same thing with him direct, that would be the shortest way. Or both might be done.

**Editor:** In her letter to James Pattison Walker, Nightingale for the first time makes the important strategic suggestion that they should not try to tackle the reform of all the stations at once, but should proceed piecemeal instead: to choose one station (or possibly two or three, not more) first, and complete its improvement in all respects. This approach would avoid mistakes that could result in the suggested reforms being judged as impossible to achieve. As the resulting debate demonstrates, the latter result was precisely what happened.

Source: From a draft letter in Dr Sutherland's hand to James Pattison Walker, Add Mss 45777 f47

[before 26 September 1864]

We have read over the minutes of your commission with very great interest, and, what is of more consequence, with a sure hope that you are laying a solid foundation for the work before you.[67] By this time

67 A possible allusion to 1 Tim 6:19.

you will have received and considered the *Suggestions* sent out from the Barrack and Hospital Improvement Commission. Their views are so nearly in accordance with yours that there is no doubt you will be able to frame plans for barracks and hospitals every way adapted for Indian climates. The antecedent improvements, so to speak, of stations, namely, their drainage and water supply, you will next have an opportunity of considering. . . . It has occurred to me whether it would not be advisable to select a station for improvement and to complete it in everything: drainage, water supply, buildings and police, and then you would see how the whole would work. Since the *Suggestions* were in hand, some of the details recommended, namely, pipe drains, constant water supply, Jennings latrines[68] and ablution arrangements, also improved cookhouses and cooking apparatus have been introduced at one or two warm climate stations with complete success. . . .

You will find nothing in the *Suggestions* in regard to the improvement of existing barracks. . . .

A great part of the time of the commission here is taken up with the improvement of existing barracks and hospitals both at home and in foreign stations, and any points of difficulty they could help you with. Generally their first improvement is in the ventilation of barrack rooms and wards because this is most easily and cheaply carried out, and probably you would find it the best end to begin with. Next they take water supply and drainage and then additional accommodation for troops and sick.

There is one point in your minutes which demands very serious attention. It would appear that many poor wretches are found dead or moribund in the streets, and that the police hospital accommodation is simply abominable. Could not this be remedied to some extent by adopting some such organization as exists at Paris, whereby the different police stations are enabled to supply medical aid, conveyance and even room for sudden emergencies until the sufferers can be removed to hospital? This would apparently be an effectual solution for the existing difficulties. We must collect and send to you all the information we can get about lunatic asylums and prisons, for it is quite clear that you are considerably behind, both in doctrine and practice, the small island of Malta, not to speak of England.

---

68 Jennings latrines consisted of a set of six, eight or ten toilets placed in a row and connected by a single hydraulic system, so that by the simple motion of a handle they were all flushed at the same time.

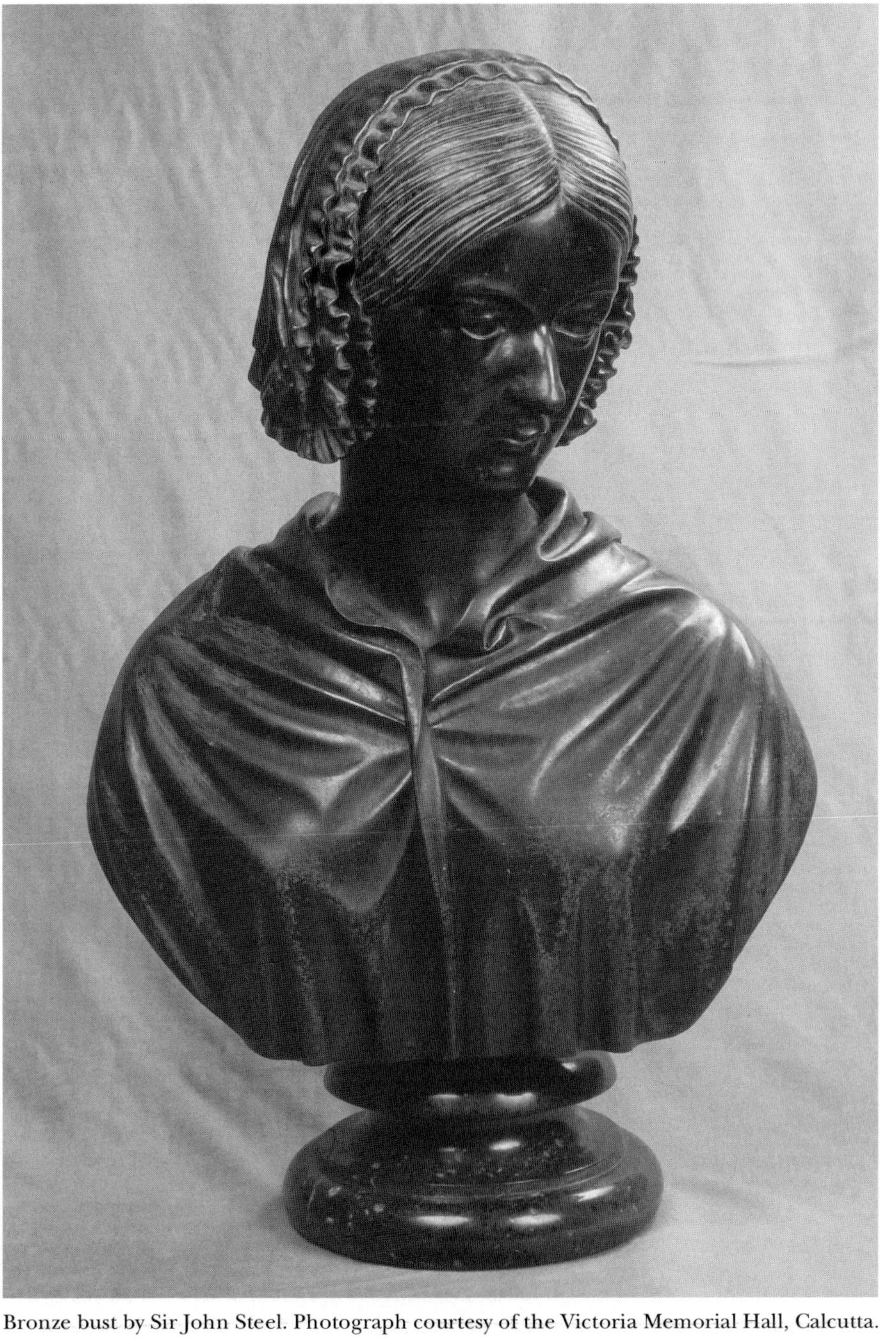

Bronze bust by Sir John Steel. Photograph courtesy of the Victoria Memorial Hall, Calcutta.

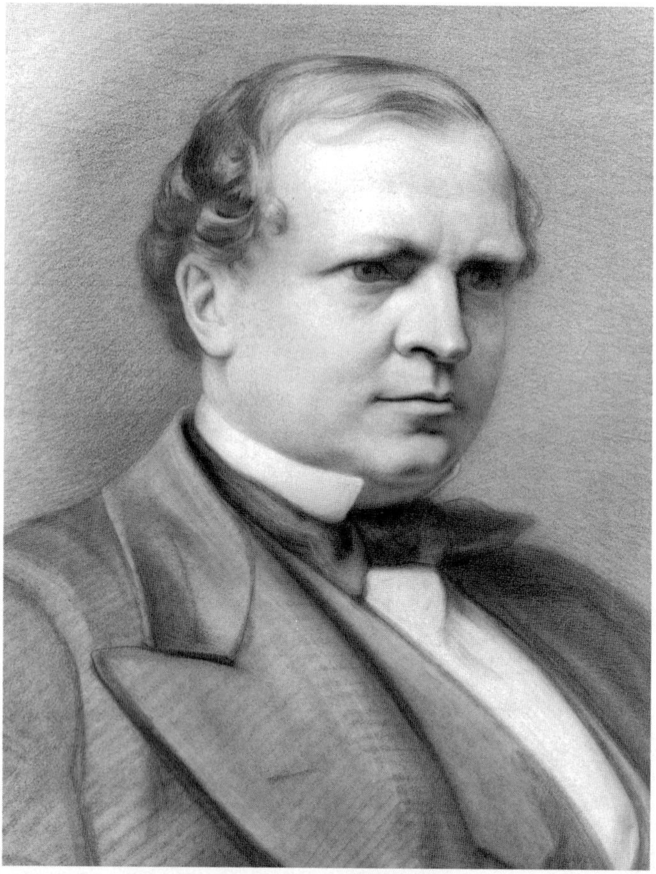

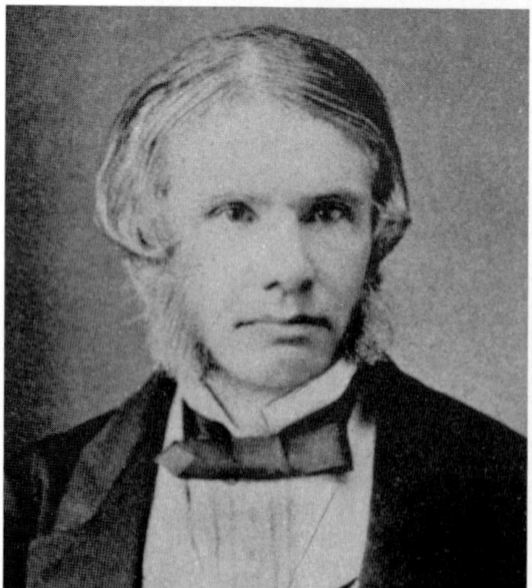

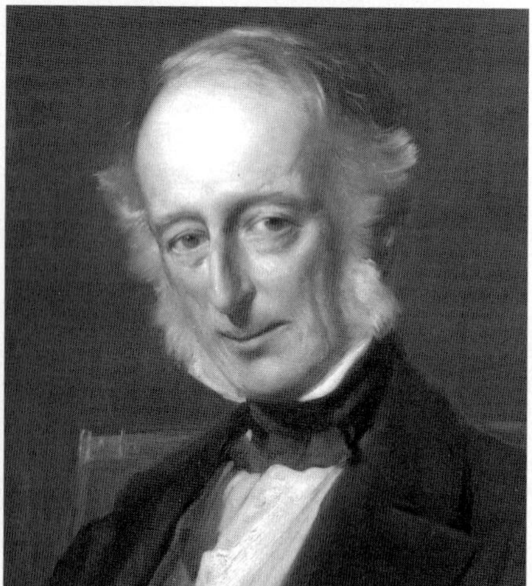

Portraits of (top) Lord Stanley, (left) Sir Charles Trevelyan and (right) Sir Charles Wood. Photographs top and right courtesy of the National Portrait Gallery, left of the British Library.

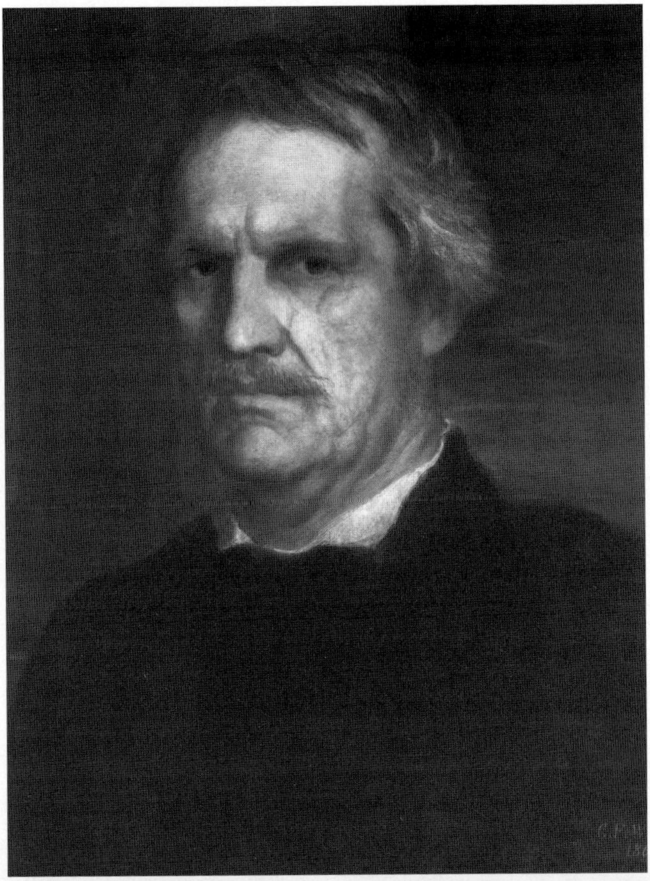

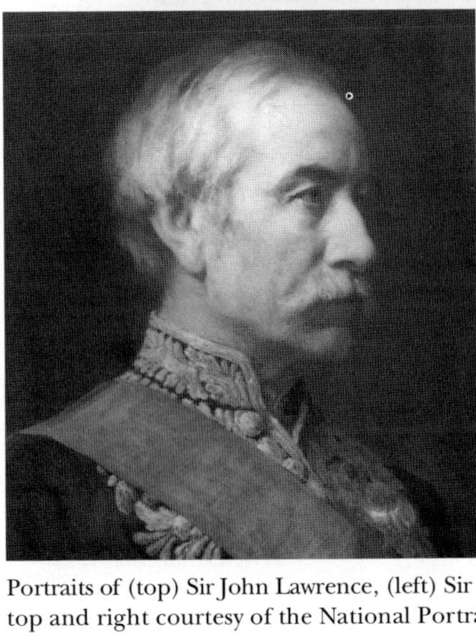

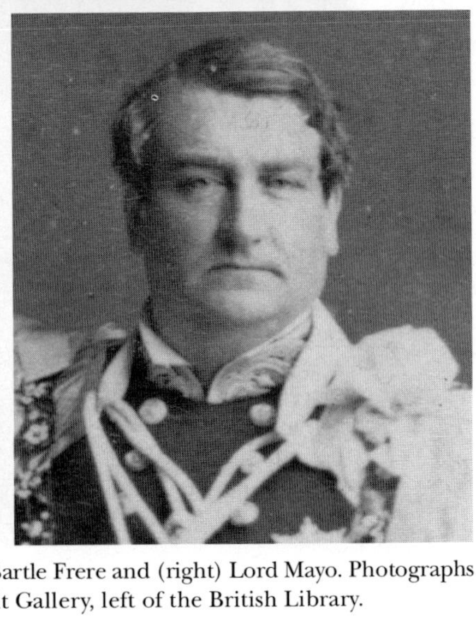

Portraits of (top) Sir John Lawrence, (left) Sir Bartle Frere and (right) Lord Mayo. Photographs top and right courtesy of the National Portrait Gallery, left of the British Library.

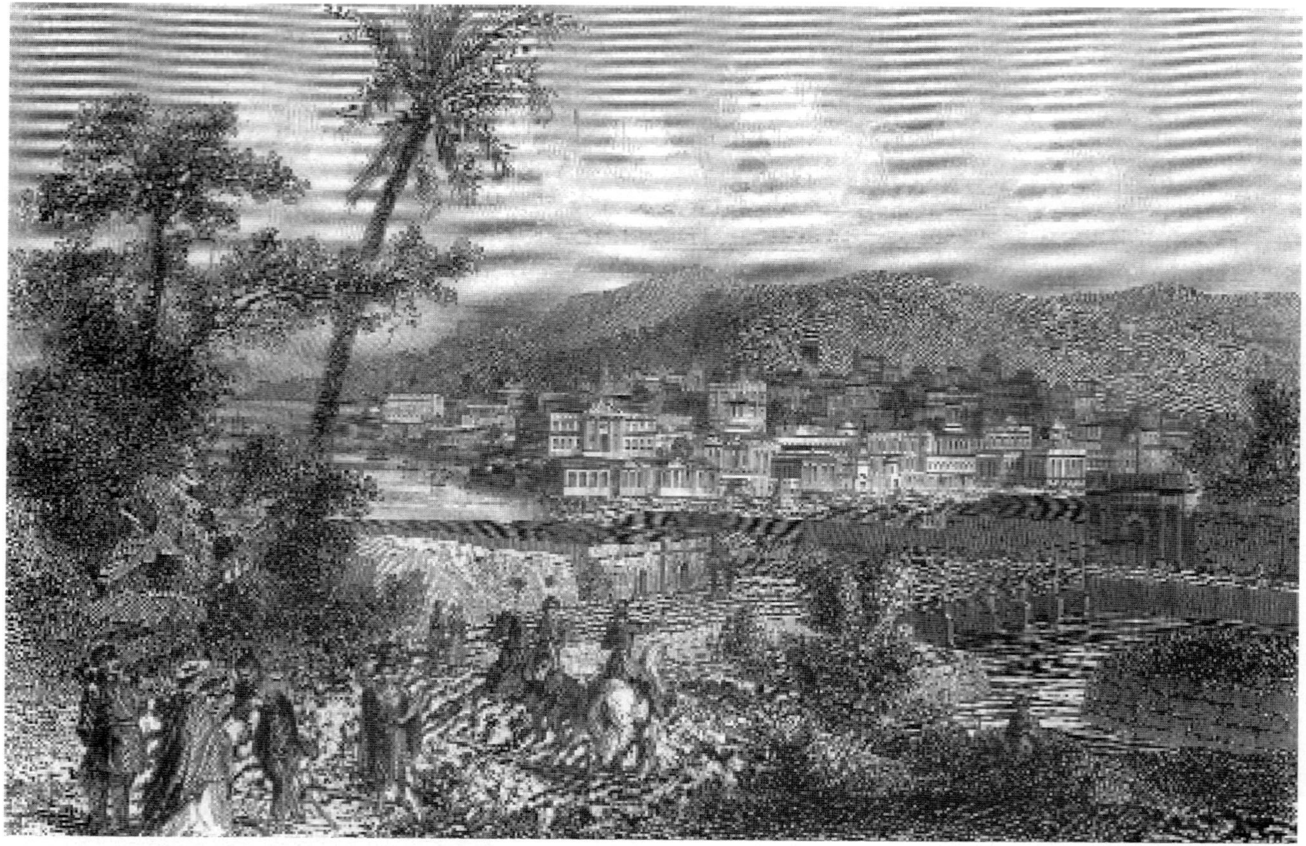

Lithograph of Calcutta, ca. 1850. Courtesy of Ronald Bayne.

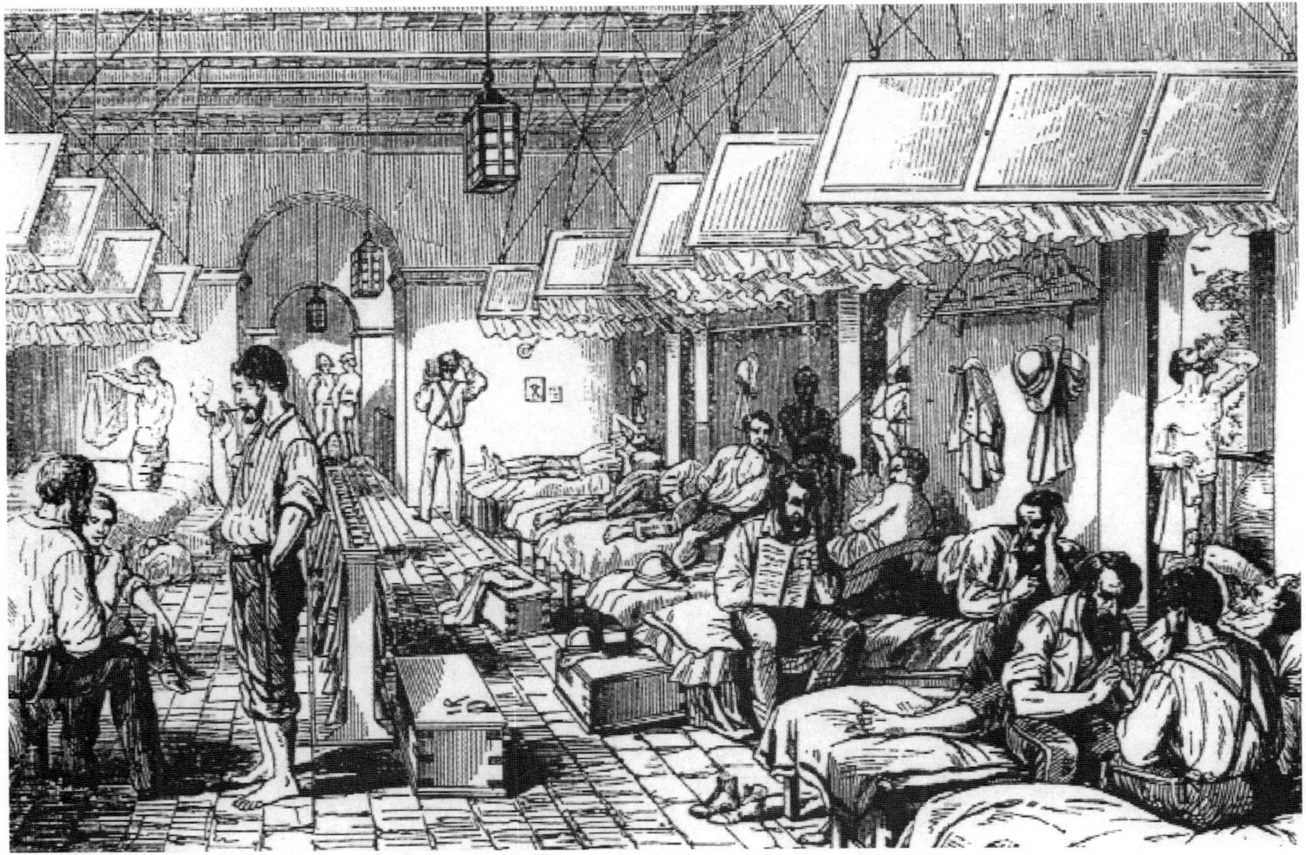

"Daily Means of Occupation and Amusement," woodcut from *Observations by Miss Nightingale on the Evidence... for the Royal Commission on the Sanitary State of the Army in India,* 1863.

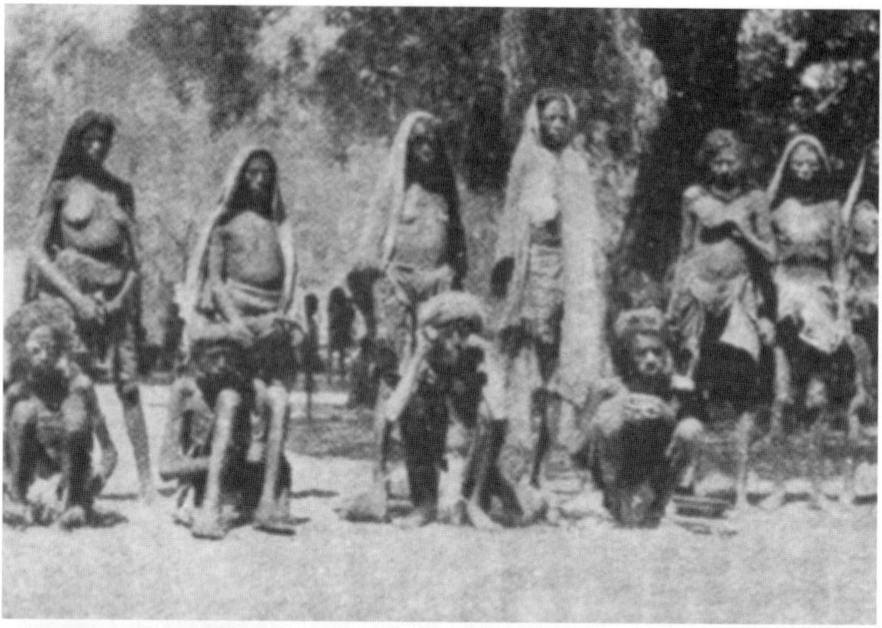

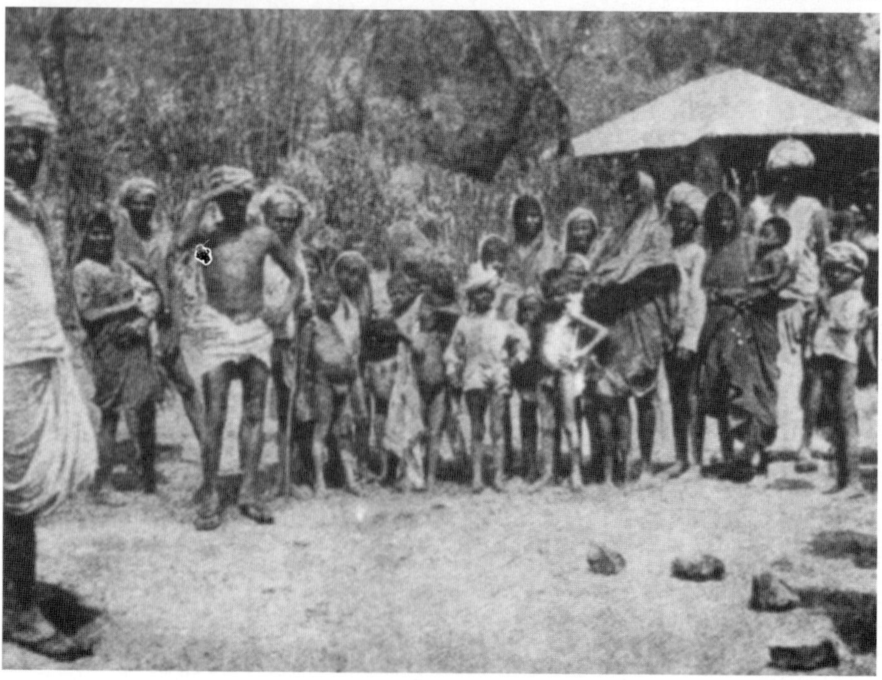

(Top) "In the Poorhouse at Nandurbar" and (bottom) "The Villagers of Valak," from Vaughan Nash, *The Great Famine and Its Causes,* 1902.

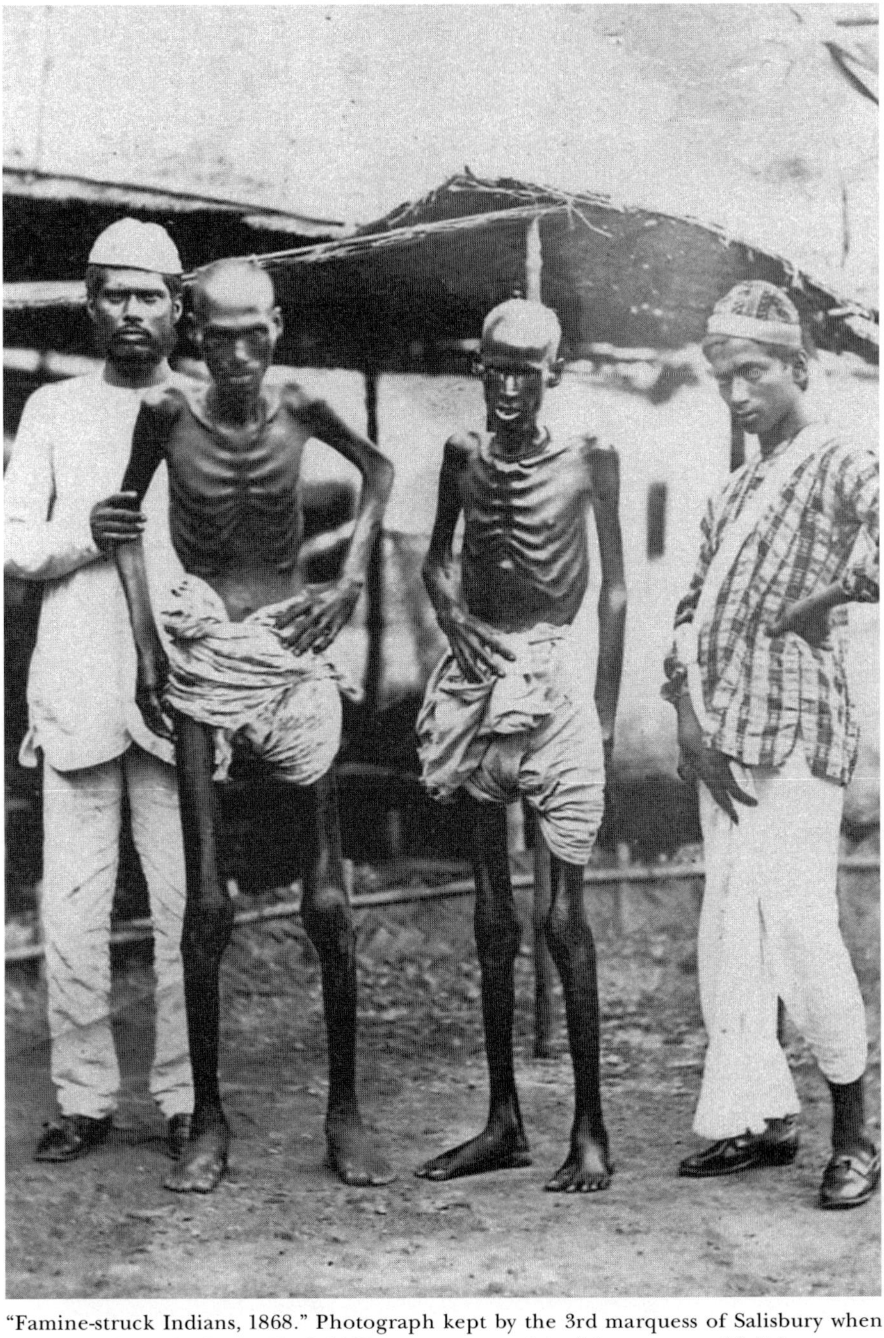

"Famine-struck Indians, 1868." Photograph kept by the 3rd marquess of Salisbury when secretary of state for India, Hatfield House, courtesy of the 7th marquess of Salisbury.

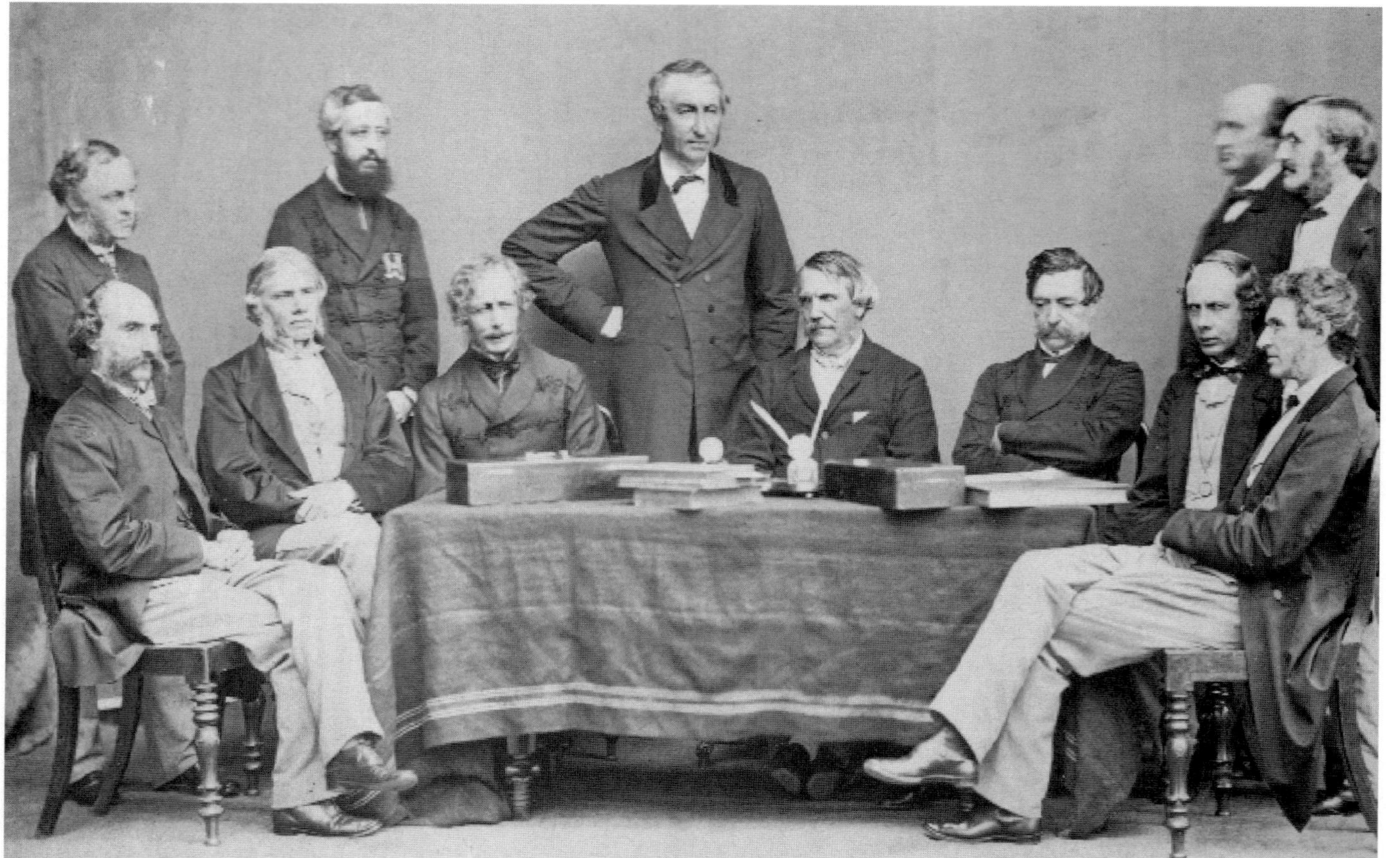

Sir John Lawrence, viceroy, with his council: seated (from left to right): unidentified, Sir Charles Trevelyan, General Sir Hugh Rose, Sir John Lawrence, General Sir Robert Napier, two men on end unidentified; standing (from left to right): Colonel Sir Henry Norman, Sir Henry Durand, unidentified, Colonel Sir Richard Strachey, unidentified. Photography courtesy of the British Library.

Source: From a typed copy of a letter to Sir John Lawrence, ADD Mss 45777 ff49-53

26 September 1864

*Private.* Your Bengal sanitary commission must be the model of the other presidency sanitary commissions. . . .

2. Would there be any impropriety in your sanitary commissions sending copies of their printed minutes to the Barrack and Hospital Improvement Commission here, through the India Office—merely for information? As far as your Bengal commission goes, these men don't want urging, they have not now to be taught. Anything which might even appear to interfere with the responsibilities of your commissions, unless at their own request, is not only undesirable, but, as far as the Bengal commission is concerned, useless. But if you saw no objection to sending the minutes for information to the War Office commission here, I am sure they would very much like it x x or, if that would be too formal and official (as regards the India Office here), if they, the minutes, might be sent to me, with permission to show them to one or two, such as Lord Stanley (our late chairman of the royal commission), Dr Sutherland, Captain Galton (of the War Office), etc., it would answer the same purpose.

The India Office here does not show now the least jealousy of the Barrack and Hospital (War Office) commission. On the contrary. One can scarcely help smiling at the small things it is glad to throw off its responsibility for upon said commission.

3. There are three glaring (though lesser) evils in Calcutta about which I know you have been employed—lesser though they are—and your attention and Dr Hathaway's have been aroused by them. These are:

(1) The police hospitals (or state of hospital accommodation) for sick poor at Calcutta. The police establishments seem about as bad as possible. Indeed the poor wretches are brought in mostly to die. The Parisian system of relief is very good: every police station at Paris has means of temporary help in cases of emergency until the sufferers can be removed to hospital. Some such arrangement with a thorough reform of the hospitals, and such additional accommodation as may be wanted, might meet Calcutta's case.

(2) The condition of jails and lunatic asylums in India. Certainly it is not for me to draw your attention or Dr Hathaway's to this. Probably he knows more about them than any man living. The reports and recommendations of one or two of the jail inspectors show that they want experience, as I am sure Dr Hathaway will agree with me. Perhaps we

might help you by sending out such reports on the subject as may be useful.

(3) The seamen at the great ports. You have already done so much, but Rome can't be built in a day. Bad water, bad food bought in bazaars and bad drinks cause a vast amount of disease and death. Self-supporting institutions, such as our sailors' homes (of which, indeed, I believe you have already founded more than one), would give the men wholesome food and drink, and lodgings and day rooms at little cost. So many men perish for want of this kind of accommodation at Calcutta, where the evil seems greatest.

Source: From an incomplete letter to Lord Stanley, Liverpool Record Office, Derby Collection 920/15/53

Hampstead, N.W.
4 October 1864

*Private.* I have not troubled you with the printed (detail) minutes which I receive very regularly from the Bengal Sanitary Commission (but on condition that they shall *not* be shown at the India Office). But these for June I will send you because they refer to subjects of (not only technical) interest—lunatic asylums and jails—which are worse in India than in any country which [breaks off].

Source: From a letter to James Pattison Walker, Florence Nightingale Museum (LMA) H1/ST/NC1/64/19

10 October 1864

*Private.* I write in haste to thank you for your important "Draft Rules for Military Cantonments," just received. I have only had time to glance through it. As a proposed sanitary code for Indian stations it shows that it has been most carefully considered with an earnest desire to make its provisions efficient (and with what a masterly hand it is done!).

There is so close a conformity in its provisions with the points in the *Suggestions* of the War Office commission which have been sent you that there will be no difficulty in arriving at an agreement.

In the War Office *Suggestions* there are some points which might be introduced with advantage into your code. With this view, might I venture to suggest that you should compare your clauses with theirs, so as to introduce into your code any additional clauses you may, on consideration, judge to be useful and practicable? Two or three points have especially struck me in my hasty perusal:

1. As to inspectors of nuisances. These are officers whose duty it is to *see the thing done* with their own eyes. This is indispensable with us

here. It may interest you to know that one of the most active "inspectors" in England has offered to the War Office commission to give up his appointments and come out to you. He says there are many others in England who would gladly lend their aid to the great work in India (not for the sake of large salaries, but simply to help forward the sanitary cause). We have referred him to the India Office. If you should want any such inspectors, you would have to apply to the India Office. And the War Office commission would try to find them for you.

2. A very important power suggested by the W.O. commission is the making of by-laws under sanction. Could you adopt this question?

3. Could not something more be said about the permanent works—granting to the local authorities certain powers of moving the government as to putting stations or towns in a complete sanitary condition (as to works of a permanent character)?

4. Could you not include the sanitary police of native towns and make some provision for introducing works into them?

These are the chief points which have struck me, not knowing the bearing of local powers in India. You may have perhaps already provided some of these powers, although I (ignorant) do not see it. You intend, as I gladly see, to send copies to the W.O. commission. They will joyfully give you every hint that occurs to them.

Source: From a letter to Douglas Galton, Add Mss 45762 ff229-33

Hampstead, N.W.
17 October 1864

There is some confusion in the Admiralty letter, about rationing on board ship, which requires to be cleared up.

1. The scale approved of by Lord de Grey for troops, women and children entirely supplants every existing scale, and is simply a substitution of one set of scales for another.

2. The proposed scales were not intended for invalids but only for healthy people. The present scale for invalids is much better than the present scale for troops, but nevertheless we have positive information that invalids arrive from India with *scurvy*. It would be necessary therefore to amend the invalid scale and this can be best done either by the former committee or by some committee specially appointed. . . .

This question affords a good opportunity for settling the kind and proportion of medical comforts for an Indian voyage. The committee should consider this; also the proposal to reduce the proportion of ale or porter put on board for from 10 percent to 5 percent of the number embarked.

Source: From a letter to John Strachey, Columbia University, Presbyterian Hospital School of Nursing C74

10 November 1864

*Private.* I am at a loss how to thank you for your kind letter, for your great exertions in the good cause in Bengal, and for the copies of interesting minutes which, through the kindness of Dr Walker, have reached me—proceedings for July; letter No. 620, by yourself of 5 September; proceedings of Madras Sanitary Commission.

I will not waste time in words but only assure you that, as far as Bengal is concerned, there are ninety-nine out of every 100 bodies in England incapable of anything like the same wise and energetic measures. And I only wish that the other presidencies were under the Bengal sanitary commissioners, as their headquarters staff.

The draft rules and regulations you were so kind as to send me are very good, and show the earnestness and skill with which you are laying the foundations of a sound sanitary service for India. You are quite right in not attempting a complete system at first. Because, without experience, this cannot be done. And from time to time things must be added, altered and amended, as the administration improves and answers its object. You contemplate chiefly the removal or prevention of easily removable causes of disease. This is perhaps all you can do at first, but, in the end, we should expect that the introduction of sanitary works would have more effect on the health, both of troops and native populations, than mere temporary measures. It was at one time thought that in London it would be necessary to avoid sanitary works and trust to cleansing solely in districts inhabited by the poorer and least civilized Irish population. But for many years it has been found that they, and even the "dangerous classes," thieves, etc., appreciate wholesome domestic conveniences with water supply just as much as the richer classes. Our experience here has been that even the most ignorant very soon learn to appreciate and use such facilities for health and cleanliness.

With regard to permanent works such as drainage and water supply of towns and stations (described in the *Suggestions* by the War Office commission), we suppose the Works Department are responsible for these, but any sanitary inquiry at a station should contemplate, as one of its results, a plan for drainage and water supply of the station. We see you refer to the dry conservancy system in your minutes. This may be necessary as a temporary measure, but you will have to do what our War Office has had to do with Aldershot, viz., to abolish the dry system after a number of years' experience, and drain the camp and apply the sewage to agriculture. Three fourths of all the camp sewage are conveyed away by drainage and 300 acres of barren sandy land have been leased to an enterprising agriculturalist, and are about to be brought under cultivation by irrigation. He will supply the whole camp with vegetables, milk, butter and a good deal of grain, grass and hay. The man will make his fortune very shortly. He has already begun his stock-feeding on land which six months ago was like the seashore.

If you could incorporate into your draft regulations any additional points arising out of the *Suggestions* and, if you would think well to send them here to the War Office commission, they would be truly glad and feel flattered, if they might give you any aid in their power to make the regulations as complete as possible.

Source: From a letter to Douglas Galton, Add Mss 45762 ff272-75

5 December 1864

This is a far more serious matter than at first sight it seems. H.R.H [commander-in-chief] and the director general seem to have some idea at last that what we have said all along is true (for there is not a bit of this correspondence new to us), viz., that the way in which the Army Medical Department has been mismanaged and treated could only end in such a "*mess*"—that vulgar word alone expresses so vulgar a state.

Of course the queen's regiments in India cannot do without queen's surgeons. And there is nothing for it at present, except withdrawing them from home or foreign service. The result, of course, will be that, until the service becomes popular, the director general must have an inferior class at home. . . .

Besides the immediate question the papers show a hazardous deficiency in the strength of the Indian medical service (British). Some time ago it was proposed to dispense with one of the regimental assistant surgeons. Such a proposal is inconsistent with the present state of things. Should you not settle the whole question, once and forever, both as regards the department itself and the number of medical officers required for queen's regiments in India?

The Horse Guards have raised the very points that we should have raised ourselves. Hitherto Sir C. Wood has been a party to the "*mess*" himself. But his recent warrant has performed his part. The War Office should now perform theirs. Your carriage stops the way.

Source: From a letter to James Pattison Walker, Florence Nightingale Museum (LMA) H1/ST/NC1/64/23

19 December 1864

On Friday night Mr John Strachey called at my house on his way to Bristol and left with me your proceedings for August and September. I was exceedingly obliged for your thought of me, but regretted the cause, I fear ill health, which brought Mr Strachey home. I did not see him, but he promised me to write from Bristol. If his health permits and his stay is long enough in England, he might obtain important information here. In the meantime, he leaves the cause in Bengal in the best hands, which are yours.

Source: From two letters to John Strachey, Columbia University, Presbyterian Hospital School of Nursing, C75 and 249, and 76

Christmas Eve
[24 December] 1864

*Private.* I could not bear to assail you the very instant you arrived in England, the more so because I fear your health is the cause of your visit here. And I dare say you wish as much as possible to forget, while you are here, the Augean stables of which it has been but one of your labours of Hercules to attempt the cleansing.

Otherwise I should have written before to thank you for giving me your address and for bringing the two months of your "proceedings" (from Dr Walker). And also to hope that it was not very inconvenient to you to come out of your way to find me here. . . .

I beg to assure you that all who know anything about the matter in England have been delighted with the zeal, energy and sound sanitary knowledge with which the Bengal Sanitary Commission, under your auspices, have set about their gigantic work, to which all that we have here is mere child's play. You have nothing to learn from us.

You have, of course, the advantage over us in local knowledge and as to the rules and methods applicable to Indian work. All we could do for you here would be to show you the working details of various departments. And the War Office "Barrack and Hospital Improvement Commission" would help you to this information, I am sure, to the utmost of their power, if you wished it and if you intend to visit London, your health permitting. They would gladly have you meet them, to see how they work, and esteem it an honour, if you would do so. . . .

We can show you completed towns, where every house is drained and supplied with water, and the sewage applied to agriculture. You could see an Indian problem solved at Aldershot, where the camp is drained, supplied with water and its sewage is being applied to agriculture. Any *practical* experience we could give you would be the best object to seek after, as in matters of *principle* you are all right. But your health must be the first thing as India cannot afford to lose the help of such men as you.

It would be a great advantage to me, if I could be allowed, while you are in England, occasionally to ask your advice upon one or two important points. E.g., would you not think it well that certain *papers*, as well as plans, such as, e.g., Colonel Crommelin's paper on the construction of hospitals, dated Simla, 15 August 1864, should be sent home *officially* for the revisal of the "Barrack and Hospital Improvement Commission"? By your kindness and by that of Sir John Lawrence or Sir C. Trevelyan or Dr Walker's, I have, I believe, received most of your printed papers about Indian sanitary improvements, also about the commissariat and about municipal powers which it is proposed to grant after inquiry. But they were sent to me privately and I could make no official use of them, except that I generally showed them, with permission, to Lord Stanley, as chairman of our late "royal commission" on the "Indian Army" sanitary state. I do not even know whether these kinds of papers are sent home by the government in India to the India government at home. I think it would be a very great advantage to both countries if Sir John Lawrence would direct all such papers involving sanitary principles of permanent importance (and involving expenditure of money) to be sent home, *before* being sanctioned (through Sir C. Wood) to the home Barrack and Hospital Commission *officially*. (Colonel Crommelin's paper on barracks, of which I have only an uncorrected proof, would be such a paper—to submit officially.)

It does not do for these things to depend on the life of one person, or the good will of another, or etc. They should be done, if at all, regularly and officially. No undue control *could* be thereby exercised by us upon you. On the contrary, as (*unfortunately* as I venture to think) there is absolute control vested, in money matters, in the home Government of India, I believe we should help you considerably in getting expenditure authorized.

I have just had a most kind note from Sir John Lawrence (Barrackpore, 20 November). I was really thinking of writing to him, by this mail, what I have just ventured to submit to you. But, as I have the advantage of being able now to submit questions to you at home, I will not write to him till I have heard from you.

New Year's Eve
[31 December 1864]

You will need all your energy to cope with the inertia in India. I wish you could lay in a good stock of health here.

To lose the opportunity of seeing you before you return to India—so little likely to occur again for me—would be to me almost as if I had not seized the opportunity, which Sir John Lawrence's goodness gave me, of seeing him before he went out as viceroy. If therefore you will be good enough to let me know when you come to London, and to let me make an appointment to see you, I shall do so, if it be only possible.

I feel so strongly, with regard to India, that what is to be done must be done now, or not at all. I mean, during Sir John Lawrence's time—in sanitary matters. We had a Sidney Herbert at the War Office—with his life, all progress passed away. So may it *not* be with Sir John Lawrence's. But I fear it will.

## Sir John Lawrence's Viceroyalty, 1865-69

**Editor:** In the letters that follow, John Lawrence no longer is seen as Nightingale's respected consultant only but as an actor in India in his own right, well placed to carry out the recommendations of the royal commission and already beginning to act on them. Nightingale placed high expectations on his appointment as viceroy. Upon assuming his post, Lawrence immediately organized the presidency sanitary commissions and, as seen above, asked for guidelines to define their precise functions, a process that resulted in the *Suggestions* of July 1864.

Soon Lawrence wanted to make changes to the makeup of the sanitary commissions, the commissions being judged ineffective. His "famous minute" or despatch of 19 January 1866 proposed various changes in the constitution of the sanitary commissions, for instance, reducing the membership of the commissions from five to two. In her previous correspondence with Lawrence, Nightingale had expressed her support for the idea that the head of the commissions "should be in direct communication with the government" (see p 525 below), creating a more effective mode of operating. The proposal to reduce the commission memberships had already been alluded to in a letter from Lawrence to Nightingale on 24 July 1865, and outlined in a paper by R.S. Ellis. Unfortunately Lawrence's despatch was lost at the India Office and was not found until May 1866. But Nightingale already knew of its content, having received a letter from Lawrence also dated 19 January, informing her of the proposed changes.

Among the proposals contained in the despatch was one that Nightingale judged aberrant, namely, the suggestion to give the post of presidents of sanitary commissions or health commissioners to inspectors of prisons, obviously no experts in sanitary matters. Such a proposal upset Nightingale to the utmost degree; she thought that the heads of the commissions should be well-qualified experts in sanitary and health matters, able to give birth to real Public Health Departments in each presidency. She communicated her polite reproof to Lord Stanley, expanding on the wide qualities expected from the presidents in the restructured commissions.

When he left the India Office in June 1866, Lord de Grey empowered Nightingale and Sutherland to write a minute in answer to John Lawrence's just-discovered despatch. Sutherland wrote a draft, Nightingale rewrote it under pressure on 19 June and Lord de Grey approved it. Nightingale's minute ended up offering a comprehensive program of public health for India, and its impact is outlined in some of the following letters. The chronology of the whole affair is hazy, but Nightingale reconstructed the essentials in Notes on Sir J. Lawrence's minute (see p 564 below).

We have, in the matter of John Lawrence's proposal of prison inspectors as heads of sanitary commissions, one of the rare occasions when Nightingale disagreed with him; the situation was delicate, Lawrence being her chief ally in India and her best hope for change. In the end she tended to attribute his mistake to a state of temporary depression. A second failure of Lawrence's viceroyalty was his lack of follow-up on Nightingale's proposal for a system of female nurses in Indian military hospitals, which had been made at his request, and which will be recounted in a later section (see p 939 below).

The present section concerns the more positive matters of moving ahead with the implementation of the royal commission recommendations, along with the imbroglio of the "famous minute." Interspersed with letters to Lawrence himself are many more to other officials and friends, in Britain and India, often written on his behalf.

Nightingale's relationship with Lawrence continued on his return to London at the end of his viceroyalty in 1869. She turned to him notably for advice in preparing material for later viceroys. Correspondence with Lawrence will continue to appear, scattered throughout this volume, and there will be a further section relating Nightingale's last contacts with him, his death and attempts to find the right biographer to write his life (see p 620 below).

Source: From a letter to William Farr, Private Collection of Susan Teagle, typed copy Add Mss 43400 f2

2 January 1865

*Private.* I thank you from my heart for your New Year's wishes. Indeed, none have touched me so deeply. They are of the true sort. It would be idle to wish me, or perhaps anyone who has seen this world as I have, a "Happy New Year." It has often seemed to me that the "good will towards men"[69] could not be what it was since it has pleased Him to take away so many of those through whom His "good will towards men" was best shown. But still, that was only in my cowardly moments. I know that His "good will" is the same. And I never despair while so able and steady a fellow worker in acting out His "good will" remains, as you are.

Do not fail to remember to send me your forms for Sir John Lawrence. We will get him to do that before this year is out. But it is not only my opinion but that of better judges than I that whatever is to be done (in sanitary, statistical and many other matters) must be done in his time or not at all. It is only his strong personal support which carries them against a host of inerts.

Poor Sir C. Trevelyan aided him, but he will never do work in India any more, though he is better at this time.

Source: From a typed copy of a letter to James Pattison Walker, Florence Nightingale Museum (LMA) H1/ST/NC1/65/1-4, copy Add Mss 45781 ff260-62

3 January 1865

*Private.* I will not let a mail pass without telling you how deeply touched I am by yours and Mrs Walker's most kind (and pressing) invitation to me, a complete stranger to you. Would that I could avail myself of yours and her great kindness! There is nothing, really nothing, on this side the grave, which I long for so much as a visit to India, nothing which would interest me so much. While others try to run away from India, I would desire more than anything else which I do desire (I "desire with desire," as the Hebrew says[70]) to go to India. I

69 An allusion to Luke 2:14.

70 An allusion to Luke 22:15.

have studied the country so much, I seem to know so well what I want to do there, that it appears to me as if I would be going home, not going to a strange country. But, alas for me, it is quite impossible. I shall never leave London, except for the grave. Even the move to the next street brings me to death's door. And I am assured that I have no prospect except of getting worse, though it appears that I must have a (family) constitution like iron, for, for nearly seven years, I have never been expected to live six months. If there were even any hope of my reaching India alive, and of my being able to go on working when there, as I do here, I believe I should be tempted to go. For my term of life cannot be much longer, wherever I am. But it is quite impossible. It is absurd for me to think of it, though I shall never forget the kindness which dictated the thought—in you and Mrs Walker—to be willing to take charge of such an invalid, an utter stranger to you. Even if it were possible, I really could not impose such a charge upon you. But it is not possible.

I may tell you in confidence that, in 1857, that dreadful year for India, I offered to go out to India in the same way as to the Crimea. But Sidney Herbert, with whom I worked for five years, all but a week, in the War Office, till his lamentable death put a stop to it. He said that I had undertaken this work, caused him to undertake it, and that I must stay and help him (meaning the sanitary army reforms). Since his death, it has been all the more necessary because all the more difficult. There is but one Sidney Herbert, there is but one Sir John Lawrence—they have no successors—you will know what I mean. What is to be done must be done in their time, or not at all. Our work is near child's play compared to yours.

Source: From a letter to Lord Stanley, Liverpool Record Office, Derby Collection 920/15/61

10 January 1865

*Private.* Sir John Lawrence's hands are so full (and yours will be so full, if you become his master) that it is at the same time a scruple and an inducement with me to bother about the relation to exist between the presidency and home sanitary commissions.

But if people are to act, they must be alive. And the difficulty of being alive in India seems one of paramount importance. May I ask whether you have had any answer from Sir C. Wood about those papers to be submitted to the home commission? I find that certain of them *have* been (or were on the point of being) sent home to the India Office. But I had better copy for you exactly what has been told me, premising that the letter is marked *confidential.* (It is always as well to consider whether the importance of the thing justifies one in perjury. I think this does.)

Sir John Lawrence "asks" his president (of sanitary commission) out there "if he sees any objection to copies of proceedings being sent home officially for the information of the War Office commission." The answer was that "far from seeing any objection, he thought it most desirable that this should be done, that the results would be in all respects good, that the more criticism the work gets the better, and if the Indian commissions are worth anything, they will always be thankful for the advice and help of sanitary authorities at home."

Sir John Lawrence says that "in these matters he is an advocate for the greatest possible publicity" and that he "will order (if not done already) that copies of all proceedings and all other papers of sanitary interest shall be sent home officially. *But there is a strong party in the Indian government which takes a different view* and which desires to prevent all publication of facts which reflect discredit on our administration" (viz., out there). "It was with difficulty obtained to circulate copies of proceedings to all the local governments and administrations in India," "the sanction for doing this was only given because" Sir John Lawrence "personally insisted upon it." x x "Colonel Crommelin's papers on construction of barracks and hospitals have either been actually sent officially to Sir C. Wood for the 'opinion of the War Office commission' (none such have been received) or are about to be sent, together with the opinions of the sanitary commission (presidency) and of the other authorities consulted, and the conclusions of the Government of India on the subject." (Why not *before* these "conclusions"? ) "We may hope that before long, therefore, we shall see such orders issued as will render it hardly possible in future that Indian barracks and hospitals should be built except according to proper sanitary principles. There is no doubt that such orders are as necessary now as they ever were. Within the last two months plans of barracks and hospitals, as bad as the worst, upon which Lord Stanley had written, have been highly approved and sanctioned by one of the best of the local governments." (F.N.: so we say.)

I shall have, in another day or two, to trouble you with another part of this same subject.

Source: From a letter to John Strachey, Columbia University, Presbyterian Hospital School of Nursing C80

26 January 1865

I thank you most sincerely for the second set of Dr Brydon's [Bryden] tables, which are most valuable, containing in addition the mortality of women and children, native troops and prisoners. I have let the Registrar-General see them. Also for Colonel Crommelin's papers on military and native hospitals.

Source: From notes, Add Mss 45836 ff23-26

[1864/65]

It is obviously of the greatest importance to derive all possible benefit from this experience in India and to provide for the following successive steps in the procedure:

1. Some competent sanitary and engineering authority must determine the drainage area and general limits within which sanitary works and improvements are to be carried out by every local authority. The reason of this is obvious: it relates to questions of outfall for drainage, the application of sewage to agricultural purposes, the deposit and utilizing of solid refuse matters, the draining and reclaiming of unhealthy ground near towns, and the prevention or removal of distant sources of nuisance.

2. The same authority should either prepare or sanction a general survey and map of the whole district, laying down the contours, levels, outfall, course of sewers and drains, streets, roads, houses, properties.

3. The same authority should prepare or sanction a general scheme of sanitary improvement, including works of drainage, water supply, paving, cleansing, opening up of streets, laying out new streets and other sanitary measures, which are to be carried out in detail and for the execution of which the local authority is to raise the required sums of money.

4. The same authority or some similar authority should inspect works in course of execution to see that they will fulfill the required object.

5. The same authority or some similar authority would have to see that the works were kept in proper and efficient repair and working order.

The royal commission proposed the appointment of the existing presidency sanitary commissions for the express purpose of giving a beneficial direction to all expenditure for sanitary purposes, whether civil or military, and the question has now arrived at this point that it will be necessary to arrange the order in which the various authorities should act.

The following questions arise. . . .

These points have been suggested by what will apparently be the probable result of entrusting uncontrolled execution of works to such local authorities as India is likely to supply. They are not put forward as affording a solution of the difficulty, but solely to show what the difficulty is, and how apparently it might be met in conformity with the inference drawn by the royal commission from past practice in India, viz., that constructive works should be executed under the Public Works Department; but you have illustrations of another method of procedure in the cases of Calcutta and Bombay, in both of which places the municipal authority has employed its own engineer as is done in England. Such a course would be most in conformity with the extended introduction of municipal authorities throughout India. But again it would be very difficult to find a sufficient number of competent sanitary engineers even to make a beginning. The way would be wonderfully smoothed if the capitals were once put into a good sanitary state. A number of engineers would be trained in the process, who might be drafted to other cities. And possibly the chief engineers of the presidency capitals might act as consulting engineers to other municipalities. There are difficulties any way and the whole case has been stated above, so far as our knowledge here extends, in order that you may have an opportunity of considering in what manner the works (described in the *Suggestions* prepared by the War Office commission) may be carried out, so far as these works are applicable to Indian cities and towns.

Source: From a letter to Lord Stanley, Liverpool Record Office, Derby Collection 920/15/66

11 February 1865

*Private.* A thousand thanks for your note.

1. The proposal to have sanitary engineers arose out of a positive statement (from India) that the requisite talent does not exist in India.

2. The functions of the sanitary commissions in India have been hitherto merely consultative (they give opinions only when asked); they certainly have not hitherto done anything in the way of inspecting and reporting on stations. If the government in India were to ask them to prepare plans for improving two or three stations, it would be found at once whether they could do the work. If not, they would apply for help from home and that help should be granted. All that we want is a beginning, plans of improvement in drainage and water supply sent home. This has not hitherto been done. The Bombay civil engineer who is doing the drainage of Bombay city is in England at

present, consulting about the works. We want similar steps to be taken with the stations.

3. If Sir C. Wood would look at para 22, p 12 of the "*Remarks*" (on Dr Leith), he would see all we want. If he thought fit to press para 22 by a minute, as he did your report, he would do all we want. I send the page, which contains all the things for engineers to do.

4. There ought to be no danger of "disputes." The questions all regard correct principles. We promise to advise Sir C. Wood as well as we can and as quietly as we can, and not to hurt his feelings the least little bit, nor anyone's else, certainly not the governor general's. We have not been aggressive, we have not been impertinent. Dr Leith attacked us ignorantly and offensively. And we put him right quietly and inoffensively. Indeed, I consider we have been models of lambs. (As for me, I have been on all fours.)

5. A very important paper has reached our barrack commission from Sir C. Wood: the views of the Government of India as to the principles of constructing barracks, that is to say, Sir John Lawrence's views on Colonel Crommelin's paper (of which I sent you a private proof to look at). (From India I hear privately that 7 millions are to be spent on barracks. And Sir John Lawrence says it will be 10 millions. Of course you know the truth of this.) This despatch from the Government of India is coming up here (I hope today) from our commission. When they have examined it, if you will allow me to claim your kind offer of a "farther consultation" (if you still have time then), there may be something to trouble you about.

Source: From an incomplete letter to Sir Charles Wood, Hampshire Record Office 334M87/1

[11 February 1865]

2. Lord Stanley's commission comes up to the reality, even in some of the best Bombay stations.

The (W.O. and I.O.) commission has now distinctly recommended a course, para 22, p 12, of proceeding to be followed at all Indian stations. And the next thing to be done would be that the presidency governments should have surveys made. Perhaps the best way would be for them to select two or three of the stations to put into proper order, then to make the surveys and send home to the India Office their reports and proposed improvements for sanction. Thus a beginning would be made.

The present position is simply this: that everybody is willing and yet nothing is done. I have heard (from India) that they have no sanitary engineers capable of making the requisite surveys. This is curious, if true. One would think there must be men in the Public Works Department. If not, I have reason to believe that we could find them men who would gladly go to India to do this work.

Should you think well to circulate the "Remarks" [on Dr Leith's Report] in India (which are, in fact, as sequel to the "Suggestions"), the W.O. would furnish copies.

I trust that you will pardon my intrusion and that you will believe me

ever your faithful servant
Florence Nightingale

Source: From a letter to James Pattison Walker, Florence Nightingale Museum (LMA) H1/ST/NC1/65/7

3 March 1865

I have to acknowledge the proceedings of your commission for November, which you have been so good as to send me. In reading 273 on the "Influence of temperate and intemperate habits," it struck me whether the data could not be obtained in the following way:

1. That a regimental list be printed containing the names of every man;

2. That a copy of this list be filled up at the canteen every day from the pegboard, showing the quantity of spirits and of beer each man has had in the twenty-four hours. Make it a current regimental return to be supplied to the commanding officer;

3. Have a medical return printed with the men's names on a similar form to be filled up on the last day of every year, showing the diseases each man has suffered from for the twelve months preceding. The returns you propose would then become of great use for comparison. Any person with statistical knowledge might extract from such tables most valuable information and a very clear view of the state of the whole case.

If our commander-in-chief (in England) were not a "snob" (which is a very disrespectful form of speech on my part) he would do all these things and get all these returns for us. But he does nothing.

*Private.* The India Office has submitted to the (home) sanitary commission (Barrack and Hospital Improvement Commission) the government papers on the principles for designing barracks in India, containing Colonel Crommelin's paper, that by the Government of India (which you were so good as to send me), the paper by your commission, etc.

Source: From a letter to Lord Stanley, Liverpool Record Office, Derby Collection 920/15/68

12 March 1865

*Confidential.* About India sanitary papers being referred to the home commission, Sir John Lawrence writes to me . . . that he *has* done what we asked, that all the sanitary papers *are* sent home; "but," he adds, "it must rest with the secretary of state to say what should be sent on to the sanitary commission. I should be trenching on his prerogative if I said more." I merely send this extract for information. I believe it was said (or supposed) that the obstacle, if any, lay "out there," not at home. I do not send it as a complaint. For we have nothing very particular to complain of just now.

I receive all the sanitary papers from India. And therefore I feel sure that the most important *are* sent us from the India Office, though after months of delay. The one upon barracks, founded on Colonel Crommelin's paper, came to the home commission two or three weeks ago, no doubt in consequence of what you said to Sir C. Wood. Our remarks on it are done and printed (i.e., the rough draft), and I meant to have troubled you with a copy. But the worshipful commission have not done their considerations upon the rough draft yet. The papers on hospitals will, I have no doubt, follow these on barracks (I received them months back).

2. General Peel "is going to attack the Herbert and other military hospitals on army estimates,"[71] I hear. Now General Peel is as much more formidable an antagonist to us than Lord Panmure, as a gentleman is more efficient than a "snob." Besides, General Peel has always behaved most generously to Sidney Herbert's memory, Lord Panmure most ungenerously (I do not mean to weary you with saying how). My object is: would you think well to say a little word for our poor new hospitals, if General Peel attacks them? in the sense of advocating the (at present) received principles of hospital construction, as set forth in your India sanitary report?

3. To return to Sir John Lawrence: he speaks eagerly, but rather despondingly, of his wish to accomplish "real sanitary improvements," of the "difficulties with which we are surrounded," and he says we

71 In fact Peel spoke for some time about lavish and increased expenditures on the army, but did not mention the Herbert or any other military hospital (Hansard, *Parliamentary Debates,* 3rd series (1830-91) 16 March 1865: 1782-88.

shall "consider" him "timid and even time-serving." (Certainly there is one thing great men don't know and that is themselves. John Lawrence was undoubtedly the only man who ever called John Lawrence a "time-server," except in the highest possible sense. For he does "serve" at the time most wanted with all his might.)

Pray burn this note. You will see that Sir J. Lawrence's letter is quite private. And indeed I am always afraid of misrepresenting him.

Source: From a letter to Douglas Galton, Add Mss 45763 ff46-47

29 March 1865

I hear that the Barrack and Hospital Improvement Commission, it is proposed, shall be called the *Army Sanitary Committee.* The two first words, Army Sanitary (*not* "War Office" Sanitary) are, I think, a great improvement in the title. But don't give up the word "Commission." I proposed it. Lord Dalhousie[72] and Sidney Herbert acceded to it. And now that it covers India, it would be very unwise to give it up. I had a tussle with Sir J. Lawrence about the word for his presidency commissions. And he gave up the word committee and has, as you see, christened them all commissions.

Source: From a letter to William Farr, Wellcome Ms 5474/84, copy Add Mss 43400 f26

29 March 1865

I have a multitude of printed papers, private, from Sir J. Lawrence's headquarters, by Indian mail, just arrived. And it really is melancholy and ludicrous to compare their assertion of well-chosen sites and stations with the facts they reveal. But they are doing their work manfully. Let us help them.

Source: From four letters to Lord Stanley, Liverpool Record Office, Derby Collection 920/15/71, 72, 73 and 76

19 April 1865

You, of course, saw the Calcutta papers (copy of report and correspondence relative to the sanitary state of Calcutta) in the form of a Parliamentary paper 22 February 1865. The experience of the War Office commission might possibly help in the satisfactory solution of some parts of the Calcutta problem, if Sir C. Wood would send them a

72 This, the 11th earl of Dalhousie, appears here mainly under his title as Lord Panmure, when he was secretary for war late in and after the Crimean War.

copy, of which they could take official cognizance, and order them to make their remarks.

2. By the India mail, which came in last night, I heard "that thirty-six square feet has (Stanley: *possibly*) been fixed as the minimum of superficial area" (for Indian jails) "and that new jails are to be constructed accordingly." "Want of money the cause." This is so very much less than the amount of area required for health even in England, that it seems as if it were the very thing in which the English secretary of state might exercise some "control," because I understand that the authorities are disposed to plead *want of experience* (of any larger area being necessary). Our prison inspectors might be referred to. But the War Office commission would do it much better and would of course consult our prison department (if referred to). I do not know whether you would think it well to interfere in these two matters yourself, by suggesting to Sir C. Wood to refer to the W.O. commission.

It is hard enough, God knows, for great public men to do their duty anywhere. But I do think it is harder and worse for them in India than anywhere else. And I know perfectly well now what Sir John Lawrence meant, when he said that we should consider him "timid and perhaps even time-serving."

29 April 1865

*Private.* In returning you Sir C. Wood's note, for which I am very much obliged, may I say that the case is this: a set of papers are laid before Parliament (22 February) containing certain statements as to the sanitary condition of Calcutta, with certain engineering proposals for rectifying the evils. Your royal commission dealt not only with the "military" points in India but with the state of towns and, amongst others, of Calcutta (inseparable from the "military" question, unless Sir C. Wood believes in the exploded superstition of quarantine).

The War Office (or home sanitary) commission was reconstituted mainly by your own instrumentality. And Mr Rawlinson was added to it, expressly for these civil matters (chiefly by the same influence). All that is required is that Sir C. Wood should send the Parliamentary paper to the (W.O. and I.O.) commission for remarks.

We think it would not be difficult to find a way out of the Calcutta difficulties, and it IS our duty to help them. I don't know that Sir C. Wood has any business with what Sir J. Lawrence or the "sanitary commission in Bengal" writes to me about "wishing for advice." These papers were, it is true, sent to me confidentially. But they are now Parliamentary papers. I think I sent them to you (in the spring of last year). I told Sir J.L. that I should (i.e., submit to you all the papers he was so good as to send me that I thought worthy your notice). I think I sent you an extract from his letter saying that he *did* wish all these papers to be referred to the "home sanitary" commission but that, having expressed that wish, it would be interfering with Sir C. Wood's "prerogative" to interfere farther, or words to that effect. I have not Sir J. Lawrence's letter before me.

I trust that you will hear "about the prisons" after Sir C. Wood has "asked" about them. The Colonial Office is putting its house in order about prisons. And it would not do for India to be left behind. The awful epidemics in her prisons are beyond parallel. . . .

P.S. It appears to me that Sir J. Lawrence and Sir C. Wood are playing at cross purposes. The former says: I *have* asked. The latter says: *if* he will ask.

F.N.

Please burn.

13 May 1865

*Private.* I am afraid you will think me very troublesome, not only that, but turbulent; "a turbulent fellow," vide Lord Panmure. And I am afraid you will also think me overeager, which is true, and unreasonable and sometimes contradictory, which I don't think is true, but apparently so. So I had better proceed at once to business.

1. I beg leave to send you a proof copy of the remarks of the Army Sanitary Commission (here) on the conclusions of the Government of India in regard to the building of barracks, which "conclusions" we received from Sir C. Wood, owing to your intervention, as perhaps you will remember, some weeks, not to say months ago. (We have accomplished our part with all our usual celerity, seeing we might have done it in as many days.) The whole subject has evidently been well considered in India, and the only points in which the (home) commission has suggested improvements are those necessary for more completely embodying the views of your royal commission. The India government has evidently profited by the *Suggestions* formerly sent out by the (home) "Army Sanitary Commission." (That is the way they choose to style themselves now.)

2. Nothing has yet been heard from Sir C. Wood about the sanitary state of Calcutta. I venture to send you (and to ask the return of) a report twenty-five years old on the same subject, exposing a state of things the father of that denounced by Mr John Strachey. But the

enclosed report is nearer the truth—on the subject of sanitary works—than the document laid before Parliament (22 February 1865). I send this *old* report in order that you may see what our case is and how old the evils are they have to deal with. From these two reports you will easily see how needful it is that the (home) Army Sanitary Commission should point out the great leading principles applicable to the improvement of Calcutta, if only they had the opportunity of so doing, afforded them by Sir C. Wood. All that he would have to do would be to send the Parliamentary paper to them for "remarks" in the usual way, and they will send as much information as they can. Sir C. Wood, if he saw fit, might then send it to India. He is aware that Sir J. Lawrence wishes it (generally).

3. You have probably received by this time Dr Farr's reply to the statements made by the Government of India about the mortality. He sent it here. And we asked him to add a little summing up. I need hardly say that, if you would wish us to add anything, we are more than ready. It was thought that, as the Army Sanitary Commission had signed the reply to Dr Leith, it would be better that this reply to the Government of India should be independent and signed only by yourself (if you approved it at least). But this is of course a matter for yourself alone to decide. We will try to alter and improve it, if not approved, as often as you think well.

4. Nothing further has been heard about the Indian jails and their thirty-six square feet per prisoner which it is proposed to give. To show in what a condition the intelligence of Indian officials is on this subject, may I say (what I dare say I have troubled you with before) that our royal engineer, who has been engaged in Turkey upon improving the Turkish prisons, says that the superficial area there to be allowed is seventy-two square feet per prisoner, or just double what Indian want of sense considers sufficient for India. The fact is that India has set up her new housekeeping with not a house over her head. She wants new jails, new hospitals, new buildings of all kinds. And she wants to be helped. God help her! and you too, I hope.

I would renew my excuses to you. But I think it more respectful not to take up any more of your time with my "sornettes" [twaddle]. So I will only say that they *are* doing a good deal—"Deo gratias" [thanks be to God] and also to you—in India.

23 May 1865

*Private.* If you saw fit, I think the true way of putting the case to Sir C. Wood is that it is not whether the "Calcutta people" desire to be improved or to ask advice. It is this: Sir C. Wood, having granted to the House of Commons certain papers exposing a state of things in Calcutta, which has brought out severe public criticism—and these things being the very things most important for the "Army Sanitary Commission" (this is the name by which they are to be called) to advise the India people about—would it not be desirable to have the sanitary (not administrative) questions simply therein raised, brought officially to the cognizance of the commission, in order that it may give its best advice as to the methods most likely to remove the acknowledged causes of disease, especially as the plans proposed are obviously by no means the best possible? (I need not tell *you* that Sir John Lawrence does wish to be informed and to ask advice, and that he has informed me that he *has* told Sir C. Wood so, because I think I have uniformly sent you extracts of his letters, and because you probably know it by much more direct means. But it is impossible for me to quote his letters, or those of the Bengal Sanitary Commission, except to yourself, or of course to ask you to quote them.)

There may be reasons of which I know nothing to prevent you from thinking it well to urge Sir C. Wood upon the general grounds stated above. I have done what I could in sending privately to Sir J. Lawrence Mr Rawlinson's opinions. But what I feel—and what I am sure you must feel much more strongly—is that it does not do to leave these vital questions at the mercy of private or accidental agency. God bless you for taking them up.

I have kept the enclosure back, because I had a question to ask of the W.O. But I need scarcely say that I have not shown it, nor your letter.

Source: From a copy of a letter to Robert Rawlinson, Florence Nightingale Museum (LMA) H1/ST/NC3/SU169/65

15 May 1865

I have this morning had a letter from Sir John Lawrence speaking with despondency of the future progress of sanitary works in India, and enclosing this article (which please return to me) from one of the Calcutta newspapers.

Does it not appear that the way in which they are proceeding with the drainage is not at all in accordance with your suggestions? But, however this may be, the matter is of such vast importance and the governor general is so good in giving me the opportunity of corresponding with him directly on all these subjects, that I very much wish you would have the kindness to write me such a letter (about this article) from the Local Government Act Office as you would have no objection to me sending out to Sir John Lawrence for their information in India.

The whole thing ought to come before your War Office commission. But I wish to save time. If you could point out tersely the errors they are committing—also the remedies—or general principles which ought to be kept in view, in a letter which I might forward, it might do much good. I need hardly say that this letter of mine to you is strictly confidential. If you could answer me, so that I might write by the Bombay mail of the 18th, it would save valuable time.

Source: Extracts from a memorandum, copied out by Nightingale with her marginal notes, Liverpool Record Office, Derby Collection 920/15/78

2 June 1865

The sanitary commission of the MADRAS presidency:

> have now been nearly fourteen months in Office and during the whole of that time have had to combat with the most determined opposition from the government. The public is kept in entire ignorance of their labours, and reports and letters are disposed of summarily and seldom acted on.
>
> What is really required is that the suggestions of these commissions should be dealt with by government on their own merits, and not referred to the quartermaster general or the commander-in-chief for their observations.
>
> In example of the mode of dealing with reports: shortly after submitting the Bangalore report a reference was made to government regarding the site for certain buildings on the "race course" at that station. A committee was ordered by government to decide the points at issue and of this committee Dr MacPherson (as president of the sanitary commission) was nominated, (officiating) during Mr Ellis's absence as a member. Dr MacPherson, etc., proceeded to Bangalore where H.E. [his excellency], the commander-in-chief, then was, and the committee ordered by government was *not* held. But Sir Hope Grant did order a committee of four military and three medical officers to report on the recommendations of the sanitary commission regarding hospitals and barracks occupied by Europeans at Bangalore. (For four days—for from three to four hours daily—the whole business was to defend the commission from the repeated attacks and innuendos of the quartermaster general's department.) Finally the committee adopted every suggestion of the sanitary commission, with the exception of one or two minor points (and their report is now before government).

> *Our only remedy must come from England.* The high officials here consider that the sanitary commissions are not authorized to do more than suggest and that it is not necessary to do more than *record* the commission's views.

[FN marginal note] This refers exclusively to the *Madras* commission. The Bombay does not *want* to *do* anything, but writes only. The Bengal has Sir J. Lawrence. But it is to be regretted that he does not make it a government office or department. Perhaps he can't.

> If such a state of matters is to continue, then the sooner these commissions are abolished, the better. The most carefully considered suggestions are set aside for insufficient reasons or for no reasons at all. Our army enjoys, as a rule, good [FN] ? health, but of the carelessness of the military authorities the sad misfortunes of the 74th Highlanders at Madras and of the artillery marching from Mhow are abundant and most painful examples.

[FN marginal note] This paper was sent me, a capital paper.

> It is now fourteen months since the sanitary commission first addressed government on the subject of selecting camps for Europeans if attacked with cholera at stations and it is little more than so many *days* since anything has been done on the subject.

[FN marginal note] The *Bengal* commission wrote to me to get them the best methods of water analysis. After much that was insufficient had been sent me by savants, Dr Angus Smith sent me a full and sufficient paper, now in the press, for them.

> An inquiry into the character of the drinking water in Madras was instituted eleven months ago at the request of the sanitary commission and they are now told that it cannot be completed until the end of this year. Seven months ago, they submitted a scheme for a Public Health Service to include registration of births and deaths: on this nothing has been done.

[FN marginal note] This too is an excellent paper. Mr Ellis hopes to carry it—the scheme.

> For twelve months certain suggestions of rules for the con[s]traint of public women were forwarded to government and have only just been adopted after the preliminary process of a committee who only interfered in minor details.

[FN marginal note] Better they never had been adopted.

> To detail all the many instances of impassiveness on the part of this government would only weary.
> Here are some of the good results of the *Madras* Sanitary Commission. At a native town some thirty to forty miles from Madras, the annual assemblage of pilgrims was followed almost invariably by the appearance of cholera, which speedily found its way to Madras. On their own responsibility and by Mr Ellis's influence, suitable measures were adopted for the conservancy of the town during the festival and for the provision of "places of convenience," the removal of cattle and the cleansing of the streets, etc. 20,000 pilgrims attended and not a single case of cholera occurred. Similar measures were, at their (sanitary commission's) suggestion, again adopted this year and with similar success. Although this was brought to the notice of the authorities, *no* similar measures were adopted elsewhere and cholera is now raging in Bellary, Sangor and other districts where disease has been introduced by large bodies of pilgrims.
>
> Without a well-planned and active Public Health Department, these unhappy occurrences can scarcely be prevented. The subject of the marching of troops has engaged the commission's attention, and certain recommendations offered on the point, but opposed by the military authorities. These latter caused by their neglect the march of the 4th M.N.I. Regiment to be made in February through the most unhealthy district of the presidency (the hotbed of cholera and fever) and when the regiment reached Secunderabad some considerable number of the whole regiment had been attacked. One European officer died.

Source: From a letter to Lord Stanley, Liverpool Record Office, Derby Collection 920/15/79

7 June 1865

*Private and Confidential.* Here I come troubling you again. But the *Madras* government is betraying us (this time). And we want you, if you thought well, to interfere, as no one else can, to bring them to their senses.

A Mr Ellis, a (kind of) cousin to Lord de Grey, was appointed president of the sanitary commission for Madras (one of the three presidency commissions inaugurated by your royal commission). He was an ignorant amateur. And his appointment made a great "row." But he set his shoulder to the wheel and worked like a man, but found he could really effect nothing and is now coming home to see if he cannot move the *home* government to do something, through Lord de Grey. (Cousin or no cousin, I don't think Lord de Grey will do much for him. But I am "a dirty bird, who fou's its own nest.")

Dr MacPherson, a man whom perhaps you will remember as writing to you "with a grievance," but quite the ablest man in India in *sanitary* administration, has been appointed, mainly by Sir J. Lawrence's personal interference, *locum tenens* to Mr Ellis for six months, as president of the Madras Sanitary Commission. Whatever energy and ability can do, Dr MacPherson will do. I think I can best tell you the difficulty by making some extracts from various letters received by last mail.

After a summary of "all that is being done, I should say *written* by the Madras Sanitary Commission, they are allowed to *write* as much as they please, but they are not allowed to *do* anything." Another letter says: "Mr Ellis, the president, has spared no pains to get up the subject and to put matters in train for action." (Mr Ellis, whom I do not know, has been kind enough to send me all his papers, which are *masterly*. But you see, he could not quite tell me what a fine fellow he was. So I prefer to quote from other letters *about* him.) "But not a single rupee is granted by the governor, who, with Colonel Herbert Marshall, military secretary to government and Colonel Scott, the quartermaster general make no secret of their opinion 'that the whole thing is bosh from top to bottom.' "

In another letter, I read that "the Madras government is doing worse than nothing, for it is laughing." "Mr Ellis's chief object in coming home is to endeavour to get some pressure put on the local authorities. If he fails, he intends to resign in disgust and return to his old duties."

"Dr MacPherson has gone over with Mr Ellis all that has been written and recommended, which substantially is what we have urged on the government for the last ten years." But "nothing has been done, because not a rupee is available, and *nothing will be done*, until public indignation *at home* is aroused and directed against the obstructions." "Mr Ellis has done much good work. He is an able man and has thrown himself with all zeal into his duties. He is fully alive to their importance but, having had much passive and not a little direct resistance, little or no good has, as yet, resulted from his recommendations. One great object he has in going home now is to get power placed in the hands of the commission to carry out at once such points as are of urgent necessity." (This is from another letter.) (I will only just add that Mr Ellis's appointment was a direct result of the recommendation of the—your—royal commission, viz., that the heads of the presidency sanitary commissions should be civilians and administrators, and *not* doctors, that the signal failure of Dr Leith, as president of the Bombay Sanitary Commission, has only justified your recommendation and that "we" have always done our little all to support Mr Ellis.)

A suggestion made to me is "either that Lord Stanley should prevail upon Sir C. Wood to write at once to Madras on the subject, in order to bring the Madras government to its senses or that Lord Stanley should move in the House of Commons for a return of the sanitary work done and the money spent in sanitary improvements in the Madras presidency since the sanitary commission was appointed." You will alone be able to decide what is best to be done. I need hardly say that it is a point on which I have no judgment at all or that I have not, in my replies, said a single word to imply that you grant me the liberty of bringing these things before you. I know perfectly well what Sidney Herbert would have done, if he had been now secretary of state for war. He would have called upon the Army Sanitary (W.O. and I.O.) Commission to furnish such queries and forms of returns as, when sent out to the Madras government and replied to, would have brought out the whole subject and facts of the case, as they now stand. But this is past praying for. And I should have a "predestinate scratched face"[73] for so much as suggesting it.

Source: From a letter to Lord de Grey, ADD Mss 43546 ff 105-08

10 June 1865

*Private.* I am afraid you will think I am interfering beyond my province. But, at all events, you will admit that I have kept the promise of a peculiar Christian "not to pray" to you "for a long time."

Mr [R.S.] Ellis, president of the Madras Sanitary Commission, is coming (or came) home; he sailed on 7 May mainly, I believe, to obtain your help to enable him to carry out his important duties in that presidency. I shall leave him to tell his own story. My story does not come from him at all.

You are probably aware that Sir John Lawrence made it one of the first acts of his government to appoint the three presidency sanitary commissions recommended by the royal Indian Army sanitary commission, presided over by Lord Stanley. Since that time, these commissions have been doing good work, but sadly hindered. But my business is now with the Madras commission and what it has done, or rather I should say, *written.* They are allowed to *write* as much as they

73 Shakespeare, *As You Like It,* Act 1, scene 1.

please, but they are not allowed to *do* anything. All speak in the highest terms of Mr Ellis (the more to his credit, because his appointment made a great "row") as having done all that man could do to put matters in train for action. But not a single rupee is granted by the governor, who, with Colonel Herbert Marshall, military secretary to government, and Colonel Scott, the quartermaster general, make no secret of their opinion "that the whole thing is bosh from top to bottom."

The Madras government is betraying us. It is doing nothing. Nay, it is doing worse than nothing, for it is laughing. What is wanted is that, from home, pressure should be put on the local authorities in India to give power into the hands of the commission to carry out at once such points as are of urgent necessity. No doubt you will, if you think fit, be able to obtain this for the commission but whether, considering the interests at stake, something more is not wanted, e.g., an inquiry, I am not competent to say. I might perhaps imagine that what Sidney Herbert would have done would have been to call upon *your* Army Sanitary Commission (W.O. and I.O.) to prepare such queries and forms, as would, when sent out from home, bring a return of the sanitary work done and of the money spent in sanitary improvements in the Madras presidency, since the Madras Sanitary Commission was appointed. Except when Sir John Lawrence's personal influence can be exerted, it is quite clear that nothing will be done by the local governments in India, until public opinion at home, and principally S. of S. for India's opinion and House of Commons' opinion, is directed against the obstructives. For there is no public opinion in India. Believe me, dear Lord de Grey,

your very faithful servant

Florence Nightingale

Of course want of money, as well as of energy, is at the bottom of the difficulty. But none but Sir John Lawrence are enlightened enough to see that a single epidemic costs the country more than all the works necessary to prevent epidemics.

Source: From two letters to Lord Stanley, Liverpool Record Office, Derby Collection 920/15/80 and 81

14 June 1865

I take the liberty of sending a copy of the remarks of the Army Sanitary Commission, in case it has not reached you, on the barrack plans which you persuaded Sir C. Wood to send to them for criticism (I think you had a proof). You will see that the requirements of your royal commission are now fully provided for, i.e., if the India government adopt the few changes proposed. And then the Indian Army will have the best barracks in the world. But indeed the original plans, the devices of Colonel Crommelin, our original enemy, the minutes of the Government of India upon them, including Sir J. Lawrence's own and Colonel Strachey's (the secretary), show how they are a hundred years ahead of what they were but eighteen months ago. I wish Sir C. Wood and the India government did but know how a single epidemic costs the country more than all the works necessary to prevent epidemics. It is like a poor *savant*, who denies himself food and fire to finish his education and ruins his constitution or dies, and then what is the good of his education? Men must *live*, first.

17 June 1865

*Private.* The man whom I mentioned to you, president of the Madras Sanitary Commission (R.S. Ellis; he was member of Council at Calcutta as I dare say you know) is come. I was asked to see him. And I did. He is a very able, energetic man and knows what he is about. He is much the best I have known of the India sanitary presidents. He devotes his six months' leave to seeing practical sanitary works in England. But that is not his main object. The most important thing he has to do is to induce the home government to settle the question of the position which the Madras Sanitary Commission should occupy with regard to the Madras government.

At Madras the sanitary commission has no direct relation to the government. It writes only to the military secretary. And this is dead against all progress. As the holding of India depends so much on the health of troops, the authority vested with the duty of looking after this should certainly be in direct communication with the government. When you desired me to see Sir J. Lawrence before he went out as governor general, in order to urge upon him the recommendations of your royal commission, I wrote a paper for him, at his request, a kind of sermon on the texts of your recommendations, in which it was proposed that the president of the commission should be minister of health for the presidency (I mention this now, in order to show that Mr Ellis's object is entirely in accordance with the views of your royal commission); at present his position is less influential than that of an officer of a London vestry. Mr Ellis proposes that the sanitary commission president should be in the position of a secretary to government, so as to communicate directly with members of government, to have the title of inspector general of public health (which word, as he says, would involve no expense).

At present the progress of sanitary works in Madras presidency is *nil,* though they have a man, in Mr Ellis, at the head of their sanitary commission, who, of all men, answers to your recommendation to put an administrator and a civilian as president (of these commissions).

Mr Ellis has carried (1) a Military Cantonments Act to give power over these, which was absolutely necessary; (2) (which is not yet carried, but on the point of being so) a Towns Municipal Improvement Bill, of which he has left me the draft—if you would care to see it. He is anxious to carry an organization of the Public Health Service for Madras presidency, of which he has also left me the draft—if you would care to see it—which would cost only £10,000 or £12,000 a year. [Mr Ellis proposes] that, in the Madras budget, from £10,000 to £15,000 a year should be devoted to sanitary works.

It is evident that the crisis is come which will decide whether the sanitary service is to be something like spirit-rapping or table-turning, or whether it is to be a real service. I do not offer any suggestions to you, simply because the way of using pressure on Sir C. Wood is a sealed book to me. Mr Ellis was to see Lord de Grey (whose cousin he is) today. I do not know whether you would think well to see Mr Ellis, whose address is: *4 York Street,* St James' Square.

Source: From a letter to Robert Rawlinson, Boston University 1/3/46

17 June 1865

*Private.* Mr Ellis, president of the sanitary commission of the Government of Madras, is in England, on six months' leave, to possess himself practically of what you have been doing in the various classes of works which have been introduced in this country. Would you kindly put him in the way of seeing what has been done in civil life in the following, among other, matters:

1. The best subsoil drainage works;
2. Specimens of town drainage, with fall and without fall;
3. Methods of constant water supply by gravitation and by pumping from wells, etc.; filtering on a large scale;
4. Specimens of house sanitary works adapted for the poorer classes (Irish labourers and such like);
5. Completed examples of improved towns, in which constant water supply is combined with sewerage and the sewage applied to agriculture;
6. Manufacturers of sanitary appliances, e.g., Macfarlane's (at Mr Begg's), Mr Jennings, Doultons, etc.

There is no end to the information you can give him. I have only mentioned a few points. Could you some day *after* next Wednesday meet him here, say at luncheon, about 2 o'clock, and go into the matter with Mr Ellis yourself, which you would do so much better than I can?

Source: From a letter to Douglas Galton, ADD Mss 45763 ff63-64

17 June 1865

*Private.* As you have no doubt heard from Lord de Grey, Mr Ellis, president of the Madras Sanitary Commission, is here and wants you to help him in every way in mastering the details of sanitary work, during his six months' leave. With regard to the military, he wants to see and to have explained: (1) your best barrack (e.g., Chelsea); (2) your best military hospital (Herbert); (3) your best military hospital *at work*; he must see the medical school, invaliding and hospital staff orderlies at work at Netley; (4) your best camp with *tenting*, draining, water supply, application of sewage, etc. (Aldershot). He wants particularly to see *camping-out* (he thought of Chalons, but is not Chalons a permanent camp?); (5) should he not assist at the meetings of your Army Sanitary Commission? He wants, in short, to see how the work is done and the results you have arrived at. I have all but promised him that you (if you can) and Dr Sutherland, shall take him to these places, to reply to all his queries, yourselves. There is no one else to do it.

Source: From a letter to Lord Stanley, Liverpool Record Office, Derby Collection 920/15/84

23 June 1865

*Private.* I am ashamed to worry your life out, but this is a question which concerns our very existence. I hear (from the War Office) that "Colonel Percy Herbert is going to attack the whole system of sanitary improvement of the army, in his speech on the question he has given notice of tonight (about Dr Sutherland)."[74] There is no one in the House who understands the sanitary question as you do. There is no one in the House who would be listened to, as you would be. Also, you know Dr Sutherland's peculiar merits (though he does think the world moves round himself). None of these royal or permanent sanitary commissions could have been accomplished without him, as you

74 Colonel Herbert objected to Dr Sutherland's salary being hidden as a per diem expense, and not voted openly in the Estimates. The government's position was defended by W.E. Gladstone as chancellor of the Exchequer (Hansard, *Parliamentary Debates*, 3rd series [1830-91] 30 June 1865:989-92.

know. *Could you defend us? tonight?* There is no time to prime any MP who did not know the subject. And if there were, he would be of no use. No one but you would have any weight. Unless General Peel would do it, who has always been most generous to Sidney Herbert's memory. But he is not sound on the sanitary point. And it would be of no avail for anyone but you to ask him, even if he were. In haste.

your very fervent suppliant

Florence Nightingale

Captain Galton, assistant under secretary at the War Office, would, I have no doubt, be in the House tonight, if you wished any information on detail points.

Source: From a letter to Robert Rawlinson, Boston University 1/3/47

24 June 1865

Would you be so good as to tell me what were the results you arrived at with Mr Ellis on the subject of the systematic surveys of stations and native towns? From all the recent documents which I have seen, this is the point in which they were most defective. I was very desirous that you should have the opportunity of going personally over the subject with Mr Ellis. Will you also tell me any points in which you think I could be personally useful in pressing the subject?

Source: From a letter to Dr Bence Jones,[75] Cambridge University Add 8546/I/171

26 June 1865

*Private.* I have a phoenix on my hands: one of our presidents of sanitary commissions from India, Mr R.S. Ellis—he was member of Supreme Council—is now president of sanitary commission, Madras presidency. He is come over to England to instruct himself in sanitary things. And I am appointed (whether with or without his knowledge I do not know) to see that he does not mis-instruct himself. I dare not ask you to take him over St George's Hospital yourself, though he is a worthy subject. But, if this is impossible, would you hand him over to the person least unsuitable for the occasion? But please remember, my phoenix is not to be perverted. False doctrine is not to be instilled into him. India looks to every man to do his duty by my phoenix.

75 Henry Bence Jones (1813-73), friend and colleague from 1853 on when he was consulting physician at the Establishment for Gentlewomen on Harley St. For a while he was also Sidney Herbert's doctor.

Source: From a letter to Douglas Galton, Add Mss 45763 ff74-77

1 July 1865

After the discussion last night about Dr Sutherland's salary, I have no doubt that we shall agree that some final settlement, one way or other, must be come to about it. You know, of course, that at the time the government asked him to go as commissioner to the Crimea, he was sanitary advisor to Lord Hanover, then president of General Board of Health and that, in order to go to the Crimea, Dr Sutherland was obliged to surrender the appointment, subsequently given to Mr Simon, with a salary of £1500 a year for part of his time only. Dr Sutherland made no bargain in complying with the request of the government to go to the Crimea. He was paid four guineas a day by the War Office for every day he was in the East. When he returned, he served on the Royal Army Sanitary Commission (Sidney Herbert's) of 1857, giving his whole time without remuneration, and holding no appointment.

When the Barrack and Hospital Improvement Commission was organized, he was asked to serve on it by Lord Palmerston[76] and Lord Panmure. No bargain was made as to salary. Three guineas a day were offered and accepted by him. The duration of the commission was not fixed. The manner of providing the pay appears to have been also undecided. The work of the commission, as you are aware and as I am aware too, is far more extensive and important now, since India was added, than it was at first. And many questions will be referred to you from India, time after time, for solution. The commission will become even more an India [Office] than a War Office one.

Considering all this, and considering the opposition of anti-sanitarians in the House of Commons, would it not be better that the government should settle at once what they intend to do? It is neither safe nor fair to let matters go on as they are. You must either, as it appears, make the appointment permanent, or fix a time within which it must cease, or make it an altogether unpaid appointment, which, of course, would be ludicrously unfair, since the other members serving on the commission and giving but a small part of their time, occupy other paid appointments. Or you must put an end to it. I have some voice in this, because I have been cognizant of the facts from the very beginning. And the future of sanitary improvements, both at home and in

76 Lord Palmerston was then for the second time prime minister, and continued to be an ally in Nightingale's causes.

India, to which I have given my life, depends mainly on the decision now taken. Should you think fit to show this letter to Lord de Grey, pray do so. Or should you wish for a fuller account of the circumstances, and the information which I should be able to give, pray command me.

Source: From a draft letter in Dr Sutherland's hand to Edwin Chadwick, ADD Mss 45771 ff65-67

[August 1865]

Now that the elections are over it appears very desirable that we should prepare for future progress in India. Our case has been before the public for about two years. It has been discussed, the statements cavilled at, some of its statistical facts doubted in the highest quarters and its results finally confirmed, not only to the letter but to such an extent beyond what we said, as in reality to form a new indictment. I need hardly tell you that what we aim at in India is the efficiency of our noble army there, the foundation of all law, order and security, and next to that the advance of civilization among our Indian fellow subjects. It is sad to think that we should after a century of power have to contest the execution of works which a Roman legion would have set about within six months of its conquest.

The Roman was a civilizer by instinct. The Briton is a merchant by instinct. What the one did the other leaves undone, and it is our duty (I need hardly say this to you) to supplement so as we can the great lack of service in this matter which all the world now knows. Except the imperfect works at Bombay, we have supplied no town in India with water. We have neither drained, paved, cleansed or built one good village even. And what is worse than all, there is opposition to all advancement on the part of not a few officials, the very fact of which opposition being itself a proof that men are thrust into offices for which they have no aptitude, and whose responsibilities they do not recognize.

Our only hope out of this is in Parliament. We have Lord Stanley there and one or two others who will help. My object in writing is to ask you if I might venture to write to Mr [John Stuart] Mill [elected MP in 1865] to ask him to consider our case and to help us to the extent he would feel himself justified in doing so from the facts. We do not ask for any particular form of help. All we want is that the work be done. We should have great confidence in anything Mr Mill might be able to do for us either openly in Parliament or privately to Sir C. Wood, but I should like to act under your advice and write to you first.

A short time ago Dr S[utherland] informed me that you had told him that Mr Mill would be glad to assist with my Indian sanitary reforms in the House of Commons or in pressing them on the Indian government. There can be no doubt of the great advantage of Mr Mill's help and we should accept it with gratitude. At present our chief reliance in the House is Lord Stanley, who has worked admirably for the cause and who, I have no doubt, would welcome Mr Mill as a co-adjutor. If Dr Sutherland's impression of your view was correct, would you be so good as inform me whether Mr Mill would be likely to render his aid, and I could then write out a statement of the present condition of the question, which would perhaps be the best way of showing what is necessary to be done. I may state, however, generally that at present our dependence is on Sir J. Lawrence, but his tenure of office is uncertain and we desire very much that the great cause of civilization in India should not depend solely on the life or tenure of office of the present noble governor general, who has always done so much for us. In India there are certainly influences which delay progress, and what we fear is that, after the years of labour we have gone through in ascertaining the facts and preparing the ground, our labour may be lost unless we can show that there are good men and true who will not stand by and see this without a protest.

Source: From seven letters to Lord Stanley, Liverpool Record Office, Derby Collection 920/15/85, 86, 87, 88, 89, 91 and 92

26 July 1865

*Private.* I have refrained from worrying you till after the elections. But your kindness obliges me to report progress, or rather no progress, a little, now. Mr Ellis, the president of the Madras Sanitary Commission, has not as yet any satisfaction out of Sir C. Wood with regard to establishing him as a kind of minister of public health and secretary to government at Madras. I have had a number of letters from India from quite different hands, all describing the unsatisfactory condition the Madras commission is in. Of these I venture to send you some extracts. You will see that they are entirely "Private and Confidential," especially those referring to Sir W. Denison's[77] "views," as when he tells his commissioners for the purpose of *removing* "stinks": "Do as I

77 William Thomas Denison (1804-71), army officer, governor of Madras 1860-66, worked for the improvement of public works, irrigation, communications and agriculture.

do, *keep away* from stinks." Though I am sure that it was intended that this information should reach you, I must not even tell you the names of the writers. The object is, I believe, to induce you to induce Sir C. Wood to write to Sir W. Denison that it would be desirable to place the sanitary commission on a proper footing as advisors of the government. Of course, I do not presume to urge you to do any such thing. But it is quite evident that this Madras commission must be put in some better position. The men know their work. The military people are ignorant and prejudiced. They should certainly adopt the principle of taking the advice of those who know the subject and not submit to be guided by those who don't know.

I think you will be glad to hear that your Bengal commission wrote to me to get them the latest methods of water analysis, and that, after some delay, your protégé, Dr Angus Smith, has given an invaluable paper, which shows for the first time the results of the labours of his whole life on this vital point (of testing water, as he did air, for organic matter). . . .

Mr J.S. Mill, since being returned, has sent us a message to the effect that he would like to serve us in India sanitary matters in the House of Commons, previously, of course, communicating with Sir C. Wood. I was rather pleased at this, as I always thought he considered the whole sanitary thing a humbug. We shall not, of course, begin "intriguing" with him without the concurrence of our head.

16 August 1865

I think the enclosed batch of minutes from Madras is rather comforting. Please to look at page 111. I recognize your hand there. You will see that Sir C. Wood has done exactly what you asked him. Please also to look at p 115 (19). It is an agreeable variety (to abuse) to find that the engineers have taken kindly to the *Suggestions* and declared them generally to be practically applicable to Indian stations.

Such a vast deal of nonsense had been talked as to the impossibility of draining India. You will find also at pp 5, 7, 123, that they are making progress in their ideas as to the possibility of making sick native soldiers comfortable. But this is a matter in which we can, of course, interfere with them but little. But what is aggravating and distressing is the manner in which all good seems to stick fast when they come to jail construction. . . . It will never be better until you have the subject referred to the W.O. and I.O. commission at home with the view of their preparing model plans. (They would of course consult the inspector of jails office here.)

I have done what I could with Sir J. Lawrence privately. But of course what is wanted is that Sir C. Wood should refer the matter officially. Then he will say that the W.O. and I.O. commission have nothing to do with civil lives. But this is the very thing which they do not say in India. They do refer civil cases to the presidency commissions, *vide* this very case. . . . How those quartermasters general do hang back from all common sense. You will see that the practical backwardness of the executive authorities continues. India would have been cured by this time, if everything *said* by the presidency commissions had only been done by the executive government. However, we have great cause for thankfulness to you and Sir C. Wood (he has been quite in a "coming-on" disposition).

This Madras commission has practical *nous* [spirit] to a remarkable degree—more so, I think, than the Bengal one. But the Bengal commission are backed by Sir John Lawrence and therefore *do* more. I am obliged to trouble you to let me have back these Madras minutes as they have desired me to reply to them. They are now engaged in reporting on Madras itself, its impure water, bad surface drainage, etc. Every well in Madras averages 5½ gr. organic and 41 gr. inorganic matter. And they have nothing else to drink. The only wonder is how they live at all. I hope we shall get Dr Angus Smith's method of analysis, when he sends it me complete, used throughout India. But they may analyze all day long and do no earthly good, of course, unless the authorities will do their part. If these will not, one would rather *not* know that one is drinking 46½ grains.

P.T.O. I think we may encourage *us* by the great progress in soldiers' workshops in all three presidencies. At Belgaum they have had a bazaar, all the articles produced by the men and their wives, and all sold. The result was most profitable, as the articles could be obtained in no other market and both buyers and sellers were equally benefited. What a reply this is to all the objections that have been made, such as "no market" for soldiers' produce.

4 October 1865

*Private.* I believe I am going to assault you again about the positions of the presidents of (Indian) sanitary commissions, with regard to government. (Mr Ellis, president of Madras Sanitary Commission, is still in England, working at this and at gaining practical knowledge. He is one of the ablest men they have.) We think that, unless they are made secretaries to government, as it were, they will do nothing. I have a private letter from Sir John Lawrence on the subject, dated 24 July, saying that *he* cannot make them so without Sir C. Wood. (He says that *his* "president" does very well because he has constant access to him, Sir J.L. That is all very well for the Bengal presidency, but not so well for the Madras and Bombay ones.)

I see that Lord de Grey means to do nothing with Sir C. Wood, though he says he does. And I believe I shall have to worry you again upon the matter.

22 October 1865

*Private.* I thank you very much for your note of yesterday. I send you a *Daily News* article, which came out while you were away. Also, a rough proof (or rather a sixth revise) of Dr Angus Smith's paper as to how to find out how much dirt there is in water, which, at Sir J. Lawrence's desire, I have had on hand—and these five mortal months too. I think Dr Angus Smith is as difficult to manage as the whole India government. He writes one thing, then he writes the reverse, then he listens to what his "nephews and nieces in Argyleshire" say (sic) and tears up the paper. (But I had it in type.) And there is now scarcely a single word in this, the sixth revise, of what there was in the first. But he is the only man in Europe who can do it. And this is well worth all the trouble. When it has reached the sixtieth revise, I shall make the India and War Offices circulate it.

But this is not what I wanted to write to you about, which is: our great matter of making the presidents of sanitary commissions secretaries to government and ministers of public health. Sir J. Lawrence has written to me that it must be done at this end, at least that his "master, Sir C. Wood," must tell him to do it. There will be no real action on the part of the sanitary commissions till it is done. Mr Ellis, who is the ablest of their sanitary presidents, is in England with this object. A paper has been drawn up (Indians are so fond of paper, as you once said) of which I hoped to send you a copy today. None of our great masters have seen it yet. If you think well to take it in hand, it will be done. If not, not. (Lord de Grey is no use with Sir C. Wood, who treats him as I treat my infant kitten. It must be playful but not troublesome.)

I mean to do myself the honour to be troublesome to you at greater length when I send this paper, if you will allow me, and also to tell you at greater length what Sir J. Lawrence said. . . .

Lord Palmerston is a great loss to our sanitary (and Poor Law) things generally. I never asked him to do a thing for the last nine years (you may be sure I did not ask him often) but he did it. He made a joke but he did it.

24 October 1865

*Private.* May I send you Mr Ellis's papers? (Mr Ellis, president of Madras Sanitary Commission, now at home, partly for this, viz., to obtain a more definite position and responsibility for these presidents, partly to make himself personally acquainted with the working of sanitary acts in this country.) When you first proposed these commissions, in the report of the royal commission, you made their position as general as possible because, without experience, you could not have done otherwise. You however indicated clearly that their duties were not to be wholly consultative. (You said: *mainly* consultative.) They have had a year's trial. And their work, from apathy or neglect of other departments, has been wholly consultative, leading in some cases to the most absurd delay and loss of time. Mr Ellis and his commission (his secretary is now in England) are unanimously of opinion that the time has arrived to change the position of the president, so that he may have a distinct personal responsibility and direct communication with the government. In order to further this object, Mr Ellis has drawn up the paper I venture to send you. (It is "*Confidential* and has not been yet shown to the I.O.) If his proposal is acceded to, he will become a secretary to government and will be assisted in all sanitary questions by his commission. In this way, progress will be more rapid and certain, and we shall escape the present danger of having the whole future of Indian civilization placed at the beck of an ignorant or indisposed governor and his departmental heads.

N.B. As to Sir J. Lawrence's last communication to me on this subject, the gist of it is that it must be done at *this* end (i.e., if Sir C. Wood would say to Sir J. Lawrence, "if you—Sir J.L.—see no objection, I—Sir C. Wood—see no objection," it would be done). Sir J.L. adds that his own (Bengal) president of sanitary commission *has* constant access to him and that this answers. We say: that is all very well for Bengal, and while Sir J.L. is governor general; it is not so well for the other presidencies. Also there is an unfortunate fact that Sir J.L. is not immortal. (What would become of us in England, if all our public works had depended on the life, personal humour and premiership of, say, Lord Palmerston?) Then Sir J. Lawrence thinks all men are like himself. He does not take into account what a "devil" of a life (excuse me) Sir W. Denison, e.g., has led us. Farther, Sir J. Lawrence asks: "What will become of the commission, if its head is made secretary to government?" We think there would be no difficulty—no more than there was in arranging the duties of the head of the "Board of

Supervision" in Scotland. But you will tell us whether this question—Sir J. Lawrence puts it as no more than a question—is answered in the paper.

Lastly, in the interview which you desired me to have with Sir John Lawrence before he left England, and when he did me the honour to ask me to put in writing the views of your royal commission and to take the manuscript with him, it was expressly stated that the ultimate position of the presidents of sanitary commissions would necessarily prove to be ministers of public health. The present question I do not prejudge but only leave it to you.

(2nd N.B.) Mr Ellis is very anxious to meet you for half an hour—if you can spare the time—not only to speak to you about this sanitary matter but about one or two other Indian subjects in which your aid is much required. He is an able man and a Supreme Council man. I have not, of course, led him to suppose that I should tell you this. He can quite well seek Lord de Grey's introduction to you. I rather mention it, because I am anxious for it myself (he would explain things better than I, who am too eager) and because, at the same time, you can quite well refuse it to me.

12 November 1865

*Private.* I particularly dislike worrying you about things which do not (and perhaps cannot) advance just at present. This is: the matter of the presidents of sanitary commissions in India and their position. I wrote to Sir John Lawrence (mail before last) in the sense you indicated. A letter, of which I now send you an extract, arrived one hour too late for me to send him by last mail. But it will go to him by the next. I have not heard the result of Mr Ellis's visit to Sir C. Wood with *your* letter. Or rather I believe Mr Ellis did not see Sir C. Wood before he left London (and had his accident, poor man [Ellis]). I am rather afraid you will be indisposed towards us by the tone of the extract I now venture to send you. But Indians, I think, always express themselves more like Irish than English.

The matter is this: Sir W. Denison's proceedings at Madras justify all we fear as to the impossibility of the sanitary commissions doing any good without a fixed position, independent of the mood of the governor (or governor general). Some time ago, the Madras commission, as was its duty to do, made an examination of part of Madras with the view of reporting on its sanitary condition, and of suggesting improvements. (I have a copy of their report, if you would like to see it.) It is signed, in name of the commission, by Inspector General

MacPherson, acting president in absence of Mr Ellis. The Madras government had, it appears, taken some steps of its own in the matter and proposed extensive and costly works, which would have required years to complete. The sanitary commission made certain *interim* proposals for improvements which, in their opinion, would do *interim* good. Without, of course, offering any opinion as to engineering merits, I think that (you will agree) the subject was one which ought to be fairly discussed and considered. The course taken was that detailed in the enclosed (private) letter (from Madras, received here by last home mail), of which we have other confirmation. This and similar steps taken by the Madras government will, it is feared, end in the resignation of the commission, unless it can have its position strengthened. They feel the proceeding as a "deliberate insult" (I am afraid of being Fenian) put upon zealous public servants by men who know little or nothing on the subject. But the end will be good if it leads to the presidents becoming secretaries to government or having some other equally authoritative position conferred on them. I worry you now merely for the sake of information as to how we are going on. The extract is emphatically private, as I need not say. And neither writer nor receiver have any knowledge of how I meant to use it.

28 December 1865

*Private.* I don't like to let anything go on in the India sanitary department without your being cognizant. Sir John Lawrence has written a despatch home (this was *before* he received Mr Ellis's paper) proposing to modify the constitution of the India presidency sanitary commissions as follows: that, as the opinions of the inspector general of hospitals, quartermaster general and inspector general of works can always be obtained by the commission or by the government, in future there shall only be *a sanitary commissioner* and *a secretary*, the latter to be a medical officer, the present "president" to become the sanitary commissioner. Whenever it may be necessary to assemble committees for any particular object, those officers, civil, military or medical, who are best up to the subject, to be associated with the sanitary commissioner.

Sir John Lawrence gives three reasons for modifying the constitution of these commissions: (1) that it is unnecessarily expensive; (2) that the several members who have other duties to perform are practically of little use; (3) that, constituted as it is, there is risk of disagreement between the commission and head of medical department or of other departments. (To this third reason, the India Office says: "The fact of the deputy inspector general being *on* the commission when his chief is *not*, and the chance of there being differences of opinion between the inspector general and the commission renders it inconvenient that the subordinate should in any way be likely to clash with his superior.")

Sir John Lawrence says farther: "Independently of pecuniary saving, there will be positive advantage to the cause of sanitary improvement."

This, in a few words, is the substance of the despatch, which farther proposes, on the occurrence of a vacancy in the presidentship, it is proposed to reduce his salary from 3500 to 2500 per month in Bengal, and to 2000 Rs. per month in Madras and Bombay, the secretaries to be carefully selected medical officers and to receive 600 per month in Bengal and 500 in Madras and Bombay, in addition to *new* scale of pay. (At present they only have 600 and 500 in addition to *old* rates of pay.) Wonderful to say, the I.O. "wished the salaries of presidents had been left alone." No action has been taken at present on this despatch. And I have obtained that the papers shall be officially referred to the War Office sanitary commission. They are already there by this time.

Upon what *they* say, and upon what *you* say, will virtually depend what determination the I.O. takes. What I strongly feel is this: we must go on the "give and take" principle. If *they* will give us the principle, as set forth in Mr Ellis's paper, of putting the sanitary commissioner in some way in connection with the finance department, let us take the modification now proposed; it is not so bad. But don't let us accept it without. (I send Mr Ellis's paper, in case you should not have a copy by you.) We have not yet seen the papers, and we cannot judge till we know the details as to how the proposed modification will work. (It appears that the "sanitary commissioner" is to be simply an advising officer.) I cannot make out that Sir C. Wood has ever seen Mr Ellis or ever read his paper or ever received your letter, given to Mr Ellis. But then he has been ill.

Source: From four letters to James Pattison Walker, Florence Nightingale Museum (LMA) H1/ST/NC1/65/20-23, copy Add Mss 45781 ff308-13

26 October 1865

We are all in confusion, because of Lord Palmerston's death. . . .

It is sad what you say about the hurry of Indians to come home. May it not be the result of the state of health which Indians suffer from the bad sanitary state of Calcutta. Bombay and Madras are not in such a hurry, I believe, are they?

As for yourself, I am afraid that cardiac and lung affections always suffer from the great altitude of Simla (do not they?) and that, though Calcutta is worst, Simla is bad for you.

I have failed to acknowledge your "No. I. Return showing the sickness and mortality, etc., military and civil population, etc. Bengal during month of –" i.e., the form, which you were so kind as to send me. It has excited a good deal of attention at the War Office and Army Medical Department here. And I send you their remarks, though fearing that you may think them impertinent.

3 November 1865

*Private.* I think you must not look at the sanitary commission as "at an end." You are doubtless aware that Sir J. Lawrence wrote a very full minute, dated 9 January, to the secretary of state here, proposing an organization for the Public Health Service in India. Some modifications will probably be proposed. But I think this is only a beginning of a great development of the service. In the meantime, let me again say how deeply grateful I feel to you for all the invaluable information, the records of proceedings and letters I have received from you. And I cannot but still regret that you have not been able to continue in the sanitary commission under its new form. Sanitary work I am sure you will do wherever you are. . . .

I may mention to you, quite privately, that we have a powerful protector in Lord Stanley (who was president of the royal commission). He will do all he can in this matter. I fear the impending renewal of political agitation will not be favourable to departmental work. Still, as Lord Stanley says himself, "we must do our best." Parliament will not be called together till January, he tells me.

It may be that, if these Ministers under Lord Russell break down (Lord Palmerston's loss is incalculable—it was *he* who dragged every too liberal measure through the Cabinet) this next session may see Lord Stanley minister for India.

3 November 1865

I have never acknowledged the "Memorandum on Hospitals" by Dr C.A. Gordon ("*our*" Dr Gordon) which you were so good as to send me. It is an admirable paper—a very good solution of the problem how far and in what manner the hospital regulations in use here are adapted for India.

26 November 1865

*Private.* I have to thank you most sincerely for sending me a copy of your "First Annual Report," which contains most gratifying evidence of the administrative energy, intelligence and earnestness of its authors and of Sir John Lawrence. The more we reflect on it, the more important does this question of the health of our army in India become. To say much, it is worthy of all of your life that has been given to it.

I showed your "report" quite privately to (General-Register Office) Dr Farr. And I send you his remarks (on the other side). I know you like to hear every opinion of any importance.

When all that you have recommended has been carried out, we shall see the results in still more greatly diminished mortality.

You have again raised the discussion regarding the estimated death rate. We consider that your points can be easily answered, especially where you have run parallels between certain home rates and yours, which do not resemble each other in the circumstances. But what is really wanted now is onward progress in the great work of civilizing and saving life. And this you are doing.

Source: From two letters to Douglas Galton, ADD MSS 45763 ff94-95 and 173-75

9 November 1865

MOST PRIVATE. *Burn.* I know nothing, except from the *Times* and yourself, about the duke of Somerset and Lord de Grey. But if the duke of Somerset comes to the War Office, our sanitary commission may be endangered just at the very time when India and Sir John Lawrence depend upon it, and INDIA work comes to it. If you will tell me the earliest information, I will do what I can about this (sanitary commission).

Lord Palmerston's loss to us is irreparable. For nine years I have never asked him anything (you may be sure I did not ask him often) but he did it. If there was anything right to be done, he made a joke, but he did it. It was he who put you where you are. It was he who put Lord de Grey where he is, etc. I wrote to you a letter I have mislaid, congratulating ourselves you are not gone yet and stating that Mr Brown was about to be minister at Peking. (I hope he will like it.)

I was very much pleased with what you said about Sidney Herbert at Bournemouth and sorry you had not time to say more. You are the only man who appreciates him now. How little his wife knows him. I wrote all this to you in the letter I have mislaid—small loss to you.

Please burn this. I hope you have burnt that letter I wrote about Dr Sutherland going abroad and the (Lord Stanley) work. It was *quite* for yourself alone.

11 May 1866

*Private.* I am very much obliged to you for your note (about Dr Sutherland). Would you please tell him today (he will be at the sanitary commission) *without making any allusion to me,* that he can't be spared, for the next two or three months, *for a longer time than seventeen days at once.* (I believe that would decide him at once not to go till the autumn, for no man on earth but yourself could induce him to do Malta in fifteen days and Gibraltar in another seventeen days. He will certainly choose to do them both together and take two months about it. But if not, an absence of fifteen-seventeen days would not damage my business so much.)

I am sure you will be within the truth if you tell him he *must* be in England (to do the business) for the next two or three months at least. But he quotes *you* to me as saying that he ought to be gone already (to Malta and Gibraltar). You are the only person who could persuade him to stay (till autumn). If *I* were to show him your note, he would only go the faster. But *you* could make him stay at once. And if the Indian sanitary business is not settled in the next two-three months, it will never be done at all. But Dr Sutherland thinks the world moves round himself, that all the India business stops till he comes back, which it doesn't.

Pray be positive with Dr Sutherland (I need not supply you with arguments, for somehow you are the only person who can make him do what you want). And put it as "business" *generally*, not as *India* business specially, to induce him to stay.

*Burn* this and, above all, deny my acquaintance, like two pickpockets in a crowd.

Source: From a letter to Douglas Galton, ADD Mss 45763 ff123-27

6 January 1865 [1866][78]

*Private and Confidential. The Presidency Sanitary Commissions.* I don't know what you know about this affair, nor how to tell it you shortly. But it is just the greatest crisis we have had since Sir J. Lawrence became governor general.

Sir J. Lawrence has written home a despatch "smashing our commissions," so said Dr Sutherland. I wrote to the India Office and found it was nothing of the kind. Sir J. Lawrence proposes to modify these commissions. And the whole matter has been referred to your War Office commission. The papers have been actually sent you from the India Office, as they informed me and as I informed Dr Sutherland. Dr Sutherland said he would desire Mr Frederick [secretary of

78 The letter was dated 1865, but the archivist seems to be right in dating it 1866 on the basis of both content and context.

the Army Sanitary Commission] to send them to me. But a week has elapsed and nothing has come. Would you take this in hand, *and make sure that the papers relating to Sir John Lawrence's despatch* concerning the modifying of the presidency sanitary commissions *are sent to me forthwith*? I would, and perhaps may write to Mr Frederick myself. But I don't like assuming this right. It is absolutely necessary that no decision should be come to till Sutherland's and Ellis's return (by the War Office commission) or judgment will go against us by default. Sutherland *assumes* that no meeting will take place till his return.

I assume no such thing. It is perfect madness of these two men to go away when the very existence of their India commissions is threatened. Mr Ellis writes to me from Paris saying that he would get off going to Algiers now, *if it were not for their instructions*, meaning, I suppose, their ladies (I find two ladies are going!!!). And Dr Sutherland, that Ellis, finding this present state of affairs to be as it is, ought to have delayed the expedition altogether (which he certainly ought). And then Mr Ellis writes to me that *I* must, at all risks and costs (by the police, I suppose) "delay decision" till their return and prevent a meeting of the War Office commission.

You see, I can't tell you the whole previous story. You probably know that our object was to get the presidents of these commissions made a kind of secretaries to government, to get it *ordered* from home that public health in India is entitled to a place in the budget and that the India Office is in earnest in wishing that the P[ublic] H[ealth] Department, civil and military, is to have a recognized position as a branch of the administration, that the head of it should be in direct communication with the government and not be impeded by passing through the offices of six secretaries.

Everything was in good train. Mr Ellis had written a very able paper upon it. I had introduced him to Lord Stanley, who was helping with all his might. Here was the moment to gain all we wanted. For we should have said, we will take your modification, if you will give us our principle. And now these two men have gone away to stare at Astley's[79] (when we know on the highest authority that all they can learn in Algeria they could have learnt at Paris). And have wrecked the whole thing, wrecked their own business, if ever a thing was a man's own business.

---

79 Hugh John Astley, consul at Algiers.

I wrote to Lord Stanley—the only thing I could do. And he has answered, a long and well-considered letter, but advising the acceptance of Sir J. Lawrence's modifications. Till I receive the papers—and while I have them—nothing can be done. *Please secure that the papers be sent me at once.*

yours most disconsolately
Florence Nightingale

Source: From an incomplete note and a letter to William Farr, Wellcome Ms 5474/98 and 99, typed copies ADD Mss 43400 ff100-02

[January 1866]

The compensation to my disturbed state of mind has been a convert to the sanitary cause I have made for Madras: no less a person than Lord Napier[80] (I managed to scramble up to see him before he sailed).

19 January 1866

*Private.* I thank you immensely for your note on determining prison mortality. It was after this wise [a] Bengal sanitary commissioner wrote to me privately for it. I said, write officially. In the meantime I asked you and you kindly sent (and I sent to them) a note on the way of determining prison mortality.

This, your *great* note, I should much like to await Dr Sutherland's return, as the Indians have got your little note. And I have written to the Army Sanitary Commission here to say so.

You shall hear I don't want them to have any important meetings till Dr Sutherland's return. But bless your heart, Dr Sutherland thinks the world moves round himself, and that all business stops naturally till he comes back, both in India and in England. He makes no arrangements for it while he is away.

80 Francis Napier (1819-98), 10th Baron Merchistoun and 1st Baron Ettrick, governor of Madras 1866-72. He paid Nightingale a visit before going to India. He was eager to implement sanitary reforms and introduced female nursing to Madras. He had been secretary to the British Embassy at Constantinople during the Crimean war. A different person was Robert Cornelius Napier (1810-90), later Lord Napier of Magdala, who met Nightingale in December 1869. He was commander-in-chief in India 1870-76.

Source: From a letter to Lord Stanley, Liverpool Record Office, Derby Collection 920/15/93

1 February 1866

*Private.* I am very grateful for your note of 29 January. I only wish we *did* "want" your help. There is no condition so desperate as that which does *not* "want" help.

The India Office is dead. We are abominably dead at the War Office. But at least we are not buried. At least we can find a paper in six weeks. At least we know whether we have one or not. The despatch of Sir John Lawrence concerning the modifying of the presidency commissions, an abstract of which was sent to me (with this I troubled you), and which the I.O. told me *was sent* to the W.O. commission for reference, hangs fire. The fact is, I believe, they (the India Office) have lost it. Anyhow, it has not reached the W.O.

On the other hand, we are always doing the most spasmodic things. They have sent a commission to stare at the French troops in Algeria (they might just as well have sent them to stare at Astley's): Dr Sutherland; Mr Ellis; the Madras Sanitary Commission president, whom you were so good as to see; and others. They have been gone a month and may be gone another month. And this just at the most important time of our year. I should not make my moan so loud but that soon people will be so busy in politics and you will be turning out ministries and upsetting powers and principalities[81] and you will be too busy to think of us when I come to claim your help.

But what I write about now is to ask you if you would not think fit to talk to Lord Napier (he was expected in town on Wednesday, yesterday, and sails at the end of this month or beginning of March) about our affair of the presidency sanitary commissions. (I do not mean as to Sir J. Lawrence's proposed modification but as to the general principle.) What we want is to have it *ordered* from home that public health in India is entitled to a place in the budget and that the I.O. should be in earnest in wishing that the Public Health Department, civil and military, should have a recognized position as a branch of the administration, that the head of it should be in direct communication with the government and not be impeded by passing through the offices of half a dozen secretaries. I believe this is, generally, your own view. Would you not think well to impress it on Lord Napier? Sir J. Lawrence has not the least idea how the governors of the minor presidencies thwart

81 An allusion to Eph 3:10.

and insult the sanitary principle. If he had, I think it would in some degree modify his view. But he thinks every man like himself. However, he has never said one word—at least not to me or so far as I know—against the above principle. Only his own virtues, as I think, prevent his seeing the necessity and force of it as we do. What he *has* said has been, generally, in its favour. But I wish he would PRESS it on the secretary of state.

Lord Dufferin,[82] I was told, declined Madras except with the reversion of the governor generalship. It seems an odd bargain for a man to make. It is said that Lord Napier expects this same reversion. You know about all this much better than I. Anyhow, Lord Napier would be a most valuable convert for us, if you would undertake him.

I only wish I could accept your most kind offer of calling upon me. But just at this time I am entirely a prisoner—even to one position—from illness.

Source: From a letter to Sir Harry Verney, Wellcome (Claydon copy) Ms 9002/3

9 February 1866

*Private. Burn.* I think that nothing had better be said to Lord Napier (especially if Lord Stanley is there) further than that I hope to be well enough to see him, Lord Napier, before he starts.

To tell you the truth, Lord Stanley wrote to me last month wishing to see me. In declining, I asked *him* to see and talk to Lord Napier. These second-rate statesmen are so queer—it would be as well now to take it quietly and not to look as if there were any active intrigue to convert Lord Napier.

I hope to be able to see him. Please learn when he goes.

Source: From a letter to Lord Stanley, Liverpool Record Office, Derby Collection 920/15/94

18 February 1866

PRIVATE. Lord Napier [Ettrick] is to go on the 23rd. He is at 24 Prince's Gate. There has been some correspondence between him and me and I hope to be able to see him for a minute before he starts. But all this would be nothing compared to your seeing him. And of course I shall not know from him whether he has seen you or not. He is clever and able but false. (I had had a previous acquaintance with him at Con-

82 Marquess of Dufferin and Ava (1826-1902), earlier governor general of Canada, under secretary for India 1864-66, governor general and viceroy of India 1884-88.

stantinople—you know he was secretary of embassy there during the Crimean War.) I shall be sorry if he becomes governor general, though it is not deliberate falseness, but half of it the falseness of genius. (He did a thing by me which is so common it is hardly worth mentioning: warned me against his chief and then took his chief's word against me and threw me overboard in the midst of my greatest difficulties. But of course he is too much of a man of the world to remember this. We are very *civil* together.) Please burn this note, the object of which merely is to tell you of Lord Napier's movements. He is reading your India report.

Source: From a letter to Robert Rawlinson, Boston University 1/4/48

13 March 1866

*Private.* I have been asked to send you the enclosed (from India) containing an extract, marked in red, from the engineer's report about the drainage of Calcutta, and to ask your opinion generally on the "insuperable" difficulties in the way of drainage, shown, as they appear to think, by their facts. . . . Who would ever have thought of building a great capital on a quicksand, and then complaining that it was unhealthy? Was it the true sons of old Leadenhall Street[83] who did this?

Source: From a letter to John Strachey, Columbia University, Presbyterian Hospital School of Nursing C85

26 March 1866

*Private.* As I am uncertain where or if this letter will reach you, I will only thank you most cordially for your very kind letter of 22 February containing too the reasons for Sir John Lawrence's minute concerning the remodelling of the sanitary commissions. You have done us a most important service thereby. For (1) the secretary of state for India here was not aware that this minute had arrived, and the India Office had been searched in vain for it; (2) he was not aware of the reasons for Sir John Lawrence's determination and against Mr Ellis's paper, and was in the act of writing to him in a different sense. I will say no more at present but only hope that you will permit me to write to you in Oudh [John Strachey became chief commissioner of Oudh in 1866].

83 The East India Company's offices were in Leadenhall St.

Source: From a letter to Lord Stanley, Liverpool Record Office, Derby Collection 920/15/95

8 April 1866

*Private.* At the risk of being a nuisance to you, I always like to let you know what is going on about your India sanitary commissions. And I think I had better tell my story through Sir John Lawrence's mouth. I have had letters from him of 19 January and 22 February, marked *Private,* but of which I shall venture to give you the substance. (Both of these letters are written after he had received Mr Ellis's paper, of which you have a copy—Mr Ellis, the president of the Madras Sanitary Commission).

Sir J. Lawrence says: "As regards the reconstruction of our sanitary organization, we are sending home to the secretary of state" a despatch "proposing a further change." x x "I have no doubt that you will see the despatch and therefore I had better not send it you." (This despatch has never arrived. I have had a sharp lookout kept for it—for which I have the means now which I had not under Sir C. Wood. It is certain it is not arrived: thus I *say.* I waited impatiently for its arrival before communicating with you. But now the Easter recess is all but over and I am afraid to wait any longer, lest I should not catch you at all.)

Sir John Lawrence says:

> We propose that, as regards the army, the president of the committee shall be a sanitary commissioner, with a secretary, working through the military department, and that in all civil matters, he shall be a deputy secretary in the home department. I incline to think that this scheme will answer very well, but, after all, the main point is the motive power, which guides and impels the whole concern. If this prove defective, no system which can be devised will work satisfactorily.
>
> A separate Department of Health, unconnected with any other, would not, I think, answer. All they do, whether in procuring funds or in spending such funds, must go through other departments. And as regards the troops, unless, at the outset, the sanitary chief can carry the heads of the military with him, nothing can be done. We propose that in each province the inspectors general of jails should be the deputy secretaries to lieutenant governors and chief commissioners on sanitary matters, and that in districts the civil surgeons should be the health officers. In this way we shall be able to organize a regular system all over India at a moderate cost. At any rate, we shall make a beginning. I hope therefore that you will be satisfied with the scheme.

(In all Sir J. Lawrence's letters, there is a tone of discouragement and sorrow. In this very letter, speaking of another thing, he says how people "in utter ignorance or in defiance of circumstances, urge" him "while they will be the first to break out in reproaches. So much for the happiness of holding a high position and trying to do one's duty." He scarcely ever writes to me without some expression of this kind. And indeed our Cabinet and governors of presidencies are full of prejudice against him. But I don't betray him, except to you. People might think him disappointed. F.N.)

The letter of 22 February enters much more into detail, still speaking of the despatch as gone (but it is not come). After speaking of "propositions" "lately sent to the secretary of state" "which will, I hope, lead to the establishment of working sanitary bodies throughout India." x x

> The great difficulty hitherto with which we have had to contend on this side of India has arisen from the fact that the Government of India, to which the sanitary commission is attached, does not itself directly administer the government. In all matters of detail, it has no more means of interfering (so far at least as civil administration is concerned) in Bengal, in the North Western Provinces or in the Punjab, than it has in Madras or Bombay. When anything has to be *done*, it must be done by the local governments and not by the Government of India, and the local governments are always jealous of interference. No sanitary advisors have been given to the lieutenant governors and chief commissioners in this presidency, although some of our provinces are, in everything but nominal dignity, more important than the presidencies of Madras and Bombay, each of which has its separate sanitary commission.
>
> According to the proposed scheme, there will be a health officer in every important district and station, and a principal officer of health at the headquarters of each of the local governments and administrations in this presidency. Under the Government of India itself, it is proposed to have, instead of a sanitary commission as at present, a sanitary commissioner, with a medical officer as a secretary *for the army*. This sanitary commissioner will also be a deputy secretary to the Government of India in the home department. In the former capacity he will act just as the president of the sanitary commission does now. The only difference will be that there will not be any paid members of the commission, except the secretary. These members have been found to be almost useless in all three presidencies. If the president of the commission requires more help than the secretary can give him, he has practically to get it from outsiders and

> not from the members of the commission in the great majority of cases. As deputy secretary to the Government of India in the home department, the sanitary commissioner will have the means of keeping up a constant supervision of the proceedings of all the sanitary officers under the local governments. According to this plan, the primary responsibility will rest with the local governments and administrations, with whom is all the power of action. I need not now trouble you with more details, but I believe that, if the home government approve the scheme, sent to the secretary of state, we shall have a really practical system of sanitary administration. x x
>
> In the minute in which the propositions were sent to the home government (this has not yet come: F.N.) it was shown that Mr Ellis ignored the fact that, in the presidency of Bengal, which comprises three fourths of India, the Government of India has (as I have said above) no direct control over the details of the civil administration. Consequently plans which may answer for a government like that of Madras are quite inapplicable here. x x
>
> Another defect was that he (Mr Ellis) misunderstood the position of our Indian secretary to government. In India this officer is not an executive minister, as he is in England. If he be a man of talent, he will doubtless practically have much influence, but he can never be the nominal head of a department. The *theory* of the Indian secretariat is that the secretary is a mere *clerk*. According to the arrangements proposed for Bengal, the sanitary commissioner will belong to the secretariat, but this will be proper because the executive work will rest with the local governments and administrations.

(Sir John Lawrence's propositions have been sent home in the shape of a very full minute of his own, concurred in by the whole council, and I hope that they may be sanctioned, for they will, I am sure, produce excellent results.)

The last paragraphs are not, as you will see, from Sir J. Lawrence's letter, but from Mr Strachey's, the late president of the Bengal Sanitary Commission and now chief commissioner in Oudh.

My letter will grow out to such an immense length that I must only add that Lord de Grey is well disposed towards us. (But he has no fight in him. And he is *little*.) I know that, if you thought well to show him a strong interest about these sanitary matters, it would do us a great deal of good. Lord de Grey has, as yet (in our matter), merely written a private letter to Sir J. Lawrence, telling him how much interested he is in the sanitary commissions, enumerating the works they have to do and hoping Sir J.L. will give them importance and will send him home a scheme for the development of the organization of a Public Health Service, etc. (I think I mentioned to you that Lord de Grey had sent Mr Ellis, Dr Sutherland and others to Algeria to see what the French have been doing there in our matters. Their report, which is not yet out, bears closely on the Indian question. It shows that it is no use improving barracks, military administration, etc., without improving stations and country round stations, so far as health is concerned. Mr Ellis sailed yesterday for India.)

The India Office swears by all his gods, if he has any, that Sir J. Lawrence's despatch or minute is not yet arrived. And Lord de Grey empowered Mr Ellis to ascertain this for himself with Mr Oliphant, who keeps the register of despatches. (It's my belief it is there all the while. F.N.) Finding this and finding that Mr Ellis would not see the despatch, in which his paper was mentioned and answered by Sir J.L., I told Mr Ellis, without of course showing him Sir J.L.'s letters, the substance of them. And he has written the four memoranda enclosed, copies of which have been sent to Lord de Grey. (I must ask you to consider all this as "private" and to return me Mr Ellis's papers.)

If, when the despatch comes, I write to Sir J. Lawrence, as he has been so good as to write to me, I think I must not criticize his scheme or Indian administration or anything of that kind, which we know nothing about, but simply go into the work to be done and the means of doing it, which we know more about in England than they do in India. I think I might go into the subject of Mr Ellis's note (enclosed) on "sanitary commissions to be retained," but not into that of the note (enclosed) on "Initiative of the Supreme Government" or "Functions of Secretaries to Government," which it would be a simple impertinence for me to go into with the governor general.

I have put off and off troubling you about all this till the despatch had arrived and till we knew Lord de Grey's view about answering it. But, as I say, the despatch being invisible and the political fight imminent, I am afraid to put it off any longer. I think Lord de Grey will answer in that sense, viz., enumerating the objects of sanitary work. Does Sir J. Lawrence think that his scheme will still answer to carry out these? If not, will he propose some further scheme?

I have made my letter of such a hideous length that I will only just mention, with regard to irrigation, that the idea has been propounded, both at home and by Lord Napier, that a clause might be put into any irrigation act (or whatever you call it) making certain sanitary restrictions, e.g., such and such conditions to be submitted to government.

Source: From a draft letter to Sir John Lawrence in Dr Sutherland's hand, ADD Mss 45777 ff75-78

[3 May 1866]

I would have replied to your letter of -- [19 January 1866] long ago, only that I have been waiting to see the despatch in which you have defined the future organization of the sanitary service in India. I have made inquiries repeatedly at the India Office and I can hear nothing about it; I shall delay no longer and shall state a few points arising out of your letter with the intention of writing perhaps more fully should it appear to be necessary to do so after I have seen the despatch itself.

Of course you will distinctly understand, in what I am about to say, that I can pretend to give no opinion whatever on the special organization required to suit the local circumstances of so vast a country as that which you rule over. You in India are far too well up to your work to submit to any interference in such matters. All I can do, and all I desire to do, is to state very briefly the objects we all have in view in organizing a new branch of the public service in India, leaving it to your far wiser heads to point out what administrative steps should be taken to secure that the contemplated objects should be realized.

At the time the report of the royal commission was drawn up the entire subject was so new that we were all of us indisposed to recommend any specific form of sanitary administration simply because such a course would have amounted to our passing a judgment on the practicability of a scheme which might afterwards have been found injurious rather than useful. We indicated the appointment of *presidency* commissions because of the vast extent of country over which the new measures would have to be applied, because we thought that a central administration would, from mere distance, be incompetent to deal with the problems.

Next, we stated what the functions of the commissions would be, and we described them as *mainly consultative.* The expression was chosen to leave you ample room for arranging details, but we were certainly of opinion that the president should occupy a position distinct from the commission, that he should have a different relation to the government, and that his commission should simply advise him in any matter he might bring before it, but that the commission should have no initiative as a body. Our view in this was to render all differences between the commission and other departments impossible. Only in order to do so and at the same time to forward the good cause, it was in our view necessary to give a distinct responsibility to the president, who would in fact become minister of health in the presidency, in which duty he would be aided by the *opinion* of a commission constituted out of all the elements necessary in order to [lead to] the formation of a trustworthy opinion.

So far as I can judge from the various papers I have seen, this arrangement has never been tried. The president and commission have been so to speak one body, without clearly defined positions, sometimes answering questions referred to it, at others taking the initiative more or less, and finally ending by getting into quarrels and hot water with various people, so that the end has come. This result always appeared to me to be inevitable from the moment that a new body was so to speak placed on the toes of all the old departments. I still think that the result would have been different if the presidents had formed so to speak part of the local governments, if they had been selected simply for administrative ability (which certainly was secured) and if their councils had been made simply advising to the presidents.

It is not for me to say whether the proposals sketched in your note would remedy the defects in the first administrative machinery. I don't consider myself at all competent to deal with such a question and I shall limit what I have to say simply to pointing out the things which should be done in order to improve the sanitary state of the civil and military populations of India, leaving it to you to decide what machinery will answer the purpose best.

The first thing in any new organization ought as it appears to me to be to get rid of the idea that sanitary administration is in any sense or manner antagonistic to anything except dirt and ill health. The originators of the movement in England did much evil, perhaps unavoidably, by saying to all public bodies, "See how dirty you keep yourselves, let us clean you." This set their back up and hence it has in part arisen that until this present time nobody in England has received Hygiea as a welcome guest. She has been turned from many a door in her time mainly by want of civility in her chaperons.

The French, who understand what administration is, have avoided this error by making hygiène part of their general administration and combining it with all the departments where its aid is required. Thus questions of hygiène arise constantly in commerce, manufacture, agriculture and public works. The French have taken hold of these and they have united all these departments under one ministry which also takes cognizance of all questions affecting health which can by possibility arise in any of the departments. The minister of health is the minister of agriculture, commerce and public works. He is an administrative officer, of course, and all questions in hygiène are sent by him to a special permanent council, the comité d'hygiène, which contains the best men in France in their several departments of medicine, physiology, hygiène, chemistry, applied arts, mechanics, architecture, engineering, etc. The office is one of high honour, besides being paid. Their reports are always acted on although their position is chiefly consultative, and even the minister gives his decision on any paper involving health questions; the health element is provided for in the reply and not separately.

In Algeria they go even further for each conseil in the dependency (there are three): one for each division besides certain selected persons contains the heads of the various departments who would have to give effect to the advice of the conseil. For instance, on the conseils are the chief of the police, the inspector of colonies (who attends to all agriculture, country drainage, etc.), the engineer of mines, the engineer of *ponts et chaussées* [highways or civil engineer], the chief of the department of public works, the principal medical officer with several officiers de santé, the general of division, etc. The presidents are the préfets.

I have given these details to show the manner in which our principles have been applied in France.

The questions with which you would have to deal in India are substantially the same as those with which the French have dealt in Algeria. You have to diminish or remove malaria by public drainage works: you have to apply irrigation so as not to be injurious and to improve agriculture (deep ploughing and draining have cured some of the worst parts of Algeria). Next you have the whole mass of questions arising out of towns and villages, cleansing, draining, water supply, police regulations of all kinds, apportionment of rates, by-laws, trades or manufactures, injuries to health, management of epidemics, management of great emergencies affecting the public health, such as inundations, pilgrimages, sanitary state of prisons, census, registration of [illeg] births, deaths and marriages, uniform direction of the Public Health Service all over the presidency, selection of sites for stations, bazaars, etc., sanction of plans for public works and buildings where health questions are concerned. I could give more details, but already I have stated enough to show that whoever undertakes the work must be a most able man and the head of a great department. It is not inspection which is wanted so much as energetic and wise direction. The head of such a department would have to work by inspectors under him it is true, but the head should be a director and not an inspector. In fact in India it looks very much like as if the entire home government and civilization of the country would fall into the hands of this new department, while all that related to justice and hanging might be done by somebody else.

The head of the department would of course require advice from the most skilled heads you could get and here a permanent council of health would be of immense advantage. The cheapest way would be to select the very best men and to pay them as the French do for every attendance, fixing these at once a week or once a fortnight unless they are called together at other times by the minister of health.

This is what strikes me as necessary and I must now leave you to think out the subject with reference to your own proposal. One thing is evident and that is that a subordinate officer would scarcely do as the head of such a department. The virtual heads in Algeria are the governor general, the governors of provinces, préfets and generals of divisions. In fact it is a special function of all the great officers of state to protect the public health or to render the country habitable. This with the French was a matter of life and death and they have reduced the army death rate from 80 to 12½ per 1000. The civil death rate is now about equal to that of France, and they can rear children quite well although all perished formerly. You would have to provide clauses in all contracts about irrigation for combined works of drainage to go along with the irrigation works.

Source: From a letter to Lord de Grey, ADD MSS 45778 ff36-37

7 May 1866

I have obeyed your desire in sending, as soon as I could, some criticisms on Sir John Lawrence's proposed machinery for public health. . . .

As to such questions as the initiative of the supreme government, the functions of secretaries, I felt it would be an impertinence, both to you and to him, for me to enter upon them. Should you however wish for any more practical suggestions before you make your decision, of course I should esteem it an honour to furnish them.

I wrote to Sir J. Lawrence on this subject by last mail and I shall write again by next mail, by his desire. Of course it would be a very great advantage, both for me and for him, if I did not say anything in opposition to your opinion. I am not afraid of your being startled by our list of sanitary duties as you know the subject as well as we do. I have indeed limited myself to enumerating what the public health machinery in India will have to do, instead of entering upon any theory.

Source: From a letter to Douglas Galton, ADD MSS 45763 ff167-70

9 May 1866

*Private.* Dr Sutherland, whenever he wants to worry me, always announces that he is going to start next Friday for some months' absence. And this he has done perpetually (about Malta and Gibraltar). But he has now stated definitively that he is going *in a fortnight,* that he does it *because of* YOUR *urgency,* that he goes over land to Malaga and so to Gibraltar by himself, *though he does not like it,* thence to Malta; consequently that he will not be back till the end of the session, that this Friday will be the last meeting of the Army Sanitary Commission. . . .

What is *certainly* Dr Sutherland's work (even more than mine) is the *Indian* sanitary work. If I were to see you, I would tell you the whole history. As it is, I will tell you that a despatch of Sir J. Lawrence's has been waiting since 19 January at the India Office (*reorganizing the whole India Public Health Service*), that Sir J. Lawrence wrote to me by the same mail about it, that it was never found till last Saturday, and then only by Lord de Grey's own hands, urged by me, that we are now doing this, that I cannot possibly undertake this responsibility without Dr Sutherland, that, for at least the next two, three, four months, this will be going on. (I am the only person left except Lord Stanley; Lord Stanley consults, he does not advise me upon this India *sanitary* affair.) If Dr Sutherland goes, I must give it up. I am not afraid of responsibility (I think my life has shown that). But I do not choose to incur responsibility which I am incapable of properly fulfilling. If you wish for more information, viz., in what way it was the absence of Messrs Ellis and Sutherland which did the Indian mischief, and what there is now to be done to repair it, which CANNOT be done in the autumn, whereas Dr Sutherland's absence in the *autumn* would not at all affect the Indian business, I am ready to give it. Please BURN this. (N.B. The India Office is thoroughly ashamed of itself for having been unable to find this despatch for four months.) Therefore do not mention it.

ever yours expectantly
Florence Nightingale

Source: From a letter to Lord Stanley, Liverpool Record Office, Derby Collection 920/15/96

24 May 1866

*Private.* Again I trouble you for no better reason than this: that you may not perhaps have time to attend to us when our affairs are farther advanced. Since I wrote to you last I became so certain from letters from India that Sir John Lawrence's minute on the Public Health Service *had* arrived that I assaulted Lord de Grey again, driving the poor man to the verge of desperation, which was attended with this excellent effect that he found the minute (I believe with his own hands) on 5 May, which had been despatched from India on 19 January. (As the India Office is, I understand, very much ashamed, not at having left a despatch unopened for three months, but at having been detected in it—all this is quite private.)

Here is the minute (enclosed). I have written to Lord de Grey, as he desired, upon it and also to Sir John Lawrence, as *he* desired. We do not think Sir J. Lawrence's proposals will meet the necessities which he points out himself, p 10, para 11 of minute (1).

To fulfill these functions, we think the inspector general of prisons would require to be a very different man. He would need to have years of practical training at home to be fit for such duty. It is true that the inspector generals are medical officers. But the duties are far from being medical. To do the work properly, a man should have a thorough knowledge of what sanitary works are. Otherwise, he would be in no position to judge as to whether certain proposed measures would be useful or injurious. The best Indian medical officers could advise on epidemic questions, but on questions involving sanitary works and expenditures, certainly not. Use them by all means to keep a general superintendence over the public health. But we must have some other officer to say. [folio missing]

As regards health questions, [the French health officer] is assisted by a special *permanent* council, the comité d'hygiène, which contains the best men in France in their several departments of medicine, physiology, hygiene, chemistry, applied arts, mechanics, architecture, engineering, etc. The office is one of high honour, besides being paid. Their reports are always acted on, although their position is simply consultative. And when the minister gives his decision on any papers involving health questions, the health element is provided for in the reply and not separately.

Of course all this is not new to you. I only recapitulate, in order to compare Sir J. Lawrence's inspector of jails and medical secretary, acting without advisors. I have not touched the army question, for it is really subsidiary to the other. And the point would be whether Sir J. Lawrence should not be asked to reconsider the whole question, with special reference not so much to inspection (the necessity for which always involves somebody's neglect) as to providing an administrative machinery capable of dealing practically with the questions.

I believe I am to hear from Lord de Grey further, before he replies to Sir J. Lawrence's minute. (He had already written a private letter to Sir J. Lawrence urging the multiplicity and importance of the sanitary objects.) I am not uneasy at not having heard yet from Lord de Grey in reply to my answer to his of 5 May. Of course, if it takes three months to find a minute, it must take three years to answer it. Would you have the goodness to return me the copies and letters (which I enclose) as soon as possible, as I shall not mention to anyone that I have sent them to you. (And *I* have to answer the India Office in three hours, if they write to me, though they can't answer in three months.)

I come now to my practical object in troubling you. You were so good as to say that, though you did not see fit to interfere with Lord de Grey, you would not object to seeing me, which I interpreted to mean that you would not object to giving me your advice viva voce, although not formally to the India Office. If you would kindly, after reading the minute, tell me whether you would not advise us in this matter of life and death for India, I should be deeply grateful. I am afraid I could not see anyone this week (for I am very ill), even if you were so good as to propose it. But I should like to hold myself at your disposition as much as is possible, knowing well how busy you are, if you will kindly think whether you could not advise us. . . .

You will see that I write in much confusion and with many interruptions. But I hope you will put the meaning into it which is not there.

Source: From a typed copy of a letter to Edwin Chadwick, ADD Mss 45771 f97

30 May 1866

Would it be of any use now my trying to interest Mr J.S. Mill in our India *sanitary* affairs? And, if so, how?

**Editor:** Chadwick responded with a letter about a month later:

> It is now a fortnight ago since I sent to Mill to ask him to see me, to show him Ellis's administrative propositions and get his opinion and, with his opinion, his support from them at the India Department. But he has not answered me on that topic. . . .
>
> From what I see and learn Sir John Lawrence has not answered well as a legislator. I propose to state points to Mill for his opinion. But as I am obliged to wait for something to arise for legislative action, so I apprehend must you. I showed Mill Ellis's letters to me and he was greatly pleased with the results stated on the inquiry. He said moreover that he had heard of Ellis before, that he had noted

him down as a man of great ability and promise. . . . I will keep you informed however of any opportunity for getting Mill's help.[84]

Source: From a letter to Lord Stanley, Liverpool Record Office, Derby Collection 920/15/97

10 June 1866

*Private.* This is only to ask whether you would like to look over the accompanying report of Dr MacPherson, of Madras. It shows how true your sanitary principles were and what results (unlooked for by Indians) have followed even the very partial application of those principles. Our conviction is strong that the 10 per 1000 which your royal commission estimated as the possible mortality of a distant future in India will be arrived at by the time the station improvements are carried out.

Pray be so good as to return me Dr MacPherson's report and Surgeon Macbeth's flysheet. I hope to be able to say next week what Lord de Grey's reply to Sir John Lawrence's Public Health Service proposals will be.

**Editor:** On 28 June 1866 a Tory/Conservative government was elected, with the 14th earl of Derby (father of Lord Stanley) as prime minister; the Liberal Lord de Grey was replaced as secretary of state for India by the Conservative Lord Cranborne.[85] Such repeated political switches made Nightingale's work quite frustrating, given that her contacts had to be recreated every time a new government appeared on the stage and that, in particular, her own political standpoint was more in tune with the Liberals. Lord Stanley became secretary of state for foreign affairs. Nightingale continued to write him, somewhat apologetically, on Indian matters, as we see in the next letter. Later correspondence shows that Lord Stanley responded to her graciously.

84 Letter ca. 1 July 1866, ADD Mss 45771 ff100-01.

85 Robert Arthur Talbot Gascoyne Cecil (1830-1903), Viscount Cranborne 1865, marquess of Salisbury 1868, secretary of state for India 1866-67, later foreign secretary and prime minister.

Source: From two letters to Lord Stanley, Liverpool Record Office, Derby Collection 920/15/98 and 99

4 July 1866

*Private.* I write to you about India, merely because I am desperate. I know quite well that you have no time to attend to us. In the universal crush, it is no use my crying over my share of it, though it comprises 150 millions of H.M.'s subjects. Had you been going to the India Office and left Europe to take care of herself (though we knew it could not be so), it would have been nothing but joy. As it is, I do think Sir John Lawrence will break his heart. And what will become of the 150 millions?

But to my work. You may perhaps remember that Sir John Lawrence wrote a minute on 19 January organizing a Public Health Service for India, that this was not found at the India Office till 5 May. With the businesslike promptitude which so characterizes us, the minute, which should reply to Sir J. Lawrence's, was not determined upon till 18 June, the very day ministers resigned. Lord de Grey then thought he could not pledge his Council to any course and postponed to submit his minute (replying to Sir J. Lawrence) to a *special* committee of five of the Council, ensuring thus that, at all events, it would be brought before his successor. (Of these five, only one would be for us. Or rather, only one knows anything about it.)

The purport of the minute was to point out what was the work to be done in India in the way of public health, what were the intentions of the original royal commission (yours), how these could only be fulfilled by a competent executive department, to prepare schemes of works and to make provision, financial and otherwise, for the execution of improvements (of which an outline was given). After showing that there should be an able *administrative* officer as the head of the Health Department, with certain permanent sanitary and engineering advisors, and others temporarily attached to answer questions, the head of the Health Department having a responsibility towards the government distinct from that of the *commissions.* The governor general was then requested to reconsider his scheme, with a view rather to the *execution* of works than to *inspection.* (And he was asked to show how he proposed the inspectors of prisons to carry out the duties enumerated.)

I have a letter from you, dated 24 May, in which you say that you "agree in thinking that prison inspectors are not the men wanted for the places in which Sir J.L. proposes to put them. You require a higher class of administrators. In the main I go with your letter." You most kindly offer to "try and be at" my "disposal."

I am not now, of course, even dreaming of claiming such a promise. What I thought of was that, if—India being your child—you could and would give the moment's pressure necessary to influence the fate of this unfortunate minute, the thing would be done. Scarcely expecting that you will have time to read this note, I have merely *indicated* the purport of Lord de Grey's minute. But I would send you a very brief analysis of it, together with Sir J. Lawrence's original minute (which you have seen before) and some details on the special (India Council) committee of five which is to consider it, if you could and would take the subject up. If not, pray don't trouble yourself to answer this letter. I shall know, by receiving no answer, that you cannot "undertake for us." And though I shall be bitterly grieved, I could not, I feel, have expected it. Perhaps, at some future time. Please burn this letter, at all events.

6 July 1866

*Private.* I cannot tell you how extremely grateful to you I am for your truly kind note promising that you will speak to Lord Cranborne on the sanitary question, and inferring that you will keep up some degree of supervision over poor India. Lord de Grey has left on record at the India Office the minute in reply to Sir J. Lawrence's of 19 January on the organization of a Public Health Service in India, the purport of Lord de Grey's minute being to ask Sir J. Lawrence to reconsider his proposals, with a view to execution rather than to inspection, the immense amount of works to be done in India being shown, the original intentions of the royal commission recalled and the probable inadequacy of prison inspectors to the task. I must not trouble you with the detail. I will only mention that Lord de Grey did *not* name the special committee, which he at one time thought of appointing, to take this minute in charge and bring it before his successor, because, as he could not have followed the proceedings of the committee, he had doubts whether it would not have been wrecking the minute, Sir Proby Cautley being the only one *positively* friendly to the sanitary question and to the public having health in general. I feel quite hopeful, with your assurance, that you will help on the matter.

We have no cause to complain of the India government; they have the very strongest desire to do what is best. But the subject is still new (even though people are tired of the very word), is no one's special business and things are apt to slip into the wrong groove. I do not know whether you would think well to suggest to Lord Cranborne to refer questions, as usual, to the Army Sanitary Commission (at the

War Office) consisting, as you know, of India Office and War Office members. We have been doing a good deal of work there for India lately, though not so much as we could have wished. (There was an idea of referring the reply to the above-mentioned minute to it. But as the minute must have gone before the regular India Council committee, after all, this idea was not carried out.)

With regard to your great kindness in offering to put me "in direct communication with Lord Cranborne" (I have not the slightest acquaintance with him), if you think I can be of the least use, I shall be only too glad. If you have been so good as to tell him who I am, I might then write to him, without impertinence, should any special case come up especially from Sir John Lawrence. Believe me, dear Lord Stanley,

ever yours faithfully and gratefully
Florence Nightingale
*Please burn.*

Source: From a letter to Lord Cranborne, British Library, Asia, Pacific and Africa Collections, Salisbury Papers

17 July 1866

*Private and Confidential.* Lord Stanley had the kindness to advise me to write to you and to tell *me* that he would tell *you* that he had "advised" me "to write to" you as I "have done to" him. This is my only excuse for what would otherwise be a very great impertinence and what I fear may seem to you such even now, viz., my present application to you on the India public health question. I know I ought to begin, "Miss Nightingale presents her compliments to Lord Cranborne." But the "third person" always becomes confused. Lord Stanley has probably scarcely had the time to tell you my long story. I fear, therefore, I must introduce myself, by saying that my apology for what you may (justly) consider an unwarrantable interference must be the part I have taken in the public health of the army in India for the last eight years, having been in communication with Lord Stanley, Sir C. Wood and Lord de Grey about it, and being now in constant communication with Sir John Lawrence and others in India on the same subject. When Lord de Grey left office, Lord Stanley, of his own accord, kindly asked whether he should "put" me "in direct communication" with you.

This is my general apology. My particular one is that by last mail I received some very pressing letters from India on the subject of the introduction of an efficient public health administration into India, which is after this wise: the spirit of the very general recommendations made by the royal commission which reported in 1863 (presided over by Lord Stanley) had never been completely acted up to—there have been difficulties and clashings in consequence. A minute (of 19 January 1866) was sent home by Sir John Lawrence proposing to connect the Public Health Service with the inspectorship of prisons. The proposal appears to have been made without due consideration of the importance and greatness of the duties; if it were carried out, it would put an end, we believe, to any prospect of efficient progress. (I think I am correct in saying that Lord Stanley concurs in this view.) Lord de Grey was deeply impressed with this defect in the scheme; he drew up a minute (just before he left office) in order to leave his views on record for you, setting forth generally the duties, and asking for a reconsideration of the subject in India, before the organization was finally decided on—of the Public Health Service. I would now venture to ask your favourable consideration for this proposal, because, on the organization of a service adequate for the object, depends the entire future of the public health in India. We commit ourselves into your hands.

Source: From a letter to Mary Carpenter,[86] British Library, Asia, Pacific and Africa Collections Mss Eur. A.110

3 August 1866

I am so overwhelmed with business that, being also entirely a prisoner to my bed from incurable illness, I have not been able to answer your kind note of 21 July as yet. I thank you much for your generous offer of doing anything for me in India but I will not trouble you. Your time is already too well filled. I shall write to Sir John Lawrence (he is at Simla, you know, till October or November) by this or next mail on your account. You have probably already introductions to him. But I enclose an envelope, which will serve as an additional one (to connect you with what I shall write).

86 Mary Carpenter (1807-77), Unitarian philanthropist. She visited India four times and agitated for female normal schools, juvenile delinquents and prison reform in India; co-founder of the Bengal Social Science Association 1867 and one of the founders of the National Indian Association, which promoted social contact between Indians abroad and British people.

Source: Undated note, not in Nightingale's hand, Add Mss 45778 f33

[c1866]

The chief points raised in Colonel Galton's letter relate to the *practicality* of carrying out sanitary reforms in Indian stations and towns in a specific manner. Now we all feel and acknowledge the difficulties, but these are of exactly the same kind as existed at home twenty years ago. The state of Indian towns generally cannot, however, be parallelled in England without going back to the Middle Ages. There is all the lapse of time therefore between the Middle Ages and the England of twenty years ago on which to work. The longer delay in civilization arose from the absence of teachers and methods. England was perhaps the last European state to arrive at the average healthiness of Europe.

Now India can be saved the whole of this long process by very simple actions on the part of the government. There can be brought to bear on the Indian question experience, talent, knowledge and power. An enlightened government can improve India in matters in which the people cannot improve themselves and would, very likely, go on in for ages. The key to the whole is first water supply, second paving, third drainage. This is the order in which civilization advanced in Europe. Society here first got rid of the water carrier, but in England solely by private enterprise. In India the government could do it. Paving was done by the municipalities, drainage chiefly by government, in the first instance. Every difficulty which Colonel Greathed points out had to be met and surmounted in Europe. No difficulty was ever experienced from the habits of the people—only from the apathy and ignorance of those above them.

As to the peculiar methods to be used, these are engineering questions. But it may be stated that, with ingenuity, many of the existing water sources available for stations and towns would afford sufficient water if economically used and if the quality were found to be good. One town at last, Bombay, has been supplied with water within a few years on a principle which cost England ten centuries to arrive at. It was transferred bodily to India with perfect success. Calcutta is being drained professedly on principles which required two centuries to perfect after England had got her capital supplied with water. Steam power is not absolutely necessary. We have yet in England one fort, Fort Pitt, which in these days of coal and steam engines supplies itself by horse labour for 500 persons from a single well and tank for water closets, water latrines, baths and every required appliance, not only for healthy people but for sick. A very great deal of water is still raised in England by windmills. I merely mention these illustrations to show what can be done, but of course in applying principles to specific cases it is the duty of the engineer to do what is best. Certainly no drainage is far better than bad drainage with insufficient water. Very likely the measures will have to be varied at different stations and to be improved and advanced from time to time, but all this will depend on the engineer.

Source: From a letter to Douglas Galton, Add Mss 45763 f256

Embley, Romsey
14 November 1866

I am satisfied that, owing to a long imbroglio of Mr Ellis, Dr Sutherland and the India Office about a despatch of Sir J. Lawrence's, the cause of sanitary reform in India has been put back for years—perhaps for half a century. Mr Ellis writes to me from India that our delay has cost "thousands of lives."

Source: From a letter to Sir Harry Verney, Wellcome (Claydon copy) Ms 9002/73

23 November 1866

Major Bartlett is doubtless an authority. Without local knowledge I can only say that we *believe* no Poor Law could be introduced into India, but only such a system as, e.g., the French have in Algeria. I could not cite this letter to Sir J. Lawrence. But, as I was writing to him on measures connected with it, I took the opportunity of asking him a question founded on this letter. . . .

The effect of the measures mentioned in the letter cannot be decided except after long experience. They have *not* had the effect he supposes here. He appears to be unaware that in Europe the "seclusion" he mentions *has* been tried, with disastrous results. But it is scarcely a question I can enter into, unless (as has been the case) it came manifestly within my duty. With regard to the Poor Law, I am of course no judge as to whether the state of Indian society would bear anything like a Poor Law. *And he is.*

Source: Notes on Sir John Lawrence's "famous minute" (of 19 January 1866) for John Sutherland, Add Mss 45752 ff 168-69

15 March 1867

As you renewed yesterday the conflict about the Indian question and directed me to believe, on the authority of Sir Proby Cautley, that a secretary of state for India would *not* do what a secretary of state for India *did* do, I must remind you of the facts. . . . *Lord de Grey empowered, in writing,* you and me to write such a minute as we desired. *Lord de Grey accepted, in writing,* the minute which we did write. That the minute did not go (to India) was entirely our own doing. We lost it by a day by our own fault.

I will give the dates, without comment (I omit your insisting upon having Mr Ellis [go] to Norwood [a resort area], the last day of Lord de Grey being in town, before Mr Ellis left England—instead of meeting him here, which was the real cause of the minute by Sir John Lawrence not being found till 5 May, when Lord de Grey found it himself).

1866: 15 June (which was a Friday) Lord de Grey writes that he empowers you and me (naming us by name) to write the minute and urges haste. (I immediately write off to you at Norwood to this effect.)

16 June Dr Sutherland does *not* come.

17 June Sunday.

18 June Dr Sutherland comes but will do nothing. Evening: ministers are beaten in the House of Commons.

19 June Dr Sutherland puts into F.N.'s hands a sketch of the minute, not written in concert with her, "for her consideration only." Lord de Grey writes *again* to ask for the minute "*at once.*" F.N. sits up all night to write it. Lord de Grey accepts the minute. For the next fortnight, ministers wavering in their seats, Lord de Grey wavering whether he shall have a committee in the India Council to despatch this minute, asks our advice. Daily messengers between Lord de Grey and F.N. and between F.N. and Dr Sutherland for a fortnight.

3 July ministers go out. Lord de Grey leaves minute in India Office *authorized by him* and for his successor.

One more thing: You have so repeatedly told me that *you had seen* a letter to me from Lord Stanley saying that he would "trust Sir J. Lawrence against us" that I must put down the dates for you. For although you made me get out of bed to find the letters and show you the dates *and you must have been convinced by your own eyes* you again renewed the same error. . . .

1866: 3 January Lord Stanley writes to me, *about quite another matter,* that he "would trust Sir J. Lawrence."

20 [19 according to Nightingale's letter of 8 April] January date of Sir John Lawrence's famous minute (*and of his letter to F.N.*).

20 February F.N. receives Sir J. Lawrence's letter [of 19 January].

5 May *Sir J. Lawrence's minute found* at the India Office.

12 May Lord Stanley writes to F.N. *that he "entirely concurs* IN OUR VIEW *that Sir J. Lawrence's proposal is wholly inadequate for the purpose and that inspectors of prisons are* NOT *the proper instruments.*"

No answer required but that you shall tell me the first Thursday in every month till Doomsday that Lord Stanley concurs in Sir J. Lawrence's minute (against us!).

Source: From two letters to Douglas Galton, ADD Mss 45764 ff56-57 and 68-71

20 March 1867

*Dr Sutherland* v. Sir *G. Stuckley.*[87] I send the enclosed (which please return) merely to know whether you have anything to suggest. The letter of Sir John Lawrence (which Sir H. Verney alludes to) is one, just received, which I showed Sir H. Verney quite casually. Sir J. Lawrence mentions that their army mortality was only 20.11 per 1000 in 1866, 24.24 in 1865. Sir H. Verney said, this would tell very much, in the House, in Dr Sutherland's favour. I always feel nervous about this kind of use, because, of course, India will say that Dr Sutherland and his commission have nothing to do with it (the decrease of mortality), though I think it perfectly legitimate to use such an argument, IF it will tell in your favour for only twenty-four hours. *What do you think?*

28 May 1867

*Private.* I want to consult you about our Indian affairs, which are "getting as drunk as they can be." I divide our misfortunes into two parts: (1) The non-foundation of any public health service, which remains, so far as I know, exactly in the state that Lord de Grey left it on the fatal 18th of June last year (you will remember), despatch still unanswered. *That* is "*same* drunk, Massa, same drunk."[88] (2) The present absolute confusion and want of responsibility in everything that is done in India as to details in sanitary matters. They don't take the advice of their own sanitary commissions, they don't take the advice of yours at home.

*Part 1.* I have spoken to Dr Sutherland over and over again about it. I regret more than anything that I have ever done or not done in all my life; that, for the last year except, of course, in private correspondence with Sir John Lawrence, Mr Ellis and others, I have not attempted to do anything about this Public Health Service. Sir John Lawrence's time is up in another eighteen months. And then we shall be able to do nothing. Dr Sutherland always says: why, Sir John Lawrence is the

87 Sir George Stuckley, MP for Barnstaple.

88 This is a possible reference to Captain Frederick Marryat, *Peter Simple.* "Massa" stands for Mister. It is also in Harriet Martineau, *Retrospect of Western Travel* 115.

chief offender. That is nonsense. Sir John L. is not aware of the consummate importance of a responsible Public Health Service. But *everything* that has been done in India *at all* for us in the sanitary line has been done by him *and by him alone.* The reason why I have done nothing at home during the last year in this has been that I have always been told: "Oh Tories will be out in another six weeks, wait till then." But Tories are not going out. And Sir J. Lawrence *is* (in 1½ years). You know how Dr Sutherland is. When he is doing Malta, Malta contains the world. And the world moves round *himself.* Yesterday I told Dr S. that I meant to wait no longer, but that, after due consultation with you and with him, I intended to do something—the more so as I have been strongly advised to communicate with Sir Stafford Northcote[89] direct. Do you know him well?

*Part 2.* What I want you to do is to give me a *locus standi* [standing], which Lord Stanley did give me with Lord Cranborne (but which I have lost by this long delay). And what I want to consult you about is how this had best be done. It appears that papers come to your commission (but which don't come to me), reversing all the judgments not only of the royal commission, not only of your commission but of their own presidency commissioners, "e.g., soldiers and sick are to sleep on ground floors, doors and not windows are to be used in construction." And that these judgments are obtained by sending the foolscap all over India to see whom it will fit, when of course it fits a great many, and then the opinion of the majority of fools is taken. The next verdict you give will be sent to the Deccan and somebody's opinion in the Deccan will be taken. Good tack [luck?]. If I were only to do my nurse training business in that way, where would it be?

It occurred to me that, if Dr S. would immediately see the subcommittee called (on these last papers), if you would then write me a letter about them (as assistant [under] secretary of state) and send me the papers? And if I were to write to Sir J. Lawrence? (That would give me a locus standi.)

*Part 1.* Still, important as this is, it is not so important as the total want of organization of any public health service in India. And I wanted to ask you: (a) *do* ministers stay in till next year? (b) should I make a statement of the case, taking it up where Lord de Grey left it

89 Sir Stafford Henry Northcote (1818-87), later earl of Iddesleigh, secretary of state for India 1867-68; Nightingale was on friendly terms with him when he was secretary of state.

last year, and bring it before Lord Stanley? I know he will only refer me to Sir S. Northcote. Or (c) would you introduce me at once to Sir S. Northcote and advise me to write to him direct? (*I* don't know him at all.) The Council of India in India and the Council of India at home are awful mistakes. (Sir J. Lawrence is constantly paralyzed by *his* Council.)

Source: From a letter to Dr Richard G. Whitfield,[90] Reynolds Historical Library, University of Alabama at Birmingham 5064

8 June 1867

I feel like a criminal for not having answered your note before about your nephew, Mr Hewlett's[91] truly magnificent work as health officer of Bombay. It is most instructive, full and graphic. The illustrations are a great addition, as it is always well to speak to people through their eyes. It is much better and more full of information than the report of officers of health in England usually are, as to what is to be done as well as what is to be observed. It is very good on the subjects to which it is especially devoted, namely, nuisances resulting from bad management and want of sanitary works. . . .

If you see your way to making the suggestions I should add—not as if it were a want in the report, because, of course, as health officer he has reported completely, but as a suggestion as to how it should be followed up immediately, before we can know really what Bombay and other Indian cities require—we must have engineering reports showing all the existing engineering defects and the plans of water supply, sewerage, house drainage and surface paving, improved streets, etc., necessary to make the cities what they should be.

We have sent minutes to this effect over and over again—not that European health reports embody the engineering points one bit more than Indian health reports do, but that Sidney Herbert established a new principle in our reportings which, had he lived, he certainly would have extended to India. He said: a report must have unity. He insisted upon the evils to be pointed out, the engineering

90 Richard Gullett Whitfield (d. 1877), apothecary and resident medical officer 1858-72 at St Thomas' Hospital.

91 Thomas Gillham Hewlett (1832-89), assistant surgeon with the Bombay Army 1854, served during the Indian Mutiny, health officer of Bombay 1868, then sanitary commissioner for Bombay presidency; deputy surgeon general in Bombay 1879. He authored *Report on Enteric Fever*. See the biographical sketch below in Appendix A.

remedies to be proposed, the constructive arrangements to be carried out, always appearing in the same report. Otherwise a sanitary report is only a report to somebody else, *that* somebody else is to examine into and report what are the essential improvements necessary.

I fear too there is a disposition in India not to take the advice of those whom she has herself constituted as her advisors, e.g., a health officer or sanitary commissioner ought to be the responsible advisor, if constituted the advisor. Instead of that, they send the foolscap round India to see how many heads it will fit—of course it fits a good many—and then they decide by the *majority* (of fools' heads). Also I think there is a tendency "to make the best of things" (not in Mr Hewlett), "to make things easy and pleasant," etc.; when I see people "making the best of things," then I know that somebody is to pay for it somewhere.

Sir Bartle Frere[92] has arrived in England and I hope he will introduce something better into our India Council here.

Source: From a letter to Douglas Galton, ADD MSS 45764 f75

10 June 1867

Could you kindly send me Sir Bartle Frere's address in London, and *what to call him?* Is he a Right Honorable? Is he already a member of the India Council here?

Source: Notes for John Sutherland on an interview with Sir Bartle Frere, ADD MSS 45752 ff179-82

[14 June 1867]

Sir B. Frere told me more in an hour of Indian administration and its difficulties and what ought to be done than Ellis told me in six months or than I learnt from Strachey in two days or from the whole India Council (secretary of state, royal commission and all) in six years. I will do my best to give you the chief points. But I am afraid, so overdone with business as I have been, that I will have no time.

The main point is that under Lord Dalhousie[93] and Lord Canning great steps had been taken to give responsibility and a certain degree of power to local administration, keeping of course the strings of the purse in the supreme government, which is and ought to be the Trea-

---

92 Henry Bartle Edward Frere (1815-84), a close collaborator with Nightingale upon his return from India. See the biographical sketch below in Appendix A.

93 James Andrew Broun-Ramsay (1812-60), 10th earl and 1st marqess of Dalhousie, governor general of India 1847-56.

sury, that under Lord Elgin this began to go back, that Sir John Lawrence has done his very best, has struggled under the *genius loci* in vain, and that during the last four years things have very much resumed their former fatal course, which I am going to describe, that things are in such a position now that *nothing* is done and that they must soon come to a *deadlock.*

The process is this: it is *all* reporting, there is *no* doing, there is absolutely no responsibility *any*where. What is done is this: a report is drawn up, say, at Bombay which, as Sir B. Frere says, is as far from Calcutta as the easternmost point of Europe is from London; it is then sent to a number of authorities in and out of the presidency government; it is then sent to Calcutta; it is referred from Calcutta to a number of authorities all over Bengal; it comes back to Calcutta; it goes through the Supreme Council; it comes back to Bombay after a period of perhaps three years, tied up with a quantity of minute restrictions, perhaps impossible to be realized; it may even happen that it has to be referred back to Calcutta a *second* time. Now a three-years officer is an *old* officer in India. And when it comes back again the old officer is changed, a new one is there, who has some new crotchet in his head. And the course of reporting has to be gone through again.

But there is something more: an active engineering officer (say at Bombay) may be ordered by Sir B. Frere during the rains when the men can't work to prepare plans. Well, the *shortest possible* time when these plans can come back from Calcutta will be just when the *next* rains begin. And so with everything.

Sir B. Frere says it has come to such a pitch that everything must come to a *deadlock.* He said in the most impressive manner, I have done nothing, I have been like a squirrel in a cage. And my heart is broken. And so is Sir R. Napier's. But, he says, my successor, Mr Fitzgerald, who is a very good man, with Sir R. Napier, might do much. But the system paralyzes every exertion.

He said there can't be three better men than Dr Leith of Bombay, Ellis [of] Madras, Strachey [of] Calcutta. But they *have done nothing.* He says, in a country like India the only thing to be done would be to have a budget, to give the presidency governments the responsibility of action *up to that sum, tie them down to* that sum, but says that work is to be done; *you* have the responsibility of it, we shall send a whip to report on the work done and to show you up if you have not done it. And *you* must report to us every year as to the work done.

Now, he says, it is just the contrary. The whip is to *prevent* the work being done till every minute detail has been reported on by a parcel of people who know nothing; the whip says to them, "the work shall *not* be done." He says they won't. He says he himself (Sir B. Frere) is looked upon as a rebel in the India Council and has been told that he must "make things pleasant." But, he says, Sir S. Northcote is well disposed. He says that when he was in the Punjab years ago it was not so, that on the contrary they were told, Get up those improved barracks in the shortest time possible, and that he himself (Sir B. Frere), when he was a little man in the Punjab and in Sind had incurred large expenditures in housing troops, and had it *sanctioned afterwards* without a day's delay. He says Sir J. Lawrence has not one good man about him and that Sir W. Mansfield[94] is the best. He says he always knew when Sir J. Lawrence had had a letter from me or even from the duke of Cambridge, for a little action took place at once.

He says there *must* be a total alteration of the system or Indian administration will become impossible. He says he (Sir B.F.) has done nothing for Bombay.

Source: From two letters to Douglas Galton, ADD MSS 45764 ff76-77 and 82-87

16 June [1867] (What a June!)

I have seen Sir Bartle Frere. He came here on Friday [13 June] by his own appointment. And we had a great talk. He impressed me wonderfully—more than any Indian I have ever seen except Sir John Lawrence. I seemed to learn more in an hour from him upon Indian administration and the way it is going than I did from Ellis in six months, or from Strachey in two days, or from Indian Councils (secretaries of state and royal commissioners and all) in six years. I hope Sir B. Frere will be of use to us. I have not yet applied to you to put me into communication with Sir S. Northcote [just appointed secretary of state for India]. Because why? Your committee won't sit on Monday, because Monday is Whit Monday, and Tuesday is Whit Tuesday, and Wednesday is Ash Wednesday, and Thursday is Ascension Day, and Friday is Good Friday, and Saturday is the drawing room, and Sunday is Sunday. And that's the way that British business is done. Now you are come back, you must send for the police and make them, the committee, do something. As for Sutherland, I never see him. Malta is the

94 Sir William Rose Mansfield (1819-76), 1st Baron Sandhurst, chief of staff during the Mutiny, commander-in-chief in Bombay 1860-65.

world. And Gibraltar is the next world. And India is that little island in the Pacific, like Honolulu. However, I think perhaps we start at a fresh advantage now with Sir B. Frere, only pray brush up your committee because we can't really do anything till your committee gives us the *locus standi.*

24 June 1867

*Private.* I send back the India papers, for which I am very much obliged. They are very important—I think the most important we have had as showing a principle. The papers say this: We, the Government of India, intend to conduct our sanitary administration on the principle of universal suffrage. And this is the first fruits of it. If you look at the authorities consulted, you will see:

1. Local governments,
2. " sanitary commissions,
3. " medical authorities,
4. " military authorities,
5. " public works officers,
6. " committees.

Then comes a summary of local authorities. Then, the conclusions of the Government of India. You will see that, by adding (Number 2) the "sanitary commissions," we have simply added *another* element of disunion and uncertainty; we have committed an immense blunder and mistake. The government consults Nos. 3 and 2. Then it consults No. 1, then No. 4, which is worse. Not satisfied with this, it must consult Nos. 5 and 6. And then the foolscap has been sent all round. And even then it does not appear to decide by the majority of fools' heads.

Could we have the least idea that this was the way business was done, or rather not done? If we had, we should have seen our (presidency) sanitary commissions a long way first before we would have recommended them (just to spoil the broth a little more with another cook).

Sir Bartle Frere was so good as to give me some conversation on this very point of administration. Nothing will ever do any good until (if they must work by presidencies and governments) each administrative authority has its own budget and its own responsibilities with an inspection from the supreme government. But this manner of referring and referring and referring is vile. And, if they had framed a procedure to hinder work, instead of to do it, they could not have invented anything better. But the question is: what are we to do?

You were so good as to say that you would forward any statement of mine to Sir S. Northcote with an introduction from yourself. And I could also get a double backing from Lord Stanley. Dr Sutherland is so very etiquette-ish that he says "but how are you to have seen these papers?" I don't know. It seems to me that the cat has been out of the bag so long that it is no use tying the strings (or untying them) now. Both Sir J. Lawrence and Lord Stanley know what my share of the business has been. (And both think that I see a great many more of the papers than I do see—now.) If Lord Stanley speaks for me at all to Sir S. Northcote, he will speak in this sense, as he did to Lord Cranborne. However, Dr Sutherland *will* have it that I must write to you to ask for the papers to be referred to me or, at least, for a letter of yours to me, not "forwarding" them but formally referring them to me. I have to write to Sir J. Lawrence on Wednesday. And Dr Sutherland will have it that *otherwise* I must say I saw this paper "*confidentially*"—I don't mind (I will say that "Broadhead of Sheffield" gave me "£15" to steal it and to blow you up, if you like it. I'm your man.)

Only, what will you have me do? The point is: in what way I could make use of the paper with Sir S. Northcote? Dr Sutherland says the paper refers to the ventilation of barracks and hospitals. I (F.N.) have to do specially with hospitals. And I object in toto to the decision of the India government. Could you (Captain Galton) get it referred to me (F.N.) for opinion on the hospital questions? I am quite agreeable to whatever you may decide. Only, I am going ahead and am not going to wait for Dr Sutherland any more (not even for my £15 reward being embezzled" out of "Mr Broadhead's accounts"). I should be rather glad if you could let me hear tomorrow—or if you would let me have the papers back tomorrow just for one day—for my letter to Sir J. Lawrence. I did nothing with Lord Cranborne and have lost a whole year—which I regret very much. But I am not going to regret bygones now, only to say that I think we have a new standing point now and must go ahead.

I believe they have a sub-committee at the War Office on Friday on these papers. I wish you would attend it and say your say. (Then, if you chose and if *you* think it needful, you might have it referred to me, as Dr Sutherland proposes. But *I* don't mind.)

### Doors or Windows?

**Editor:** Nightingale took to heart the matter of ventilation of barracks by means of "doors" or "windows," as she shows in this next set of letters (see p 580 below). She thought that to decide in favour of doors was to jeopardize the entire cause of sanitation in India. The main point of the following letters, however, has to do with the nature and function of the presidency commissions.

Source: From a draft letter to Sir John Lawrence, ADD MSS 45777 ff98-101

[26 June 1867]

A paper has been confidentially shown to me containing the decision of the Government of India on a subject which involves the entire question of hospital and barrack ventilation. It is a letter with enclosures dated 1 April (No. 61) 1867, as to the relative merits of doors and windows for barracks and hospitals for European troops in India. I should have contented myself with reading and returning it, had it not been for the very serious nature of the consequences likely to follow from it not only as regards the ventilation of the new barracks but as regards the whole future of sanitary administration of India.

1. As regards the ventilation of barracks and hospitals, evidence of the highest character laid before the Royal Commission on the Sanitary State of the India Army had been shown that the method of ventilating barracks by doors had been productive of two very serious evils. (1) The direct infliction of disease on men while asleep by exposing them to draughts and this more especially with cases of disease in hospitals, which are often aggravated and probably rendered incurable by want of attention to the manner of ventilating the wards. (2) The infliction of the plague of darkness both on barracks and hospitals. The R.C. very properly recommended that the bad old system of ventilating by doors should be put an end to. And the A.S.C., to whom was remitted the duty of putting into a practical form the suggestions of the R.C., prepared draft plans of both barracks and hospitals for your consideration in India, which plans were based on the assumption that improved lighting and ventilation were to form part of them. Had this not been the case I have reason to believe that the plans would have been modified. The recommendation of the A.S.C. with regard to doors and windows is placed at the head of the enclosure in the letter referred to.

The meaning of the recommendation is to me perfectly clear. It does not lay down an iron law to be applied in every case. The commission in their suggestions give their proposed plans with the method of ventilation everywhere required. And they recommend that windows shall be introduced instead of doors when local circumstances admit of the change. These circumstances or conditions are clearly indicated in the evidence given before the R.C. There are many stations in India which, at one season or other, have a great difference between the day and night temperature. And at all such stations open doors are perfectly well known to be dangerous to health at night. At all such stations it is evident that while there should be sufficient ventilation this should be supplied without the slightest risk of checked perspiration. . . .

On the other hand, there are no doubt stations in India where there is a still atmosphere with a tolerably equal temperature between day and night. And, wherever this exists, common sense would point out that the less obstruction to movement in the air at night the better. In such cases, open doors might be necessary. You will see then that it is impossible to have standard plans founded on one rigid system for the great variety of climates which India presents.

2. The next point—and it is one of the very gravest importance—is the method by which the conclusion in the letter referred to has been arrived at. I find, e.g., that after H.M. had appointed a royal commission of the most competent men she could find to deal with the India sanitary question, after that R.C. had examined the most competent witnesses at command and made a general recommendation on the evidence thus obtained, after the A.S.C., to whom the subject was referred, which commission consists of experts specially appointed "for giving advice on all structural questions in which the health of the British Army was involved," had distinctly recommended that windows should be introduced instead of doors wherever it could be done, it appears that the Government of India remitted the question to the following authorities: local governments and administrations, local sanitary commissions, local medical authorities, local military authorities, local public works officers, local committees. Thus a question which was one of pure administration, viz., the adaptation of a principle to suit local circumstances, is sent abroad over the whole of India to be dealt with by those who may or may not have any knowledge of the subject—a kind of administration, so to speak, by universal suffrage. And the worst of it is that the decision of the Government of India does not even represent the result of the ballot.

I need scarcely say that the slightest consideration of this proceeding is sufficient to show that so long as it exists, anything like real sanitary progress in India is impracticable. You are perhaps not aware that, at the Constantinople conference, the benefit of our rule in India was called in question and that it was stated that, to the neglect of the public health in India, was due the epidemics of cholera which devastated Western Asia and Europe. . . . What you want in India is a competent Public Health Service, advised from home on special questions for a time at least. The decisions of this service (?) should be accepted and acted on and administrative provision made for giving effect to them to help you in the application of [illeg].

You apparently want really authoritative sanitary advisors together with a scheme of sanitary organization extending over the whole of India. But whatever you do, I should strongly recommend that this voting be never resorted to on any such questions. Better leave India without any provision of the P.H.[S.], tell us that there is none and ask us to organize one, than have recourse to such expedients. [the rest in Dr Sutherland's hand] You will never do any good until you have either one administrative public health authority for the whole of India with its own budget, or if you must [breaks off].

Source: From notes/draft letter to Lord Stanley, Add Mss 45781 ff198-201

[10 or 11 July 1867]

The enclosed paper [on doors and windows] was sent to me by Captain Galton from the War Office for my opinion on the questions regarding ventilation raised in it. But, on going over it, it was easy to see that questions were raised by this paper not only of the gravest importance regarding the future health of soldiers in barracks and of sick in hospitals, but involving the whole question of sanitary administrations in India, to such a degree that I have felt compelled to send it to you as the president of the India Sanitary Commission in order that we many consider what had best be done to save the cause in India from administrative ruin. . . .

You will see that, notwithstanding the opinion of the royal commission and of the Army Sanitary Commission expressed in their *Suggestions,* the Public Works Department had tacitly given the go-by to both and had adopted doors alike for barrack rooms and hospitals irrespective of local position and climate, thereby exposing both healthy and sick men to a large class of diseases well known to have been the result of this door ventilation previously carried out by this same department. . . .

I need scarcely point out that, with such a method of doing business, which amounts simply to administration by universal suffrage, anything like progress in sanitary reform is impossible. We have come to a deadlock through a vicious system of administration. In dealing with all health questions we require an active zealous executive, having sufficient knowledge, enlightenment and funds. Up to the present time, we have made no progress. The sanitary commissions have been so ill-arranged and so altered that you will see, by these documents, instead of being the sanitary advisors of the government, they are merely another element of discord and disunion thrown into the system. And the question now for us is: what should be done? All the best men are either out of the sanitary commissions or they are dead. And now appears to be the time for reorganizing the whole sanitary administration.

Would you be so good as to take the whole matter into your consideration and let me know whether anything and what can be done? The sanitary part of the question comes before the Army Sanitary Commission at its next meeting, which will be on an early day. In the meantime I am informed that the sub-commission to which the matter had been referred had decided unanimously against the Government of India [the rest in Dr Sutherland's hand] and in accordance with the views of the royal commission, as well as the medical officers in India to whom among others the question was referred, namely, to ventilate irrespective of either doors or windows, and to use doors or windows or both according to local requirements of climate.

Source: From a note for John Sutherland, Add Mss 45752 f187

16 July 1867

Lady Napier[95] has written to me that she is in England, returning to India next week, and asking to see me to communicate a message from her husband and ask for mine in return. She comes tomorrow afternoon.

Source: From notes for John Sutherland after Lady Napier's visit, Add Mss 45752 f202

[ca. 26 July 1867]

Lady Napier: Ellis is afraid of me and does not dare to come home. He says, if he is deluded away to Norwood again, his life is not worth ten minutes' purchase. Pycroft [?] is leaving India. Arbuthnot, chief secretary, is to have Pycroft's place on the Council. Ellis is offered the chief secretaryship but awaits my concurrence. Lady Napier did not know of [Duncan] MacPherson's death; she brought me this letter from Ellis: Oh no, he refers to Europe. I *have* heard from him and I

95 Wife of Lord Napier and Ettrick, governor of Madras 1866-72, who was to report on 22 September 1867: "My wife had taken an active interest in the Magdalen Hospital, the Lying-in Hospital and the orphanages of various kinds" (Cook, *The Life of Florence Nightingale* 2:170).

have alas seen Lady Napier. And I have also heard from Sir B. Frere; Captain Galton says the jealousy is of the Army Sanitary Commission, that our paper must dwell as exclusively as possible on the mode of procedure to be deprecated in India, as little as possible either on the disregard of the Army Sanitary Commission or on the door and window [issue]. He also says that it is essential to obtain Sir B. Frere's support as Sir S. Northcote is quite sure to show our paper to the Council.

Source: From three letters to Douglas Galton, Add Mss 45764 ff89-91, 92-94 and 95

16 July 1867

*Confidential.* Here is my letter, or rather a draft of it, to Sir S. Northcote at last. And I beg you to be so kind as to go over it and criticize it. Lord Stanley, I believe, spoke to him on Saturday. My letter to Sir J. Lawrence has been gone nearly a month. And therefore if we are to do anything with Sir S.N., the sooner it is done, the better. If we are to do anything will depend mainly, I fancy, on whether *you* can get Sir S.N. to give his consideration to it. I feel tolerably certain that nothing has been done with Lord de Grey's minute at the India Office (you remember 18 June 1866). Because I think I should have been quite sure to hear of it from Sir J. Lawrence, for Sir J.L. [has] always written to me on these subjects, as e.g., "such and such a despatch went from me, Sir J.L., on such and such a date."

If Sir S. Northcote does take me into consideration at all, I particularly wish that no blame to Sir J. Lawrence should be implied by me, because *everything* that has been done for us has been done by Sir J. Lawrence himself.

However, I leave my letter for your criticism. (I could not get Dr Sutherland to do more than this. You may take the horse to the water, but you can't make him drink. He had mounted his imagination to think that Lord Stanley would strike out a new plan of Public Health Service for us—as if it were physically possible for a man at the Foreign Office to do that now—Lord Stanley's letter to me was much more than I had expected, instead of less.) However, I only mention this in case Dr Sutherland should have spoken to you. I think we all three think it better to ask for a reconsideration of the whole subject on the basis of the minute we drafted for Lord de Grey (18 June 1866). Will you kindly go over this my draft and suggest any changes or additional points which may strengthen it?

The more we think over it, the more deplorable it seems. (Lord Stanley's promise on Friday was that he would speak generally to Sir

S. Northcote about the matter.) Your sub-committee has decided unanimously against the Government of India. You must make the general committee adopt the decision and send it to the India Office, with as strong a letter as you can without doing mischief by raising jealousies. But indeed everybody seems to me to be jealous of somebody else. And without exactly knowing why, I think Sir S. Northcote is jealous of Lord Stanley's interfering. (How different all that used to be under Sidney Herbert.) . . . I hope in this recourse to Sir S. Northcote as a last hope. Hope was green and the donkey ate it (that's me).

24 July 1867

CONFIDENTIAL. Your note of 16 July has been growing into a mustard tree.[96] (1) I rewrote my letter to Sir S. Northcote in obedience to your invaluable advice. (2) I have twice seen Sir B. Frere, in consequence of your hint to "make *him* safe" because "the Council are jealous." He claims to be a connection of yours. (Except Sir J. Lawrence, I have never seen any Indian who impressed me so much.) . . .

He immediately took our matter in hand, ferreted out Lord de Grey's minute (you remember) at the India Office and what had been done since (there have been a despatch on it from Lord Cranborne and one from Sir S. Northcote in April. Neither has in the least improved or even altered our position). Sir B. Frere was of opinion that my letter to Sir S. Northcote should go in, therefore, exactly as it is *now*, as altered according to your orders. (I showed it him.) He offered to take it with him and give it himself into Sir S. Northcote's hands. I thought it as well to wait for this reason: the famous "doors and windows" paper is here; this should go in from you (with your minute) to the India Office, so that Sir S. Northcote may, if he sends for it (my letter is founded upon it), be able to see it at once.

I shall see Dr Sutherland tomorrow. I shall send in then the "doors and windows" paper to you (after he has suggested anything he wants to suggest). And you will, I hope, aid and abet me in my letter to Sir S. Northcote, in which I have mentioned you as fathering my letter. This I shall send through Sir B. Frere, as I could not well refuse his offer to take my letter himself, although, "my son, my beard is white,"[97] I feel more hopeful now than I have done for a year past.

96 An allusion to Luke 13:19.

97 A possible allusion to "The Treason of Ganelon," in *The Song of Roland* viii:23.

It is an immense thing for us to have Sir B. Frere "safe" for us on the Council. (If we could get a Public Health Department in the India Office to ourselves with Sir B. Frere at the head of it, our fortunes would be made.) At all events, we have now a certain channel, both of information and of support, at the India Office, in him. Many thanks for the hint.

P.S. Sir B. Frere rather wished me to send the "doors and windows" paper (WITH my letter) to Sir S. Northcote through him. But that would be contrary to all order, would it not? . . . I think I shall send my revised letter to Sir S. Northcote for you to look at again tomorrow, if you will be so good.

July 1867

Sir B. Frere, whom I saw again yesterday, renewed his offer to present the letter and I really felt that I must give way and it is going to him today. I have stated to Sir S. Northcote that you would communicate to him on the subject. Which you could very easily do in sending back the "doors and windows" paper. I have restrained my letter solely to the administrative point and have not said a word about your War Office commission. I entirely agree with you about this.

Source: From a draft letter to Sir Stafford Northcote (secretary of state for India) in Dr Sutherland's hand, ADD Mss 45779 ff82-92

25 July 1867

My apology for writing you on a matter intimately affecting the health of Her Majesty's British troops in India is that I took part in the royal commission of inquiry into the sanitary state of the army, and that ever since that time I have been lending what little aid I can lend to the improvement of Indian stations, hospitals and the like. On this subject I have been in frequent communication with the authorities both here and in India, and thus it happens that a short time ago my opinion was requested by Captain Galton on certain proposals made by the Indian government for using doors in every case where we would use windows as a means of ventilating both barracks and hospitals, thereby exposing both healthy and sick men to grave risks from a method of ventilation which had been directly condemned by the royal commission as well as by medical officers serving in India.

The subject is one of the very greatest import to the future healthiness both of barracks and hospitals in India, for the proposal of the Indian government, if carried out, would simply be to increase the risk of disease and death at all stations where there are rapid changes of temperature. The matter was referred to the War Office Sanitary Commission (letter 1 April 1867) and will, I have no doubt, come before you with their opinion in proper time—as to the relative merits of doors and windows for barracks and hospitals for European troops in India.

My present object in writing is not to discuss this matter but rather to ask your consideration of the means by which the decision of the Indian government was arrived at. . . . In doing so it will be necessary to go back to the history of the matter.

The royal commission recommended the appointment of three commissions of health, one for each presidency. . . . The authorities in India . . . at last broke up the commissions, retaining I believe the name without the constitution recommended by the royal commission and proposed to make the duty of inspector of health a part of the duty of inspector of prisons. . . .

The recent occurrence which has led me to write to you has shown that the whole affair has gone to ruin and that if any good is to come of the royal commission over which Lord Herbert and Lord Stanley presided some immediate action is necessary. I will now state the case in a few propositions:

1. The royal commission recommended certain principles for ventilating barracks and hospitals.

2. These principles were approved and sent to India in a detailed form for local application to suit local circumstances by the India Office on the recommendation of the Army Sanitary Commission. . . .

3. The government in India, instead of proceeding to apply the principles by the assistance of these health commissions, sent the whole subject abroad all over India. . . .

The great question now is how to put the India Health Service once for all on a satisfactory footing. This was the point raised by Lord de Grey. It can only be done after thorough consideration of the problems to be met.

These late papers have merely shown that those who feared the prospective ruin of the health question in India from the delay in working out any public health service at all, as also in working out an efficient responsible constitution for the sanitary commissions in India, had unfortunately too much reason for their fears. And these occurrences afford the best possible reason for taking up the question again. It is in the hope of being able to aid in this that I have now ventured to address you. I have already written to Lord Stanley, who was one of the presidents of the royal commission, and he kindly said that he would speak with you on the subject.

Source: Letter, Add Mss 50036 ff283-89

London
25 July 1867

*Private*

Sir [Right Honorable Sir Stafford Northcote, MP]

I should be afraid of thus venturing to address you but that I believe Lord Stanley has already kindly spoken with you about the matter. Captain Galton also promised his co-operation.

My apology for writing to you on a matter intimately affecting the health of H.M.'s British troops in India is that I took part in the royal commission for inquiry into the "sanitary state of the Indian Army" appointed in 1859 by Lord Stanley, when he was secretary of state for India, and presided over first by Sidney Herbert and then by Lord Stanley.

Ever since that time I have been lending what little aid I can to the improvement of Indian stations, sanitary service, hospitals and the like. On these subjects I have been in frequent communication with Sir John Lawrence and the authorities both in India and here and have received papers both from India direct and from government offices here.

A short time ago I thus saw a paper entitled "Public Works Department, Letter 1 April (No. 61) 1867 as to the relative merits of doors and windows for barracks and hospitals for European troops in India," in which the different constructive arrangements on this point are entered into. My present object in venturing to trouble you is not to discuss this matter but rather to ask your consideration of the *means* by which the decision of the India government was arrived at. And these I will state in as few words as possible. But in doing so, it will be necessary to go back to the history of the matter.

The royal commission which, after four years' hard work, reported in 1863, recommended the appointment of three commissions of health in India—one for each presidency—to advise the local government on all questions referring to the health of the country. These commissions were appointed by Sir John Lawrence (2 February 1864) immediately after he went out, in accordance with a despatch from Sir Charles Wood (Military No. 297, 15 August 1863), which however was not acted upon till Sir J. Lawrence became governor general in the following January.

The authorities in India have not however followed up this measure by other measures essential to give it practical effect. They have not adopted any organized system of procedure by health officers, as was recommended by Lord Stanley's royal commission, and such as we have in this country. (There are officers of health connected with the municipalities of Bombay and Calcutta but no *government* health officers.) There is, in fact, no sanitary organization properly so-called. And, at last, two at least of the presidency commissions have been broken up (to save cost), retaining however the heads and secretaries and the name, though without the constitution and organization in detail recommended by the royal commission and without substituting any other constitution, which increasing local experience might have pointed out as more efficient.

In a minute by the governor general and the other members of Council (9 January 1866) it was finally proposed to make the duty of inspector of health a part of the duty of inspectors of prisons. (This minute was, unfortunately, mislaid in the India Office here and could not be found for Lord de Grey, till he found it himself on 5 May 1866.) The matter was under Lord de Grey's consideration just before he left office. And he has left on record in the India Office (end of June 1866) a minute embodying his views as to the necessity of reconsidering the future organization of the health service in India.

We are not aware whether, during subsequent ministerial changes, any action has been taken with regard to this organization of a more efficient health service. But recent papers have shown that the whole matter has gone to ruin and that, if any good is to come of the royal commission, over which Lord Herbert and Lord Stanley successively presided, some immediate action is necessary at home.

This particular case may be put (as an illustration of the whole) in a few propositions.

1. The royal commission recommended certain principles for ventilating barracks and hospitals.

2. These principles were approved and sent to India in a detailed form—for local application—to suit local circumstances by the India Office as *Suggestions in Regard to Sanitary Works Required for Improving Indian Stations* (15 July 1864). These *Suggestions* were prepared at the request of the Secretary-of-State-for-India-in-Council, conveyed in letters dated 8 December 1863 and 20 May 1864, which again were written at the request of the Indian authorities.

3. The government in India, instead of proceeding to apply the principles, by the assistance of their three health commissions, sent

the whole subject abroad all over India to the following authorities: (1) local governments and administrators, (2) local sanitary commissions, (3) local medical authorities, (4) local military authorities, (5) local public works officers, (6) local committees, all over Bombay, Madras, Bengal, N.W. Provinces, Punjab, Straits, British Burma, Central Provinces, Oudh, Mysore, Hyderabad, Rajputana, Central India; the foolscap wanders collecting opinions on the universal suffrage principle.

As already mentioned, the effective constitution, such as it was, of two of the presidency sanitary commissions had been broken up so that they no longer represented the recommendation of the royal commissioners, nor indeed do they responsibly represent anything now, except a new element of discord and disunion, a new element of uncertainty. And none of the other authorities to whom the question was sent have any knowledge of it, except the medical authorities.

It is the nature of this procedure which has alarmed all who take an interest in the future health, civil and military, of India. We feel that it is impossible, with such a course of proceeding, that good can ever come. (It is not only that "too many cooks spoil the broth." It is that actually many of the "cooks" invited to make the "broth" are not "cooks" at all—no more "cooks" than are railway clerks or boards of guardians.)

As it is, all sanitary progress in India is impossible. And the great question now is how to put the India Health Service once for all on a satisfactory footing. This would indeed be a noble service for a secretary of state to render to India. This was the point raised by Lord de Grey. Might I venture to suggest that reference be made to his minute again?

The character of the organization required can only be decided after thorough consideration of the problems to be met. These last papers have merely shown that those who feared the prospective destruction of the health question in India, from the delay in working out any public health service at all—as also in working out any efficient responsible constitution for the sanitary commissions in India—had but too much reason for their fears. And these papers afford the best possible ground for taking up the whole question again and for giving to the secretary of state some effective control and the means of knowing what is being done to protect the health of India. It is in the hope of being able to aid in this that I have taken the courage to address you. I had already written to Lord Stanley as the surviving president of his own royal commission. And he kindly said that he would speak with you on the subject. Pray believe me, Sir,

ever your faithful servant
Florence Nightingale

Source: From four letters to Douglas Galton, Add Mss 45764 ff96-97, 98-99, 102 and 103-04

26 July 1867

*Private.* "Excuse haste and a bad pen." Today my letter to Sir S. Northcote went in, under the patronage of Sir B. Frere, as amended by you. I have been so immensely hurried about various things that I can only enclose to you a copy of what has gone in, and beg for your cooperation with Sir S. Northcote, as you kindly promised, and as I have stated in the *letter.* Please return me my copy. It is only sent to show you what has gone. I hope it will meet with your approbation. Sir B. Frere renewed his offer to present the letter himself. And I really felt, with you, that I must accept. If you would communicate with Sir S. Northcote at once, or on sending in the "doors and windows" paper, it would be very desirable. I don't think you can justly accuse me of being too "sanguine." As for our having an India Office Public Health Department under Sir B. Frere (if we ever could get it, which we shall not) that would be the only way *of really getting things referred to you* for *your opinion.*

The moment I can, I will write you word [as to] what have been the intermediate despatches between Lord de Grey's minute and this time. And also what, if anything, comes of this. . . . Mr Ellis is "too much afraid" of me to come home, too "much afraid" of me to be ill (what an exemplary man!) and is to be made "chief secretary to government" (Madras) if I "permit." This will help us much. Lord Napier is inclined to give us a Public Health Service and to appeal home about it. Lady Napier is in England and brought me this word. Dr MacPherson is dead (Madras), Dr Leith has been dying (in England) but is (this morning) better. He is Bombay sanitary commissioner.

F.N.

*Burn.*

30 July 1867

*Private.* I send you the enclosed note, merely for you to see the exact position in which the matter is. If I don't hear soon from Sir S. Northcote, I shall begin again, through you and through Sir B. Frere. But I should like to be guided by you *as* to the time. (I am afraid of pressing the matter while they have this fag end of the Reform Bill[98] still in hand) for fear of being forbidden to press afterwards. Will you talk to Sir S. Northcote? Have you talked to Sir S. Northcote? He *had not* seen Lord de Grey's minute. That is India Office all over.

I am told they are in a great fright about this Orissa affair and "really" think that "something" must be done (about Indian administration), which gives us a favourable opportunity. I have read the Orissa papers. Simplicity and direct action, these are the two things wanted. Hindus are not English. And, even if they were, simplicity and direct action are two good things.

Sir C. Beadon's[99] defence is pitiable. But the fault is in the system of administration. The governor general sits at Simla like a great hen and lets all his chickens scratching all over India. And, if there is a grain of corn too deep for them to scratch up, he gives a dig with his claw to help them; that is all. Lord Dalhousie and Lord Canning had made a step towards better administration. Lord Elgin let it all slip back. Sir J. Lawrence has struggled (in vain) against the dead weights around him.

31 July 1867

*Private.* Sir S. Northcote wrote to me last night. I will send you his note and my answer (to criticize, please) if possible this afternoon. But my reason for writing now is to ask you *not* to see Sir S.N. till you have seen these two letters, as he is all astray on one point and it would be important to us to reserve (as a party reserves a debater) you to answer him on this point.

31 July 1867

*Private.* I send you Sir S. Northcote's note and my proposed answer (a sentence of Dr Sutherland's about the dreadful diseases caused by doors, *would* come in like King Charles the First.[100] But I steadfastly

---

98 Presumably the Representation of the People Bill, which gave the male working class the vote.

99 Sir Cecil Beadon (1816-81), governor of Bengal 1862-67.

100 On 3 January 1642 Charles I (1600-49) found the doors of Parliament locked when he arrived with armed soldiers to attempt to take away MPs impeached for supporting Parliament against him; he was tried and beheaded at the end of the Civil War 1642-48.

resisted him. We are getting so excited about doors. But we shall insist upon having in "Registrar-General's List of Diseases" next after "Cholera," "*Doors,*" but immediately before "Delhi Ulcers," whom poor fellows I do so miss after having seen them there for two years off your committee's List of Subjects. However, though I have no doubt the men do die of "doors," I think they die more of something much worse than "doors." Orissa certainly did not die of doors.) You will see that I have taken advantage of your hint about urging a section of the Council being devoted to health matters. I shall *not at all* mind rewriting my letter, according to your criticisms (as I ought to have a copy of my letter especially for Sir B. Frere). I do not propose showing my letter to him beforehand or sending it by him, as there is mention of him in it, unless you expunge it. I would either send it by you, if you advise it, or direct by hand to Sir S. Northcote.

I am so busy. I saw a deputy inspector general from Madras, by Lady Napier's particular desire. And today I see a Parsi from Bombay, by Sir B. Frere's, which makes me incoherent.

*If* you approve, I propose to send with this letter to Sir S. Northcote, a copy of Sutherland's Algerian report.

Source: From a draft letter to Sir Stafford Northcote in Dr Sutherland's hand, Add Mss 45779 ff102-04

[after 30 July 1867]

[Reply to Sir S. Northcote's letter of 30 July 1867] I entirely agree with you that in carrying out any measures for protecting public health due regard should be paid to local information and peculiarities. This is in fact indisputable, but the principle applies to details rather than to great leading sanitary works. The question which occasioned my writing to you was precisely one of this nature. It regarded the application of a great general principle to suit local circumstances and the gist of my complaint against the method pursued by the government in India was this, that instead of proceeding to apply the principle to suit local circumstances they threw the question broadcast over all India to all classes of persons, and after having got opinions, especially from medical officers who understand the points, the government in India passed a minute in the teeth of the advice they had asked for, and determined to apply an iron rule to the almost infinite variety of circumstances to which ventilation has to be applied. And as a certain result of this decision, if carried out, we must all look for the continuance of certain diseases among the troops, which are perfectly well known to have been occasioned at certain stations by the very kind of door ventilation which the government has decided should be applied to all.

But more than this we object in toto to the method of application of principles which the Government of India has adopted in this case, simply because it is known to be intrinsically mischievous, and because we have a decision of a royal commission, presided over by Lord Stanley and Lord Herbert, which points out what the administrative principle ought to be. These health commissions were recommended and appointed . . . officers of health and executive authorities. Health questions in India comprise two classes:

1. Those of military stations and the populations about them.

2. Those of groups of population where there are no military stations.

Both have to be provided for. Both require authorities to administer under the advice of the commissions on all special questions and also laws and regulations to be administered. Both require inspection. Both require funds. And what is of great importance, the India Office here should keep its hand so over the work in India that it should know almost by every mail what is being done to improve stations and people, and it ought to be able to check the work and to report annually to Parliament. Even in Algeria this is done and the reports are published annually to show the progress in well-being and health of the entire community, civil and military. Almost every case of disease is reported, at least of special diseases. Why should we not do this for India? The practice since the report of the royal commission was published has been nothing more than playing with one of the greatest questions of our foreign empire. Those who interest themselves in these subjects know that we, the English people, are rotting out everywhere because we will not learn what the natural laws are which we must obey in order to live. Look at Bermuda, Demerara, Mauritius as recent examples and to India itself. Recurring epidemics are the result solely of want of civilization and neglect in applying remedial agencies. It is not as if the questions were new. Everything is known. There is one thing only wanting, which requires to pervade all government offices having anything to do with foreign possessions, and that is "intelligent doing." There is no question of the kind so great as this Indian question. I have reason to know that we have made the natives *think* more about it than we have been able to get government to *act*. Now is the time to begin. . . .

If I might suggest anything, it would be that the subject should be considered here before Sir John Lawrence is written to. I have been in the habit of communicating with him and have written on this very point, but what we really want is not so much to deal with the present case as to enter on a new phase altogether and to organize a health service once for all. It is not a difficult matter to do and it requires to be done. It ought to be considered just as much in the Estimates and also as much a part of the current work of the Secretary-of-State-for-India-in-Council as any other part of the public service. You have members of council of large Indian experience who thoroughly understand the whole subject.

Source: From a letter to Sir Stafford Northcote, ADD Mss 50036 ff295-301, draft partly in Dr Sutherland's hand ADD Mss 45779 ff102-08

31 July 1867

*Private.* I am very much alive to the great kindness of your note of 30 July. And it would be most ungrateful of me to press for a decision now at such a moment of pressure of business. But I do not. What I venture to say now is suggested by a passage in your very kind note. And it is only written (now) in the hope that it will be taken into consideration *when the time* comes for your taking the whole subject into consideration (of the India Public Health Service). In carrying out any measures for protecting public health in India, you most truly say that due regard should be had to local information and local peculiarities and even to local "habits and prejudices." It is just because we had this principle so intensely in view that we have been so confounded by the turn that things have lately taken. The principle, it is needless to say, applies rather to details than to great leading sanitary works.

The immediate question which occasioned my writing to trouble you was precisely one of this nature. It regarded the application of a great general principle to suit local circumstances and the gist of the whole outcry I am making (against the method pursued by the government in India) is this, that, instead of proceeding to apply the principle to suit local circumstances, they threw the question broadcast over all India to all classes of persons. And after having received opinions from all manner of persons (including medical officers who understand the point), the government in India passed a minute in the teeth of the advice they had asked for and determined to apply an iron rule to the almost infinite variety of circumstances to which ventilation has to be applied.

But, more than this, we venture to object to the method of application of principles which the Government of India has adopted in this case, because it is known to be intrinsically mischievous and because we have a decision of a royal commission, presided over by Lord Herbert and Lord Stanley, which points out what the administrative principle ought to be. Three (presidency) health commissions were recommended and appointed. And, connected with these, there were to have been officers of health and executive authorities. Health questions in India comprise two classes: (1) those of military stations and the populations about them; (2) those of groups of population where there are no military stations. Both have to be provided for. Both require authorities to administer under the advice of the commissions on all special questions and also laws and regulations to be administered. Both require inspection. Both require funds. And, what is of great importance, the India Office here should keep its hand so over the work in India that it should know, almost by every mail, what is being done to improve stations and people. And it ought to be able to check the work and to report annually to Parliament. (Even in France this is done as regards Algeria. And the reports are published annually to show the progress in well-being and health of the whole community, civil and military; almost every case of disease is reported, at least of special diseases. These are noble reports—I wish I might venture to send you some. I take the liberty of sending you the Algerian report by a commission sent out from our War Office and might well excite our ambition to "go and do likewise"[101] for India.)

The practice now in India has been little more than playing with one of the greatest questions of our foreign empire. Because people must live in order to work. And a secretary of state for India who really set about this great question might save as many lives as the first Napoleon[102] destroyed lives. (It is a melancholy fact that we English die out everywhere, because we will not learn what the natural laws are which we must obey in order to live, e.g., in Bermuda, in Demerara, Mauritius and in India itself. It is a miserable thing which constantly comes before me in my small way, when called upon to send out trained nurses to our foreign possessions. We can't depend upon the offspring of Europeans living, the girls to be trained, say, as nurses, no, not even the boys to supply our drummer boys. We must be always importing from England, and this only to die.)

---

101 An allusion to Luke 10:37.

102 Napoleon Bonaparte (1769-1821), emperor of France 1804-15, for Nightingale the "arch fiend" whose military campaigns caused thousands of deaths.

Recurring epidemics are the result solely of want of civilization, of neglect in applying preventive agencies ready to our hand. It is not as if the questions were new. Everything is known. There is one thing only wanting, viz., "intelligent doing." There is no question of the land so great as this Indian health question. I know from educated natives themselves that we have made the natives *think* more about it than we have been able to induce government to *act*. And now is the time to begin. Great hopes have been entertained since you have assumed the secretaryship of state. (But, above all, I would not be understood to be worrying just now for action this minute.) If I might venture to suggest, it would be that the subject should be considered here before Sir John Lawrence is written to. Sir John Lawrence's great kindness to me has enabled and encouraged me to write to him (privately) on all these sanitary affairs, and I have written to him on this very point (this famous "doors and windows" paper).

But what we really want is not so much to deal with the present case as to enter on a new phase altogether and to organize a health service once for all. What we really want is reconsideration and reorganization—reconsideration on the part of the secretary of state, of course in conjunction with the governor general and the presidency governors afterwards. It is not a difficult matter to do, only it requires to be done. And it ought to be considered just as much in the Estimates and (if I might take the great liberty of saying so) be considered also just as much a part of the current work of the Secretary-of-State-for-India-in-Council as any other part of the public service. At this moment there is a member of council just come home from India [Sir Bartle Frere] and of large Indian experience, who thoroughly understands the whole subject.

I am afraid that it will require a very large measure of your indulgence to enable you to pardon, if you do pardon, this long letter. I scarcely venture to say that, having had this work well "*grimed in*" to me from the beginning, I should esteem it the greatest favour to be allowed to communicate with you on the subject, at any time or in any way least inconvenient to yourself.

Source: Notes for John Sutherland, ADD Mss 45752 ff211-15

14 August 1867

Sir B. Frere says that now is the time to attack Sir S. Northcote; that if we don't do it this autumn, we shall not do it at all; that Sir S. Northcote is willing but weak, very hardworking and conscientious, but always anxious to be *safe*; that he won't do anything revolutionary;

that he is anxious to do something; but that the whole thing turns upon my seeing him personally and that I must make his education like a baby; that he is far more hardworking than Lord de Grey but has far less insight and perception than Sidney Herbert (which of course I knew); that he would like me to write, offering to see him; that he, Sir S. Northcote, is only going to leave London for ten days this autumn and he, Sir B. Frere, only for two days; that they don't go into their new office till 15 September and that in short he, Sir B. Frere, thinks these next two months are the time for work.

Sir B. Frere says the two debates have only unveiled their excessive weakness and confusion; that Lord Cranborne [secretary of state for India before Sir Northcote] is full of splendid fallacies; that he is energetic, imaginative and that when he talks about the confusion of Indian affairs in the House of Commons he positively foams at the mouth. Sir B. Frere says it's all very well to talk of a despot viceroy or governor being the right thing. Yes, it's the right thing if he can have twenty wazeers [viziers or ministers in a Muhammadan government] in his Cabinet behind him, and cut their heads off if they don't give good advice, but what they want is not more councils but more counsel, counsel from men who know something about it. That we talk about India as they talk about Europe: a man remembers something about Devonshire in his youth and he thinks Spain and France are like it, or he talks about Shields or Wapping and thinks England is like Shields or Wapping. So, he says, we talk about India. A man may know twenty things about India and he may not know twenty other things.

He says the stuff that has been talked about, the failure in Orissa;[103] it's not the men, but the system is like if you have a bad mariner with bad barometers who can't foresee or provide for the storm which wrecks his ship, which a better mariner could provide against; it's no use saying, It's not the man but the system. What you must do is to give the man better training. Then he went into more details.

He said Lord Elphinstone [governor of Bombay 1853-60] first, at Bombay, saw and acted upon the absolute necessity of reclaiming the marshlands; I did what I could. But now we can't sell the lands we reclaim, we've *too much* land. Well, they can't see that it's a matter of health, not of market. And we've got the subject up now at the India Office.

---

103 Publication of the Report of the Famine Commission (Bengal and Orissa) is discussed below (see p 704 below).

Then about the barracks: you must be cautious with Sir S. Northcote. If you say every man must have [so many] cubic feet and then multiply that by the men, it mounts up to such a sum that the council snub Sir S. Northcote (who really doesn't know anything about it) at once. What you must say is, do the worst first and find out which are the worst.

Lastly, he said that he was quite sure the "doors and windows" paper *had* attracted Sir S. Northcote's attention in my letter. For, last Thursday, at the council, when it came up, he, Sir B. Frere, was prepared to stop it and bring it forward instead of its being lost with the other papers, but that he (Sir S. Northcote) was beforehand with him and brought it forward. And it is to be discussed today. He says the council is quite sure to go wrong.

Lastly, he said that I must begin Sir S. Northcote's education, that I must have him here as soon as possible and go through the principal points with him since Sir J. Lawrence's accession. Lastly, he said that the state of the India Office is inconceivable, that just the routine of the old East India Company, the worst part, has survived the wreck, that there has been no master hand to create *any*thing, that *no*thing *has* been created and that they are just wading and waddling on and doing *no*thing.

(And I'm sure he thinks that Sir S. Northcote is *not* the master hand which *will* create anything. Lord Cranborne, he says, *was* a genius but then he positively "foams at the mouth.") He is quite shocked at the indifference of the House of Commons. He says the speeches were good but the few MPs who were there sat like gulls and only stayed "to defend Sir S. Northcote if he were attacked; that the Manchester school[104] and people who live by commerce on manufactures relating to India, and the country gentlemen who have sons and relatives making their fortunes in India *ought* to be there, taking part in or at least interested in the debate." But devil a bit does one of them care.

Sir B. Frere told me (by the way) that Lord Elphinstone had been the first to bring a water supply to Bombay. It was thought excessive but the people drank and washed to such a degree that the only fruit of Lord Elphinstone's supply has been to show that what was thought excessive is wholly inadequate. . . .

---

104 The Manchester school supported free trade and non-interference by government in the economy.

[Questions to Sutherland] You said I was to show Sir S. Northcote my papers to Sir J. Lawrence. I have hunted them out but there's no one but Frere I could trust. My son, my beard is white. Sir B. Frere said I was to show Sir S. Northcote all the papers I showed him. Now shall I?

I always feel with a secretary of state that they are so jealous of each other. If I show Sir S. Northcote any other secretary of state's letters, he will think I shall show his. If I show him what we have done for Lord de Grey, he will think I shall show any future secretary of state what we do for him. Shall I ask him to let me see Lord Cranborne's despatch?

**Editor:** A new India Office Sanitary Committee was formed in November 1867, with Sir Bartle Frere as its prime mover. The committee functioned only to the end of 1874, but was an important force at a time when the India Office, the Army Sanitary Commission and the presidency commissions needed to be given firm direction.

Source: Notes on a conversation with Sir Stafford Northcote for John Sutherland, Add Mss 45752 ff216-19

[after 20 August 1867]

Well, I've won this: a department [sanitary committee] in the India Office for our business: Sir B. Frere, president, Sir H. Anderson, secretary with an assistant secretary. He mentioned Sir [Thomas] Erskine Perry and General [William E.] Baker as members.

I think he [Northcote] will [do it] because I spoke strongly about it. But he said first there was an immense jealousy of the Army Sanitary Commission and it would not do to have Sir Proby Cautley on both, Sir P. Cautley consulting himself. Then he said, quite of his own accord, that he understood and admitted that the department with Sir B. Frere at its head should consult the Army Sanitary Commission. And I said we looked upon the proposed department as a controlling authority and upon the Army Sanitary Commission as a consultative. Sir S. Northcote says, that's a perpetual rub and sore.

Sir S. Northcote was very confidential. He says he is going to make constitutional changes and actually asked me my opinion. I lilted up with my budgets and responsibilities for local governments. And he was quite agreeable. He says, Should you not leave drainage, water supply, etc., to local governments, and barracks to the supreme government?

He asks whether it would not be better not to have those grand, permanent buildings at all, whether buildings to be pulled down every thirty years are not better in a climate where the very walls get saturated. He asks, Is there not danger of any building in India getting polluted in thirty years? I told him that.

Sir S. Northcote is going away today, but comes back the week after next. He spoke with great feeling of the Orissa business [famine]. He said they tell us we could not save all but we did not try to save any. We were actually told that no famine was expected, that there *was* a fever, but not the result of famine. He is very well-intentioned but he has not the elements of sanitary [knowledge].

He asked me why I said there was no organization, no government officers of health when there were sanitary commissioners. And I was obliged to explain from the beginning, that officers of health are not sanitary commissioners. He is a man of very much the same style of mind as Lord de Grey, none of the rapid unerring perceptions of Sidney Herbert, none of the power of Sir J. Lawrence, none of the power and keenness of Sir B. Frere. But he is *very* well intentioned and, I think, has great industry and also perseverance. I believe he will carry out exactly what he consents to do.

He took away Sir J. Lawrence's minute and my criticism upon it (to study). *That's* not the minute. No, it was written on 5 May 1866 here, when Sir J. Lawrence's minute was first found. He is intent upon making great constitutional changes in India so as to localize responsibilities.

Lord Napier appears to be badgering him to death; he is always writing for something; he has sent him home an account of the success at Conjeveram; he has told him his next letter will be about hospitals. Aye, I said, and his next letter after that about Public Health Service.

Then *I* began about nurses and he said he was pestered by private people with their philanthropic schemes about India (like Miss Carpenter, he said). I said I'm not a philanthropic person. It's *they* who are pestering me to give them nurses. I sit here like a stupid Paged [Panegea?] and say, Well, well, give me money and I'll see what I can do for you. He said the India Office at home was rather a controlling power as to expenditure, that *they* did not propose to the governor general to spend but rather checked him. He said they had had no proposals, he believed, from [the] governor general or any presidency governor to spend about nurses. I said, Will you favour it if it comes? He said, Yes, I'll do more than that, I'll write to Sir J. Lawrence about it.

He talked a great deal about jails. He said the mortality was "monstrous." I don't know that he saw how afraid I was of him. For he kept his eyes tight shut all the time. And I kept my eyes wide open.

I went fully into the question with him about sending royal engineers to be educated. I showed him Captain Tulloch's report. But I told him he must not expect to find another royal engineer who would make so good a one. He said he would talk the whole matter over with "Clinton."[105]

Source: From a letter to Sir Bartle Frere, in John Martineau, ed., *The Life and Correspondence of the Rt Hon Sir Bartle Frere* 2:39

21 August 1867

Sir Stafford Northcote came here to see me on Tuesday of his own accord, which I think I owe to your kindness. We had a long conversation, much more satisfactory to my hopes than I expected. I think you have imbued him with your views on Indian administration more than you know. We went as fully into the whole subject as was possible in an hour, seeing that India is rather a big place. But what I write now more particularly about is this: he proposes to have a committee in the India Office expressly for this (sanitary) work. I told him that we want the executive machinery to do it (in India) and the controlling machinery (at the India Office) to know that it is being done. If he will do this our fortunes will be made. He proposes yourself as president.

Source: From a letter to Douglas Galton, ADD Mss 45764 ff108-11

22 August 1867

CONFIDENTIAL. I saw Sir S. Northcote on Tuesday. He came of his own accord, which I think I partly owe to you. The result is—that is, if he does as he says—that there will be a controlling committee at the India Office (for sanitary things) [India Office Sanitary Committee] with Sir B. Frere at the head and Sir H. Anderson at the tail [as secretary], and your War Office committee as the consulting body. (I suspect that you will get a great many more references from Sir B. Frere than you do at present from Sir P. Cautley.) As to the Public Health Service, I told Sir S. Northcote that we want the executive machinery in India to do it, and the controlling machinery at the India Office to know that it is being done. The work of the controlling committee will really be introducing the elements of civilization into India.

Sir S. Northcote said something about having General Baker and Sir E. Perry on as members and an assistant secretary to Sir H. Ander-

105 Lord Clinton (1834-1904), Conservative MP, briefly Parliamentary under secretary for India.

son (I wish I could choose the members as I did in Sidney Herbert's time). But I have the greatest faith in Sir B. Frere and he asked me to let him bring Sir H. Anderson here. So we shall have the chairman and secretary on our side. I liked Sir S. Northcote but he appears to me to have much the same calibre of mind as Lord de Grey. He has none of the rapid unerring perception of Sidney Herbert, none of the power of Sir J. Lawrence, none of the power and keenness of Sir B. Frere. However, we have no time for moralizing. When you see Sir S. Northcote (he is coming back to town week after next) please back me up all you can, though, of course, you will not betray me.

*Confidential.* Sir S. Northcote talks about "talking it all over" with Lord Clinton. And that alarms me, though, of course, it is necessary. Who was Lord Clinton? And does he know anything about it? But my principal reason for writing to you now is this: I went as fully as I could with him (Sir S. Northcote) into this, that no time should be lost in sending royal engineers intended for service in India, to examine and make themselves acquainted with improvements in sewerage, drainage and water supply of towns, and in application of sewage for agriculture, and with improvements in barrack and hospital construction, etc., as carried out here. Now, there is no one but you who can properly advise Sir S. Northcote in this matter. Pray do so. Do you know Lord Clinton?

Please destroy this letter, when read and acted upon.

Source: Notes on a conversation with Sir Bartle Frere for John Sutherland, ADD Mss 45752 f229

22 September 1867

I am going to Lea Hurst[106] but I will tell you what Sir B. Frere says for *you* to do. Sir B. Frere says that the next fortnight will decide our fate; that it is *not* at all certain that the committee will be appointed [the India Office Sanitary Committee was approved in November], *unless* we keep worrying Sir S. Northcote; that Sir S. Northcote comes to town tomorrow for two days, but that he has enough subjects before him to take *weeks,* if they were to be considered properly, which they will not be; that he then goes to Manchester and then to Balmoral; that our letter ought to be before him *there,* when he will have a little time; that if we let it stand over till Cabinets begin in a month's time,

106 Nightingale's letter to her father, W.E. Nightingale, 4 October 1867 shows that she did not go, ADD Mss 45790 f353.

or till the reform and Parliament begin again, we are lost; that he proposes we should write Sir S. Northcote a letter, summing up and reminding, reminding him *also* of the committee and explaining also in words which he will read Mr Ellis's plan to be tried in Madras. He says, upon this depends not only whether the committee will be at all, but, what is far more problematical, whether it will be allowed to be of any use at all. That then, when the committee is appointed, he shall ask us to draw up a plan of procedure.

Source: Notes from two interviews with Sir Bartle Frere for John Sutherland, ADD MSS 45752 ff230 and 231-35

[ca. 22-26 September 1867]

Sir B. Frere says that as Sir J. Lawrence's despatch refers only to Bengal and provinces, we ought to say either in our private letter to Sir S. Northcote or elsewhere that we hope something will be done for Madras and Bombay and that we ought to send him Ellis's paper with abstracts from his letters. He is going to send back our whole concern this morning.

26 September [1867]

Sir B. Frere was here two hours [25 September]; he has no alteration to make in the letter to Sir S. Northcote, which he would wish to go to Balmoral on Saturday or Monday. He thinks that a letter ought to go out without delay from Sir S. Northcote to Sir J. Lawrence (without even waiting for the appointment of the commission) on 3 October and he thinks my letter should reach Northcote in time to prompt this. But he thinks it is of the utmost importance that *we* should privately write to Sir J. Lawrence on 3 October asking him to inquire into the Peshawar. Sir B. Frere says not. Sir B. Frere says that they are now (at the India Office) granting £400,000 for *works at Peshawar*, that, so far as they know, these plans contain not one of the sanitary conditions which we require. They won't. Certainly. But Sir B. Frere says that, when he said something, he was told that Lord Cranborne had made this promise, that Peshawar was to have the £400,000 for works alone for the cantonment of Peshawar, that no inquiry was to be made, that the plans would not come before the India Office at all. Well, it's going to be done; it's sanctioned by Lord Cranborne. Sir B. Frere says that he knows of his own personal knowledge, that Sir J. Lawrence will do that for me which he won't do for the secretary of state. He thinks we might interfere successfully about Peshawar. Sir S. Northcote is not going to decide at all.

Lord Cranborne *has* decided we *shall have* that committee but not till November. And Sir B. Frere told me all about that. He knows Peshawar and Mian Mir well and he gave me a long account of the cantonment of Pune, which he says will do just as well for Peshawar. He says that Pune is as we know a town of 90,000 people, that the cantonment grew up *below* and under the prevailing wind of Pune, that the interval became filled up with another town of 30,000 people, that the drinking water was supplied by a river into which the whole drainage went, that they had always cholera or something else, that Sir Jamsetjee[107] at last said he would pay a fabulous sum to give them good drinking water, that the river was dammed up (to make a reservoir) by the military engineer, that the dam gave way, that the river was dammed up by a civil engineer and the dam gave way.

It was then asked how the native engineers made tanks and it was then done according to their plan and the dam did not give way, but that the whole drainage was still allowed to run into the river; that Dr Leith remonstrated, that they made a plan and estimate and sent it to the supreme government. That they said it was too dear, that they made another, that, in the meanwhile, it was found out that they could irrigate a ground of 90 miles at a remunerative cost of from 5 to 20 percent, that *this* was referred to Calcutta, that then they said *that* came under the head of irrigation loans and they must have a new and minuter estimate for *that*; that Sir B. Frere said, Well, the estimate is for £200,000, make it £205,000 if you will. But let us have it; the *least* return will be 5 percent. This has been going on for nineteen years. And *it has been up to this moment* lying at just the same point that it has been for nineteen years. Sir B. Frere told me exactly that about Mian Mir. He says it might be remedied but that nothing has been done. He says so and he says Sir J. Lawrence is not only trying to drive over the heap of stones (like the hackney coachmen) but to break them, all by himself and he can't.

Sir S. Northcote has appointed a committee on the Orissa business which holds its first meeting today. Sir B. Frere is on it. He says, the only proposition that has reached them to make 40 millions of uncivilized starving people into 40 millions of civilized people is to have two

---

107 Jamsetjee Jeejeebhoy (1783-1859), Parsi merchant and philanthropist, founder of schools and hospitals. First Indian national to be knighted 1842, he was made baronet in 1858. His descendents took the same name as second, third, etc., baronet.

commissioners and ten stipendiary magistrates. He says that everything must come from Sir J. Lawrence, that Sir J. Lawrence would do for me what he won't do for Sir S. Northcote

Sir B. Frere says it is of the utmost importance that Sir S. Northcote should write to Sir J. Lawrence by next mail before the effect of our letter to him of last mail has gone off. He says it will be effective in the same way as telling a drowning man to swim. Sir B. Frere says that Sir J. Lawrence is about India exactly as England is about Ireland, trying all kinds of every imaginable specific but never going to the root of giving India a good government.

He says, with regard to all those things, the refusing a guarantee of 5 percent to railroads when no one knows that the possession of India may not turn upon being able to throw in a few hundred men from Karachi and such things as the supply of water to Pune when there is a certainty of remunerative return in irrigating ninety miles of land. If you ask, Well, who is it who prevents these things? The answer is, Nobody. The answer is, There is no one to shake the financial minister and say, You find us this money somehow, for we must and will have it.

Sir B. Frere says that it would be highly advisable if I could only get Lord Stanley to say to Sir S. Northcote, Well now, this was a subject which interested me very much—do look it up now.

Only Galton never does anything for me but criticize *my* letters (for which I am very much obliged to him). For the matter of that, Galton does less for me than Lord Stanley. For we do know that Lord Stanley spoke for me both to Sir Northcote and to Lord Cranborne.

Sir B. Frere says that Lord Cranborne may possibly be the next governor general or the next secretary of state, that he is a very dangerous enemy and ministers would gladly do something for him and that it would be most desirable if we could get hold of Lord Cranborne now.

Sir B. Frere still thinks that we ought to write to Sir J. Lawrence and tell him that we understand large sums are about to be expended on Peshawar as a cantonment and stronghold and have such and such sanitary considerations been attended to. *He* says we ought to apply to Sir J. Lawrence. The expenditure was sanctioned by Lord Cranborne. Sir B. Frere says they can do nothing farther (he has tried) but I could.

You stated [Dr Sutherland] (in this which Sir B. Frere has seen) that we have no hint in *any* document as to the cause of the disease. Now, you say, that we have a hint as to the causation (in those papers). That's just what he says. Well, Sir B. Frere says I ought to ask for that. He said so on the grounds in this letter.

Source: From a letter to Sir Stafford Northcote, ADD MSS 50210 ff63-68, draft ADD MSS 45779 ff114-18

28 September 1867

*Private.* I have no apology for again writing to trouble you, none but the extreme urgency of the business. And therefore I may as well not attempt any apology. You have no doubt received the same deplorable accounts of cholera in the N.W. Provinces as I have from Sir John Lawrence.

Up to the date of the last accounts, several companies of the best soldiers in the British Army had perished at and near Peshawar, the regiments losing as many men from cholera as usually fall in a great battle. We have besides had a great many papers (after Indian fashion) on the subject, which show that the sanitary arrangements are just as unsatisfactory now as they were years ago and that there is no reasonable hope of anything really efficient being done, unless there be established a properly constituted Public Health Department at the India Office and in India, as a recognized branch of permanent administration. On this general subject, printed papers sent to me from India, in answer to my own letters, all show that, whatever has been done in the way of improving the public health, has been done by fits and starts and without any system. It is true that barracks are being built and that some stations are being improved. But these things do not constitute public health administration any more than building houses in London. For example, why are Mian Mir and Peshawar so deadly to regiments quartered there? It is not the first time that these catastrophes have happened. Men have been perishing by cholera year after year. And we who have been asking and receiving deluges of information, both public and private, on this matter, cannot nevertheless at this moment give an opinion as to the causes of unhealthiness at either station. No document in our possession gives the slightest hint as to what steps have been taken to remedy the unhealthiness.

Surely the most costly of all administrative proceedings is to send these strong Highland regiments into districts of [a] country where the causes of unhealthiness ought to be perfectly known, when no efficient steps are taken to remove them. Years ago we were told that at both stations the troops died because they had no wholesome water to drink. The late experience would show that the same deficiency exists still. It is obvious that such calamities ought not to recur, neither in the army nor in the civil population.

Our present position is simply this, that four years ago the report of the royal commission was sent to India, that everything promised fair in the first instance, that the beginning of a public health administration was first made and then unmade, before the administration itself was organized. Something has been done on no definite system and without any defined responsibility so that in all probability (to quote my nursery) "all the queen's horses and all the queen's men" could not find out who or what was to blame for either Mian Mir or Peshawar. In Madras presidency alone was any definite method proposed for organizing a Public Health Department, viz., by officers of health and inspectors, acting under the presidency commission. But it was first discouraged, then rejected. And the head of the commission, Mr Ellis, who proposed the plan, was so disheartened that he intended to resign because he could do no good (which was not exactly true). He is now secretary to government at Madras.

This great question being now in this position, Sir John Lawrence, who has done the very best he could under the circumstances, will be home in a year or little more. And there will be no security that the work, which he has been doing his utmost to forward, will make progress for a single day after he has returned, that is, *not unless* there is some executive machinery in India to do the work, and some controlling machinery here to know that it is being done.

We have now ample experience to guide us as to what should be done. The first step towards improvement is (what you kindly informed me that you proposed) the public health committee at the India Office. It is perfectly true that you cannot improve the public health in India except by local action in India, in the places where causes of disease exist. But your committee would forward the systematizing of local effort. And, as its head possesses a perfect command of the whole Indian subject, he would be able to advise on all administrative points connected with the reform of stations, bazaars and towns while he would also aid in the consideration of methods of procedure, sanitary laws and all the machinery (so requisite) which may be proposed in India for the future improvement of the country. All persons in India having any public health function to perform would know that their proceedings were watched by a special department of the India government (nothing stimulates them so much). And such things as have happened at Peshawar could scarcely pass without rigid scrutiny and discovery of the causes and their ultimate removal.

As Mr Ellis is now secretary to government at Madras, would it be possible and advisable to allow him to make a trial of his health organization (by districts, officers of health and inspectors, followed by the execution of works and measures) with such modifications as farther consideration may have enabled him to make in the plan in Madras presidency? This would bring us farther administrative experience. But what we really want is a thoroughly comprehensive organized system of proceeding. The things *to be done* are all laid down in the report of the royal commission, over which both Lord Herbert and Lord Stanley presided. And the time has certainly now come when Indian administrators should take this great subject in hand and define the *methods in which* these things *are to be done.*

This certainly is a most favourable moment, when we have a governor general who only waits for the secretary of state in order to do it, and a secretary of state who is ready and able to guide and sanction the governor general in doing it. It is a combination which we have never had and may never have again.

Source: From an incomplete letter to Sir John Lawrence, Add Mss 45777 ff142-43

September [1867]

The improvement of stations, barracks, hospitals and other military establishments would, I apprehend, go on as at present.

With reference to this subject, Colonel Crommelin's letter has afforded us a great deal of pleasure: It is indeed a great thing for us that the Works Department in India and we here should be so much at one on these questions that we differ only in a few details. Permit me a remark or two on this subject.

Colonel Crommelin says that he does not understand an observation of mine that the barrack plans suggested by the Army Sanitary Commission would have been different had they been arranged for doors instead of windows. I only meant that, as the ventilation had been arranged with special contrivances for increasing or diminishing it according to circumstances, and as the arrangements had been made contingent on the introduction of windows which could be closed to prevent draughts, these ventilating arrangements would have been different if the doors had to have been left open and some contrivance would have been introduced to have protected the men from the doors themselves causing blasts of wind.

Nearly every barrack in Algeria has only one door per room and no door opens upon the outer air. Their plan is not a good one. But the men are certainly preserved from diseases incident to changes of temperature.

The effect of these changes both in barracks and hospitals is a purely medical and not an engineering or military question. And their results on health is matter of purely medical evidence.

The medical authorities cited by Colonel Crommelin are not adverse to us, because one of them states that draughts are not injurious "ordinary care being taken to avoid them," which is just what soldiers don't take. The other authority says that he does not consider draughts to be so injurious, "except in the case of men coming into a room in a state of perspiration," which is just what soldiers *do* do in most Indian barracks.

Here in England, in all our barrack improvements, we have had to consider soldiers' habits. We cannot be always dragooning them.

Source: Notes for John Sutherland on Sir John Lawrence and Lord Cranborne, Add Mss 45752 f241

17 October 1867

Sir J. Lawrence's postscript: The important part is the P.S. In it he says that the secretary of state does *not* support him. Now the S. of S. says Sir J.L. has only to propose and it is done. Lord Cranborne "foaming at the mouth" says (about irrigation?) he never can make out, when the S. of S. is all anxiety to sanction and the governor general is all anxiety to do, why it is not done. That is just what the G.G. says to me (I am not a big enough man to "foam at the mouth"). He says *he* is willing. The secretary of state says *he* is willing. Why is it not done?

I believe the answer is there are two supreme powers: India government in India, India government at home. But there is a higher power than either and this is English jobbers, men who have neither money nor principle but only wit. I believe this is the true answer to Lord Cranborne. For example, in the works at Rio de Janeiro, ditto at Malta, but for English jobbers, the works might have been done at one tenth the price. For example, the British Railways have spent 700 millions and are paying (some of the greatest who are insolvent) their dividends out of borrowed money, money not earned.

We are given up to bribery and corruption. For example, at this moment it is quite uncertain, at the metropolitan board of works, whether, in the Thames embankment, there has not been the same jobbery. About India: I often think that I, a fool, rushed in where angels feared to tread. Government in India must take these great works into its own hands and not leave them to "private enterprise."

Source: Notes for John Sutherland on a conversation with Sir Bartle Frere, Add Mss 45752 ff242-43

22 October 1867

The [India Office Sanitary] Commission is actually appointed—I have seen the letters of appointment. And it enters on functions on 1 November: Sir B. Frere, chairman; Sir E. Perry, P. Cautley, Mr Arbuthnot, Captain Eastwick (the best), Sir H. Anderson, secretary. Sir B.F. says that there is a nasty prejudice expressed in the very letter in which he received his appointment by Sir S. Northcote, against the royal commission and the Army Sanitary Commission. He came to me, knowing that Sir S. Northcote was coming here, to ask me to explain to Sir S. Northcote the real state of things. Sir B.F. says there is not the slightest difficulty about it. He says Sir J. Lawrence has written a despatch which neither Sir S. Northcote nor he have yet seen (such is the state of disorder at the India Office), that it is of the utmost importance I should see it, that he is told Sir J.L. has asked for a Public Health Service with a central responsible authority, that Sir J.L. has since telegraphed, asking for an immediate answer, that he wants me to say to Sir S. Northcote (telegraph at once): "We accede to your proposal; we will send you a despatch mentioning the heads of what is to be done and await your answer as to how." That he thinks it of the utmost importance that *we* should see this despatch. . . .

Sir B. Frere says that Sir S. Northcote should in his despatch summarize the past history and then call on Sir J. Lawrence to point out the methods by which the past history can now be developed and organized and extended into practice. But he wants us both to initiate and to revise the despatch. He says the first thing is to find out what Sir S. *Northcote* proposes to do, what he has in his mind.

Sir B.F. says that the court of directors [of the Company] always managed in this way. If one local government proposed some scheme, they sanctioned it; they then wrote to another local government, such and such has succeeded, if you wish to do likewise, adapt it to your own varieties, and we will sanction it. He told me a good deal, *without* wishing it to be embodied in the despatch.

He says, there must be a central responsible authority in Bengal, North West Provinces, Punjab, Madras, Bombay, that this should be the president of [the] sanitary commission, that all officers of health should report to him, but that it should be left to Sir J. Lawrence whether this man should be one of the secretariat (to which he, Sir B.F., acknowledges that he sees some objection. He says the man will get overwhelmed with routine business), or whether he should be a man to stand at the governor general's or governor's elbow, to have a day every week to bring all his business before governor or governor general. He (Sir B.F.) thinks this the best plan. He says the president in Bengal should be the superior deity of the other presidents. He says this man in *each* local government should decide as to whether the execution of works or rather the funds should come from the central government or from the municipality. That nearly every city has its municipal act now, though some are very bad, that it will be either the public works or the municipality which will have to do it. He says nothing can be easier.

He says that the vaccination people (who have been improved and educated) might be improved (instead of being cut down, as is now the case) to be officers of health of the districts. He says the president, the centre man, ought however to be rather an inspector general than a director general. He says that the small towns should have a civil surgeon, in some cases a native surgeon, as officers of health. He says that the natives are very much coming on in engineering, that at Bombay they have lately developed a college to teach native engineers not only surveying but real sanitary engineering and that this will develop native engineers. Then he says that hitherto the fatal difficulty in India has been that no one had any idea that there was any necessity (e.g., in an outbreak of cholera) to do anything but look after and report that all this look-aftering and reporting ended in nothing; no works were undertaken to prevent another cholera, that the great business of the India Office committee will be to call upon them: What is going to be done? What *has been* done? and to publish it yearly.

Source: Notes for John Sutherland on a conversation with Sir S. Northcote, ADD MSS 45752 ff244-45

23 October 1867

Now you're going to be good aren't you? For I *am* so tired and feverish. Sir S. Northcote said he came for two things:

1. Because he wanted to announce Sir B. Frere's [India Office Sanitary] Committee in the India Office tomorrow (today) where it meets with some opposition from Ahriman[108] Ross Mangles and he wanted me to coach him as to how to put it, that is, how to arrange the connection with the Army Sanitary Commission. In this I think I showed him there was no difficulty. I think he was satisfied.

108 Ahriman, the spirit of evil in Zoroastrianism.

He read over the names, but very fast: they were these: Sir B. Frere (I think I settled), General Baker, Sir P. Cautley, E. Perry, Captain Eastwick, Sir H. Anderson. He wanted to know whether Sir P. Cautley should remain on the Army Sanitary Commission.

2. He wanted to ask us what answer should be made to Sir J. Lawrence. And I have got his despatch here. I don't like it very much. But since that, Sir S. Northcote has had a private letter from Sir J. Lawrence, which he read to me, saying that there was the utmost urgency, because of the state of country villages. Sir S. Northcote has given me the despatch and begs us to give him the points for an answer.

I should tell you Sir S. Northcote thinks of sanctioning this with any suggestions we may make for Bengal and the Central Provinces only and then of asking Lord Napier to do Ellis's scheme. I wrote it out and sent it to Sir B. Frere with a letter. He said, with regard to Ellis's memo, "If he has in any way modified his view, you ought to give him the benefit of it, because we Indians never look again at any of our memoranda without wishing to add or alter something."

I have therefore looked out Ellis's two letters which bear upon it. Here they are.

Source: From a letter to Sir Bartle Frere, in John Martineau, ed., *The Life and Correspondence of the Rt Hon Sir Bartle Frere* 2:39-40

25 October 1867

I think, if you will allow me to say so, that it is very important for us now to begin well—to fix the points of what the organization proposed has to do—and then to call upon Sir J. Lawrence to fix the best methods of doing it.

We might never have such a favourable conjunction of the larger planets again: You, who are willing and most able to organize the machinery here; Sir John Lawrence, who is able and willing, provided only he knew what to do; and a secretary of state, who is willing and in earnest.

And I believe nothing would bring them to their senses in India more than an annual report of what they have done, with your comments upon it, laid before Parliament.

Source: From a letter to Sir Stafford Northcote, Add Mss 50210 ff72-75

30 October 1867

*Private.* I have kept the papers which you were kind enough to leave with me much longer than I intended and, I am afraid, longer than you expected. But I have tried to do carefully what you desired, by the light of what you said. And I now venture to send you the result of my cogitations.

I return the despatch of the Government of India relating to the sanitary inspectors and, in considering the whole subject raised in the despatch, I have found it to be impossible to deal with the one question of inspection, simply because if you were to sanction this and say nothing more, we should be just where we were when the original commissions were appointed, i.e., you would be sanctioning the advising element only and leaving the executive element out of the question. I need not say what this would lead to.

I have therefore ventured to trouble you with two papers. Paper No. 1 gives the heads of the whole subject seen from the administrative side. In Paper No. 2 I have ventured, as you permitted, to put down what might be the heads of a despatch on the subject. Of course I know not how far these heads may meet with your concurrence. But if, after you have considered the subject, you thought well to let me see a rough draft of what you might consider it advisable to send to India, I need scarcely say that I should esteem it a favour to be allowed to look it over in order to see that it covers our ground as far as possible. (And I would not keep it such an inordinate time as I have kept this despatch.)

As Sir John Lawrence's despatch applies only to Bengal and Provinces, it might be said that similar measures are equally required for Madras and Bombay. If you thought well, after your new committee have seen Sir J. Lawrence's despatch, to send a telegram, it might approve of proposed appointment of sanitary officers as inspectors general to do duty under civil governments as proposed in despatch 152, 16 August 1867 as a part of a sanitary administration for India. A despatch will be sent on the whole subject. I will not take up a moment more of your time with apologies for my lengthiness, as it is the subject which is important and not I. . . .

I think that I possibly may, in a few days, unless you forbid me, take courage and send you Mr Ellis's paper (and make you a very short abstract of his views) concerning a sanitary administration for Madras presidency, as it is possible that you might think well to sanction it, if urged by Lord Napier, as an experiment for Madras.

Source: From a letter to Douglas Galton, ADD Mss 45764 ff114-15

10 November 1867

*Private.* Sir S. Northcote has formally appointed his public health committee at the India Office. And it will meet for the first time on Monday (tomorrow): Sir B. Frere, chairman, Sir P. Cautley, General Baker, Captain Eastwick, Sir E. Perry, Sir H. Anderson, secretary. I am afraid that you do not approve, but I expect good work out of this committee. The fact is the irritation and jealousy (as regarded the War Office sanitary committee) was so perpetual that we scarcely made any way at this end. Indeed we had come to a deadlock. Sir B. Frere, who is completely above all that sort of thing and who is very anxious to consult your committee, instructed me how to proceed about it. And I think we shall be in a better position than before. We could hardly have been in a worse. Sir B. Frere's committee will keep a hand over the question in India, so that we shall now have official means of calling people to account and of reporting to Parliament. I believe that Sir P. Cautley and Sir R. Martin will remain on your committee as before and that in future the India Office committee will send formulated questions to you instead of papers. In this way the grudge will be done away with.

The next thing is to reply as quickly as possible: would you think well to have a standing sub-committee for Indian work, by whom these questions might be at once taken up and, as soon as the sub-committee had finished its report, a general committee might be called and the reply sent to the India Office at once?

ever yours

Florence Nightingale

*Is* Colonel Greathed put on the Council of Education?

Source: Notes for John Sutherland on an interview with Sir Bartle Frere, ADD Mss 45752 ff259-60

23 November 1867

I have been so hard-worked and my cares are more than my hairs. Sir B. Frere says the [India Office] Sanitary Committee (I mean to call it department) sits now every Monday. Today it takes our despatch in hand. He says it will then come before the India Office on Thursday.

Sir S. Northcote who is (he says) a very good judge as to what will pass the gate, doubts whether our whole despatch will pass the I.O. on Thursday. He thinks it better to proceed by steps to adopt Sir J. Lawrence's proposal first and then to creep on. *But,* he says, if the committee of this morning should strongly recommend to go for the whole thing at once, he will try it on Thursday.

Well, Sir B. Frere hopes that he's got the Bombay drainage referred to Rawlinson. He says that he is sure Sir S. Northcote means me to see the despatch before it goes but that, if it does not go the whole length, he STRONGLY recommends us to lose no time but write immediately to Sir J. Lawrence and ask HIM to INITIATE the rest.

Sir B.F. says that at present, the I.O. send him (the public health commission) all the papers they are bothered with and want to get rid of. They have got a most curious set of papers about fever in the Ganges Delta and at Goa and Canare [Cannanore?]. He told me the contents and asked me whether they should be sent to you. I said Yes, if without jealousy. I told him so: to ask for observations, even if not for opinion, to send all the papers for observations or remarks (for a minute which will guide them).

They have got the Hardwar fair papers and he asked me whether . . . I did not tell him of Sir J. Lawrence's letter. He says that Lord Napier has a little the credit of writing finding-fault minutes and going *no farther.*

He says it is quite impossible to describe how entirely the Government of India is running to a government of detail. He says Massey[109] is worth nothing—Lord Elgin inaugurated all this government of detail. He says, under Lord Dalhousie and even under Canning, the governor general really reigned, that he said to his council, You disagree with me, shall I record your dissentient minute and send it home? They sometimes said, Yes but more often, No. The consequence was that the G.G. really governed. Lord Elgin did not make AN ATTEMPT at governing. He had not an opinion of his own.

Source: From a letter to Sir Stafford Northcote, ADD Mss 45779 ff133-34

29 November 1867

Telegram [to the Government of India]: it might approve of proposed appointment of sanitary officers of rank of deputy inspectors general to do duty under civil governments as proposed in despatch 152, 16 August 1867, as part of a sanitary administration for India. A despatch will be sent on the whole subject.

I will not take up a moment more of your time with apologies for my lengthiness, as it is the subject which is important and not I.

---

109 William Nathaniel Massey, successor to Sir Charles Trevelyan as financial member of the Government of India 1863-68.

Source: From a comment on a letter from Sir Bartle Frere of 20 March 1868, in John Martineau, ed., *The Life and Correspondence of the Rt Hon Sir Bartle Frere* 2:41

[after 20 March 1868]

I find nothing to add or to take away in the memorandum (sanitary) [memorandum/despatch for Sir John Lawrence]. It appears to me quite perfect in itself, that is, it is quite as much as the enemy will bear, meaning by the enemy—not at all the Government of India in India, still less the Government of India at home but—that careless and ignorant person called the Devil, who is always walking about taking knowledge out of people's heads, who said that he was coming to give us the knowledge of good and evil,[110] and who has done just the contrary.

It is a noble paper, an admirable paper—and what a present to make to a government! You have included in it all the great principles—sanitary and administrative—which the country requires. And now you must work, work these points until they are embodied in local works in India. This will not be in our time, for it takes more than a few years to fill a continent with civilization. But I never despair that in God's good time every man of us will reap the common benefit of obeying all the laws which He has given us for our well-being.

I shall give myself the pleasure of writing to you again about these papers. But I write this note merely to say that I don't think this memorandum requires any addition.

God bless you for it! I think it is a great work.

Source: From a letter to Julius Mohl, Florence Nightingale Museum (LMA) H1/ST/NC1/68/11

Lea Hurst
Matlock
22 September 1868

Sir Bartle Frere is come back. And it is he who advises me what to do in this provoking India business. The great point is to get a sanitary administration, including towns, villages, bazaars, etc., established before the end of Sir John Lawrence's reign. It is not so difficult as people think. For, as you know much better than I, the village organizations are there, ready to our hand. But of course it would not do for us at this end to advise a great sweeping uniform measure over that (small and compact) country we call India.

110 An allusion to Gen 3:5.

There is a great want of ability—somewhere. The three chief presidency sanitary commissioners (whom we established) keep sending us home schemes and plans on paper. But they still ignore the real practical matter, viz., who is to do the duties laid down and who is to find the money. Each is almost as great as the other on the subject of looking after other people, but neither the one nor the other have pointed out who these other people are to be, what they are to do, not who is to pay for it. To sweep India would be after all an easy matter if they had the least ability in dealing with these simple questions. But in "sanitary" things a "masterly inaction" does not do—on the contrary, they require the most energetic action not to get worse. These things don't settle themselves or, like Talleyrand's[111] letters, answer themselves, but are engaged in less dirty subjects.

Source: From a draft letter to Sir John Lawrence in Dr Sutherland's hand, Add Mss 45777 f172

[1868]

It is a mistake to suppose that natives take little interest [in] or would object to pay for improvements. The cost of the sanitary service at Congeeveram was gladly borne by the natives. The pilgrims at Hardwar gladly paid a tax to help the expenses incurred by government for the sanitary arrangements and one of the officials argued from this that they would gladly pay for the town and village improvements. Lately a severe marsh fever, due to want of drainage and bad agriculture, broke out in villages near Calcutta. It was pointed out to some of them that they might improve the public health by cultivating the ground. They grasped at the idea and began immediately. . . . The central government must lead the way in all these improvements. There is nothing to show that the natives would not readily follow.

111 Charles Maurice de Talleyrand-Périgord (1754-1838), variously bishop, supporter of the French Revolution and foreign minister.

Source: From a letter by Sir Bartle Frere to Sir Richard Temple,[112] copied out by Nightingale, Add Mss 45780 ff131-32

India Office
14 October 1868

*Private.* By this mail you will receive a copy of a Blue Book on Indian sanitary matters up to the end of 1867. It is as you will see not quite complete as a précis, but it gives all that is officially on record here and some important papers, which you perhaps have not seen. Let me especially beg your attention to pp 14 to 17.

I know that your financial labours will not diminish your interest in these matters, and your aid is now especially needed because all men do not feel as strongly as, I am sure, you do, that the best way to save the public revenue is to spend a good deal of it in saving the lives and the health of industrious and money-making morals; and you will not, I am sure, be deterred from helping to save life and health, merely because it costs money.

But what I want you immediately to do is to get Sir J. Lawrence to take the decisive steps necessary to put the work on a proper footing before he leaves. The Blue Book will show you how much has been done and how much proposed since he went out, but you will see that everything is in a transition state and that, unless something be done to give fixed and definite form to the Sanitary Department and make it a regular recognized part of the administrative machinery, things may revert pretty much to the state they were in before the Crimean War.

There is now a Sanitary Department in this [India] Office, but I cannot learn that the Government of India has noticed this fact, which was conveyed to them in a despatch dated in November last. . . .

You can understand why I do not write to Sir John direct, but this is a subject which much concerns the credit of his administration, as well as health and life, and on which, I am sure, he feels very deeply; if you could discover where the hitch is and remove it, you would prevent the labour and thought he has bestowed on the subject being wasted.

---

112 Sir Richard Temple (1826-1902) had a long career in India before becoming a member of the viceroy's council in charge of finance 1868-74, lieutenant governor of Bengal 1874-77 and governor of Bombay 1877-80. In 1880 he embarked on a political career in England. He wrote several books on India.

A parting resolution by the Viceroy-in-Council, reviewing what has been done and is being done, might be drawn up in laying down a course of proceeding for the future. The expense of the executive which is required to give effect to what all wish to do is the only difficulty I can think of, and if you could wind up the resolution by a promise that a special assignment should be made for this purpose in the forthcoming budget, there ought to be no more excuse for inaction. The local governments ought to be able to tell you by telegram what they will want. Or Strachey for Bengal, Ellis for Madras and Bell (Colonel) for Bombay could at once name to you a lump sum which would suffice to start with in each presidency and you could fix something less for each of the other administrations.

But much of the expense will of course be done by the municipalities. I need not tell you how much will depend on leaving much latitude in details to local judgment.

Source: From a letter to Sir Harry Verney, Wellcome (Claydon copy) Ms 9003/51

4 November 1868

To undertake anything *at all* that will bring down any correspondence upon me is past my power. I have more painful cares at this moment than any one human being can or ought to undertake. I am pressed to that degree by Lord[113] and Lady Mayo's departure (*she* too has just been here) that I can hardly breathe. . . . I don't think either Mr Mill or Mr Chadwick or many other men have used me well about many things. They make me take no end of trouble for them. They never do anything for me. Mr Mill has never helped me about India. Then they both of them often say to me, "Give me your name" and leave *me* to bear all the correspondence which *invariably* in my case follows upon it.

Source: Note on sanitary engineers for John Sutherland, Add Mss 45753 f102

[5 November 1868]

He [the sanitary engineer?] might ask each governor, lieutenant governor, chief commissioner and each chief sanitary officer either by letter or orally: "What special reports have you on the sanitary measures required in any large city or district under your charge? What are the

113 Richard Southwell Bourke, Lord Mayo (1822-72), viceroy and governor general of India 1869-72, a moderate Conservative; he was assassinated by a Wahabi supporter in 1872. Lord Mayo was active in promoting schools and hospitals, and in improving means of communication (roads, railways and canals) better to serve famine areas.

measures recommended and approved by you for improving its sanitary condition? Have these measures been carried out, and if not why not?"

They would probably plead deficiency of men or deficiency of money. If so, the government should provide properly trained engineering officers, as they have done in Captain Tulloch's case, whom they sent to England on purpose. If they want money, it would have to be found.

Source: From notes on health officers and staffing of commissions for John Sutherland, ADD Mss 45753 ff111 and 158

[c1868]

The thing seems to be in a nutshell: it is wholly a question of persons. If you had more Hewletts than one, you would say, Put the executive power into the hands of the medical officer of health. If you had more Tullochs than one, you would say, Put the executive into the hands of the executive engineer. But as to putting such power into the hands of a Goodeve, a Farquhar,[114] a Murray, a Hunter,[115] or *any* or *all* of the now numerous Indian doctors who have been sent to me or have corresponded with me, you might much better put it into the hands of Temperance [Nightingale's maid].

As to putting it into the hands of a Parkes,[116] a Farr, a Rumsey, a Sir J. Watson, or any or all of the Crimean War doctors whom I know, you would get out of them a discussion upon contagion and nothing more. Parkes is totally unfit to give even the elementary knowledge Hewlett requires [breaks off]. He's [Hewlett] unique. He's like his

114 Sir John Lawrence's physician.

115 William Guyer Hunter (1827-1902), born in Calcutta, received a commendation 1854 for his work during a fever epidemic, army medical officer in Bombay 1850, principal of Jamsetjee Hospital 1876 and professor of medicine at the Grant Medical College, sent by the Indian Medical Board to Egypt to investigate the cholera epidemic 1883, which he denied was imported from India but rather was due to unusual weather conditions; his report emphasized sanitation instead of quarantine; defended his opposition to germ theory at the Sanitary Conference in Rome 1885; supported Nightingale and Galton's work on village sanitation in India for Tropical Section of 8th International Congress of Hygiene and Demography at Budapest 1894. See Mariko Ogawa, "Uneasy Bedfellows" 676-80.

116 Edmund Alexander Parkes (1819-76), professor of hygiene at London University and Army Medical School at Netley, regarded as the founder of the science of modern hygiene; friend.

uncle, Mr Whitfield, who can scarcely write English but who is and remains the only hospital man who has the least inkling of the real portée [import] of the question of health of hospitals.

[ca. December 1868]

Sir Bartle Frere has put into a general minute what we said about Dr Hewlett, that Bombay officers of health must have executive powers. If this does not succeed, he will write a special minute about Dr Hewlett and he has indoctrinated Mr Scobell, the legal remembrancer and financial advisor of the Government of Bombay, who is just going out, upon the position Dr Hewlett should have.

He wishes us to go forward with a training scheme for officers of health for India to be submitted to him privately and then to be sent *officially* by the Army Sanitary Commission to his department at the India Office, while they are in their present favourable temper.

Well, he says, take care not to put too much into the answer to *that* despatch, for fear of not securing the first point.

Source: From notes on Sir John Lawrence's papers, Add Mss 43546 ff125-27

6 February 1869

*Private and confidential.* All this time, Sir John Lawrence had been busily urging forward (1) general improvement in *stations*; (2) extension of *barracks* and hospitals, both in building the new and improving the old; (3) *water supply*. This is being carried out for Calcutta and about to be carried out for Madras; (4) *drainage*. That of Calcutta is being carried out. Lord Napier of Madras and Mr Ellis of Madras had sent home a very promising young engineer officer, Captain Tulloch, to see the latest and best drainage operations in Europe. Captain Tulloch made wonderfully good use of his time and was so successful that, on his return to India, he was snapped up by the enterprising Government of Bombay. His plans seem likely to be accepted both at Bombay and Madras. They are very good. (F.N. would send Lord de Grey Captain Tulloch's drainage report of November 1868. But it is of course technical.)

There are now here a multiplicity of papers on all points of the subject, some of them administrative and *in transitu*, such as regarding the duties to be discharged by the local sanitary commissioners and their relations with the sanitary commissioner with the Government of India, some of them, reports of progress such as report on the sanitary administration of the Punjab for 1867 [the list of papers continues]. . . .

F.N. would gladly send all or any of these documents to Lord de Grey. But they are so voluminous that she does not like to do so without special desire. She has therefore indicated by the above list what they are and the general advance of the question. The accompanying Blue Book is the only *general* document that has been issued by the I.O. This is the first year's issue. It is to be annual.

Source: From a letter to Lord de Grey, Add Mss 43546 ff119-21

6 February 1869

*Private and confidential.* If I could, I would write the "History of a Minute" [Lord de Grey's minute of June 1866] in the same way as the Egyptians wrote the History of a Soul in all its different transmigrations in hieroglyphics on their temples; how this minute had really grasped the entire subject of social reform in India so far as connected with the state of agriculture and the public health; how the constant Tutelary *Genius,* Sir John Lawrence, had apprehended this; how Lord Cranborne, with all his great abilities, had not; how a "sanitary department" was formed in the Council of India expressly for the purpose of cultivating this minute; how Sir Stafford Northcote reproduced this minute; how the great Oracle of Delphi, the *Times,* without knowing it, selected this minute, the epitome of the India sanitary question, as being one of the most important papers on the principles of Indian administration; how this minute fructified not only for sanitary work but in many other directions, so that it would have been worthwhile being S. of S. for India to have done nothing else but put such views on record; how it is the pivot of a record of progress in India to be proud of.

Much, however, remains for this minute to do, e.g., in initiating a better prison system, and in extending public health works for natives as well as troops. I enclose the first year's of an *Annual* Report to be issued by the I.O. ("Memorandum" [*on Measures Adopted for Sanitary Improvements in India Up to the End of 1867*] [in *Social Change in India*]) which is by no means complete or even a summary of all that has been done, on account of the want of official reports; but taking it as it is, it is a marvel in its way and will be improved year by year.

New principles have taken root. And the minute must give its care and guidance to see that they flourish and bear fruit. It is not so much among the troops now, for really what Sir John Lawrence and the minute have done for them is marvellous, as it is among the native towns and villages that we want a wise progress, the spread of sound principles and of knowledge to be inculcated and extended by the minute.

The extraordinary success of sanitary measures at the fair of Hardwar, where the annual crowds of pilgrims are so enormous that they might well baffle all precautions, at the pilgrimage of Conjeeveram

(Madras) and this not only with the perfect concurrence of the natives but with their willingness to *pay* for these measures: these and similar examples show how great and hopeful a work may be begun among them, even to realizing the fact eventually that India, which is more fatal to the natives now than the worst parts of Europe are to the European natives, may become as healthy as the best parts of Europe to European natives, and that India is no more necessarily fatal to Europeans than this their own home.

The minute will no doubt farther comprise in its history the zealous part it took in initiating the work. During the whole period of Sir John Lawrence's reign, he has been so good as to be in constant communication with me on all the subjects of the minute (indicated in the other paper). He is not, as you know, a sanguine man and he scarcely does himself justice either in what he has done or what he has set on foot, though he is extremely sensitive to others doing him injustice. He has entered warmly into all the views of the minute and has done all he could to forward them. There have been, and there are and will be great difficulties and opposition. And the habits of vast native races cannot be changed in a day. But his own personal weight and interest have done a very great deal. And India owes a vast debt to him in this matter as in many others.

*Private.* I trust that his successor will do something also. I was not in the least acquainted with Lord Mayo, but he wrote to me to ask to see me and we, in November 1868, discussed as well as we could in so short a time the points for progress, and I also, at his desire, drew up some on paper for him. He is extremely well disposed to sanitary and agricultural improvement. That there is no sanitary organization as yet for villages is one of our great deficiencies in India.

I have drawn up a very bald and meagre Note on the progress of things (sometimes backwards) between June 1866 and January 1869 and enclosed it in another envelope with the I.O. Blue Book in question, which very likely you have already, with a supplement of the *Times.* I imagine you so busy with papers of another department that I have not liked to send you a great mass of illustrative documents which I have, many of them sent me by the kindness of Sir John Lawrence without your specially desiring it.[117]

---

117 Ff 122-27 contain a detailed "note on the progress of Lord de Grey's minute (left at the India Office in June 1866) on the sanitary service of India from June 1866 to December 1868."

Allow me again to thank you for all the good you have done us which, believe me, dear Lord de Grey,

makes me your ever obliged and faithful servant

Florence Nightingale

Source: Note on Lord de Grey for John Sutherland, ADD Mss 45753 f186

[ca. 16 February 1869]

I could wish I could have shown you my letter to Lord de Grey, but I did not like to delay it. You know he is [lord] president of the council and that is why he wishes to see all those papers about quarantine and cholera. It is a most favourable opportunity of getting hold of him. I tried to use it.

Source: From two notes for John Sutherland, ADD Mss 45753 ff195 and 192

[ca. February 1869]

Do you wish to hear about Galton? He has written to me in answer to mine, yielding and saying he *will* attend if summoned, but saying that he does so only to delay the doom of the Army Sanitary Commission, which he looks on as doomed; [as long as] Cardwell[118] and Northbrook[119] are there, nothing can save it.

[end February 1869]

I must now write to Sir B. Frere. It isn't the "class of" officers he wants to know—he suggested that himself—it is their powers and duties, what we should suggest to put into their second annual memorandum.

It is a fortnight since he was here and he begged me to write or see him as soon as possible. I told you that I told him every word of this. I told you that he said we were to say what we should suggest officers of health were to do in India.

Source: From a letter to Robert Rawlinson, Boston University 1/4/56

2 March 1869

*Private.* I have received lately very strong complaints from the India Office on the dilatoriness of the Army Sanitary Commission in sending in their answers and minutes. This, I am sure, is in no way to be attributed to you or Dr Sutherland. And I believe I know where the

118 Edward Cardwell (1813-86), secretary of state for war 1868-74.

119 Thomas George Baring, Lord Northbrook (1826-1904), governor general and viceroy of India 1872-76.

fault lies. But I wish it could be remedied. The India Office is dilatory enough in itself.

Source: From a letter to Frances Nightingale and one probably to her also, Wellcome (Claydon copy) Ms 9003/94 and 102

8 April 1869

All the offices ask me for advice—I give my advice—my advice is masterly. I tell them what to do and they don't do it. Or rather I am like the French journalist who says that he has uttered eight millions of truisms in the last ten years; so have I, that it is more tiresome to teach truisms than to relate murders, which Tacitus[120] says is tiresome—so I think—and that not one of the eight millions of truisms has benefited one of the eight millions of his readers. That is just my case, always excepting India.

Sir John Lawrence, in his grand simple way, said: "You started the royal commission, you initiated the public opinion which forced Sir Charles Wood to take up sanitary works, which he did not believe in, *as a policy*. And now there is not a station in India where they are not doing something." But I shall be wearying you.

6 May 1869

It is now thirteen years that I have been in the service of the government offices and, during those thirteen years, I have left London *once* before the House was up (viz., last year). And then a great disaster was the consequence. There have flown three years since I have had this house, thanks to you. And the first year, 1866, I could not leave London till *18 August*, the second year, 1867, I could not leave London *at all*. The third year, last year, I came to Lea Hurst the first week in July—the first time that I have broken loose since 1856—and we lost an important India Office step in consequence, owing to the inevitable delay of sending papers backwards and forwards.

## Later Contacts with and the Death of Sir John Lawrence

**Editor:** Nightingale and Lawrence remained in contact after his retirement as governor general and return to London in 1869. She saw him from time to time and continued to be impressed with his person and character, notably with the fact that he took on the (humble) post of member of the London School Board. Lady Harriette Lawrence often

120 *Annals* 16:16.

wrote letters for her husband and hence was at least in indirect touch with Nightingale. Letters to him regularly included comments about or for Lady Lawrence. In 1864, when he was beginning his work as viceroy in India, Nightingale wrote: "I think with the greatest satisfaction upon your reunion with Lady Lawrence and (some of) your children" (see p 212 above) and later she rejoiced "to think that, by this time, Lady Lawrence and your daughters are with you to take care of you. And I do not at all agree with you (nor, I am sure, do they) that it will be 'a sad sacrifice to them.' It is anything but a 'sacrifice' to be with you" (see p 214 above).

In a lengthy letter to her friend Mme Mohl, Nightingale compared Lawrence with Sir Bartle Frere, "two men so unlike, yet each so roundly perfect in his own." Frere and Lawrence would never understand each other, and Nightingale had given up the "slightest attempt" to effect an understanding, but "each is too much of a man, too noble, too chivalrous, to denigrate (dénigrer) the other." After this praise, however, came a statement of the "great faults" of his government, "the greatest of which was Caesarism." Lawrence could not see that, while an authoritarian approach was necessary in the period of Lord Dalhousie, during the process of conquest, it did not do for governing 200 million people in peacetime: "He could not delegate power to the local governments. The centralization was something inconceivable. . . . Sir J. Lawrence tried, with his indefatigable industry and powers of government, to do all the business in his own room for a country bigger than Europe." Yet he had "left his mark on India . . . set India on a new track, which—may his successors follow." She regretted that the new Government of India gave more power than they had to Lawrence to the new governor general, Lord Mayo, who did not "know a Sikh from a Bengali."[121]

On Lawrence's death in 1879 Nightingale mourned the loss of her hero and remembered his nobility. Lady Lawrence visited Nightingale after her husband's death to describe his last days and death.[122] There are eight surviving letters of Nightingale to Lawrence's private secretary, Louisa Gaster (below), thanking her and Lady Lawrence for sending mementos of him, commiserating on their mutual loss and answering Gaster's questions about an appropriate biographer to write his life.

121 The full letter is in *Women* (8:569-71).

122 Letter to Sir Harry Verney 5 July 1879, Wellcome (Claydon copy) Ms 9007/248.

Source: Notes on Sir John Lawrence for John Sutherland, Add Mss 45753 ff235-36
[ca. 3 or 4 April 1869]

In the first place, when I see him again I see that there is nobody like him. He is Ramesses II of Egypt. Gladstone and all the ministers are rats and weasels by his side. He says that Lord Mayo must hear the reports of the new medical sanitary inspectors of provinces, that he must consult the local governments what taxes can be laid on the people to carry out their recommendations and so go on gingerly.

He says that much has been done for the soldier, but still the soldier has not had *that* done for him which induces him to spend his money otherwise than in drunkenness, that drunkenness has diminished but not so much as it ought, that the fatal plan of paying the 2d. [pence] a day in lumps, of paying batta in lumps, of paying them for road-making in lumps. Though many soldiers do put into savings banks, still a great bulk of the money is spent in beastly drunkenness. He says this money ought to be given either in pension or, leaving a certain choice to the soldier, in increased pay.

He is quite against the short time system and the reinlisting system. He says people don't know the Indian soldier who talk in that way. He says why don't you get recruits? Because the soldier when he comes home deters others from enlisting by his wretchedness; *he* is the inducement which *prevents* decent young men from enlisting. He says the man takes his run home, he spends his money in drunkenness, he reinlists, he spends that money in drunkenness. How short-sighted, he says, is this short system talk? It's a system, he says, to enlist the scum of the earth.

If a decent man does enlist, he gets on, he gets made a clerk, he does not come home; why, if there is a man fit to get on, he *does* get on in the army. But the scum come home scum and are fit for nothing. They can't go into civil life, they become paupers and Sir C. Trevelyan talks nonsense.

Then, he says, about married men, what nonsense you talk. The men marry half-castes or quarter-castes and these women are very good women, much better than your soldiers' wives. They have their allowances and their children have allowances and they get on very well. Then you think it's a favour for them to come home. Why, they come home, they have no allowances and the woman turns prostitute for a living.

Lord Dalhousie, he said, asked me whether the men who distinguished themselves should have their names posted up on the church doors in England. "I think" (I said), "you had much better do something for them." Then they will be an advertisement to other men to enlist, when you want recruits. Now your time-expired men are an advertisement to other men *not* to enlist, when you want recruits.

Source: From a letter to Frances Nightingale, Wellcome (Claydon copy) Ms 9003/93

4 April 1869

Yesterday afternoon Sir John Lawrence spent with me. He had just come from the queen, from the presentation to her as a peer, but he did not mention this. I think he is a little more simple, modest and grand than ever. When I see these grand old fellows from India, how the English ministers of the present day dwindle into mere rats and weasels in comparison. Sir John Lawrence is like a Roman Caesar of the noblest type—say Titus or Marcus Aurelius.[123] He went off in a thick drizzling east wind fog and would not even let a cab be sent for.

Source: From a letter to John Strachey, Columbia University, Presbyterian Hospital School of Nursing C94

14 May 1869

Although it is a thousand years and a half since I have heard from you, still I hope that we have interests enough in common for me to write to you, not as a stranger.

I have had the very great pleasure of seeing Sir John Lawrence since his return (I don't like to call him by his new title yet—his old is so one and the same with our noblest history of India). He was good enough to come and see me in my sickroom. He does not look a day older. And I hope there are long years of service for him yet. He may still do so much good for India here, even without office. I always think of him as of the most *impressive* man I have ever known (though I have known many in a very eventful life). . . .

I am not so impertinent as to deal in praise. Mr Gladstone says that praise always implies something patronizing and that we ought to approach as pupils, not as praisers. And when I think of the immense work you and Sir John Lawrence have done in inaugurating the sanitary work all through India—a problem so immeasurable that we have nothing like it in England—I feel most deeply that it is not for me to approach with praise but with reverence.

However, I had almost left, womanlike, the most important thing to the end. And that is, the organization of a sanitary executive on

123 Titus Flavius Vespanasius (39-81 CE, emperor of Rome. Marcus Aurelius (121-80 CE), Roman emperor and Stoic philosopher.

which, we understand, you are engaged. This would be the crown to your arch. We hear, from time to time, of the administrative progress you are making in public health work. But we have heard but little of the results of the questions you sent some time ago to local governments about points of sanitary executive. If you have time to write a line—and great men have always time—it would interest me exceedingly to hear the result of this; also, how the administration of your sanitary rules is to be carried out.

Source: From notes on an interview with Lord Napier of Magdala on 14 December 1869, in Cook, *The Life of Florence Nightingale* 2:175-76

[December 1869]

When I look at these three men (though strangely different)—Lord Lawrence, Lord Napier of Magdala and Sir Bartle Frere—for practical ability, for statesmanlike perception of where the truth lies and what is to be done and who is to do it, for high aim, for noble disinterestedness, I feel that there is not a minister we have in England fit to tie their shoes—since Sidney Herbert. There is a simplicity, a largeness of view and character about these three men, as about Sidney Herbert, that does not exist in the present ministers. They are party men; these three are statesmen. S. Herbert made enemies by not being a party man; it gave him such an advantage.

Source: From a note/draft on Sir John Lawrence, Add Mss 45777 ff206-07

[14 January 1879]

I feel it such an honour to be allowed to call myself, even in the humblest degree, one of your followers. May I without impertinence lay my homage at the feet of Lord Lawrence for his splendid and patriotic part in heading the movement against the Afghan War? Though a majority, appealed to by the meanest and most claptrap of motives, has been successful this time against a minority higher both in light [right] and honour (a minority is not always in the right, but at least the right must always begin by being in the minority), yet immense good has been done not only by interesting the people of England but by making the meanness and the impolicy of charging the cost of the Afghan War upon poor dumb India more difficult to carry out.

The great Indian officials returning home do not in general interest England about India. Especially does an ex-viceroy think he has "a responsibility": he is afraid of being an "agitator." He *has* a "responsibility" indeed, but is it not that of interesting England in India? You cannot interest the India Office unless you interest the people of England. You cannot interest even Parliament unless you have a majority or a strong minority of the people of England at your back. How nobly India's statesman Lord Lawrence has fulfilled this duty history will tell.

Source: From a letter probably to Sir Harry Verney, Wellcome Ms 9007/246

1 July 1879

O what a loss. O the pity of it—the pity of it. To all India as to me. I received a letter from him [Sir John Lawrence] the day *after* his death, dictated but signed by himself, sending me Indian reports he had read and wished me to read, all marked and the page turned down where he had left off. Precious remembrances, though as remembrances not needed, but precious as what he wished me to do. God and he had not forgotten me.

O that I could do something for India which he saved and for which he lived and died. I am glad you have offered to go to the funeral, though I hope it will not overdo you. I am glad it is to be at Westminster Abbey, that all may see and be inspired by his greatness—the greatest man of our age. "Unselfishness and firmness," an Indian official said to me, "that could not be surpassed," and his voice broke down with tears.

I am in great trouble. Diphtheria in the house, doctor four times a day, trained nurse. I forbid everyone coming to the house. It is my little cook. Last night he came prepared to perform tracheotomy. But it was not needed. . . .

I have an article in *today's Good Words* on Bombay famine.

Source: From eight letters to Louisa Gaster [Sir John Lawrence's private secretary], Wellcome Ms 5475/1 to 8

30 June 1879

I cannot thank you enough, I cannot thank you enough. Those precious signs of him—the signature in his own hand, the reports he had read and wished me to read, the place where he left off—they have hardly been out of my hands since. O India for which he had done all, would that I could do something for her. O poor Lady Lawrence—poor daughters—and yet not poor, rich beyond all—for they have had, have still the greatest hero of our day—the vice gerent not only of an earthly sovereign but of God, the recreator of whole races—yet humble and simple, as became the servant of God, which he so truly felt himself to be and of which he was one of the highest in all time. O how he will be missed.

And who will write his life? None can do it but those who have lived as he lived. But he will be with us still; he is living, not dead, *living* more than ever. May his spirit be with us! as Christ promised us that His would be;[124] he followed in so many ways the steps of our great Master—he is now in the presence of God for which his whole life had made him fit.

He was so good as to come to see me (about sanitary things) just before his hurried departure from England for India in December 1863. He spoke of Lady Lawrence—*she* knows *how*—of the little babe unborn and of his children, his youngest. Then all about India—he had the blue eye and tender expression in it of a girl of sixteen and the brow, the head of the ruler of nations, the statesman, the general—a greater never ruled.

I can write no more. God bless and support Lady Lawrence and his children. There is not in all the world who can feel with them as I can. O may not his body lie in Westminster Abbey, where all may see and be inspired by his greatness. And may I say how *you* are to be envied for all you have done for him? May I write again?

yours overflowing in grief and sympathy
Florence Nightingale

30 July 1879

How good of you to remember the photographs for me. Even you cannot imagine how I have looked and longed for them. They were like a message. And even you cannot imagine how deeply sorry I am that I cannot see you this morning, as you so kindly offer.

This is the month of matrons to me, of seeing all our trained matrons. And I shall miss the divine strength of hearing all about *him*, who *was so strong*, from you. Alas! we shall miss him more and more every day, what must it be for Lady Lawrence?

Kindly *promise*—you say you will be in London again in three months—*to let me know* and promise me *a visit*. I shall look forward to it. My memory of him will be as fresh, my feeling of his loss ever increasing, as any. O what can we say about such a loss? There are no words. I have dried the rose which came from his coffin. His books are ever before me.

I will write again. The "message" of the photograph. God bless you; *do not forget* that I shall be longing to see you again. May I say:

124 An allusion to John 16:4-13.

write down *now* all that about his last days, his last years which you knew so well—all that you remember of him: it will be so valuable, so precious.

"How are the mighty fallen in the midst of the battle!"[125] God continue his work in India. God bless you and God bless Lady Lawrence and his children.

ever yours in him
Florence Nightingale

31 July 1879

I cannot thank Lady Lawrence enough for the photographs. May I try and say to you what they say to me (I think they say it more plainly even than when first I saw them, before the body of our hero was laid in Westminster Abbey). I have never seen anything so beautiful or so holy in the holiest pictures of the old masters. If it had been an old picture, we should have said: how far art transcends nature—the lips slightly parted (like those of a child in a rapture of joy in first awakening) with a childlike joy at entering into the presence of the Heavenly Father whom he had served so nobly and so humbly, the poor eyes looking down but as if they were looking inward into the soul to realize the rapture of surprise that is there; God for the first time dwelling in him in His fullness, like Milton's "And joy shall overtake him like a flood";[126] the face so worn, "it behoved Him to have *suffered* these things that He might enter into His glory."[127] What words those are! Here it was the joy *arising out* of the long trial, the toil, the cross out of which came the crown, the expression that of the child-soul rising spiritually out of the worn-out body shuffling off the "mortal coil"[128] and passing into the immediate presence of God. The subject is almost too sacred to write about. "My father, my father, the chariot of Israel and the horsemen thereof'[129] as they bear him away from us into the Immediate Presence of God. We see the path of light left behind and we ask, Upon whom has fallen the mantle? *Upon whom?* It shall not be "her last great man," sad India now deplores.

Who shall write his life? I think so much of that—that he may *not* be *the last.* You cannot think how little he is known in England and

125 2 Sam 2:25.
126 John Milton, "On Time," in *The Journey with Jesus: Poems and Prayers.*
127 An allusion to Luke 24:26.
128 *Hamlet,* Act 3, scene 1.
129 2 Kings 2:12.

how the little curs here have barked and bit round the heels of the noble lion! And now he is gone to undertake yet greater labours, to bless more worlds in the service of God.

I could not but write a word of thanks to Lady Lawrence today. Did I know where you were going, I would venture to write again; there is so much to say. You cannot think how I deplored not being able to see you, but one cannot throw aside duties to do honour to the man who was above all the man of duty. In haste to catch you before you go, with the precious photographs and his books ever before me at my bedside.

yours ever in sorrow but not in sadness
Florence Nightingale

That account was so infinitely touching which you gave about his having left nothing behind him, and the old shoehorn. You know, his was an ideal character: it was the ancient Roman, the hero saint, the chivalrous knight and statesman, and the anchorite of the first ages of Christianity, all in one with the tender husband of domestic life. If he had been a youthful lover instead of a viceroy going to his empire, he could not have spoken of her differently than he did to me in December 1863.

F.N.

Lea Hurst
Cromford, Derby
30 August 1879

I am *always* thinking of the question, as you put it, as to who could best write the life of Lord Lawrence, a "memorial" I think of more importance than perhaps any other or than anything the world could have said to it at this moment. And I have been making inquiries.

I am afraid what I have to suggest, if indeed it could be of use, has been delayed too long to be of any. The first thing is, what are the materials? The despatches he wrote from the Punjab, especially at the time of the Mutiny (I suppose, to the governor general), must be absolutely priceless. (The duke of Wellington's despatches could not be of so much importance.) These, I believe, have never been published. Would they be at the India Office or at Calcutta? Or both? And have they been asked for? As to the correspondence, you are making a list of it. The next thing is, what does Lady Lawrence propose? I supposed that the entire life could not be published at once, because parts of it must bear so hard on persons still living or lately dead. I venture to think that the great deeds of his viceroyalty would receive better justice some ten or twelve years hence. But what I hope will be brought out at once WITHOUT ANY DELAY is, not the whole Life, IF that cannot be done, but a biographical sketch of his government of the Punjab, especially at the time of the Mutiny. There is scarcely any deed of history, ancient or modern, to compare with this—the winning over the Sikhs to save the empire, the denuding himself of help and the having so converted our late fierce enemies that he could send *them* to *save* us. "Lord, here am I: send me,"[130] has been said by many (like Isaiah). *But he* could say, "Lord, here are *they*, send *them*."

This is what everybody can understand and reverence, what everybody would read, what would stir up no hideous controversies "o'er the grave where our hero we buried."[131] But *all* would reverence. I earnestly hope that those despatches are forthcoming. And there must be those still living who could add the most striking and telling personal facts, among them Mr Arthur Brandreth. But alas! how many are dead!

The next thing is, who is to do it? Has Lady Lawrence thought (1) of the *dean of Westminster*?[132] One drawback is that I believe he had not the good of being much acquainted personally with Lord Lawrence; the other is that he is very much occupied. The materials must be placed within easy access to him. But if he undertook it and was inspired by his subject he would make something like a worthy representation either of the whole life or of the Punjab epic. (2) Then there is *Mr Theodore Walrond,* the C.S. commissioner. He wrote Lord Elgin's life. Lord Lawrence's life is on the heroic scale and should have a hero to write it. But where are the Indian heroes who shared his labours and who are also writers? Who survives? Mr Walrond has judgment and in the selection among correspondence and despatches, perhaps good judgment is as much wanted as good writing. If he undertakes it, he should write the whole life. (3) Then there is *Mr Froude.*[133] He would do it well but he is so plastic one never knows what line he will take. (4) I confess that, if the dean of Westminster is not to be had, *Mr George Trevelyan* is the person I should like to see write the life. What

130 Isa. 6:8.

131 Charles Wolfe (1791-1823), "The Burial of Sir John Moore after Corunna" line 4. Sir John Moore (1761-1809), lieutenant general, was killed at Corunna in Spain when trying to stop the French.

132 Arthur Penrhyn Stanley gave the funeral sermon at Westminster Abbey.

133 James Anthony Froude (1818-94), historian and editor of *Fraser's Magazine.*

he writes would be read. And he is capable of enthusiasm. But he is very busy. (5) If he cannot be had, what would Lady Lawrence think of *Sir Charles Trevelyan, not* to write the *life* but to write the Punjab part of it? He has a true feeling of Lord Lawrence's great career. If the Punjab could be elicited out of him, it would be done with the just enthusiasm of a friend. (6) Of other Indians, there is *Colonel Malleson.*[134] What would Lady Lawrence think of him? The sketch he wrote of Sir John Lawrence was infinitely below the mark (published seven or eight years ago, or more, in a volume with sketches of Sir B. Frere and others). But he is known as a writer. (7) Colonel Sleeman[135] was a good writer but he is dead, is he not? Cannot you think of some Indian writer who is not dead? who would and could do some justice to the subject? and who personally took part in his life? or even one who could be a Johnson's Boswell? (8) Lastly, there is, in default of a more experienced writer, *Sir Arthur Hobhouse.* He is painstaking and conscientious; he is an earnest supporter of Lord Lawrence's opinions on Afghan policy.

I pray God that someone may be found not wholly unworthy of the subject. Why are there no Plutarchs[136] now? no Thucydides?[137] Lord Lawrence would be a finer subject for such an historian than Pericles[138] was for Thucydides. I cannot think but what someone will be raised up to do it.

I trust I shall see you again in London this autumn and must ask your forgiveness for not having written sooner. It is not for want of thinking of him whom we have lost and of those he has left without him.

I had to come down here (in Derbyshire) to take charge of my dear mother. This is always "neck or nothing" to me. Last year it was "neck," this year it is "nothing," that is, it was a nervous fever with ninety hours of sleeplessness. But I must not trouble you with my troubles. God speed the work of making John Lawrence known to *this* world as he is to God and heaven and the saints and heroes gone before.

---

134 George Bruce Malleson (1825-98), sanitary commissioner for Bengal, then India 1866-68.

135 Sir William Henry Sleeman (1788-1856), soldier and administrator in India, best known for his suppression of the thuggees or religious murderers in India.

136 Plutarch (46-120?), Greek biographer and philosopher.

137 Thucydides, Greek historian of the fifth century BCE.

138 Pericles, Athenian statesman, orator and general of the fifth century BCE.

Lea Hurst
Cromford, Derby
20 October 1879

The prayer is ever before me that this great man's life may be made an inspiration for generations to come, as well as the thought of Lady Lawrence which does not leave me. But I have hesitated to write because you kindly promised that you would let me "know the result" whether "the despatches written by Lord Lawrence from the Punjab" were "forthcoming on application." I feared to appear impatient. Possibly Lady Lawrence and her advisors may already have come to a decision as who shall write his life. The materials, as you have shown, are ample. I think matters stand on a very different footing now than they did before the appalling events at Kabul [second Afghan War of 1878-80], which one is almost glad he did not live to see, proved his unerring knowledge and forecast in so terrible a manner. I mean that people are much more disposed to read the great lessons of his life now.

Who is to write them? You asked me about Professor Bryce, "whether he would do justice to a work like this." He is an extremely able man, but I believe he neither could nor would undertake it. I have questioned intimate friends of his and mine, who have the highest admiration for him, but they say he is too busy and scarcely the man for the work. You ask, would Mr G. Trevelyan undertake it? I cannot but think that he might and be inspired by it; he is writing, I understand, the life of Fox[139] now but as that has waited so long, it might wait longer. And were Mr G. Trevelyan to see the wealth of materials so grand and so ample before him for *such* a life, I do believe that he could not resist. And his father, Sir C. Trevelyan, though without writing, might contribute materials.

The friends who thought that Professor Bryce would not undertake it suggested the Rev Stopford Brooke, who wrote the life of the Rev Robertson.[140] I merely mention the name. I do not know that Mr Stopford Brooke has any Indian knowledge and can scarcely conceive that he would "get up" such an immense subject.

Another person who has been suggested to me is one known, I believe, to Lady Lawrence: "T.C. Saunders." He is a clever, dexterous

---

139 Sir George Otto Trevelyan (1838-1928), historian, author of *The Early History of Charles James Fox*, 1880.

140 Stopford Augustus Brooke (1832-1916), author of *The Life of Frederick W. Robertson*, 1865.

writer, indeed, I am told, much the cleverest of the men suggested, writes well in the *Saturday Review* and has some knowledge of Indian things.

It appears as if these men stand as desirable writers of the life (I entirely agree that it would not do to forestall *the* "life" by a short biography. I only thought that a sketch of his Punjab action during the Mutiny might be published at once and his "life" later. But I am no judge of these things), in the following order: first Mr George Trevelyan, next Mr Theodore Walrond, then Professor Bryce, then Mr Saunders.

Still I cannot help thinking that one of his own disciples, one to whom he was guide and friend, one who has followed in his steps in Indian administration—that great career—would still be the best person to write his life. And if Sir Richard Temple would undertake it and is good writer enough, he would be the man.

I thank you most heartily for having shown me this beautiful letter. I did not know he could write such a one and I return it most gratefully. Probably the momentous question has been settled already of who is to be the writer. I pray God that this great and unique life may be worthily done. You, I trust, have written down ("committed to writing" expressive words: our memories are so treacherous) all the precious details of his last weeks and months and even of his last years.

I suppose Lady Lawrence is now expecting home Mrs Cunningham: that will be a renewal of grief but a comfort to both. Possibly Lady Lawrence has returned to London. Fare you all very well, very well, in the highest sense.

God has blessed his great deeds. May He bless them yet further.

No blacker cloud hangs over us than the dread that this second Afghan War will force "retrenchment" in all *good* things. It is a crisis almost as great as the Indian Mutiny for future good or ill. And we have no John Lawrence to ride the storm.

20 November 1879

I have been so ill and knocked up on my return that I have hardly been able to sit up. But I am almost appalled to think that you will be gone in a fortnight. I hope that you will kindly be able to give me twice an hour before that going abroad.

How I do feel for Lady Lawrence and wish that I could do the least little thing for her. And how this Life of him clings to my thoughts! Could you kindly settle, any day *after* tomorrow (Friday), to see me at 5 or if more convenient to you at 4? With the warmest sympathy,

ever yours sincerely
Florence Nightingale

25 November 1879

*Private.* You asked me to think over who could be of use in contributing information or help to Lord Lawrence's Life. *Sir William Muir* you have already. *Sir John Strachey* would contribute a chapter on sanitary matters. Lord Lawrence inaugurated sanitary reform and sanitary organization as viceroy in India and Sir John Strachey was his first appointment. I have always known Sir John Strachey as an enthusiastic disciple of Sir John Lawrence. Should he be otherwise now, I should still apply to him because you do not want *partisans* on either side: you want honest men who will give information. Colonel Crommelin would contribute information on Lord Lawrence's barrack reforms. Lord Northbrook says that a *Mr Jenkinson* (I believe he is some relative of his) would give information and assistance; he did not say particularly on what subjects. (Lord Northbrook is warm in his admiration of Lord Lawrence and would I have no doubt help.) He mentioned that Sir Arthur *Hobhouse* "with Jenkinson's help" might be of use, but is too much of a partisan and not earnest in religious matters. You certainly know both men. He also mentioned a *Gordon* (I do not quite know what Gordon he means), I believe he said commissioner of Mysore. He spoke of *T.H. Thornton, D.C.L.* Is that the Mr Thornton of the India Office (I know *him*) or the *Dr Thornton* of upper India? I see you have a "*Mr E. Thornton*" on your list. There is a *Mr Elliott,*[141] the secretary to the Famine Commission, just come to England. Everybody seems to think he would be of use. All I have seen of his was most able. He too was of upper India but he did not know Lord Lawrence, did he? (Was his grandfather resident of Lahore?) *Dr* [William Guyer] *Hunter* is also spoken of as able, but I am sure his sympathies are not right.

These are all the people I have to mention just now as likely to give information. I am quite sure you know them all better than I do, excepting perhaps *Sir John Strachey* and Lord Napier of Magdala. Have you thought of the last? He had much to do with Sir John Lawrence in the Punjab and afterwards. Lastly, as an advisor people think a great deal of *Morley*, of the *Fortnightly* (editor),[142] "who writes like Defoe"

141 Charles Alfred Elliott (1835-1911), Indian civil servant.

142 John Morley (1838-1923), later viscount, editor of the *Fortnightly Review* and the *Pall Mall Gazette*, a follower of John Stuart Mill.

(Mr Elliott's *History of the Mysore Famine* of 1877 reads like Defoe) as a man to *consult with* for good writers, in case you fail in your present search.

May God speed you! I do not think my letter of this morning *or this* will be of any present use to you, but at least I am trying to do my best for as holy an object as ever was pursued. Did you ever think again of *Mr Theodore Walrond*? In haste, believe me,

ever faithfully yours and the cause's

Florence Nightingale

*Most Private.* Most singularly my brother-in-law, Sir Harry Verney, calling on Lord Northbrook this morning and talking about a life of Lord Lawrence, met his nephew, Mr Henry Cunningham, at Lord Northbrook's. Pray do not think if you hear this that I have been consulting Mr Cunningham about this sacred matter. I should not weary or despair in this Quest of the Holy Grail, that is, the very best man who can be found to undertake it. The work will be so extremely interesting and inspiring, and if done by such a man, will add so much to his reputation that, if you find *present* difficulty, some good man, *now in India, who served under Lord Lawrence,* might ask to be entrusted with it. Surely some good man will offer if time is given.

F.N.

27 November 1879

I was very glad to receive your kind note. Do you know it has so strongly struck me that you ought to be the private secretary, so to speak, of anyone who wrote Lord Lawrence's Life, as you were of him whom we have lost during the last years of his life, that I felt aghast at your going abroad and almost hoped that the Life would not be written till your return? No one could give the help but you as, apart from other distinguished characteristics, you have had such extraordinary opportunities of personally *living* Lord Lawrence's *experience.* Nothing can replace that—specially in his case, who was an individuality without a parallel.

The writing of this Life is an event unique in history, as he was unique in history. And it would seem as if everything should be made to work together for that to be done as well as possible. I shall hope to see you before you leave England. I am very much overworked, but I would put off everything to see you once more. I may be no longer here in this world when you return. Friday and Saturday and Tuesday and Thursday I am afraid I am quite full of engagements.

It is very good of Mr and Mrs Bosworth Smith to wish to see me. It is very many years since I have been able to see two people together—

not even my sister and her husband. And my doctor tells me to talk "only half an hour every other day," which is simply impossible. I have not seen anyone for years but with long-standing claims of business upon me who, including the trained nurses, are numbered by hundreds. But if it would do the least good for me to see Mr *or* Mrs Bosworth Smith some afternoon that he or she would fix the week *after* next at 5 or at 4, I would. I am afraid I am quite "full" till then.

I have written thus much to show that my "poverty and not my will" consents[143] to putting off the visit. But I cannot fancy that I should be of any use, because overwork prevents my taking up such a subject as this in the only way that is deserving of it.

I do not know of any "detailed account" of the Jullundur time. That is the *worst* of the *best* of it that there never was any great man who was so little written of—even his despatches not published.

I think there must be two Thorntons, that is, three. (1) Thornton "of the India Office" whose initials are, I think, W.T.; he writes on Peasant Proprietorship; (2) Dr Thornton (T.H.) of upper India (L.L.D.) who is, I think, the man Lord Northbrook recommends; (3) your Mr E. Thornton.

Godspeed. I wish I could help more.

Source: From a letter to Sir Harry Verney, in Cook, *The Life of Florence Nightingale* 2:45

17 February 1893

How many touches—short but sweet—I could add to the book![144] The real tale of Sir J. Lawrence's appointment as viceroy will never be told. During the only ten days left to Lawrence before he started, he came to see me. How kind it was of Lord Stanley; he came like a footman to my door and, without giving his name, sent up to ask whether Sir John Lawrence was coming. The interview was one never to be forgotten.

Source: Notes on Sir John Lawrence, Add Mss 45845 ff220-21

23 February 1899

Three most delicate and lovely pure white cyclamens reflected on the black coat and stern face of Sir John Lawrence's portrait [which Nightingale kept in her room]. How like, how figurative of the life of the original, his attention and tender regard to the prejudices as well

143 Shakespeare, *Romeo and Juliet*, Act 5, scene 2.

144 C.U. Aitchison, *Lord Lawrence.*

as welfare of those he ruled over. He would not eat beef though ordered by his doctor (he had had the fever six times) because the cow was a "sacred animal." (It is in neglecting these things that we lose our influence with the natives.) And his reward was that in the Mutiny he had the most valuable information the great native chiefs (who wished to remain loyal to us), through their wives and Lady Lawrence, could give. He held his province in the hollow of his own hand and sent all his troops to Delhi which was then in the hands of the mutineers. "Jan Larens," said the natives to me, is worth 30,000 troops and 30,000 troops would be worth nothing without him.

## Lord Mayo's Viceroyalty

**Editor:** Richard Southwell Bourke, Lord Mayo (1822-72), held the office of chief secretary for Ireland before Disraeli appointed him to succeed Lord Lawrence as governor general and viceroy from 1869 to 1872. He practised a policy of non-intervention and secured the friendship of the ameer (emir) of Afghanistan. He was especially active in the fight against famine (see p 708 below) and cholera (see p 897 below). During his administration the finances of the country were substantially improved and the first general census was undertaken 1870. He founded the Mayo College of Ajmer. On 8 February 1872 he was stabbed to death by a Pathan convict at the Andamans while on visit there.

Source: From a letter to Julius Mohl, Woodward Biomedical Library A.11, copy Wellcome Ms 9086/19, draft Add Mss 43397 ff330-31

21 November 1869

I find that every year, taken upon the last four years for which we have returns (1864-67), there are, in the Home Army, 729 men alive every year who would have been dead but for Sidney Herbert's measures, and 5184 men always on active duty who would have been "constantly sick" in bed. . . . In India the difference is still more striking. Taken on the last two years, the death rate of Bombay (civil, military and native) is lower than that of London, the healthiest city of Europe. And the death rate of Calcutta is lower than that of Liverpool or Manchester! . . . But this is not the greatest victory. The municipal commissioner of Bombay writes that the "huddled native masses" "clamorously invoke" the aid of the "health department" if but one death from cholera or smallpox occurs; whereas formerly half of them might be swept away and the other half think it "all right." Now they attribute these deaths to "dirt, foul water and the like," and openly declare them "preventible." No hope for future civilization among the "masses" like this! I wish the Privy Council were as intelligent and progressive as the "Bombay masses." But it is not.

Source: Notes on Sir Bartle Frere's visit for John Sutherland, ADD MSS 45754 ff33-34

4 December 1869

Sir B. Frere was here for three hours. They are writing and telegraphing from India every week to abolish something, for the sake of saving a few hundred thousands on which the security or the welfare of the empire depends:

1. The police,
2. The education policy of the last fifteen years,
3. The public works, such as (a) the Karachi harbour, (b) the Godavari River, both of which were nearly completed—and all that money is to be wasted,
4. The barracks,
5. The sending out of medical officers from Netley.

He told me a great deal on all these points. But I can only tell you the last. He says that they have telegraphed home that, having abolished thirty regiments, they have thirty medical officers to spare. And they don't want any from Netley for at least a year. It is on this last point he wished to consult us.

He says that the expense of medical officers is after all very small, that they *always* want medical officers in India, that they have always had a *deficiency* of applicants, that, now that we have got them ready—twenty-five (I understood) *from*/at Netley—it appears to him destruction to stop this supply even only for a year and to make an uproar for nothing.

But he wants us to give him arguments to convince the duke of Argyll.[145] He says: if only ten were sent out, that would be better than stopping the supply altogether. . . . He is *quite* sure it comes from Lord Mayo. The proposal to send no more doctors has not come from the India Office. Sir B. Frere had heard all that and he was perfectly aghast at the director general's ignorance. I spoke with Sir B. Frere

145 George Douglas Campbell (1823-1900), duke of Argyll, Liberal Cabinet minister; he was secretary of state for India 1868-74.

about that. He says no papers have as yet reached the India Office. But, again, he was perfectly aghast at that proposition.

He says (this is a cognate subject only) "the way to make an Indian medical officer is this: to have him for five or ten years at the presidency hospital, then to have him for at least ten years at a large native town, seeing the native diseases which after all are very different from the European, and then and not till then he begins to make a good Indian medical officer."

"We have not too many, we have too few medical officers," he says. "If you were to double the number out there, you would have too few. And the D.G. knows nothing about it." *I* did not mention the D.G. at all to Sir B. Frere. But *he* spoke of the whole thing as of their ignorance inspiring terror in him.

He read over [John] Strachey's letter most attentively. He says it is sound as far as it goes. But he says Strachey forgets that he and his cousin [rather: brother] (Colonel Strachey) are the two men who have done the most in India to carry "standard plans," hard and fast measures, measures drawn by plummet and line, over every population in India, however different. He says Strachey forgets that we begged and prayed to be allowed to put up in Pune and the Deccan, where the winds are terrific, where the ground is rocky, one-storeyed barracks, that we were *ordered* to wait; Sir Robert Napier was *ordered* to wait till a 3rd-class engineer, Colonel Crommelin, an ordinary man such as you can find anywhere, sent us "standard plans," which we were to use and no other and which were extravagantly expensive. However, he says, Strachey's is a good letter, only somewhat tardy. And he advises us to answer it cordially and immediately, and to say also that as economy has come at last, it would be better to proceed with individual inquiries into the requirements of individual towns and stations, to offer them an engineer and then to draw up plans of improvements.

Source: From a letter to John Strachey [at the time financial member of the viceroy's council], Columbia University, Presbyterian Hospital School of Nursing C92

10 December 1869

*Private.* I cannot thank you sufficiently for your most kind and interesting and instructive letter of 10 October which is just as important on the side of sanitary economics as a sanitary report is important on the side of health.

We entirely understand what has occurred and we deeply sympathize with the difficulties which surround progress in India. But even with the present revenue deficiency, there is really nothing to fear. With such able statesmen as you are to adapt and to originate, no position is really more hopeful for a country than the one which induces a government to look carefully to their existing obligations and existing expenditure so as to adjust both wisely. A great fault of our national character has always been to substitute principles for details. It is so much easier to settle all questions (or to pretend to settle them) by a single stroke of the pen!! But such a way of doing things ruins a business, as we all know. And it ruins a government just as much, to say the least! I am sure that, great as your difficulties are, they will, as you point out, only make the good day more sure to come. You have *150* millions of people behind you whose lives and security and trade and commerce you have to provide for. The inducement is greater than fear. And your careful consideration of the various interests and questions at stake will throw the necessary caution and light into your future proceedings.

So far as concerns our great questions of the health of troops, we more than agree with every word you say. Both the royal India sanitary commission and the present standing Army Sanitary Commission (late "Barrack and Hospital Improvement" Commission) had no other idea but to arrive at the soundest general principles, leaving to you in India to originate the best applications of them in detail. We have all along felt with you that we must "*go on* unto perfection."[146] Towns and stations are, as you know from your own great experience, very like patients. They have not all the same disease. They don't want all the same medicine. A careful diagnosis must be made of the complaints of each town, station, barrack or district. And it would be mere useless extravagance, as you say, to apply the same expensive medicine to the complaints of all diseased cities or stations. We cannot improve the health of all groups of population by any one procedure. Individual inquiries into the requirements of stations must be made and then plans of improvement drawn up.

We have often thought that if you thought well to command the services of a thorough sanitary engineer and health officer (for which office medical knowledge *per se* is not of much use) you might put your stations—one at a time and the worst first—into their hands just as we put sick under clinical care, and your officers might report to

146 Heb 6:1.

you: "Such and such a station is ill of such and such a complaint, and the remedies are so and so."

This is what we are at the present time doing here. We have had our barracks not only examined, and their symptoms stated, but we have had the symptoms classified according to their importance. The most pressing are to be dealt with first. Double-storeyed barracks will, as you say, no more cure all your stations than single-storeyed barracks. Ornamental and extravagant barracks will cure none. Measures which are *immediately* and urgently required and measures which may be allowed to stand over can be determined by a thoroughly competent inquiry.

If you had this inquiry made from yourselves, this would determine where first money *must* be spent to save a greater loss, where delay may safely be made till there is more money to spend. A great part of your death rate in ordinary years comes from certain stations and not from others. This is always a guide. Your statistics are a matter of intense interest to us. They indicate very decided improvement for all ordinary seasons. And this result corresponds with that obtained for our foreign—not Indian—stations generally. Your danger is now, as your knowledge which is far greater than mine tells, from *epidemic* seasons.

Our hope is that the cholera inquiry, if duly carried out, will tell you *what to do*. Your influence is all-essential to OBTAIN FACTS. (If one could joke on so vital a matter, one would say: fine every doctor who upholds or starts a theory. There is not one which is more philosophic than witchcraft. All theories are only the cloaks of ignorance—the surest sign of mental incapacity. Instead of drawing conclusions first and observing afterwards, let them collect *facts first*, and sacrifice theory to fact.) As for your barrack requirements, the first thing is to arrive at an enlightened military knowledge of what is wanted, to decide this, then to put the requirements into the hands of the sanitary and engineering authority to be properly embodied. As you say, it would have been much cheaper to have adopted the construction advised by the Army Sanitary Commission generally—also perhaps their row construction.

You are doing a most hopeful thing in occupying your attention with the general question of country drainage in Bengal. It is in Lower Bengal that the great epidemic problem has to be grappled with. Lower Bengal is, I suppose, the endemic centre of India. This, you will say, is only a theory. But at least it expresses one fact, viz., that of all parts of northern India, cholera and fever are most apt to appear there. There (as elsewhere), after the epidemic has assumed a certain intensity, it spreads and flies about like an incendiary lighting up the conflagration wherever there are materials ready to catch fire. However much the North West may be improved, cholera and fevers will remain indigenous in Lower Bengal. But, should you ever succeed in draining that huge swamp and clothing it with crops, we shall hear little of cholera—I would you had a ministry of agriculture!

The world's thanks are due to you for the amazing improvement in the health of Calcutta. Taken on the last two years, the death rate of Calcutta has been lower than that of Liverpool or Manchester. (I fancy that the Calcutta works might have been more cheaply done, might not they?) I am sure that the deficient revenue will not in the slightest degree lead any statesmen in India into the enormous mistake—committed by us here before the Crimean War—of saving a few thousands to incur an expenditure of as many millions in order to replace troops prematurely cut off by preventible disease.

N.B. If you should think well to initiate any such inquiry as that mentioned above into individual stations and wished for a royal engineer of great sanitary experience to help to conduct it, it might be possible for us to find you one. . . .

Since writing the above, I have looked at the propositions of the *Royal Commission on the Sanitary State of the Indian Army*, also at the *Suggestions* of the standing Army Sanitary Commission (called, till lately, the Barrack and Hospital Improvement Commission), also at their reply to Dr Leith. They all agree, as you say, in recommending a course similar to that stated above, similar to what the presidency sanitary commissions, which had too short a life [they were replaced by "health commissioners"], intended, viz., for you to conduct these very local inquiries and to recommend the measures necessary for removing the several disease causes, pointedly adding that barrack building must not be considered as *the* remedy for unwholesome stations. It is only *a* remedy—and a remedy, only where required.

You will now, I am certain, be taking up the question anew, in which you have already done so much, on its economic side, effect even more good than you have yet effected and at a much less proportionate cost. I will not make a letter already too long longer by apologies, but only thank you again for your inspiring letter and remind you that "la reconnaissance n'est qu'un vif sentiment des bienfaits futurs."

Source: From a letter to Sir John McNeill, Florence Nightingale Museum (LMA) H1/ST/NC1/70/SU161, copy Add Mss 45768 ff236-43

8 February 1870

Might I ask you to glance over this good-natured but startling letter from Lord Mayo [viceroy 1869-72] (which I received just after I had the pleasure of seeing you)? Startling, because it shows that not one of the men, from Lord Mayo downwards, understands the question. (I shall not answer Lord Mayo till I have seen Dr Cuningham,[147] as he desires.) I know Dr Cuningham by correspondence. He is a good, excellent man, who has gone head foremost into all the "theories" against which we have warned them, but who is clever and candid and now acknowledges that he "knows nothing"—a great step in knowledge.

The causes of the failure in the healthiness of the "new barracks" we could tell them, every one. Yes surely: I remember your Memorandum on preparing the ground. We made great use of it. Also you will perhaps remember that we sent them our *Suggestions*—asked for and approved by the India government here, asked for and approved by the Government of India there—on water supply, drainage, sewerage, stational improvements, every kind of matter affecting the public health. And the government sent a copy to every official whom it concerned. And this is the result. We have greatly succeeded in native and civilian health. The military alone is *stupid.* Should anything suggest itself to you as to what questions I should ask Dr Cuningham, as to how I should fix him to stating (to us) the objections to the "new barracks," etc., would you kindly tell me?

It was hardly necessary for me on Sunday to put in words to you how much I am discouraged. As for the War Office, one may say that they have "crucified" Sidney Herbert afresh, and "put him to an

147 Dr James M. Cuningham (1829-1905), sanitary commissioner for Bengal 1869-75 and for the Government of India 1875-85, surgeon general. He became a member of the reorganized Army Sanitary Commission in 1890. He authored two books on cholera in which he took an anti-contagionist stance. Nightingale often misspelled "Cunningham" when referring to J.M. Cuningham, thus creating some confusion since two other persons involved in health questions had similar names. D.D. Cunningham of the Indian Medical Service belonged to the team that investigated the causes of cholera in 1878 and concluded to a "telluric" origin of the disease. Henry Stewart Cunningham (1832-1920) was an India expert in Madras and Calcutta, and member of the Famine Commission 1878-80. All three seem to have opposed the "contagionist" view of diseases in the 1880s. The right spelling has been restored as much as possible.

open shame."[148] The sticking up a man's statue in the courtyard,[149] and destroying his work within, is an organized hypocrisy which Jesuits might envy.

India is after all our best hope. But, when the work there does not progress it retrogresses. For me to see you is at once the highest hope and the deepest pain. It reminds me of days when a great career was just begun, when great works and great purposes seemed so prosperous, when the goal seemed in view. Now, all our hopes seem blasted and all our plans destroyed. But it reminds me too of your patient courage and devoted endurance, in a long life of successful sacrifice to the good of our country. And, though it will not be given *me* to see of the fruit of my toil, of the travail of my soul, yet who am I that I should complain?

Source: Draft letter to Lord Mayo for John Sutherland's consideration, Add Mss 45754 ff124-28; the actual letter is found below (see p 905 below)

23 March 1870

*Lord Mayo.* Present *aspect of public health question in India.* Too great a tendency in India to invent first principles. Field of India enormous, like working at a continent.

Barracks:

1. Too hot.

a. plaster and whitewash outside to protect walls from sun radiation;

b. fill the tall verandah arches with the venetians [blinds] to protect the room walls. The lofty arches are right enough, but the upper part of the arch of the verandah should be filled up with broad wooden jalousies admitting of adjustment to let in light and keep out sun, or spaces between pillars even then filled up.

These two remedies can easily be tried at any station and a comparison made of the effect in temperature, ventilation and comfort with other blocks.

2. New barrack building alone will not cure the sick, lower the death rate or guarantee from epidemics. So much enters into the improvement of a station besides the actual putting up of a new house! The four things essential to health on which it depends:

---

148 An allusion to Heb 6:6.

149 A statue of Sidney Herbert was erected in the courtyard by the War Office; after Nightingale's death it was moved to Waterloo Place next to hers.

a. a thorough drainage of ground occupied by station;

b. an abundant supply of pure water distributed over stations;

c. healthy principles of barrack and hospital construction, *including means of employment,* exercise and recreation;

d. improved sanitary police of stations, bazaars and adjacent native towns.

These four things in reality [function as] *one* as regards health. To omit three and build one is to spend much money with little hope of money's worth. For on (a) the condition of the surrounding native population and (b) the water supply drainage, etc., depends very much whether we shall have epidemics or not.

Whether it is necessary to construct new barracks and what their construction shall be must be determined on the spot after competent inquiry into the general sanitary condition of the station where it is proposed to build.

The *construction* of the new barracks does not appear to have had anything to do with cholera, fever or other disease in these buildings. The construction may even have lessened the sick rate, for there are plenty unfortunately of causes of sickness undealt with, which lie outside the towns altogether, e.g., Allahabad.

What is the condition of the neighbourhood of these barracks? the filthy towns where cholera flourishes almost perennially, where there is neither drainage nor wholesome water—and this close to the new barracks. All the barrack building in the world would make but little difference in the epidemic susceptibility of troops exposed to malaria day and night—more especially during sleep.

Is Allahabad a solitary example and exception? Are there not instances of new barracks suffering from foul ground covered with filth by work people and others? Nusterabad nuisance directly produced cholera.

In India improved construction, sufficient space and ventilation, upper-floor sleeping rooms where necessary, have no other object than to remove the depressing constitutional influences of foul air, and to enable the men to resist other disease causes not themselves connected with the barracks.

3. Such causes require to be attacked always outside the barracks, sometimes outside the cantonment, and it may be at a considerable distance from its boundary. Filthy towns and bazaars, or foul native houses and inhabitants *inside cantonment* boundaries, or too close to them, are constant sources of danger. Of course the only real safe-

guard is to keep such population out of cantonments and at a safe distance to leeward. This is not always possible. And for civil purposes troops must be near civil populations. Then, either the native population must be put under efficient sanitary police, or the troops (and natives too and civilians too) must suffer.

4. No difference of opinion as to men sleeping as far as necessary above level of ground. Principle applicable to all climates and countries. Only question in India: amount of elevation must be determined by local and climatic inquiry on the spot.

5. Whatever the height of sleeping room is raised above ground, great principle must never be overlooked: in Indian climates, men cannot be always in the same rooms, inhabiting the same rooms day and night with safety. (If they do, floors and walls get impregnated with "men," as in European climates is the case with hospitals constantly inhabited.) Their day and dining rooms must be separate from their sleeping rooms. And there must be means of occupying the men at trades, remunerative work or reading or exercises, instead of lying on their beds, thinking of cholera for perhaps eighteen hours out of the twenty-four.

And there must be commanding officers who will devise, support and encourage such remunerative employment, such active industry and recreation among the men as will *pull* them off their beds by force of interest. Such things have been done and may be done again and done more extensively, although of course there is much talk about impossibility and difficulty. Si, c'est possible [yes, it is possible].

Road-making in India has cured the troops engaged in it. Elementary principle of physiology that men eat and sleep solely to lay in a store of force to be expended under the action of the will. If the force is not expended in healthy production, it will be expended in unhealthy or diseased products. Half the diseased predisposition in India among the men arises from "lolling" on their beds.

But men can't *will* themselves active. They must have the necessary room and appliances, the necessary means and inducements for work and recreation in order to have the requisite means of cure. If the lower floors of barracks are furnished only with a bench or two; if they have neither fittings nor punkahs [fans], of course the men won't go into them; if there is nothing to do in them, of course the men will do nothing in them.

If these appliances are necessary, they must be had. If not had, the men must suffer. Anyhow there is no saving, for men in India cost more than tables, tools or punkahs. But all the workshops and appliances in the world will [be] of no use unless the officers see to their use; the men's health [is] of more importance to the state than the officers' difficulties.

6. Every man should have his bed, whether on or off duty, whether in barracks or in hospital. One principle to give by regulation *every bed* its quota of space, whether occupied or not. A soldier's bed is his home, the only home he has; he ornaments it with his little pictures and things. And no good was ever done to a Briton by destroying his notion of "home."

At cool hill stations or at damp, changeable, other stations, the barrack room should always have its fireplace for use or comfort.

7. Gardens. Almost every regiment should supply itself with vegetables, a prime element of healthy diet in India.

8. India is rather short of pumps. I will make India a present of a pump (ex[ample] maire, "il a doué sa commune d'une pompe" [he endowed his municipality with a pump]) provided I am not thrown into my own well by the bheesties or coolies whose trade I shall have damaged. Might not steam pumps, forcing pumps, answer as well in Indian as in European latitudes? We do not here depend upon "natural headworks" [?] nor upon water carriers.

Source: Notes on a meeting with James W. Cuningham for John Sutherland, Add Mss 45754 ff129-30 and 132

26 March 1870

Dr Cuningham, as you said, wanted to see me. But when he came he had no "administrative plan." Nothing to propose but—what do you think?—that young Chadwick[150] should be adjoined to him. I said I had no idea he was experienced enough. He said you had recommended him. I said, ask Dr Sutherland again.

He says the new barracks at *Morar* are all masonry. New barracks at *Allahabad*, Peshawar, Rawalpindi, Jullundur, Umballa—married quarters—Sabathu, Mussoorie [are] in red brick. He says plastering and whitewashing will make them very glaring. He says the large staircases which Lord Napier likes are ducts for foul air to the whole building, as in hospitals.

---

150 Osbert Chadwick (d. 1913), son of Edwin Chadwick. In 1898 he was appointed the first Chadwick professor of municipal engineering at University College, London.

I mentioned Major Gordon to him. He asked me to send out books through Smith and Elder to him. He says it takes six-eight months to get books sent out official way.

He asks, Would it be best to begin with Allahabad as a station?

I am very sorry to say that each time I have seen Cuningham, I have hope less from his ability. You get all out of him at first.

*Dr Cuningham:* he says that he does not think, if civil sanitary engineers are sent out from England, that you can put the time under a year when they can be useful. He says, you can hardly tell how useless a man [will be] till he has learnt something of the language and the ways. He must be his own foreman in so many things, making materials, etc.

He says he hardly thinks there is any real difference, in saving *time*, between sending from India engineers home to learn and sending from England engineers out to learn India. I told him I thought six months in England would do for an Indian engineer. But he was to ask you.

Source: From a letter to Robert Rawlinson, Boston University 1/5/59

11 February 1871

*Private.* A propos to the "attempt to provide sewers and drains to remove rainfall" at some stations in India, could you give me some information as to a rather unlucky reference which was made to the India Office about an engineering scheme of the kind said to exist at Kanpur, but which it seems does not exist? The India Office applied to you, i.e., the Army Sanitary Commission (in accordance with a request they received), about this Kanpur scheme of sewerage. You wished, I believe, to be able to raise the case. But when the inquiry came to be made, no data could be found for the statement, though the data were said to be in one of the India papers sent for perusal by the I.O. to the A.S.C. But every effort at both offices failed to trace the document, it is said. Now the person who made the reference and the request to the I.O. was I (F.N.). And I did so on the strength of a document and a request which I received from the Army Sanitary Commission (about the first week of last December), the gist of which was as follows: that a case in point (viz., the cost of engineering sanitary works) "came up privately at the last sub-committee meeting," that an engineer at Kanpur had 300 acres to sewer, that he proposed to construct sewers of so costly a character as to carry away when only half full half an inch of rain per hour, etc., that, in order to prevent an enormous and quite useless expenditure and to prevent in dry weather the sewers from distilling fever and cholera, the I.O. should require oversight of these municipal plans?

Upon the faith of this statement and view I applied to the I.O. (in obedience to a request I received) and had not an idea that the "subcommittee" had not all the facts before them in black and white in an authentic form satisfactory to themselves as to correctness. (For I have made it a rule through life to make applications, especially to government offices only in such case or where I myself had such facts in a form to satisfy both sides as to their authenticity.) And I "proposed" to the I.O.—still in accordance with the document I had received—that "oversight of municipal plans" should be required, on the ground of this flagrant instance of the Kanpur plan. And now I am told that no such "instance" exists.

*You* will understand, I am sure, that, knowing your great accuracy and wide information, I should apply to *you* to give me the facts, as far as is possible, about this Kanpur plan.

Source: From a letter to James M. Cuningham, Wellcome Ms 5482/87

31 March 1871

*Private.* I cannot help writing to you à line by this mail, though it must be a hasty one, to say how truly grieved I was to hear of your illness, a matter of the deepest regret, as your recovery, which I trust is perfect, must be of sincerest congratulation to us all.

With regard to the chief subject of your letter, viz., its scheme, our own view has always been from the very beginning that all medical officers (civil) paid by the state for any purpose, should be fit and also available, for all purposes. We would include, so far as we know, not only vaccinators but all civil surgeons throughout India. They should all pass, so far as we can judge, under the sanitary commissioner; they should report to him and execute his instructions.

Sir C. Adderley's royal commission here has recognized the propriety of making all Poor Law medical officers in England sanitary inspectors. This royal commission have included it in their report and have placed the whole sanitary administration, including Mr Simon, the Privy Council medical officer, not under the director general (which is what you fear for India) but under the president of the Poor Law Board. This is a great reform.

Of course circumstances differ so widely between England and India that, where we speak positively in England from our own experience we can only collect from India the best experience we are able to command from the best Indians. But your scheme will have, so far as we can see at present, our best support.

(I see that you say, in your letter to Dr Sutherland, that "to make him (the local sanitary commissioner) head of the medical civil officers of the province" would be to "abolish sanitary work altogether, for he cannot possibly do both." This is undoubted.)

I had meant, before this, to write fully my opinion in detail (which is one only of admiration and encouragement to go on and do more) on your last annual report on your devotedness to our great cause, and also about your opponents: "the more difficulty, the more glory." But again I must put it off. . . . [rest of letter on Franco-Prussian War]

Source: From notes on War Office Add Mss 45843 f26

May 1871

In all the government work I have done, in both the royal commissions which I conducted, in Sidney Herbert's five years of War Office work 1856-61 (during those five years, S. Herbert came to me day by day. And we organized every practical step together), in Sir John Lawrence's Indian work, I have always been responsible for acts as well as for opinions, i.e., I not only "got up" the data, statistical, administrative and practical, brought out the evidence and except in one instance wrote the reports, but I organized the standing commissions, departments or other mechanism[s] which were to carry out the conclusions or recommendations or "opinions" when they were laid down. (The reason why royal commissions are become a sham and a stone of offence is that they don't do this. They simply report.)

## Reorganization of the Army Sanitary Commission

**Editor:** The Army Sanitary Commission (A.S.C.), along with the presidency commissions, was intended to be a central instrument in the implementation of the royal commission recommendations. The threatened abolition, then reorganization of the A.S.C., from the late 1860s caused major concern for Nightingale and her team. As reported above, its initial formation as the Barrack and Hospital Improvement Commission in 1858 followed the first royal commission under Sidney Herbert. In 1865 it became a joint commission of the War Office and the India Office, and was given the important function of monitoring the sanitary improvements in India related to both public health and the army, to examine critically the progress reports sent in by sanitary authorities in India and to give advice as to all sanitary aspects deemed relevant to the Indian situation: barrack and hospital construction, cleaning-up and inspection of stations, diet and hygiene of soldiers, civilian conditions as they impacted upon the army, sickness and mortality statistics, town and village sanitation, ways of dealing with famines and epidemics, etc.

The responsibilities of the A.S.C. were heightened in periods of famine and epidemics, but not everybody saw its relevance, placed as they were so far away from the "field" where the real decisions ought to be taken. Doubts were expressed as to its ability to meet the challenges set by Indian circumstances and to the expenses it occasioned. Sir Bartle Frere's return from India in 1867 made people in London more acutely aware of the shortcomings of the A.S.C. in its relation to the India work in general and to the presidency commissions in particular. That is why, in the following material, the presentation of the debate around the function of the A.S.C. begins at the time of Frere's return to London.

The A.S.C. suffered with recurring problems of jurisdiction, efficiency, raison d'être and precise function, while awareness of the need for changes in the A.S.C.'s structure grew over the years. One seemingly minor change that was contemplated consisted of striking out the salary of the only paid member of the commission, Dr Sutherland; doing so, it was feared, would destabilize the entire commission and wreck the work initiated by Sidney Herbert. Nightingale's interventions with Lord de Grey, who took up the case, were effective in stopping the proposed elimination of Sutherland's salary. At least she could say: "We are safe for the present" (see p 655 below). It was still felt by Nightingale's group that the role of the commission in determining sanitary policies was important and was to be upheld.

Debate on the reorganization of the A.S.C. raged in the 1880s as Dr Sutherland's retirement and replacement were considered. Dr Sutherland retired in 1888 and Dr Thomas Gillham Hewlett was favoured as his successor, but he died prematurely. Thereafter the danger arose of the A.S.C.'s complete abolition. Further adjustments were called for and suggestions put forward. All this led, through ups and downs, to a reorganized commission in 1890, structured in such a way as to respond more adequately to the needs of the army at home and in India, and to those of the Indian nationals themselves. In fact Nightingale remarked at that time that the A.S.C. had "really more to do with the native population of India than with the army" (see p 674 below).

At the same time, presidency sanitary commissions were being replaced by a central executive sanitary board in each province, which were to work along with district boards and municipal committees. This took place in 1888. The staffing of those boards evidently became a serious concern, as did their financing, but their establishment indicated a further move toward giving more responsibility to Indian nationals.

Details of this entire evolution are presented in the following letters and notes. The process began early in 1869 with Nightingale consulting Dr Sutherland, then enlisting Lord de Grey's help before addressing the secretary of state for war, Edward Cardwell. The correspondence deals with important administrative problems, but is also interspersed with material concerning individual persons (e.g., Sutherland and Hewlett).

Source: Notes for John Sutherland, Add Mss 45753 ff181 and 178-79

[ca. 31 January 1869]

It was worthwhile for you to come out, perhaps. I suppose you know that everything is going *by the board* in the new estimates, the Army Sanitary Commission, yourself, the Army Medical School. I do not mean to take the responsibility of doing anything unless you share it and wish it. I could also write to Lord de Grey, asking him to state what has been done. It's no use talking nonsense now. Everybody knows that I have been working with you for twelve years. There are several things to be done.

I could write to Sir B. Frere and ask him to speak to the Indian work. I could write to Lord Stanley and ask him to speak to the work under him. I could write to Gladstone (whom I know a little) and who asked me (in 1861) to draw up a statement of Sidney Herbert's work.[151] But then I should have liked to ask Sir Harry Verney to take my letter (and he, most unfortunately, is ill at Embley). I could ask Sir Harry to go to Cardwell [secretary of state for war], whom he is much attached to, and take a letter from me. But Sir Harry is at Embley. I never saw Cardwell but once at S. Herbert's.

[February 1869]

Lord de Grey, Lord Stanley and Sir B. Frere would at my request fill up and state the work that has been done [by the Army Sanitary Commission] under their eyes. But Cardwell and Gladstone are perfectly ignorant. Cardwell and Gladstone would say: we are not going to

151 Letter 9 August 1861, in *Society and Politics* (5:430-34).

destroy the Army Sanitary Commission. Then I should say, Dr Sutherland and they would say: *Is* Dr Sutherland the Army Sanitary Commission?

Well my dear soul, you've only to say the word. I am so weary of all the responsibility of the correspondence with Sir J. Lawrence being thrown upon me and the irregularity of the help given me, that, if you do but say the word, I believe I would throw it all up, let this house and throw myself into private hospital and nursing business.

Source: From a letter to Lord de Grey, Add Mss 43546 ff113-16

1 February 1869

*Private and confidential.* I may perhaps be allowed to invoke you about a work which was yours, quite as much at the India Office as at the War Office. And that is: the Army Sanitary Commission. I am told at the W.O. that they are about to destroy the Army Sanitary Commission by striking out of the estimates the salary paid to Dr Sutherland (whom you will remember) and so to rid themselves of the man of all others whom they could least spare. I believe that you will think this almost as great a loss to the public service and almost as desirable to prevent as I do.

You will perhaps remember one of the last minutes you wrote at the India Office 18 June 1866 (Dies Irae [Day of Wrath]) [resignation of Liberal government] about the sanitary service in India, and a kind note you wrote to me afterwards upon it. After an immense delay, Sir Stafford Northcote, in April 1868, wrote a despatch to India, almost exactly embodying the contents of your minute. Also, we have now a sanitary department of our own at the India Office, with Sir Bartle Frere at its head. And we have done a good deal of work. Of all this Dr Sutherland has been the life and soul as he was of the Royal Commission on the Sanitary State of the Indian Army which reported in 1863 and which led to the extension of the Army Sanitary Commission to the India Office. (I would gladly draw up for you a little sketch of what has passed in the sanitary line at the India Office, since you alas! left it in 1866, with an appropriate chorus of printed documents, if it would not be troubling you too much.)

I need scarcely mention to a minister of your experience that, if the responsible member, whose business it is to carry on all this procedure, is struck off, it will all fall to the ground. But my object in now troubling you is simply to ask advice. I have no right to apply to Mr Cardwell, whom I have not seen for twelve years and who would not remember me. I knew Mr Gladstone once and occasionally since Sidney Herbert's death; he has told me, in some friendly way or other, that he remembered my work with Sidney Herbert. But please to understand, I have no claim upon his acquaintance. I have written the enclosed draft letter to *somebody* merely to state our case. Would you be so very good as to advise me upon it, what to say and to whom I should say it? It even occurred to me that, upon the ground of you yourself having, in two offices, presided over the sanitary work in general and Dr Sutherland's in particular, it might possibly, without your seeing any inconvenient interference in it, be within the bounds for you to present my letter yourself. At all events, there is no one who could, if he would, give me better counsel how to act in endeavouring to prevent the wreck of that great work for which Sidney Herbert gave his life and for which you have done so much.

Source: From a draft letter in Dr Sutherland's hand and a copy of a letter probably to Edward Cardwell, Add Mss 45753 ff182-83 and Add Mss 45801 ff188-89 (both written on the same day)

1 February 1869

I have heard of certain projected changes in the War Office which will so completely reverse the work initiated by Sidney Herbert and bring us back in the army to the bad old times that I cannot refrain writing you about it. It is stated that, among the reductions about to be made in the W.O. . . . [some concern the] Army Sanitary Committee, which is a public health committee for troops in India as well as for troops in other parts of H.M.'s dominions. Now I am the last person who would stand in the way of real economy. I would say, Let everything which cannot prove its necessity as well as its usefulness cease to be a charge on the public. But let us be sure, before the step is taken, that the charge to be abolished cannot justify its own continuance, and that the persons who deal with it are competent to judge. . . .

I feel myself to some extent responsible and to some extent struck at personally in these proceedings. I have been a prime mover in advising H.M.'s government to adopt the improvements which have been carried out, and just at the time when we are laying the ground of an entire reform in India in all its sanitary arrangements—carrying out there Lord Herbert's great principles—I now learn that somebody or other is destroying them. I write simply to ask that these things be considered and that justice be done to the great principles which have raised, as we all know, the credit of the British Army out of the slough into which it had firmly fallen and into which it is evident that there are some who without knowing it will land the army there again.

1 February 1869

*Private and confidential.* I have heard of certain projected changes in the War Office which will so completely reverse the work initiated by Sidney Herbert and bring back the sanitary state of the army, even in India, to the bad old times, that I cannot refrain from asking to be allowed to write to you a few words about it.

It is said that, among the reductions about to be made in the War Office estimates, the Army Sanitary Commission, which is a public health committee for troops in India as well as for troops in other parts of Her Majesty's dominions, is to be brought to an end by cutting out of the estimates the salary of the paid member, Dr Sutherland (all the other members being already in receipt of government or Indian pay).

Dr Sutherland has been the responsible worker and advisor of the Army Sanitary Commission since he was specially requested by Sidney Herbert, by Lord Palmerston and subsequently by Sir George Lewis to undertake this work. . . .

The agency which it is now proposed to cripple and destroy was set on foot by a royal commission presided over by Sidney Herbert, for the express purpose of remedying defects which all admitted to exist. Its necessity moreover was subsequently confirmed by the recommendation of the Royal Commission on the Sanitary State of the Army in India. The question is: is this committee answering or not answering its purposes? Are the purposes so completely fulfilled that the agency may cease? This is the question suggested by a real economy.

May I venture to say, not indeed for vainglory, but to justify me for speaking at all, that I have been cognizant of every step and every procedure, and have seen these procedures result in the reduction of army mortality to one half and in some cases to less than one half, that mine has been the private correspondence with Sir John Lawrence and other high officials in India by which they have been so very good as to keep me informed of every step taken in applying the principles of improvement in stations and barracks in India, involving an ultimate outlay of ten millions.

To proceed ruthlessly to destroy the progress of this work—and this by persons who know little or nothing about it—can hardly be intended just at the time we are laying the ground of an entire reform in the sanitary arrangements of India, for the people as well as for the troops. . . .

May I hope not to be thought presumptuous in asking simply that these things shall be considered before striking off the member of the standing committee who has done its work, as can be testified by many ministers and officials.

Source: From a letter to Douglas Galton, ADD Mss 45764 f131

3 February 1869

*Private.* Many thanks for your note. As you say, we are safe for the present. Lord de Grey *had* spoken to Mr Cardwell and has engaged me to write to Mr Cardwell, which I suppose I must do. Lord de Grey has written me a nice note, which I will send you as soon as I have answered it.

Source: From a letter to Lord de Grey, ADD Mss 43546 f117

3 February 1869

*Private.* I have just heard from the War Office that "the Army Sanitary Commission has been ordered to *stand* in the Estimates as hitherto and that it can be discussed *during year*" so that we are safe for the present. I cannot doubt that we owe this to your kind influence. And I make haste to write, not only to save you farther trouble for the present by announcing the fact about the estimates, but to thank you for all the good you have done us and to beseech (as tradesmen say) a continuation of your benefits for the future.

Source: From a memorandum, ADD Mss 43546 ff137-39 and 150-55, draft ADD Mss 45778 ff70-72

November 1869

Memorandum regarding sanitary progress at home and foreign military stations and in India in conformity with the principles and recommendations of the Army Sanitary Commission.

There are two classes of sanitary questions connected directly and indirectly with the army.

1. The questions regarding sanitary works properly so-called involving inquiries, plans, specifications, sanitary details and general structural improvements of barracks, hospitals, stables, quarters, including ventilation, warming, cooking apparatus, drainage, water supply and means of cleanliness. Questions of this class have come under the Army Sanitary Commission for report and recommendation. The works have been carried out by the Works Department at the War Office.

2. The questions specially connected with the personal hygiene of the soldier, including diet, clothing, duties, epidemic diseases, etc., together with the practical efficiency of the various sanitary appliances provided on report of the Army Sanitary Commission. These questions come directly under the Army Medical Department. They

are quite distinct from the points of construction referred to, nevertheless any matters involving sanitary works would come before the commission for discussion and report.

The following statement of progress refers solely to the work of the Army Sanitary Commission.

The royal commission of 1857 (under Sidney Herbert) reported that the soldier suffered greatly from preventible diseases and preventible mortality. It traced most of this to the excessive amount of tubercular and miasmatic diseases prevalent among troops on home service and it recommended the appointment of a commission for the purpose of investigating the subject and reporting on remedial measures. This recommendation was the origin of the "Barrack and Hospital Improvement" Commission, of which Sidney Herbert was himself the first president. At the close of 1861, Sidney Herbert being then dead, and questions daily of a more extended character coming before the commission, it was reconstituted by Lord de Grey (Sir G. Lewis being then secretary of state) with the quartermaster general as president under its present name, "Army Sanitary Commission."

Two years later, 1863, after the Royal Commission on the Sanitary State of the Indian Army, under Lord Stanley, MP, had presented their report, the S. of S. for India, Sir C. Wood, in communication with the S. of S. for war, Lord de Grey, finding it essential to have the help of the Army Sanitary Commission for initiating improvements in India, added two members to the commission to represent the India Office. And, as many questions regarding larger works of drainage and water supply were now coming before the commission, the chief engineering inspector of the Local Government Act Office was added. In this way the Army Sanitary Commission was constituted as it now exists.

The work of the commission has thus become extended by degrees from the improvement of home stations to the improvement of foreign stations, and finally to India. Apart from the Indian work, it may be stated generally that the commission by reports and published documents has already laid the basis for improved sanitary works at every station where there are British troops.

In India the details founded on the principles laid down by the commission are worked out by the local authorities, while the plans have been submitted to the commission by the S. of S. for India. At all home and foreign stations the action of the commission on the details has been more direct. The following is a brief sketch of the work already done at home stations. . . .

One word about India. The report of the Royal Commission on the Sanitary State of the Indian Army, together with the immediate action of the India Office, of the Government of India and of the Army Sanitary Commission in tracing out the practical course of proceeding, has already produced results—as is known to Lord de Grey—which could scarcely have been anticipated. The most recent reports show that, over the whole of India, the sanitary officer is at work, inspections are made, requirements are pointed out, barracks and hospitals are being improved or rebuilt on improved plans, embodying the recommendations above mentioned. Improved sanitary appliances are being introduced. The great capitals are being drained and supplied with water. And in a few years the whole face of that country will be changed. The Calcutta authorities state that anyone who has been absent from that city for two or three years would scarcely know it now, and the report which arrived from Bombay a short time ago contains the following passage which is more hopeful for the future civilization of the country than anything which has been recorded since it came under British rule. . . .

The latest work of the Army Sanitary Commission has been preparing the "Instructions" (copy enclosed) for a great inquiry into *cholera* which is now proceeding. The first answer to the cholera inquiry has come in. And the first result is apparently to destroy the prevailing theories that cholera is caused by "germs" or fungi, and to point at the same time the probable cause of the mistakes in this vital matter.

The commission will have to reduce the reports as they come in so as to arrive at the results, with the view of being able to recommend, from the experience thus obtained, measures for saving human life in India and elsewhere.

The work is second to none which has been undertaken by the commission. Up to the present time the whole question of cholera and of epidemic and epizootic diseases has been in the hands of theorists. Men have been anxious to arrive at correct principles for managing these diseases, but through their theories have arrived hitherto only at disaster. The attempt is now being made in India to ascertain *facts* by the help of the instructions issued by the commission. When these facts are obtained and reduced into practical shape we shall for the first time have solid grounds to go upon in preventing and managing epidemics. And it is needed, for already, since the beginning of this present year, the reports which have come in show that the British Army serving in India has lost from cholera nearly an entire battalion.

These facts show, although only very generally, the nature of the work hitherto done by the Army Sanitary Commission. This commission was invested with the duty of giving practical effect to the conclusions of two royal commissions on the sanitary state of the army at home and in India. Its work has hence been strictly practical. It has studiously avoided all merely hypothetical discussions and has dealt solely with well-ascertained disease causes. The results to health hitherto obtained have more than justified this method of proceeding, while great practical and administrative improvements have been gradually introduced over vast areas of country in such a way that there is every probability of the progress already made being not only maintained but extended—not without the hope of the improvements reacting on the slower progress incident to our home administration.

The future work of the Army Sanitary Commission should consist in extending the improvements already begun and to so large an extent carried out by the successive secretaries of state for war until every cause of disease at home and foreign stations is removed. The work in India must be done in India and great improvements in the executive will have to be made in that country before the public health is safe. The importance of this point may be estimated by what has been said in France with reference to the Suez Canal interests. It was stated that Bombay was so deadly a place that the trade would have to be removed from it to Suez.

All these facts show the importance, which however is scarcely doubted, of having a *skilled* advising body capable of affording guidance to these improvements at the beginning. And almost every sanitary paper received from India shows that practical help is still necessary from home to prevent mistakes.

There is, besides, the constant danger of retrograding towards the bad old system which made our British Army a byword for mismanagement in its sanitary arrangements. The constant changes which take place in our great public offices tend to deprive the public service of the help of men who have mastered and who appreciate the principles of such improvements. And hence the necessity for not only gaining new ground but for keeping what has been already gained.

**Editor:** Through the 1870s the Army Sanitary Commission survived. Its presence seemed to be a necessary fixture of the War and India Offices, but its structure remained inadequate and its function ill-defined. In the 1880s debates on its reorganization raged and came to a head when Dr Sutherland's retirement was being considered.

Source: From a letter to John Sutherland, ADD Mss 45758 ff179-81

17 December 1883

PRIVATE. *Burn.* There are but two objections to your (and our) plan about the Army Sanitary Committee.

1. There is not the slightest probability or possibility, as far as I know, of "Captain Galton" being "appointed in your place." He does not think *if* he will accept it, because he knows this. Also, no one would attend to him, IF he *were,* because he is a royal engineer, not a doctor.

2. Alas! alas! The committee is a "War Office committee," as we all know. But that does not "prevent" its "clashing" with the Army Medical Department. They simply ignore it, that is all. Has anyone since Irving "consulted" you? Does the War Office ever "refer anything to you as a committee"? No secretary of state has any idea of its difference from the Army Medical Department. If you resigned, he, the secretary of state, would, IF he did not dissolve the Army Sanitary Committee altogether, consult the director general and appoint an army medical officer in your place. This is *as far* as I know, of course. Dr Cuningham told me distinctly that he *would* accept your post, IF it were offered him on his return. This seems the only chance. The India Office would, I think, appoint him.

I can say nothing about the War Office. There is no one there with any of Sidney Herbert's traditions. Sir R[alph] Thompson [Parliamentary under secretary of state for war] is quite useless. Pray think again and inform.

Source: From a letter to Sir Richard Temple, Wellcome Ms 5483/40

7 November 1885

I am encouraged by your old kindness for me to believe that you would be so good as to consider the desirableness, which we sanitarians feel very strongly, of appointing to the post (which will now be immediately vacant) of surgeon general to H.M. forces in Bombay, your old friend (may I say?) deputy surgeon general Dr Hewlett, though of the Indian Medical Department, and, if you think well, of pressing it upon the secretary of state for India, without whose confirmation it cannot be made. Captain Douglas Galton will kindly furnish you with the circumstances. . . .

I have still your invaluable minutes and reports which you were kind enough to leave with me. They shall be returned to you whenever you wish. Had I thought that there was the least chance of your being at leisure enough to be in London, I would have hoped for the pleasure of a call from you.

Source: From a letter to John Sutherland, ADD Mss 45758 f223

20 July 1886

I grieve exceedingly for the state of your health. As for your remarks about the Army Sanitary Commission: what else have I been painfully doing (among all my other business) for the last two years, and am *still*? The possible collapse of the Army Sanitary Commission is ever on my mind and heart. During the political earthquakes of the last eight months, still continuing, no permanent interest can be expected in those who are so little permanent. The subject excruciates me. I wish you better with my whole heart.

Source: From a letter/draft/copy to Henry Yule,[152] ADD Mss 45807 ff219-22

14 September 1886

Private *and Confidential.* The point which I wished to consult you about, which comes out of your kind note of September relating to Dr Sutherland's "intended retirement," is: would you think it possible or desirable to try to reorganize the Army Sanitary Commission when this event takes place? so as to give it more executive power, not indeed directly, but by public opinion and secretaries of state. Do you contemplate the Army Sanitary Commission as a part of the *India* Office with, say, Dr Hewlett of Bombay or Dr Cuningham as Dr Sutherland's successor? And do you think it would thus have the weight of your present Army Sanitary Commission?

Might I ask what you think of the possibility of so reorganizing the Army Sanitary Commission as to obtain a living force to be exerted by the highest authorities at the War and India Offices, so that it should be strong enough to strengthen their hands by having public opinion at its back, in giving money and executive reality to what it, i.e., you recommend?

As you are good enough to think that I could help in obtaining a successor to Dr Sutherland at the "expense of the India Office" and back you in your good "fight," I would write you a short note in the

152 Sir Henry Yule (1820-89), Royal Engineer, member of the Council of India 1875-89 and of the Army Sanitary Commission till 1888, mostly referred to as Colonel.

sense of what follows, if that is what your kindness means. Dr Sutherland did so much work viva voce with executive officers coming to consult him that it is difficult to find all the evidence in the department of his utility and of the absolute necessity of a successor to him.

The reviews and criticism of Indian sanitary matters furnished in the annual Blue Book, of which Dr Sutherland has hitherto been the real author, have been of the greatest importance. But it is little known how native authorities in India, e.g., the native heads of municipalities, attach such value to these reviews that they actually obtain the reports from London before they are sent even to us in England, and use them literally and to the best effect.

What is required is no doubt executive work, but without the criticism the executive work would have gone on upon wrong lines or not at all. And there never was a time when so much activity has been awakened in India, more especially among the natives. And therefore when continuing the work done hitherto by Dr Sutherland was so important, abandoning it would be such a serious evil.

Source: Letter, Florence Nightingale Museum (LMA) H1/ST/NC1/86/7

Sir Harry Verney's
Claydon House
Winslow, Bucks
14 September 1886

*Private and confidential*

Dear Sir Thomas Crawford[153]

You have kindly talked to me more than once of your wish that the Army Sanitary Commission should be strengthened, especially as regards the work which you have so much at heart: the sanitary work of your own department (British and Colonial) and not only the Indian work, that it should have the power of *calling for* all reports (even "secret minutes" or whatever they are called) coming within its competence and that it should be made strong enough to influence the secretary of state for war to give the money and the *executive* reality to what you recommend. And it recommends in short that it should be reorganized to strengthen your hands and to be what it was intended to be at first.

We had eagerly hoped and expected that you would have been yourself the president of the reorganized Army Sanitary Commission

153 Sir Thomas Crawford (1824-95), principal medical officer in India 1880-82, director general of the Army Medical Department 1882-89.

and would have led its work yourself. But you cut this ground from under our feet—the last time I had the pleasure of seeing you. You spoke then of who should be its president, how it should be made a strong commission and who should succeed Dr Sutherland, whom you had so often kept at his post, but declined yourself to be the president. About this last, Dr Sutherland's successor, you mentioned Dr Hewlett or Dr Cuningham. You also spoke of the great necessity of the secretary of state for war himself taking the commission and its business in hand and giving it a living life, as Sidney Herbert did (war ministers change so often now that they seem not to have time to take anything in hand). Is it true that the crisis is approaching and that Dr Sutherland's intended retirement is about to take place? (He did not seem to contemplate *immediate* retirement.) Is it true that the War Office does not intend to give him a successor? And that, if the duty has to be maintained and if a fit man can be found, it will have to be done at the expense of the India Office, which will doubtless make considerable opposition to this, in the bad state of the finances of India?

Now, we must ask you what is to be done. You will say, most truly, that as for the Army Sanitary Commission, as a part of the India Office having the weight of the present Army Sanitary Commission, it simply cannot and the commission, instead of being strengthened, will have been weakened. How to obtain a living force to be exerted by someone in authority at the War Office? We look to you to tell us. Pray believe me, dear Sir Thomas,

ever your faithful servant

Florence Nightingale

Source: From a letter to Frederick Verney,[154] Add Mss 68884 ff174-75

17 November 1886

I am very sorry, but tomorrow (Thursday) I am entirely engaged in a most disagreeable affair, trying to save the Army Sanitary Commission. They are trying to abolish it and undo the work of thirty years. Secretaries of state are worse than Leipzig doctors.[155]

---

154 Frederick W. Verney (1846-1913), son of Harry Verney.

155 Lettice Verney, daughter of Captain Edmund Verney and niece of Fred Verney, was ill in Leipzig.

Source: From a copy of a draft letter to W.H. Smith,[156] ADD MSS 45807 ff240-41

10 January 1887

*Private and confidential.* Your extreme kindness to me and the favour you did me in desiring me to write to you on subjects connected with our conversation make me bold to obey your desire, notwithstanding that the event we most dreaded has happened [election of a Conservative government] and you are no longer at the War Office.

*Army Sanitary Commission.* You were so good as to say to me that you desired (1) to reconstitute the Army Sanitary Commission so as to do its work as a commission; (2) to give it work to do. Would you think well to impress on your successor [Edward Stanhope[157]] the uses of the Army Sanitary Commission which induced you to think/consider that it would be wise to have a *working* commission? . . .

The importance of revivifying and utilizing the Army Sanitary Commission and the facts of its not being utilized could be illustrated by many more instances, if you thought well to speak of it to your successor. But you yourself are the best advocate and illustrations are needless and only troublesome to you.

Source: From a letter to Douglas Galton, ADD MSS 45766 ff3-4

5 February 1887

*Private and confidential.* Hearing nothing of you, I thought you were gone to Florence. Have you heard of any further proceedings or resolutions of the War Office or other authorities in referring to the Army Sanitary Commission and connected matters? Colonel Yule writes to me that he "can learn nothing certain, but his *impression* is that the intentions regarding the maintenance of the A.S.C. are *not* favourable; nor can I ascertain what is likely to be the course in regard to the supervision or review of Indian sanitary matters should the A.S.C. cease to exist. But I doubt greatly its being in accordance with your views or with my own." I cannot sum up in a note what has passed on my side since I last saw you. Suffice it to say my letter to W.H.S. [W.H. Smith] was written and sent but, by the fatality which attends all they do, arrived an hour before Lord Iddesleigh's [secretary of state for

156 William Henry Smith (1825-91), secretary of state for war 1885-86, then first lord of the Treasury. Nightingale likened him to Sidney Herbert for his effective commitment to soldiers.

157 Edward Stanhope (1840-93), Parliamentary under secretary of state for India 1878-80, secretary of state for war 1887-92.

foreign affairs] death. It received a beautiful answer, promising to do all he (W.H.S.) could.

Source: From draft letter to W.H. Smith, Add Mss 45807 ff254-55

26 February 1887

Only your extreme kindness could pardon me for asking a question now of your overburdened time. I hesitate very much to trouble you. But the time is passing and steps practically irrevocable may be taken to make a future for the Army Sanitary Commission impossible.

The India Office will do nothing or perhaps worse than nothing till the War Office does *something*. You will remember that you most kindly said to me that you desired (1) to reconstitute the Army Sanitary Commission so as to do its work as a commission, (2) to give it work to do.

Might I ask whether you thought well, as you so kindly wrote about the middle of January, to impress on the War Office, on your successor, the uses of the Army Sanitary Commission and to influence him to make it a *working* commission, or whether you would think well now to say anything to interest him in it. If you would wish it, I should be glad to save you trouble by discussing it with Mr Stanhope. But any word to be powerful with Mr Stanhope must of course come from yourself.

Source: From seven letters to Douglas Galton, Add Mss45766 ff12-15, 16-17, 20-21, 22-23, 24-25, 26-29 and 30-31

6 July 1887

*Private.* I wrote to Colonel Yule and he appoints *tomorrow* (Thursday) to see me. He says he has "no information" on the "plans or prospects" of the "Army Sanitary Commission" and "looks to" us "for it." What am I to say to him about Dr Sutherland?

2. This is however the less tangible thing I drew from Mr Henry Cunningham with some difficulty, and even now what he says is far from precise; *what he wants* is: (1) *an official with the local governments in India,* who has time, knowledge, independence of character, appointed to make a *searching critique* of the sanitary reports of each of the municipal and public bodies. He says, as we know, that now *any* secretary or clerk out there makes these "critiques" for the local governments entirely without knowledge. He recurred strongly to the vague character and disregard of recent facts in Dr Sutherland's "memos" and general carelessness which, you know, has often painfully struck me. (2) *An independent body*—independent of the Government of India which does not wish to be brought into hot water—whose func-

tion shall be *to have the control of municipal bodies,* consisting of experts, engineers, doctors, etc. (*local government board*), that is to say, *an authority under the law in India* for this purpose, without embroiling the local administrations. He very wisely wished to leave such questions open as [to] the *numbers* of such a board and whether *one* or *more* boards. He was less sweeping and, though not very practical, still more so than the first time I saw him: less vituperative, less Payne-ified,[158] less "scientific," which I attributed to your influence.

3. About the Army Sanitary Commission he wishes, as we all do, that it should be entirely reconstituted. He says that Dr Sutherland's memos are so little searching as to be entirely useless—besides being so long after date—that they actually do harm, that they take no notice of the most terrible evils, and he pointed out several gross errors or omissions, as he did to you. It is not "the thing" for *me* to go over this. He wishes that "we" (i.e., himself and I suppose the other is Dr Payne) "should be called before someone here," who? to slate what is wanted "in the body" (Army Sanitary Commission) "here" and what changes are wanted in India. But how is he to be "called"? They don't want to hear. . . .

I shall have to guide me, with Colonel Yule, the notes I took from you on Saturday. Would you be so good as to read and *give me your opinions of these* [notes] *from Mr H. Cunningham,* especially his *1st and 2nd* sheets . . . and let me have them *by 10 tomorrow morning* (Thursday), please.

9 July 1887

I should be very thankful if you would kindly give me a line telling me the impression Dr Sutherland's and Mr Henry Cunningham's interview yesterday (Saturday) made on you. Colonel Yule came to me on Thursday according to appointment. He was, as usual, most anxious to be helpful. He took down all my principal questions, culled from you and Mr H. Cunningham, and will send me answers. And I lent him Mr H. Cunningham's report on Calcutta health. His general remarks were that no impulse for a local government board in India would come from *here,* that the India Council here would oppose any plan involving the taxation of the *people* for sanitary works and this would be a reason against the loans, he says. Though Dr Sutherland might not resign at once, yet Colonel Yule was decidedly of opinion

158 Dr Arthur Payne, surgeon general; he worked at recruiting nurses for India.

that *we should be ready with a plan for reorganizing the Army Sanitary Commission.*

Claydon House
Winslow, Bucks
17 July 1887

*Most Private.* I am more than ever distressed that I left London yesterday, i.e., had to leave it, when I might have stayed longer, had I known. I enclose you Mr Cunningham's letter which followed me here. I cannot make out whether it was written after his "breakfast" with you or not. This makes an important difference. Please return it me and say nothing about it.

2. Particularly I deplore being away because you see he asks me to write to Lord Cross.[159] I think I could have *seen* Lord Cross and usefully. To write to him would only be to add another "minute" to put into the hands of another private secretary. Still I will write if you approve and if you will tell me the gist of what I shall say. (But I do regret not having seen Lord Cross all this time. It was neglecting an opportunity.) I shall *not* touch on the "note on the (contagious disease) condition of the army," as Mr Cunningham wishes.

4. You see that Mr Cunningham entertains a very different idea of the "memo" he is called upon to write from what Colonel Yule (whose letter I sent you) does. You see that Mr Cunningham says "a memo on the general question of improved sanitary administration" [while] Colonel Yule, much more wisely, says, "on the *evils* of sanitary things and those of sanitary administration." (I have simply answered Mr Cunningham, accepting his offer to send me the "memo" "to see before it is sent in to Colonel Yule." But I *must* have *your* views, please, upon it too.) You will then have seen it. Tell me what to think and what to say of it.

[July 1887]

If I write to Lord Cross—rather, I think, I ought to follow up what passed between Lord Cross and me in the winter [see letter of 2 December 1886 in *Social Change in India*], when he did all we asked and all bore fruit. (It was chiefly though not altogether about Bombay. And much of it was in direct opposition to some of Mr Cunningham's views, such as I took down in pencil and sent to you.)

---

159 1st Viscount Cross (1823-1914), secretary of state for India.

7 August 1887

PRIVATE. Today I am almost sorry to tell you that Mr Henry Cunningham's short "Note" [on sanitary issues in India] has come, about fifty-sixty folio pages, which I read through without changing position or stopping. It is very ably done, like everything he writes. But I am almost glad to tell you that I think there is no chance of its being moulded into any form that can be of practical use, so as to be the substance of a despatch, till it has been very fundamentally revised by all of us, which can hardly be before October (?). (He says in his letter that he is going "to give a lecture on the subject to the Sanitary Institute in London in October in which" he will "be able to deal with the subject more fully." I do not think *we* shall "be able to deal with" his "Note" "fully" before that.)

A few of the things in which I think he is *raw* are as follows. He starts on the assumption that the mortality of the army in India had an average of 69 per 1000 *up to the time* of the royal commission. . . .

I have never answered Colonel Yule's letter, which I showed you rather more than three weeks ago. And I scarcely know how to answer it, for I suppose he does not know that I am to see Mr H. Cunningham's memorandum. I want you to advise me about this. Also whether the sending in of Mr H.C.'s paper may properly be deferred till say October. Also whether you have seen this paper. I will finish this letter tomorrow. *Nothing* more opportune or important has happened to us these many years than Mr H. Cunningham's arrival or than this paper as a beginning of operations. It is providential as an *impulse* to us. Let us make use of it and of him!

26 August 1887

*Private.* Mr Cunningham's manuscript. Sanitary. India. Mr Cunningham is still very eager, as I am, about the despatch from the S. of S. here to the Government of India, of which he was to write a draft *when* he heard from Colonel Yule. And this draft he promised to send me *before* sending it to Colonel Yule. But nothing apparently is being done. I now send you such of my notes as I have had time to write out on Mr Cunningham's paper, with which he concurred (the scratches on the backs are memos of our conversations which I have *not* had time to write out). Please *read and return.* Mr Cunningham being one of the reconstituted Army Sanitary Commission is an essential, just as it is an essential to have a reconstituted Army Sanitary Commission. Mr Cunningham was very eager that I should write to Lord Cross. *That* is useless. But I shall be back in London on 7 September. And as it seems the House will not be up till the 15th, I could see Lord Cross if anyone else has "steam up," viz., you and Colonel Yule—Mr Cunningham *has* "steam up." . . .

I think Mr Cunningham's information very important as to the useless character (from want of knowledge of present evils) of Dr Sutherland's memoranda. . . . The reason why I want you, if you possibly can, to read the enclosed (*im*perfect) notes in which Mr Cunningham concurs (I did not *show* him the notes) is that they will avail to *modify* the "despatch," of which *you* must *modify* the draft.

26 August 1887

I send you some extracts from the Bombay sanitary commissioner's recent illegible letters (private), which are important as answering your questions that I sent him and as bearing on Mr Cunningham's paper. See our query answered which Colonel Yule could not answer; see also the necessity borne out described by Mr Cunningham (and also by Dr Sutherland) of a sanitary executive board in India. But see also the absolute necessity of sanitary orders from the *secretary of state here*, and there must be a (reconstituted) Army Sanitary Commission here to direct the S. of S.; see also Mr Cunningham borne out about a young under secretary doing the government resolution on the sanitary reports; see also that the Army Sanitary Commission here *must* have power to CALL FOR papers and plans.

N.B. I think *Dr Hewlett must* be Dr Sutherland's successor on the Army Sanitary Commission next May; he is coming home. I wrote to Mr Hewlett, as you desired, urging him to make this, his last annual report, as full as possible. He could not do it. But the next annual report will contain remarks of his. And he *asks* us to *tell* him "*the points*" we want his "*opinion*" upon. PRAY, GIVE THEM ME.

Source: From a letter to Henry Yule, ADD Mss 45807 ff277-80

15 September 1887

*Private and confidential.* First, allow me to send you the letter of Mr [Henry S.] Cunningham on sanitation in India in the *Times* of 9 June. . . .

3. Let me thank you again for your most useful and magnificent present of the glossary of Anglo-Indian words. But I always wish you had been kind enough to write my name in it.

4. You are making progress with the subject of our conversations. Lord Cross, if I understood him aright, has given orders for the preparation of a kind of draft despatch, to be forwarded to him in a week or

two; but has not yet quite made up his mind what is to be put in it. You of course know a great deal more about this than I do.

Lord Cross was good enough to ask me to write anything for his consideration within the next week or two anent [regarding] particularly the personnel, the powers (and where the funds were to come from) of the executive proposed sanitary boards for the three presidencies. He staggered me very much, though he was more than well disposed towards the boards, by saying that the government could not borrow *in India* except at enormous rates of interest, that if they borrowed *in England*, there was the depreciation of the rupee to reckon with and that he did not suppose the municipalities would be willing to pay the difference of the exchange.

This is so very different from what the Anglo-Indian world supposes and especially from what Mr Cunningham rests upon that we must rather alter our line of argument. *What are we to say?* Upon all other things connected with our wishes he was most favourable.

(You will understand, I am sure, that all this is strictly between you and me and indeed the fact of Lord Cross having been here at all.) Kindly tell me what it is desirable that I should know, if I am to write to him. . . . *Burn.*

Source: From a letter/draft/copy to Lord Cross [secretary of state for India], ADD Mss 45807 ff289-90

September 1887

The absolute necessity of the government making a step, even if only a small one, seems obvious. If all that is desired cannot be done now, from financial and other difficulties, if an executive with full powers, including that of authorizing the borrowing from government at low rates of interest, cannot be given, may there not be an executive with modified powers? If all that is wanted cannot be done with the municipalities at present, owing to the great cost of works, may not the villages be taken in hand, where the cost is certainly *comparatively* small, the gain enormous, sanitary, *economical*, in enabling the people to have health to work . . . and taken in hand immediately, not all India at once but choosing your field?

For an executive there must be a sanitary engineer and a sanitary commissioner. There is an extremely limited number of sanitary commissioners from whom to select, probably only *four*; of sanitary engineers, only *one* or possibly two. I am not neglecting the cause of the cities.

Source: From seven letters to Douglas Galton, Add Mss 45766 ff55-56, 62-64, 67-68, 71-74, 75-78, 102-04 and 113-14

10 South Street
28 November 1887

The despatch is now being written. Dr Sutherland has, as you possibly may not know, been in extremis. He is now slightly better but I believe it is impossible that he will ever do another day's work. . . .

Something must be done about the Army Sanitary Commission at this end, as you said yourself, in consequence of the changes of the W.O., even if it were not for the "great change" preparing for Dr Sutherland.

5 May 1888

Private. I have scarcely heard of you, much less seen you, since before Christmas. But all this time this affair of the sanitary *despatch* from the secretary of state for India to Government of India has been hanging fire owing to poor Colonel Yule's inability, and it has only now reached the secretary of state's table. And the reorganization of the Army Sanitary Commission, far more important, seems to have dropped altogether.

From the direct source we know that poor Dr Sutherland will never do another day's work, though apparently he is not thinking at all of resigning. . . . *Could you kindly tell me*—I am too blind to read newspapers—*how it stands now with army estimates? Is vote for Dr Sutherland's salary, etc., passed?* . . .

2. You see that Colonel Yule speaks only of "maintaining the duties *here*" (i.e., *I.O.*) and nothing at all of the W.O. Yet the "duties" *at the W.O.* were a very large part of the reorganization scheme. I should greatly deprecate what he, Colonel Yule proposes, as far as Sir J. Fayrer[160] is concerned; and indeed as far as he himself is concerned. He does not at all recognize that the *Army Sanitary Commission must be reorganized* or fall and is, besides, poor man, "hors de combat [unable to move]." . . .

3. *Mr Hewlett* is coming *home* from Bombay (retired) *this month*—in the full vigour, mind and body, of his long experience and enthusiasm. We have no one at all to compare with him in practical knowledge and keen interest, whether we want him at home on the *Army*

160 Sir Joseph Fayrer (1824-1907), president of the Medical Board of the India Office, joined the Army Sanitary Commission in 1893. He authored *Inspector General Sir James Ranald Martin* and *Recollections of My Life.*

*Sanitary Commission* or in India for the proposed *sanitary executive*[161] (which by the way is being stoutly opposed by the I.O. Council). It would be a sin to let *Mr Hewlett* fall out of our ranks. We have no one like him. . . .

For the last two months and more, I have been quite laid aside, beginning with pleurisy, etc. I have but once been able to leave my bed to have my room "done," as the housemaids say.

8 May 1888

*Private. Reorganization Army Sanitary Commission.* The way seems opened for a real reorganization [of the Army Sanitary Commission]. As you say, if the Army Sanitary Commission is to exist, it must be reorganized. It does *not exist* now. It has no real authority with the departments.

We have now a director general, A.M.D. [Army Medical Department] [Sir Thomas Crawford] (we might not have again) who is cordially anxious not only to refer "all his own department's reports to the reorganized A.S.C. but that it *should* have real "functions," as you say, and authority. . . . It is a great plunge, after Dr Sutherland has been in it for thirty years and more.

13 May 1888

*Private.* Reorganization of the Army Sanitary Commission. You know of course, what I heard yesterday, that poor Dr [J.M.] Cuningham, the *ex*-sanitary commissioner with the Government of India, arrived in England from Australia two or three days ago to have the surgical operation of lithotomy performed on himself. Probably he will never be the same man again. Dr Sutherland has always looked on *him* as his successor. While acknowledging his (Cuningham's) superiority in the literary line, i.e., in drawing up reports, to the other two men, Hewlett and Cornish (these three, Cuningham, Hewlett, Cornish,[162] were the three mentioned to me by Sir T. Crawford as being those among whom he would wish that Dr Sutherland's successor should be nominated and that *you* should be *chairman*), I think Cuningham immeasurably inferior to Hewlett in everything else (and *now* certainly, poor

161 Parallel to the reorganization of the Army Sanitary Commission, the presidency commissions were being reformed and, in 1888, were replaced by a Central Executive Sanitary Board in each province.

162 William Robert Cornish (1828-97), sanitary commissioner for Madras 1870-78, author of several reports on famine and cholera in the Madras presidency.

fellow). And Cuningham is so unpopular. Hewlett has a *practical "go"* in him, which none of the others have, and such experience *practical.*

*You were quite right* to say what you did about *Cornish.* He has done, it is true, a good work in Madras (it was he who gave me the famine statistics which I published in the *Nineteenth Century* ["The People of India"] and was scolded for my "exaggeration" as never man was scolded by the India Office. And it turned out that the statistics were *under* the mark). But Dr Cornish is not so *sound* as Hewlett and is inferior to him. He is "not," as you say, the "right man."

2. But is the "Home Army" to be vested in the same man as the "Indian Army" if home reports are to go in to the Army Sanitary Commission, as Sir T. Crawford proposes, and *as they ought,* in the same way as Indian reports? Can they be? In that case, I should unhesitatingly say: of the three, Hewlett would be the best for the "*home*" purpose. But none of them have good experience for it. But did you not think of having *two* men, one for each army?

3. Is Dr Sutherland to have a retirement pension? at least a "consideration"?

4. His "statement" is finished. . . . He had been advised, I don't know by whom, to draw up a sketch of his services for the last forty years and has done so.

19 May 1888

*Private.* From Dr Sutherland I have received to my joy (unasked for) a letter to show to the authorities, recommending *Dr Hewlett* in the most unqualified manner as his successor. . . .

*Private.* [Colonel Yule] adds: "Without the concurrence of Galton, I doubt if we can do anything to the purpose." Except as concurring in this last, I have really no opinion, further than that I want *both,* the Home Army and India Army, to be "served" by the Army Sanitary Commission. . . .

*Despatch* to Lord Dufferin [viceroy]: Nothing can be less hopeful than the prospect. The draft despatch is still, I believe, with Sir John Gorst[163] to whom Lord Cross sent the papers. I am asked both to see the latter and to write to Lord Dufferin. But Lord Cross is out of town here and Lord Dufferin is "out of town" in India. Procrastination has been fatal to us.

---

163 Sir John Gorst (1835-1916), lawyer, Parliamentary under secretary of state for India.

8 July 1888

*Private.* Can you, O can you tell me anything about Mr Stanhope and the *reorganizing the Army Sanitary Commission*? (Both Mr Cunningham and Dr Hewlett have seen Lord Cross and are well satisfied with him.) But I cannot find out that anything is done! And here is July!! And Lord Lansdowne[164] is in London!!! And he must be enlisted in the cause!

13 July 1888

PRIVATE. I had a long Indian sanitary talk with Mr Hewlett yesterday. He only asked two questions about himself: (1) Whether it would prejudice his chance of being appointed to the Army Sanitary Commission (upon which his whole heart and mind are fixed, but not more than ours) to take a post on the Local Government Board. I assured him it would not. (I had your authority.) And I believe he will send in his official letter today. (2) Whether it would be more than a few months before the Army Sanitary Commission matter was decided, to which I answered we could not tell.

Source: From a letter to "Cousin Arthur" [Clough],[165] Boston University 2/23/A3

17 July 1888

I have a terrific interview on Thursday with an Indian sanitarian [Mr Hewlett], who wants to be on the reorganized Army Sanitary Commission, but not more than we want to have him, for in twenty-five years in India we have no one his equal for vigour, experience and knowledge of and influence with natives. But the terrific nature of the interview is, how can we promise an appointment which rests with TWO secretaries of state?

Source: From a draft letter to Lord Lansdowne, ADD Mss 45778 ff181-84

19 July 1888

PRIVATE. In answer to your remarks about the Army Sanitary Commission here, which seemed to say what have I to do with urging them (it?) and directing, and what has it to do with practical sanitary reforms in India, I think I did not explain (because I had already tres-

---

164 Henry Charles Keith Petty-Fitzmaurice, 5th marquess of Lansdowne (1845-1927), Liberal politician who had served previously as under secretary for India and war, governor general of Canada 1883-88, viceroy of India 1888-94.

165 Arthur Hugh Clough, Jr (1859-1943), son of poet A.H. Clough and Nightingale's cousin Blanche Smith, an executor of Nightingale's estate.

passed too much on your time) that its name of "army" is a misnomer, that the Army Sanitary Commission is really far more to do with the native population of India than with the army. . . .

If Mr Hewlett, sanitary commissioner of Bombay, who has returned to England, is appointed (as successor to Dr Sutherland, the acting member who has resigned), as those who know best desire, you will have in him a man whose heart and mind and experience are in India as his service has been for so many years, and whose knowledge and influence with the natives is beyond the common. . . .

It is needful to increase the usefulness of the Army Sanitary Commission by not limiting it to reviewing annual reports sent to it, which makes these annual Blue Books really two years old, but to have questions referred to it from the Governments of India and the India Office, and for the Army Sanitary Commission to be able to ask questions in return. . . .

I shall hope to claim your generous offer to see me once again before you leave for your kingdom. Success to your great work. Godspeed.

ever your faithful servant
Florence Nightingale

Source: From two letters to Douglas Galton, Add Mss 45766 ff125-27 and 129-33

5 August 1888

*Most private. We* must decide "if it is necessary for" Mr Hewlett "*to apply*" for Dr Sutherland's appointment "*and when.*" This is the way the question is put to me. You will see that it is impossible for me to take the responsibility upon myself of advising him *not* "to apply" or "to apply." "Dr Cornish *is* trying for it and others." I do not know whether formally or not, whether to the secretary of state for India or to whom?

I cannot possibly take the responsibility of advising Dr Hewlett *not* to apply. Sir Joseph Fayrer states that "Dr Sutherland had resigned and that he, Fayrer, did not think that the appointment would be filled up." Probably it will *not* if there is no reorganization of the Army Sanitary Commission. But the "others are trying." . . .

You will remember that, upon your authority, though of course I did not give my authority, I advised Mr Hewlett "to *keep quiet* for the present." Do you think that "*present*" is now gone? And that he had better enter the lists?

The filling up Dr Sutherland's place really depends, I suppose, upon the reorganization of the Army Sanitary Commission. But people are *not* waiting for that. And Hewlett must not be left out in the cold, either for the work's sake or his own.

The matter is so important that, though I was trying to get off to Claydon at once, I would gladly, if *you could see me* on *Wednesday afternoon* on your return to London, stay *till Thursday*, in order that you should advise me upon Hewlett's course more than you would do by a letter.

Claydon House
Winslow, Bucks
28 August 1888

*Strictly private.* The Government of India "resolution," of which a telegraphic summary appeared in the *Times*, has reached me from Simla in a letter dated 1 August. No doubt you have seen it. . . .

It gives us the "*executive* agency" (it is expressly stated that it is to be "more than consultative") in each province a sanitary board composed of:

1. An officer of administrative experience;
2. The sanitary commissioner (who *is* there?);
3. A sanitary engineer P.W.D [Public Works Department] (query: is "he" there? is there *one*?);
4. Non-official members appointed by local government;
5. *Ex officio* members (some commissioners of division and district officers are rather terrible in their ignorance and apathy).

The sanitary board is to have the control and supervision over sanitary works, whether in urban or rural areas and is to be the *executive* agency through which the government is to work in the sanitary department. The provincial sanitary boards are to communicate with the sanitary commissioner with [the] Government of India (pity he is not a better man, this seems to me fatal) (possibly later a sanitary engineer is to be associated with him). . . .

The "resolution" "considers favourably" the question of *loans* to *local bodies*, and the authorizing of a "provincial loan fund" to enable local bodies to raise funds for sanitary improvements on "less onerous terms," and says that on this point the Government of India's "decision" "will not now be long delayed" (probably not longer than 1888). It alludes to the Act XI of 1879. The "resolution" refers particularly to *village* sanitation and, as an Appendix, gives the *Army* Sanitary Commission's remarks, March 1879: "Practical hints for sanitary improvement of smaller municipal towns, of *villages*." (It alludes to the royal commission report of 1863.)

I do not want to analyze, rather to seek information from you: what are its bearings, etc., especially its bearings as to the reorganization of the Army Sanitary Commission; such a resolution making the *home* machinery doubly important, the sanitary advisors of the Government of India being so far behind the present day in knowledge. . . .

*Private.* I end as I began: how much action, or how little, will come out of this "resolution," how much will remain "all talk"? *How can the Army Sanitary Commission be so reorganized as best to prevent its becoming "all talk"?* (The "resolution" is curiously like his excellency. Whoever drafted it must have an intimate knowledge of his character and style.) I feel rather curious to know what effect the "resolution" will produce at the India Office, whether it will be simply shelved both in England and India, or whether Sir John Strachey and Sir John Gorst will eat their words (which are in print). I presume sacred and mystic bodies like the India Office Council never look foolish.

As to India, of course much will depend on Lord Lansdowne whether it will be "vox et praeterea nihil" [words and nothing more].

**Editor:** Nightingale had visits from Lord Lansdowne in July, then 28 October 1888 before he left for India as viceroy.[166] They talked about the Army Sanitary Commission, as becomes clear in the correspondence below with Henry Yule and Lord Ripon. Nightingale continued to seek Lord Ripon's help.

Source: From a note on a meeting with Lord Lansdowne, Add Mss 45778 ff185-86

28 October 1888

A curious and terrible book might be made of how we have tried to benefit the natives and sunk them deeper than they were before. Debt, ruin, irreproachable courts of justice . . . comma bacilli,[167] refuse so bad that comma bacilli cannot live in it.

Lord Lansdowne objects to A.S.C. because sanitary things so "purely local" can be treated only on the spot (not so: sanitary principles the same everywhere, then we should have Indians of thirty years' sanitary experience as working members on A.S.C., *and* India has done nothing for twenty-five years by herself).

166 Described in a letter to Douglas Galton 29 October 1888, Add Mss 45766 f173.

167 Seen in a microscope, the cholera bacillus was shaped like a comma.

Lord Lansdowne impressed by Lord Dufferin's scheme of executive boards being cumbrous and expensive and by the thing to be worked, I presume, by the old collector.

Source: From two letters (of the same date) to Douglas Galton, Add Mss 45766 ff169 and 170-73

29 October 1888

*Private.* Could you kindly bring me a brief *written* answer to Mr Hewlett's difficulty? and return me the papers? (I could never make extracts from his letters again.)

I send you the opinion of Cuningham and Co. on the A.S.C. in the *Pioneer.* I for my part should be very glad to have Cuningham on the A.S.C. About the A.S.C. I had some conversation with Lord Lansdowne.

29 October 1888

*Private.* Here is a very serious matter and even more serious than Mr Hewlett thinks. He has received the enclosed extraordinary "resolution" (the "young civilian" is revenging himself). Mr Hewlett is fully aware of the great blow it will be to sanitary reform in western India. This resolution is circulated to all collectors and every municipality. It will make the natives doubt the correctness of the advice which Hewlett and Co. as the sanitary advisors of the government give them. And it will greatly discourage his successor and I am afraid has already done so. "Du reste" [moreover] Hewlett and Co. have an ample answer to it. But who will read the answer?

These would be the heads of the answer. As to the *foreshore*: Lord Reay[168] has forgotten Hewlett's letter No. 2112 B dated 13 July 1885 (a copy of which both you and I saw) in which Hewlett drew Lord Reay's attention to the state of the foreshore in Bombay in nearly the same words. Dr MacCatter, the zealous health officer of the port, brought this again to notice last January or February, and how nothing had been done by the port trustees.

Hewlett sent this report to government but it was returned "unread as government did not wish to have the reports of subordinate officers."

2. Hewlett was obliged to say what he did about those plans being submitted to the superintendent engineer. He has convincing proofs

168 Donald James Mackay, Lord Reay (1839-1921), governor of Bombay 1885-90.

of his assertion about those plans, "but I left that letter of mine *regarding the* General Post Office in Bombay with Sir Douglas Galton, who promised kindly to read it. I don't know whether he has had time. But that will show whether I am right or wrong. Let the original plans and all correspondence on the subject be sent home. I am quite willing to abide by experts here."

3. All his previous five masters, including Sir S. Fitzgerald, Sir P. Wodehouse, Sir R. Temple and Sir J. Fergusson, have always encouraged his reports.

4. At p 40 of his Annual Report for 1876 and at p 133 of that for 1884 he gives his opinion/experience on "the ignorance of the officers of the Public Works Department regarding sanitary engineering" almost in identically the same language and makes the same recommendation.

5. To the remarks about Colonel Ducat's and his action they have a complete answer. Now *what would you advise him, Hewlett, to do?* He wants to bring it to the *notice of Lord Cross.* He will at all events bring it to the notice of *Sir James Peile*[169] at *the I.O.*

As for the "personal" account of the visit to the "Deccan village" and the "Gujarat town," it is the best thing Hewlett or any sanitary commissioner has done. The whole extent of the mischief which he is not aware of or has forgotten embraces this.

I gave a copy of his proof on Bombay villages (which you have) with his desire and with Henry Cunningham's sanction . . . to Lord Lansdowne when I saw him in July. Lord Reay, so Lord L. tells me, is his particular friend. I have indicated to Lord Lansdowne Hewlett as the only thorough sanitary commissioner they had now in India. (This was of course only in answer to Lord L.'s questions about sanitary commissioners there and A.S.C. here.) Lord Lansdowne sees Lord Reay of course straight upon his arrival at Bombay.

I saw Lord Lansdowne again yesterday and not having been able to take your advice first I said, in the course of conversation, a very few words about this imbroglio. But what can one say? It is not anything that Hewlett has said or done professionally that has stirred up this wasp's nest (which I fear may be fatal to him). It is his having stirred up the enmities of the "young civilian."

---

169 James Braithwaite Peile (1833-1906).

Source: From two letters to Lord Ripon (of the same date), ADD MSS 43546 ff224-25 and 226-33, typed copies ADD MSS 45778 ff150-53

13 November 1888

PRIVATE. Will you excuse this hastily written letter, the fruit of years of interest in these things? If you could see your way and thought well to speak to Lord Lansdowne about the reorganization of the Army Sanitary Commission, to which I believe Lord Cross is still favourable, and perhaps about Lord Dufferin's scheme, if you approve it, it would be doing us a great service.

N.B. Why should Lord Dufferin's executive boards be "expensive"? Of the members I suppose only the sanitary commissioner (and he is paid already) and a sanitary engineer, would have to be paid. I know I need not ask your kindness to make no reference whatever to me or to any words I may have written here, but to consider it all as *strictly between ourselves.*

13 November 1888

*Private and confidential.* No. 2. I did not send my first letter, because the events upon which I wished to consult you have succeeded each other so rapidly, and some of them are very curious. I now only send No. 1 *for reference.* And will you pardon me for writing another?

Lord Lansdowne kindly came to see me in July. He was most favourably disposed to these objects we have at heart, but specially well disposed to village *native* agencies, to panchayats and the like, to local self-government, etc., which I attributed to his having had the advantage of seeing and hearing you. He has now been to see me again and has sent two others to see me (he leaves England on Thursday next). It is upon what I have learnt from them and others during the last *fortnight*—and all of it is *strictly private*—that I now wish, if I may, to trouble you.

1. Already the Government of Bombay is in revolt against the "sanitary resolution of the Government of India 27 July 1888" (enclosed in the other envelope). That is, I do not know how far *the governor* is pledged to this. And it has not committed itself to a word on paper, so far as I know. But it *condemns the proposed executive boards* as "cumbrous and expensive" and it condemns at once the "Resolution of the Government of India" for proposing too much and too little. . . .

3. *Army Sanitary Committee.* You will remember this, which grew out of the Barrack and Hospital Improvement Committee appointed by Sidney Herbert in 1859—and of which he himself was president—to carry out the recommendations of the Royal Commission on the Sani-

tary State of the Army. By a minute of yours (1862) all plans of new barracks and all important alterations were referred to this committee and other questions were also referred to it by the S. of S. for war. A vast improvement in the health of the army resulted.

In 1863 the committee was reconstituted, as you will perhaps remember, by adding two India Office representatives, in order that it might report on the causes of disease and the remedies, in pursuance of the recommendations of the royal commission appointed in 1859 "to inquire into the sanitary state of the army *in India*" and presided over successively by Sidney Herbert and Lord Stanley (Lord Derby). It became the present Army Sanitary Committee. All Indian sanitary reports—civil, native and mofussil [countryside], as well as army—are sent to it for criticism and suggestion. And its Indian business far outweighs of course its home and colonial army business.

Dr Sutherland has been the working member ever since its very beginning. He has now resigned on account of ill health. The Army Sanitary Committee was now to have been reconstituted and to receive a new vitality. But it seems doubtful whether it will be reconstituted. *Mr Stanhope—all this is strictly private*—is quite impressed with its necessity but admits the decided hostility of the royal engineers and department of I.G. fortifications. He asks if a sanitary officer, attached to the quartermaster general (who is the present head of the Army Sanitary Commission) as a substantive part of his staff, would not suffice. But is it not necessary to have *not a lining* [bandage?] but a regular permanent body outside the regular administration as our sanitary representative? especially for India.

Mr Stanhope says he is attached to the doctrine of *personal* responsibility and does not like the system of so many committees. But how to keep personal responsibility and give it the weight that a few good men of knowledge and experience would give it, is your question, is it not? Mr Stanhope then asked about India. At present India cannot be safely left to her own arrangements because she has neglected for twenty-five years to adopt measures recommended by royal commission. Yet if she NOW gives vitality to Lord Dufferin's scheme (N.B. *it is doubtful if she will*, e.g., Bombay) she *ought* in a few years to suffice for herself.

*Lord Lansdowne* has not considered the subject but somewhat demurs to an Army Sanitary Commission, "because sanitary things are so 'purely local.' " (Not so. Are not sanitary principles the same everywhere? The *local* conditions are to be considered and there would be an Indian sanitary commissioner, just come home, of twenty-five years' Indian experience on the committee. *And* India has done nothing for twenty-five years *by herself.*) Lord Lansdowne liked the idea of an *adlatus* [seconded person] better at the I.O.?

But if you abolish the Army Sanitary Commission as a committee and put an individual to do the work, do you not lose the weight that a committee consisting of eminent sanitarians gives? Would you think well, if you approve, to speak to Lord Lansdowne about this? of course with no reference to me. Lord Lansdowne is somewhat impressed by Lord Dufferin's scheme of executive boards being "cumbrous and expensive" and that the thing should be worked, I presume, somewhat after the fashion [of the Bombay Village Sanitary Bill].

Source: From a draft/note to Henry Yule, ADD Mss 45809 ff49-50

17 November 1888

When I saw Lord Lansdowne, he was fully convinced of the necessity of an "Indian expert," but not of an Army Sanitary Commission. I believe I am expressing your views when I say that an expert, a kind of adlatus [ . . . ] without the weight given by a commission of experienced sanitarians, a body as it were external to government, would have little influence in important matters, or at least it would depend entirely on the man to whom he would be adlatus.

A sanitary commission is not a society. It is a commission or a committee. To such a body, which requires practical sanitary experience of value, Cuningham would lend no weight.

**Editor:** The following letter appears to be by Nightingale but is signed by Sir Henry Yule. Its style and content are hers and it certainly contains her views, as the letter of 2 February 1889 (below) makes clear.

Source: From a letter in Nightingale's hand, signed by Henry Yule, ADD Mss 45778 ff164-65

22 January 1889

(Nightingale's hand:) *Strictly confidential.* No. 2. Arrangements for future reviews at home of sanitary proceedings in India. At present I feel quite unequal to writing anew upon this subject, but I desire in the most earnest terms to draw attention of the Secretary-of-State-in-Council to what I have written on the matter in the paragraphs added at the end of my minute of 10 December 1888. I regard such reviews of sanitary progress in India, as were drafted for so many years by Dr Sutherland, as of the highest value and I think that a moderate expense should not be grudged for the maintenance of such a system.

*Now that the War Office has decided upon abolishing the sanitary committee and to lend us no aid in the maintenance of this system,* I think we should provide for ourselves an officer of the highest competence that we can find to keep up these periodical reviews. There are several such officers now available, who have belonged to the Indian sanitary service. I may name Dr Payne and Dr Hewlett, either of whom would admirably perform this duty. Whether it would be desirable to reinforce such an officer by a committee of members of this office, whether of the council, of the secretariat or of the medical department, I will not venture positively to say, though I incline to think it would be very expedient to do so. It is well to divest such reviews of a personal character as far as possible. No expenditure would be involved except a salary of perhaps £400 a year for the sanitary expert, and some small outlay on copying.

I can add no more except to commend this matter very seriously and strenuously to the favourable consideration of the Secretary-of-State-in-Council and to repeat my strong conviction of the importance of what I urge, now that my fourteen years' connection with the sanitary department is coming to a close.

Source: From two letters to Douglas Galton, ADD MSS 45766 ff213-14 and 223-24

16 January 1889

STRICTLY CONFIDENTIAL. I am not a little appalled at what I have to tell you of the information received by Mr Hewlett from Sir Ralph Thompson.

> [quotation in another hand] He yesterday had an interview with Sir R. Thompson, who told him that the secretary of state for war had written to the India Office to say that he (Mr Stanhope) proposed to abolish the Army Sanitary Commission altogether and to let India make her own arrangements. He [FN hand: Mr Hewlett] stated to Sir R. Thompson that this would be a most fatal step, that the European Army in India consisted of about sixty thousand men, that it was difficult enough with present conditions for sanitary officers to get any money out of the government for improvement of barracks, etc., and the only way, hitherto, had been to get the matters brought to the notice of the Army Sanitary Commission, who thus afforded a most useful check, as the Government of India felt compelled to carry out suggestions.

[FN: Mr Hewlett writes:]

> Sir R. Thompson listened most kindly to what I had to say, and said that I had undoubtedly made out a strong case and that he would mention the matter to Mr Stanhope. On this I said, "Shall I send you a letter on the subject?" to which he replied "he would be very glad, if I could." I am therefore going to be very busy writing a memo pointing out the great "assistance the Army Sanitary Commission have been and could be, and also pointing out that the sanitation of the towns and villages, although principally affecting the civil population, really affects the military element in no slight degree, as it is there these sad epidemics of cholera spring up, and by improving the general health of the people, you will certainly improve the general health of the British soldier. . . .

[FN resumes]

> I do trust . . . this decision of Mr Stanhope's is not final. Will you, when you have done with with your election, take it up?

1 February 1889

*Strictly private.* The *India Office* says: "The committee have proposed that a letter should be sent back to the War Office saying that they acquiesce with Army Sanitary Commission being abolished, at least that they have nothing to say against it, but they hope that if the *War Office* appoint an expert that he may do *Indian* work for the India Office."

Source: From two letters (the first partially dictated) to Thomas Gillham Hewlett, Woodward Biomedical Library A.67 and 68

24 January 1889

I was very much obliged to you for your two successive letters giving me important information, both about the threatened curtailment of the sanitary department in Bombay, and yet more about the Army Sanitary Commission. I will write further about these; in the meantime, may I ask you what news you have of the famine, or the scarcity, said to be impending in India?

yours faithfully

Florence Nightingale

[FN hand] *Private.* Have you any news of the result of your letter to Sir Ralph Thompson at the W.O.? I should like very much to see a copy of it, as you kindly offer.

*Strictly Private.* I have this bad news from the I.O. "Two points I wished to get the secretary of state to notice in writing to India—I found it not practicable, as there was no basis for his action—viz., the

Ahmedabad scheme and the Bombay rebuke of Mr Hewlett. The secretary of state must not do evil that good may come, and it would be evil if he did (which he would not) intervene where no report from India gave him constitutional ground, and where it would be manifest [continued in the next letter]

25 January 1889

that he was intervening on some private representation."

I am afraid, *re* Army Sanitary Commission, that the I.O. accept as final the W.O.'s abolition of the A.S.C. They are however "putting before secretary of state" "about arrangements *in loco* Sutherland."

Source: From a letter to Lord Ripon, Add Mss 43546 ff234-38, draft Add Mss 45778 ff154-63

2 February 1889

*Private.* No. 3. We are now in a discouraging crisis at both War Office and India Office, which looks as though it would end in a defeat of your (and Sidney Herbert's) sanitary arrangements and measures, unless you could think well to intervene with your powerful help, founded on knowledge from the beginning. The present crisis is this:

1. The War Office has decided *to abolish the Army Sanitary Commission* . . . "and *to lend the India Office no aid in the* maintenance of that system," viz., "the system" of such reviews of sanitary progress in India as were drafted for so many years by Dr Sutherland and which were "of the highest value," especially in the sanitary education of leading natives in India. The War Office appears to have written to the India Office to this effect. But it is thought that the matter must be still under discussion. No notice whatever has been received by the members or by the secretary of the Army Sanitary Commission or any intimation that they are being "*abolished.*"

A very strong minute has been written by a member of the Council of India, dated 22 January, to be put before the secretary of state, "about the arrangements *in loco* Dr Sutherland," saying that they (the India Office) should provide for themselves in case of the War Office carrying out its intention of "abolition." An officer of the highest competence they can find, to keep up these "periodical reviews," etc.

Such an officer is now at home, retired in his full usefulness, viz., the deputy surgeon general, T.G. Hewlett, who belonged to the India sanitary service and as sanitary commissioner did such admirable duty for so many years, including the great famine, in Bombay presidency. . . .

2. The *Government of Bombay* has asked its surgeon general to reduce the "medical budget" by 1,25,000[170] Rs including the *sanitary department.* It is thought that two deputy sanitary commissioners (out of six!!!) may go, that eastern and western Gujarat may be united and that the overworked sanitary commissioner (of the whole presidency) may hold a district!! It was hoped that the Bombay sanitary department had so far weathered the financial storm. And Lord Dufferin kindly wrote to me that he had saved that sanitary department from any reduction. . . .

I can only lay bare our imminent dangers to you, to you who have guided or instituted all these things almost from the first—before Parliament meets—without venturing ever to suggest what you might think well to do.

Source: From two letters to Douglas Galton, ADD MSS 45766 ff226-27 and 229-30

8 February 1889

*Strictly private.* Sir T. Crawford says, "the question (of the Army Sanitary Commission) is, I believe, still in abeyance." If this is true, something may still be done.

16 February 1889

*Private. Burn.* Interview with Lord Ripon satisfactory inasfar as he wished to do what we proposed (he said he wished he had known all this earlier). . . . [He] asked me for the *original instructions* of *Sidney Herbert* to "*Army Sanitary Commission.*" I have written to Mr Frederick for them. Can you give me any suggestions about this to give him? (I was rather sorry he asked for them, because I suppose S. Herbert's instructions were less full than his, Lord Ripon's own? and it was not then the "Army Sanitary Commission.")

Source: From a letter to Lord Ripon, ADD MSS 43546 f246, draft ADD MSS 45778 f169

22 February 1889

*Private.* How can I be grateful enough for your great kindness and your efficient exposition of the need of the Army Sanitary Commission (reorganized) to Mr Stanhope, which no one could make with as much force as yourself, of course. Might I hope that you may be able to see Lord Cross about this matter (which, as you said, concerns India even more than home) before you go into the country.

---

170 Rupees are written as follows: one lakh means 100,000 or in digits 1,00,000 Rs. The present case can be expressed as one lakh and 25 hazaar.

I do not presume to urge the importance of it. It is you yourself who have taught us. Pray believe me,

ever yours faithfully and gratefully
Florence Nightingale

Source: From a letter to Douglas Galton, ADD Mss 45766 f243

10 April 1889

It would be of the greatest consequence to know whether there is any chance of the War Office deciding before Easter if it means to reorganize the Army Sanitary Commission. I have put off—unwisely, as it appears—writing to diverse people on the subject till then. And now it seems unwise to write until the War Office has made up its mind

Source: From a draft letter to Henry Yule, ADD Mss 45809 f133

30 April 1889

*Private.* It was understood some little time ago that the secretary of state for India would be disposed to appoint a commission at the India Office if the War Office did not reappoint theirs (the Army Sanitary Commission). Might I ask what is the case about this? Have you anything you would advise me to do? I defer troubling you with other questions till I know that they would not be disagreeable to you.

Source: From a draft letter to Lord Cross, ADD Mss 45809 ff137-39

3 May 1889

*Confidential.* Your extreme kindness to me in matters that lie so near my heart as the sanitary interests of India encourages me to endure once more to trouble you with a question: Might I trespass upon you so far as to ask if you have decided yet what steps are to be taken to preserve some control over the sanitation of India?

It would take some time to bring Lord Dufferin's proposal, the sanitary "Resolution of the Government of India" (Simla, 27 July 1888), even if it be carried out, into working order in the several presidencies and provinces. Until it is in working order, you are doubtless retaining the important power of using some means to criticize sanitary reports from India such as was afforded by the Army Sanitary Commission and quickening these means too. At this moment it is more and more important in India, instead of less.

But it is impertinent of me to be suggesting considerations to *you.* I believe I am only echoing your own views in saying that an "expert" would be a bad substitute for the reorganized commission at the War Office, which should include as heretofore representatives of the different aspects of sanitary questions: medical, engineering, general and especially Indian, and that the commission should actually meet and discuss together the matters referred to it. Also that their proceedings should be expedited, especially as regards India. But that a solitary "expert" at the War Office should be permitted to exercise the same supervision over Indian as over imperial service reports would be a fatal mistake and can come to nothing. The W.O. "expert" may be quite without Indian experience or the capacity to review Indian conditions. And your view, which I believe was understood to be that, if the W.O. were to abolish the Army Sanitary Commission, you would yourself appoint one for India, is surely the right and the only one.

Forgive my intrusion and impertinence. It is your own kindness that is in fault. I need hardly say that it would be my highest privilege if you could spare half an hour and would be so very good as to make an appointment to see me some afternoon on these matters and give me your verdict. But I am not so utterly unprincipled as to expect it.

Source: From a draft letter to Sir Thomas Crawford, ADD Mss 45772 ff83-84

3 May 1889

*Confidential.* How deeply do I regret that your term of office is at an end. You have been a great and true friend to us. And we shall, I fear, miss you much. Especially as you were so absolutely in favour of continuing and even increasing the powers and the work of the Army Sanitary Commission, your retirement may, it is to be feared, affect its prospects. You are persuaded . . . of the necessity for it in India. Might I ask you what ARE the prospects of the A.S.C? at home? and also, if what you mapped out is not to be carried out at home, what steps ought to be taken to preserve control over the sanitation of India?

It would take some time to bring Lord Dufferin's proposal (of last July), even if it be carried out, into working order in the several presidencies. Until it is in working order, there can be no doubt that it is most important to retain some means of criticizing the sanitary reports from India, such as was afforded by the A.S.C., and to quicken these means too. But it is impertinent of me to be suggesting consideration to *you.* Lord Ripon, Lord Wolseley[171] and I know I am only echoing your own views in saying that an "expert" is a bad substitute for the commission at the W.O. and that the reorganized commission should

171 Garnet Wolseley (1833-1913), created viscount for conquering Egypt, led the attempt to rescue General Gordon.

embrace representatives of the different aspects of sanitary questions, medical, engineering, general and especially Indian, and that the commission should actually meet and discuss together the matters referred to it. Also that their proceedings should be expedited, especially as regards India.

A solitary "expert" at the W.O., who might be quite without Indian experience or the capacity to review India conditions, would be a fatal mistake if meant as a substitute for the commission. Better that the I.O. should have a commission of its own than this. There is I suppose a most formidable antagonist to the employment of army sanitary officers in the field. Does this antagonism hinder the reorganization of the Army Sanitary Commission?

I need not say with what pleasure (and pain at losing you at the W.O.) I should see you again if you would be so very good as to make an appointment.

Source: From a draft letter to Henry Yule, Add Mss 45809 ff145-48

13 May 1889

*Private and confidential.* I cannot thank you enough for your most kind letter. Amid our deep regrets that we lose you at the India Office, I cannot but rejoice at what you are good enough to tell me about your pension and your health, and I trust that it will yet farther improve with your well-earned comparative rest. May it be so!

You are so good as to say that I may write to you about India Office affairs before you leave. I trust that you will be able to say something to Lord Cross about having an Army Sanitary Commission for the India Office if Mr Stanhope does not reorganize his. Who after you will help the cause at the I.O. and who of the I.O. ought to be your successor at the Army Sanitary Commission, if there is to be one? And if unfortunately there is not, to whom is our cause to look in the I.O. to do what you have done? Give us your advice and know we may depend upon you to recommend and explain the cause to someone at the India Office and instruct him!

I think I did not trouble you with a letter I was asked to write to the Bombay leading native associations about the village sanitation bill, which I find has been translated and favourably commented on in the Bombay (not government) *Gazette.* But I have not heard what the finally revised bill is to be. It is in the charge of Sir R. West,[172] who was

172 Raymond West (1832-1911), vice-president of the Royal Asiatic Society, author of *A Digest of the Hindu Law of Inheritance, Partition and Adoption.*

good enough to call upon me when in England. I hope you will not trouble yourself about this or about what I am going to say, unless you have something particular to tell me. It is all about Bombay presidency. You were good enough to interest yourself about the water supply and drainage schemes of the president of the municipality [and of the sanitary commission] of Ahmedabad, Mr Runchorelal Chotalall.[173] You have often said besides that there are no government engineers in India to whom sanitary structural works could be entrusted or I should hardly venture to say what I am about to say. They are waiting for the sanction for borrowing 1½ lakhs for sewering a corner of the city; Mr Runchorelal is not strong enough by himself to get the municipality to pass a resolution to have a skilled engineer from England. The Bombay government has offered their engineer at 2½ p.c., who is said to be "admittedly not competent." And he has been accepted.

It has been suggested (not by me) that the viceroy should be asked to lay down a rule that no money would be sanctioned, or that permission to borrow money on loan would not be granted to municipal bodies, unless the Government of India approved of the engineer to whom the work would be entrusted. But would not this be asking the viceroy to interfere in what is strictly provincial business? Please say [what you think].

Source: From a draft letter to Lord Lansdowne, Add Mss 45778 ff200-01

21 June 1889

I feel, even more than you can, now that I am presuming upon your great kindness. That kindness and my intense interest in the subject of sanitation in India must, if anything can, plead my excuse.

Might I ask what is the position of the sanitary boards proposed in Lord Dufferin's minute/resolution of the Government of India of 27 July 1888. It would of course take some time to get these boards even if organized into working order in the several presidencies. Might I ask you to be so very kind as to empower someone to tell me whether any such boards have been carried out? There was some objection made to them in Bombay. Yet last month at the India Office it was given as a reason for abolishing the Army Sanitary Commission "that sanitary boards were being organized under the India government resolution mentioned above." And I believe that on 21 Febru-

173 Runchorelal Chotalall (1823-98), president of the Ahmedabad municipality, member of the Bombay Legislative Council.

ary the discontinuance of the Army Sanitary Commission was notified to you from the India Office.

Am I too presumptuous in asking for information from the highest authority as to the position of these sanitary boards in India?

Source: From a letter to Sir Henry Acland, Bodleian Library, Ms Acland f156

25 July 1889

*Absolutely private.* For the last twelve months I have been exceedingly tried about the Army Sanitary Commission, which was to be reorganized, in which reorganization Mr W.H. Smith, while at the War Office, took the deepest interest. It has now been abolished, simply by default—let to slide. . . . The matter is of such immeasurable importance to India that you will excuse me for mentioning India's grief—I cannot speak about it. Nothing can be done now.

Source: From two letters to Douglas Galton, ADD Mss 45766 ff263-64 and 265

11 August 1889

*Private and confidential.* The plot thickens. By the last post last night I had a long answer from Lord Lansdowne re sanitary boards, etc., in India, also enclosing a short memo he had had drawn up. I subjoin an abstract on another sheet.

You will see that three local governments (Madras, Bengal, Central Provinces) make the board to consist of sanitary commissioner and sanitary engineer, *special* or otherwise. We know that they have *no sanitary* engineers. And now appears to be our time, if we could work it.

1. The Government of India is now addressing secretary of state at home to sanction the MADRAS appointment of sanitary engineer. Who is he? BENGAL: the special sanitary engineer (who is he?) is not even to be a whole-time officer; the Government of India is pressing it. CENTRAL PROVINCES: the engineer is not even a special, merely the SUPERINTENDING engineer, who is as a rule entirely *non*-sanitary.

As to the sanitary commissioners of each province I must get hold of their names correctly; you see, owing to the sanitary commission having lived at Norwood of late years, I have none but private information. And Indian sanitary commissioners never know each other. My melancholy impression is that they are nobodies. Lidderdale, an invalid, is I think still the Bengal one. Lord Lansdowne says I shall "frown" because they are so "slow." I think they have been too quick. It seems to me that the very best Army Sanitary Commission at home with the very best ex-Indian sanitary working number is vitally necessary. . . . (I am very glad you made me write to Lord Lansdowne.)

12 August 1889

*Private.* 2. It occurred to me how valuable a man Sir T. Crawford would be on the *Army Sanitary Commission.* He and Mr W.H. Smith were the only men in the administration who thoroughly understood and wished to carry out the objects for which the A.S.C was intended. But I suppose it would be contrary to etiquette to have an ex-director general. He would be invaluable in the place of -- ? who is there now. . . .

3. I write to Mr Hill this morning at the I.O. for the names of India sanitary commissioners and engineers. But I am afraid he is absent on his holiday.

Source: From a draft letter to Sir Ralph Thompson, ADD Mss 45809 f205

24 August 1889

Sir Douglas Galton has telegraphed to me from Paris suggesting that, as in your note to him of yesterday's date, you had told him that Mr Stanhope was so kind as to wish to see me to "talk over the future of the Army Sanitary Committee." . . .

Most gladly will I see Mr Stanhope *any* afternoon that he will be good enough to fix beforehand *after today.* And I will gladly put off my departure from London till afterwards. I am obliged to ask for an appointment because I am an overworked invalid. 5 P.M. or 6 P.M. would be my best time. But I am sure you will kindly understand that I would make Mr Stanhope's time mine any afternoon.

Source: From two letters to Douglas Galton, ADD Mss 45766 ff267-71 and 283-84

Claydon House
10 October 1889

*Quite private.* 4. I have heard nothing directly from Mr Stanhope who is busy at his guns. But *confidentially* and indirectly, I heard that the Army Sanitary Commission *is* likely to be revived, that the hitch has been that everything is now vested in the quartermaster general and that the Army Sanitary Commission does so little work now except for India; but that it will probably be reorganized and other besides Indian work given it; that if Sir R. Buller[174] would say he wanted it, it would be done directly.

174 Sir Redvers Buller (1839-1908), major general, quartermaster general.

24 October 1889

Private. Sir Henry Cunningham has sent me the proposal for a "Sanitary Indian Institute here" which he says he has sent you and you alone. He asks to see me about it *this* week. I *must* see you first, please, to know what you think. . . .

It makes me quite sick to see this proposal, when they raved so against the Army Sanitary Commissioner and Sir H. Yule, when I found from Sir Charles Bernard that they had converted him to the same view, when we have lost Hewlett and when I know from you how unwise a "proposal" you think it, and when I know what are the people they have to work it

But we must not throw cold water upon it. Could it be made a branch of your Sanitary Institute? For us the first thing is to have the *Army Sanitary Commission* reorganized. And I can only think of you for home matters, Dr Cornish for India, upon it. Dr Payne, whom Cunningham recommends, is clever but untrustworthy like a half-caste, always "I" is No. 1. And Hewlett's bad temper was an angel's while his is a devil's. Please let me talk over the "proposal" with you *tomorrow* if possible, if not, *Saturday*.

Source: From two letters to Sir Thomas Crawford, Florence Nightingale Museum (LMA) H1/ST/NC18/89/18 and 90/3

3 December 1889

*Private.* Long ago you kindly promised me a visit but have never kept your promise. Sir Douglas Galton tells me that you are considering a point for me, viz., who should be Dr Sutherland's successor, we having lost Mr Hewlett, and whether there should be two, one for India and one for home, and who? Might I ask you kindly to let me know, if possible, by tomorrow (Wednesday)? If I could hope to see you tomorrow at 3:30 or 4, I should be delighted, but at such short notice how can I expect it?

13 March 1890

You have probably seen the enclosed pamphlet, which was the last thing Mr Hewlett did. The I.O. sent out copies to the Government of India (and, I believe, to the presidency governments). Do you think well of it as being *practicable*? I have more copies if you should wish to give any.

Source: From a copy of a letter to Sir Robert Rawlinson, Florence Nightingale Museum (LMA) H1/ST/NC1/90/130

13 March 1890

*Confidential.* I have two, if not more, most kind letters to thank you for, which I do from my heart. You saw that Mr Stanhope brought forward in the House of Commons on this day fortnight his plan for spending four millions on barracks and camps (*not* in the Estimates) and for the reverification [revivification] of the Army Sanitary Commission.

Might I ask you (in strict confidence) whether you could recommend either Colonel Tulloch or Colonel Ducat for the *sanitary engineer* whom it is proposed to put on the commission? And if either of them would take it? (Their knowledge of India would of course be very useful.) It is very difficult to find such a man among the royal engineers who would do all the work of the Army Sanitary Commission. *You* know (none better) what the qualifications needed are, so I need not mention them. He is to give his *whole* time to the commission, as I understand (as Dr Sutherland did).

Source: From a letter to Angélique Lucille Pringle,[175] Edinburgh University, Pringle Letters (162)

8 November 1890

I will tell you a story of a man, a hero, like Gordon[176] in character, who for thirty years in India was our guide and instrument [T.G. Hewlett], whose death, last October, has greatly increased all our work and difficulties, both Indian and War Office.

Source: From a letter to Douglas Galton, ADD Mss 45767 ff56-57

22 April 1893

*Private.* Queen's India cadetship asked for by Dr Hewlett's widow. Would you kindly suggest what is to be done? I know you thought as highly of Dr Hewlett's India work as I did. I do not know Lord Kimberley[177] as I did Lord Cross, though he has done some good things

175 Angélique Lucille Pringle (1846-1921), lady superintendent at the Nightingale School, St Thomas' Hospital, London.

176 Nightingale's friend, "Gordon of Khartoum," General Charles George Gordon (1833-85), killed in Sudan on 26 January 1885. Correspondence in *Society and Politics* (5:490-512).

177 John Wodehouse (1826-1902), first earl of Kimberley, Liberal politician, secretary of state for India 1882-85, 1886 and 1892-94, then secretary of state for foreign affairs 1894-95.

for us since he has been in the I.O. In fact, I do not know him personally at all. Would you be so very good as to draw up a sketch of what ought to be said and of Dr Hewlett's labours, *whoever* is to tackle the secretary of state?

## Sanitary Conditions in Prisons

**Editor:** This topic, though little developed by Nightingale, belongs as an appendix to her concerns with the army and public health care. The high mortality rate in prisons has already appeared in several letters as instances of sanitary neglect that called for reform. There are obvious parallels in sanitary conditions and overcrowding between barracks, prisons and other institutions like asylums. Mary Carpenter was one of the persons who provided Nightingale with concrete information on prison conditions in India.

Source: From two letters to Douglas Galton, Add Mss 45762 ff224-25 and 234-35 (both written from Hampstead, N.W.)

3 October 1864

*Private.* I don't know whether you know of the correspondence between Sir J. Lawrence and the Bengal Sanitary Commission and me about the state of their lunatic asylums and jails, which is worse than that in any country which has lunatic asylums and jails at all. They send me their printed minutes but on the express condition that they are *not* to go to the India Office. Else I should just refer them to your Barrack and Hospital Commission. Would you (since Sir J. Jebb's[178] death, I have not the same means) get me a list of all the reports published by the *Prison* Board, marking those which have reference to prison construction, and regulations as to cubic space, etc., and send it me as soon as possible. Of course whatever we send out must be sent out through your Barrack and Hospital Improvement Commission. And the India Office must be brought in somehow, since it holds the purse strings and the expenditure required will be immense.

I think you will have to send out Gordon, royal engineer of Constantinople, who knows how all that can be done in jails for a precisely similar people, to reform the Bengal jails. The *Times* has got hold of

178 Sir Joshua Jebb (1793-1863), surveyor general of prisons and member of the council of the Nightingale Fund.

the subject and given us great help in its articles. But I did not furnish it with its information. However, it makes our path much easier.

20 October 1864

I sent back today by hand the Pentonville report sent you by Captain Ducane. This is one of the reports I want. Will you have the goodness to send me a copy (for Sir John Lawrence) as soon as you can, and also any *reports which contain authorized prison rules, especially for the guidance of governors and of inspectors of prisons*?

The commissioners in lunacy (who were applied to by me at the same time) have sent me long ago all their reports which I wanted and marked too, and they are already speeding away by her majesty's *Book-post* to Sir John Lawrence (for we found it would be too slow an affair to wait for your Barrack and Hospital Improvement Commission).

Source: From two letters to James Pattison Walker, Florence Nightingale Museum (LMA) H1/ST/NC1/65/9 and 18

26 April 1865

I was in hopes to have sent you your (water supply) analysis questions, answered, by this mail. But my learned men are so dilatory. However, I will not delay to thank you for all the rich store of information, which touches me so deeply, that you have been kind enough to send me. I feel so much what you say about your inspector general of prisons, Mr Woodcock, whom you call the first of Indian sanitary reformers, so justly. What a great work he did and at how great an expense to his own peace of mind. Indeed we ought to be very grateful to him. It is hard enough, God knows, for public men to do their duty anywhere. But I do think it is harder in India than anywhere else. So much the greater honour to their memories, be they living or dead.

In regard to jails: the diminution of overcrowding, with the increase of superficial area, has been the result of progressive experience. Every climate has its limit. Thus, for Turkey, the inspector, who is at present in England, informs me that 72 sq. ft. are allowed, both in cells and in common rooms. This Turkish experience is probably the nearest to yours. One would think the recurrence of epidemic disease in Indian jails a sufficient reason for increasing the space. If you have any prison in which epidemics prevail, your area is too small. If you have any exempt, your area is sufficient. Increase your area and cubic space, until cholera, dysentery and fever disappeared *epidemically*. Of course ventilation and cleanliness are inferred. Prison epidemics in England have been taken as the test of sanitary condition. Formerly they killed prisoners, jury and judges. Now they have ceased to exist in prisons. This is your Indian test.

You have the reports on prison construction and prison regulations by Sir Joshua Jebb (he was the great prison sanitary reformer in England, of whom I should speak as you of Mr Woodcock, both as to his sacrifices and to the unworthy return made him). The best plan for a tropical prison I ever saw was for Malta (for a new prison there) by a Mr Inglott, of Malta, a man who has a perfect genius for that kind of thing. The Colonial Office (of course this is entirely in confidence) is now "girding up its loins"[179] to clean out *its* house too, with regard to its prisons. It has instituted an inquiry. And India must not be left behind.

If these kinds of questions in India could be referred for an opinion to the home sanitary commission, we might back you up with our experience. It is a wonder that men do not learn—both from these dreadful epidemics and from their absence, when conditions are improved. Lord Stanley is at this hour (again, this is in perfect confidence) applying to Sir Charles Wood to refer to the home sanitary commission for an opinion both on the jail question, and on the question of Mr Strachey's most able Calcutta paper, which, as you are aware, has been made a Parliamentary paper of, and presented to the House of Commons on 22 February.

I must again thank you for your invaluable statistics (eight forms). I am quite touched by your having taken Dr Bryden's duty, which, I think, is very magnanimous. And I only hope that you will do your very best to keep your health and Mr Strachey's too. For, as I shall tell him, it will not do for sanitarians to die. Martyrs used to do good by dying. But, in these days, martyrs *must live* to do good.

The statistics are very good indeed—very cheering—and give a great deal of invaluable information. Let the absence of epidemics become a permanent condition. You will succeed in this at last. A large part of your diminution of death rate is due to absence of epidemics, specially of cholera. No higher reward can be wished you than that you may become able to depend upon, in future, this absence of epidemics. (We must not boast in London. Typhus has become more prevalent the last two years and is always trying to raise its head and burst out *epidemically*. So much the more shame for us, in a temperate climate.)

179 An allusion to 1 Pet 1:13.

I cannot close my letter without recurring again to the honour which must be paid to you for undertaking Dr Bryden's work. I do trust it will please God to preserve Sir John Lawrence's health. I conceive there has scarcely ever been a time in history when so much depends *for good* (often it has depended for evil) upon one man as the head. Sir C. Trevelyan's breakdown in health is a great misfortune. Mr Massey, however, comes out with the highest possible desires (and ability) of seconding Sir John Lawrence and doing India good service. . . .

N.B. I am quite aware that one of Sir John Lawrence's first acts was to appoint a commission to report on the whole question of Indian jails within a month, on which commission you were; that the several governors were desired to send in their requirements and their "bill" for their own provinces, in obedience to the recommendations you then made; that Madras and (I suppose) the other governments *have* sent in theirs, which, I suppose, have been approved. (Was it in reference to these that you complained so justly that so small an allowance of superficial feet had been asked for?) How very glad I should be, if we could help you about these things. Could you send us a copy of your report (viz., of the commission on jails above mentioned) and of any administrative papers appertaining to it?

25 September 1865

I have received all your enclosures, I believe, including one on the present defective method of calculating prison death rates. And as you are so very kind in wishing everything to be submitted to you—which is worked out on your subjects in England—for your consideration, I venture to send you a memorandum by Dr Farr, of the General Register Office, with whom I have been always greatly associated in work. The object is not to obtain the *absolute* mortality, which is scarcely possible, but to obtain a result which will be comparable with other results similarly obtained.

You will think that I am never going to send the method for finding out the amount of "*dirt*" in water. All I can say for myself is that I have myself revised it six times through the press, that my learned men are always making fresh additions, which worry the printers very much and me still more, but which are quite worthwhile, for the paper is quite a different thing in worth, since it was begun more than six months ago. I do hope this is the very last revise, and to send it you now very soon. . . .

I am going to take the liberty of sending you tracings of plans of a small prison about to be erected in one of our (hot-country) colonies, which we think a sanitary model of its kind for warm climates.

Source: From a typed copy of a letter to an unknown recipient [Mr Inglott?], Royal Malta Library Ms 396, Wellcome Ms 9085/18. See another part of the letter in *Public Health Care* (6:526)

3 October 1865

I am sure you must have thought me very ungrateful not to acknowledge sooner your kind letter of 31 August and also the plans of the female prison you propose to establish at Malta. As soon as these arrived, I had two copies made, one of them for Sir John Lawrence in India and one is for your own Colonial Office.

I hope that this plan will be imitated, with modification, throughout our country's dependencies. For hot climates it is the very best I ever saw. It was shown here to the president of one of Sir John Lawrence's three (Indian) sanitary commission[er]s, who is now in England [R.S. Ellis]. And he bespoke a copy for each of these sanitary commissions (Bengal, Madras, Bombay).

I hope therefore your trouble will not have been in vain but that your plans will extend as far as the queen has possessions, or alas has jails (which is the same thing).

Source: From a letter to Lord Stanley, Liverpool Record Office, Derby Collection 920/15/90

28 October 1865

*Private.* I received some little time ago from India the enclosed manuscript about fifty-one jails in Bengal lower provinces. The facts are so very startling that I feel inclined to trouble you with it.

It is true that we rely upon no statistics which we receive, even from headquarters in India—they continually contain blunders. It is true that they are themselves so aware of this that quite lately I received a request to get them a method of computing jail mortality statistics from our General-Register Office, which I have done (not yet received in India). But even if you put a pound of salt into this paper, it is sufficiently appalling.

It is not that cubic space is the only sinner. It is that the whole management and laws of Indian jails require to be entirely raked up and set to rights. *Could not Indian prison returns be moved for in Parliament?* I must, please, ask you to make no use of this identical paper, but to return it to me. This kind of paper does not, I believe, reach Sir C. Wood. And I once erred in this matter, for which I repent in sackcloth[180] (but

180 An allusion to Matt 11:21.

as I am luckily a "*female* criminal," I shall have "1097 cubic feet" to repent in).

Source: From a letter to James Pattison Walker, Florence Nightingale Museum (LMA) H1/ST/NC1/65/21

3 November 1865

*Private.* I have seldom been so struck by anything as by the "extract from" a letter, No. 247 dated the 8 May 1862, from the inspector general of jails, Lower Provinces to, etc.," which you were so kind as to send me. (I am aware I have acknowledged it before.) I believe I could give you a help towards furthering the object you have so much at heart, viz., providing a remedy.

Could you send me any later information in such a form that we could use it here? Everything relating to this subject is of immense importance to the future of India and also of our colonies.

Should you be so kind as to grant my request, would you, in sending figures, be so good as to state the precise manner in which the statistical results are obtained? In other words, how you get the percentages of mortality? We should also have the chief groups of diseases.

Source: From a letter to Douglas Galton, Add Mss 45763 f105

7 December 1865

Do you think you would be so good as to have three more copies made for me of the enclosed Malta prison? Of the two you were already kind enough to make for me, one is gone to the Colonial Office and one to Sir John Lawrence direct. But you see India is rather a big place and one is now wanted for the inspector general of prisons, North West Provinces, who builds all the prisons there—at least his subordinates do: one for Madras presidency, etc.

Source: From a letter to James Pattison Walker, Florence Nightingale Museum (LMA) H1/ST/NC1/65/27

18 December 1865

I sent you, by this, a plan of the Malta (female) prison which we consider the best for hot climates we have yet done. Perhaps you will like to show it to your friend, Mr Stewart Clark, the inspector general of the North West Province prisons. It may not be quite suited to India. But your acumen would see at a glance how it might be adapted. The facility of supervision, the opportunity it gives to the prisoners of sleeping in the open air, the facility of ventilation, the power of multiplying the units to any extent (if a larger prison is desired) are what we prize. (I sent a copy direct to Sir John Lawrence.)

Source: Notes from an interview with Sir Bartle Frere for John Sutherland, Add Mss 45752 f201

[ca. 5 July 1867]

Sir B. Frere says "Miss Carpenter did much good." He says the jails *were* like D. Dalgetty's horse:[181] when he had been taught to live on one straw a day, he died (the jail mortality from starvation—excessive).

Source: Notes on an interview with Mary Carpenter for John Sutherland, Add Mss 45752 ff250-51

[August or October 1867]

I had Miss Carpenter here for two hours yesterday. She is always a great deal too much for me, but she certainly told me yesterday much that was useful.

She says that it is perfectly useless for the Indian government to go on as they do now about building prisons. She says that there is a prison just built at Coimbatore or Ootacamund (I forget which) at I forget what enormous cost for 1000 people on the model of Pentonville, that in *each* of these cells there are four or five prisoners, that there is no water supply, no privies, no hospital, no sanitary arrangements, no sufficient ventilation, and yet that the Government of India make use of the fact of their having built these prisons at enormous cost to say that they can do nothing more. That a *better* prison might be built, *she* says, at no cost at all, just of huts for the prison cells. She says that the council of engineers which sits at Calcutta on the prisons is the destruction of everything good.

She says that a *Dr Wiehe*, whom Sir B. Frere employed about prisons (Bombay presidency), is a very good man. She also praised Dr Mouat, but says he has no influence with the council of engineers. But, she says, they *will* put four or five into each cell made for one. She says, they *have*, at Ootacamund. She says never. She says Dr Wiehe has published an excellent report.

She says the mischief done by putting female prisoners under male warders, a practice universal in India, though denied by Sir J. Lawrence, is incalculable. She says, "What Dr Mouat says, that hecatombs are yearly sacrificed in Indian prisons to preventible disease, is the exact truth."

181 An allusion to Sir Walter Scott, *A Legend of Montrose* chap 14.

Source: From a draft letter to Sir Bartle Frere in Dr Sutherland's hand, ADD Mss 45780 f180

[1868-69]

I have often had it on my mind to talk to you about the awful mortality in Indian prisons. It crops out in all your papers: fever and cholera, cholera and fever and the doctors, with one or two brilliant exceptions, knowing nothing about how to analyze [or] to treat ordinary disease manifestations and, because they are so, laying the blame on the old devil contagion just as firmly in this country. Old women were burned because cattle died of bad treatment. Can nothing be done in this matter? Could you at the India Office not take it up and deal with it? A century ago we in England were so well up in jail fever that we could kill not only prisoners, but witnesses and judges at trials, I believe we once killed a lord mayor. Thanks however to Howard[182] and next to Sir Joshua Jebb and other prison reformers our prisoners go out better in health than they came in. Here is a noble field for reform in India. Who will lead?

182 John Howard (1726-90), whose *State of the Prisons*, 1777, inspections and reports led to considerable penitentiary reforms.

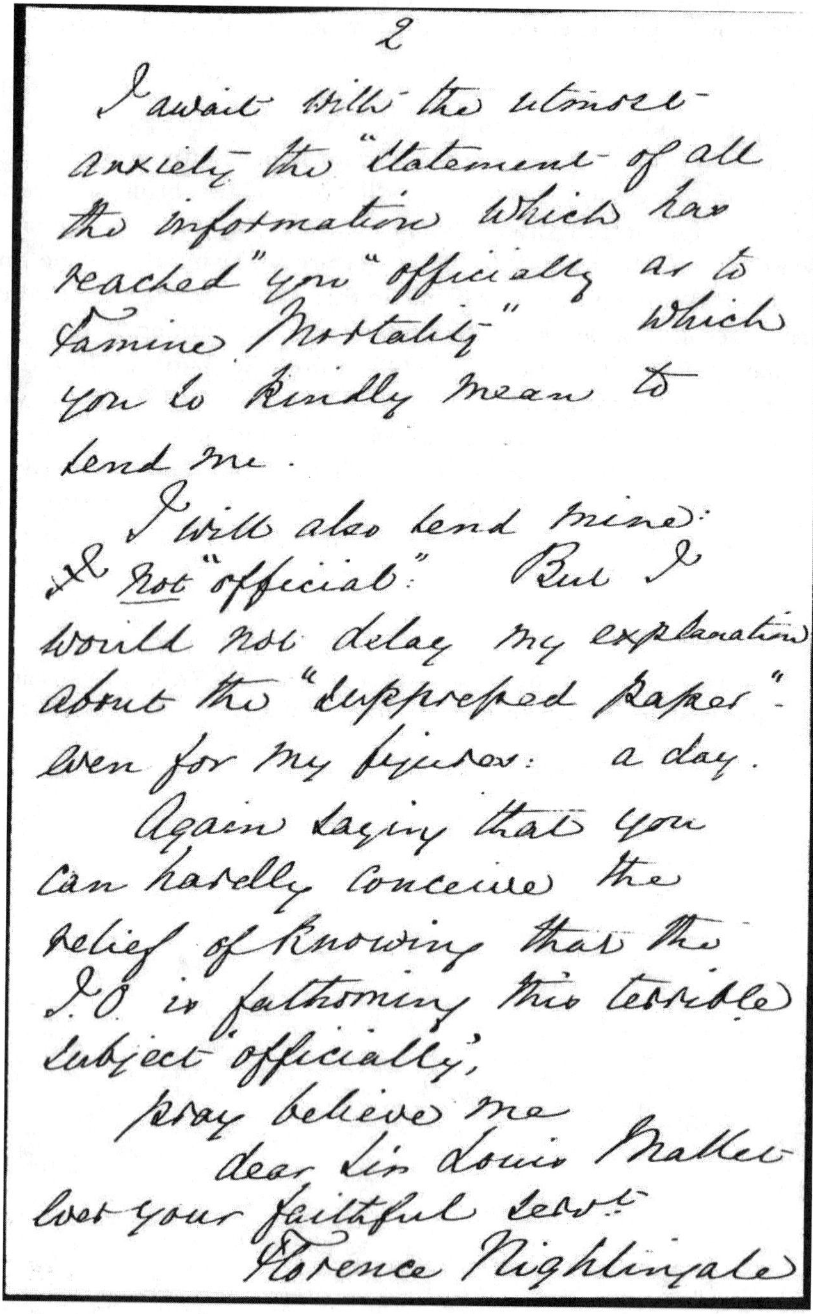

2

I await with the utmost anxiety the "Statement of all the information which has reached" you "officially as to Famine Mortality" which you so kindly mean to send me.

I will also send mine: & not "official". But I would not delay my explanation about the "Suppressed Paper": even for my figures: a day.

Again saying that you can hardly conceive the relief of knowing that the I.O. is fathoming this terrible subject "officially";

pray believe me
dear Sir Louis Mallet
ever your faithful servt.
Florence Nightingale

Nightingale letter to Sir Louis Mallet, Mallet Collection, held at Balliol College. Reproduced courtesy of Alfred Mallet.

# Famine Prevention and Irrigation

The implementation of the recommendations of the royal commission on India, especially through the newly created sanitary commissions, did result in improved health and reduced mortality for the British Army in India. As we have seen, Nightingale next took on the health of civilians, and considerable progress was made in reducing preventible mortality in that massive population. Improvements in infrastructure, such as sewers, canals and drainage systems, benefited the entire population, of course, but offsetting those gains in public health were periodic famines.

Famines were mainly occasioned by prolonged droughts and the failure of monsoon rains, but sometimes also by excessive monsoon rains[1] and floods. Famines left "the affected population relatively defenceless against infectious disease."[2] Food crises led to elevated mortality. In the second half of the nineteenth century in India, the period of British rule coinciding with Nightingale's work, an estimated 29 million people died of famine. Nightingale herself referred to the estimate of a major famine roughly every ten or eleven years. There were many famines across India between 1861 and 1908: in 1861-67 there were famines in the North West Provinces, Bengal, Bihar and Orissa; in 1876-79 in Bengal, Bihar, the Deccan, Oudh, Bombay, Madras and Mysore (the "Great Famine"); in 1896-97 in Oudh, Bengal, Punjab and the Central Provinces; in 1899-1902 in Punjab, Rajputana and Gujarat. There was also plague in Bombay in 1896-97. As during the terrible Irish "potato famine" of 1845, food was exported from famine districts while people were starving. Nightingale often cited Ireland as an example in trying to persuade W.E. Gladstone to take as strong a leadership role on India as he had on Ireland, even to lead a new liberal approach to India as he had to Ireland, but he never did.

1 See Ronald E. Seavoy, *Famine in Peasant Societies* 263.

2 Arup Maharatna, *The Demography of Famines* 7.

The Orissa famine,[3] which culminated in 1866, was the first to occur after Nightingale started to work on India; it had a strong impact on her and increased her sensitivity to the problem (see p 709 below). The early stages of the famine coincided with the intense period of data collection and analysis for the royal commission. It evidently worsened in 1866, to kill an estimated million people—a rough estimate since there was no census then. The worst part occurred during John Lawrence's viceroyalty but there is no correspondence between him and Nightingale on it. There was occasional coverage of the famine in the press in England, and occasional mentions in Parliament. Lawrence himself was active in famine relief, a point made in the inquiry put into place by the British government in 1866. The governor of Bengal, Sir Cecil Beadon, was ill during the worst period and went to the hills. He accordingly was exonerated by the inquiry, but one must wonder about a government structure that would fail so badly on account of the illness of a foreign official.

The commission of inquiry's lengthy report was published in August 1867.[4] Nightingale read it and from then on famine prevention became a major concern. Before 1867 it seems Nightingale was simply not aware of the seriousness of famine in India. The first clearly dated mention of famine in Nightingale material occurs only on 30 July 1867, in a letter to Douglas Galton. Beadon's defence she described as "pitiable." She faulted Lord Elgin's administration for the inability to act quickly; Lawrence "struggled (in vain)" against the "dead weights around him" (see p 586 above).

The dominant political philosophy of the time was laissez-faire liberalism, or a principled rejection of active intervention by government in the free market economy, a policy with which Nightingale and social reformers disagreed. The famine commissioner, Sir George Campbell, himself related in his memoirs that the members of the Board of Revenue "held by the most rigid rules of the driest political economy, and had the most unwavering faith in the 'demand and supply' theory." They "rejected almost with horror" the proposal to

3 See Bidyut Mohanty, "Orissa Famine of 1866: Demographic and Economic Consequences."

4 East India (Bengal and Orissa Famine). Papers and Correspondence Relative to the Famine in Bengal and Orissa, Including the Report of the Famine Commission and the Minutes of the Lieutenant Governor of Bengal and the Governor General of India, in *Parliamentary Papers* 31 May 1867.

import grain, so great was their "zeal for free trade and supply by private effort."[5] Lord Cranborne, then secretary of state for India, similarly denounced the doctrine in a speech, both of course after the fact.

The first item below is an undated draft letter to Lord Cranborne. We do not even know if the letter was sent, but it refers to "his able speech," which could be his magnificent denunciation of the handling of the famine he gave in the House of Commons 2 August 1867. There he roundly condemned the Indian and even more so the Bengal government's mismanagement, citing the ample evidence of impending disaster given them, but the lieutenant governor, Beadon, had argued that "proof should be undoubted . . . the certainty complete that the people were going to starve before the slightest step could be taken to relieve them." He explicitly blamed the political economy doctrine, "systematically misused by unintelligent officials," who left the laws of political economy to work themselves mechanically while hundreds of thousands starved." He raised the issue of "despotic government" and even racism. Officials in India did not regard the "lives of their coloured fellow subjects with the same sympathy . . . zealous and quick affection" as those at home, and he called on members of Parliament to correct all abuses and set an example on that point. Cranborne also exonerated John Lawrence, describing him as having accepted the evidence set before him, such that he would have had to have acted directly contrary to it to intervene. If he had not had the council he had, "several hundreds of thousands who were now dead would have been alive." The speech includes as well cogent points on the absurdity of officials managing India from the hills, at a great distance, for months of the year.[6]

Salisbury's own memoirs, written ten years later, give further background, citing the warning he received from a former governor general, Lord Ellenborough, the day he took office, warning of "indications of a terrible famine" and urging him to "to take measures in time." But he was "quite new to the subject and believed that if any precautions were necessary, the local government was sure to take them, and so "did nothing for two months." By then it was too late, for the ports of Orissa were closed by the monsoons and could not be

5 Sir George Campbell (1824-92), governor of Bengal, in *Memoirs of My Indian Career* 2:157.

6 Hansard, *Parliamentary Debates* 2 August 1867:808-14.

used to bring in supplies. It was said that "a million people died," while the governments of India and Bengal had taken "in effect no precautions whatever. . . . I never could feel that I was free from all blame for the results."[7]

It took time for the colonial powers to give famine serious attention and vigorous response. The above-mentioned points were a response to the famine commission on Orissa famine appointed in 1866, which reported in 1867. Another commission was launched in 1878 and reported in 1880; James Caird[8] was on this commission and thanks to him some of Nightingale's arguments (such as her insistence on irrigation as a means of preventing famine) were reflected in the report. Unfortunately the report was played down by officials, who manipulated its statistics to obscure the problem. The officials' criticisms had to be rebutted. However, the report made evident that not only was irrigation important in the production of foodstuffs and the fight against famine, but drainage and safe water were also necessary elements of public health, all aspects mirrored in Nightingale's published writings and letters. Much of her correspondence focused on mortality statistics, for the British government minimized the death toll by inadequate means of data collection (who collects the data when the registrar is dead?) and frankly evasive categorization (deaths by disease were not counted as famine deaths).

Indian famines prompted the search for causes and remedies, as well as for immediate relief. Nightingale and her team pursued a number of interventionist strategies. The famine itself offered, as she put it, a "favourable opportunity" for intervention by the government, but it was "in a great fright" about it (see p 586 above). There is much writing on this especially in the mid-1870s, both articles and correspondence. She worked notably with Sir Arthur Cotton,[9] the builder of great irrigation works, towards means of preventing famine. Her three-part article, "A Missionary Health Officer for India," 1879 (in *Social Change in India*), deals with famine and the relief work done particularly during the "Great Famine" of 1876-79. Famine continues

7 Andrew Roberts, *Salisbury: Victorian Titan* 85.

8 Sir James Caird (1816-92), English representative on the Famine Commission.

9 General Arthur Cotton (1803-99), commandant of engineers, Madras, and an enthusiastic builder of canals. He was the author of *Public Works in India*, 1854, and *The Madras Famine*, 1877.

to be a major concern in *Social Change in India*, indeed with another "great famine" in the last years of the nineteenth century.

The horror of famine took Nightingale away from such issues as nursing and hospitals to those of food production, transportation and government. Her analysis of the social causes of famine in turn, we will see, prompted greater support for Indian self-government. The need for increased agricultural production suggested a greater recourse to irrigation and scientific agriculture (topics that shall be taken up further in the next volume). Obviously it was not just the lack of food in a particular area that caused famine, for in a well-functioning social system food could be brought in. Adequate transportation (canals and railways) had to be part of the solution, with a political structure that would ensure that they were used in a timely way.

Widespread poverty meant the absence of a buffer against famine. Poverty became for Nightingale a key issue to investigate and it was imperative to determine its causes. In the course of understanding the causes of chronic poverty, issues of land ownership and taxation had to be pursued. Again the search for solutions to famine led to an analysis of social structure and political decision making. It became clear that money needed in the recovery from famine was being diverted, for instance, towards paying for army forays into Afghanistan (1878-80). Again this raises the issue as to who the political decision makers were.

Nightingale became aware that there were two kinds of famine, a grain famine and a "money famine." Peasants' money was drained into the pockets of the landlords, which left the ryots unable to procure food stuffs or to build up stocks for hard times. Money needed for public works in order to get income into the hands of producers was diverted to other uses; thus people who had to plant the next crop were without reserves. The letters, notes and journal articles Nightingale wrote throughout these famine years address this complex of interconnected matters. The urgent need for famine prevention led her to the great challenge of social reform in India, the focus of the next volume.

The presidency sanitary commissions appointed in the various provinces from 1864 had a special role to play in this context beyond promoting public health. One of their many functions was precisely to devise strategies to fight against famine and to assist in relief provision. Gradually, "without formally violating the precepts of free trade, the government began to take on greater responsibility for famine relief and control. . . . Irrigation received some state support, though, to Cotton's dismay, considerably less than the railway system developed in India in the post-Mutiny decades."[10]

In 1873 Nightingale's article "Life or Death in India" explored death rates and healthy irrigation measures. Nevertheless, due to the peasants' traditional conservatism and, without unjustly blaming peasants for their lack of social and political power, "Indian subsistence culture" resulted in merely "marginal food surpluses in normal crop years" and made people "vulnerable to famines" when there were "successive poor crop years."[11] That is why increased state responsibility for famine control was called for and was shown, for example, in the drafting of the Indian "famine code" of 1880, which offered "guidance as to how administrators might anticipate famine by responding to the first signs of impending distress . . . and how they should act to alleviate suffering, if necessary by providing gratuitous relief to needy villagers in their homes as well as on public relief works."[12]

The central role of the sanitary commissioners, or "health missioners," in the fight against famine and in the work of famine relief, was emphasized by Nightingale, especially in her 1879 articles. However Lord Mayo, viceroy from 1869-72, had already done his share in the battle against famine. He wanted India to have not only more schools and hospitals but also more roads, railways and canals, so that famine areas could be reached more quickly.

At home it was felt that the monitoring of the Indian situation remained essential if real progress in sanitary matters and public health was to take place. However, imperial managers were too often satisfied with mere lip service to the cause. At the time of the 1880s debates over the reorganization of the home Army Sanitary Commission, the institution central to all sanitary work in India, Nightingale worked hard to influence the shaping of the new body that emerged in 1890 and which she found important for the effective control of all sanitary measures in India.

The last famine to occur in India was the Bengal famine of 1943; in that year 3.5 to 4 million Bengalis died from starvation and related

10 David Arnold, *Famine: Social Crisis and Historical Change* 114.

11 Ronald E. Seavoy, *Famine in Peasant Societies* 284. Seavoy's claim that peasant societies are ruled by an "indolence ethic" is criticized in David Arnold's *Famine* 57-59.

12 David Arnold, *Famine* 114, see also 125-26.

diseases after the Japanese invasion of Burma cut off supplies of Burmese rice and the colonial economy failed; moreover, British administrators insisted on the continued export of Bengali grain despite food shortages in order not to disturb the sacred forces of the market. Famines ceased to occur after Indian independence in 1947 and the establishment of a multiparty democracy, lending credence to the argument that major famines do not occur in democracies, even when they are very poor, because they bring failures of social policy under public scrutiny. [13] It is therefore significant that famine in India persisted as long as the raj did, British power being unable or unwilling to take effective measures against it.

Source: From a draft letter to Lord Cranborne, ADD Mss 45779 f7

[after 2 August 1867]

As the session of Parliament is approaching, it has occurred to me that you might possibly afford most valuable assistance in advocating those administrative reforms which are necessary for giving effect to public health improvements in India. I was impressed with this on reading your most able speech on the Orissa famine. We know perfectly well that the public health service is just in as great a chaos as was the Orissa administration and that at the present time there is just as little personal responsibility in the former as there was in the latter.

Crowds of people have died in India since the Orissa famine from cholera, including many of her majesty's troops. It would be just as difficult to fasten the responsibility of those deaths on the right man as it was in the case of the Orissa famine. The prevention of famine indeed has always been an important part of Public Health Service.

The subject is too long and too important for a letter. But such is the interest I feel in it and so high do I estimate your influence in obtaining a public health code for India that, weak as I am, I should be very glad to have the opportunity of discussing the subject with you when you could conveniently do so.

---

13 See Amartya Sen, *Poverty and Famines: An Essay on Entitlement and Deprivation* and *The Argumentative Indian: Writings on Indian History, Culture and Identity*, and Amartya Sen and Jean Drèze, *Hunger and Public Action.*

## "Life or Death in India," 1873

**Editor:** This paper was written by special request for the Social Science Congress held in Norwich in 1873; it reviewed the progress made in the field of sanitary reforms since 1863 when Nightingale had presented a similar paper, "How People May Live and Not Die in India" (see p 184 above). Much had been achieved; much more remained to be done. The paper contains a bitter attack against the zemindar class, which Nightingale held responsible for people's poverty and misery: such attacks would be increasingly voiced in her dealings with Indian matters. An appendix published the next year, "How to Make Irrigation Healthy," deals expressly with famine and the means to combat it through well-engineered irrigation. Nightingale sent out copies of the paper to influential persons; for instance, following the paper below is a letter to Lord Salisbury, at the time secretary of state for India, asking him "to glance over this little pamphlet which I have just printed" (see p 746 below). Sending out her papers to friends and experts was usual practice on her part.

Source: Florence Nightingale, "Life or Death in India," a paper read at the meeting of the National Association for the Promotion of Social Science, Norwich, October 1873, with an appendix on "Life or Death by Irrigation," also titled "How to Make Irrigation Healthy" (London: Spottiswoode & Co. 1874)

The paper was also published as "How Some People Have Lived and Not Died in India" (without the appendix), in *Transactions* of the Association for the Promotion of Social Science 1873, ed. C.W. Ryalls (London: Spottiswoode & Co. 1874) 463-74.

It is also found in *Report on Measures Adopted for Sanitary Improvements in India, from June 1873 to June 1874*, together with abstracts of sanitary reports for 1872, forwarded from Bengal, Madras and Bombay, printed by order of the Secretary of State for India in Council (London: Eyre and Spottiswoode, printers to the Queen's Most Excellent Majesty 1874) 48-64.

On a former occasion I ventured imperfectly—for India is immense, while a paper is small—to bring before the association how people have died and not lived in India, how people may live and not die in India. I used some of that great body of information brought together by the Royal Commission on the Sanitary State of the Indian Army, which was at work during four years, 1859-63, and was presided over, first by Sidney Herbert—whose statue still stands before the War Office as a witness in favour of progress—then by Lord Stanley, now Lord Derby. Ten years have elapsed, during which most of the sanitary proceedings which have been initiated and their results have passed (on paper) through our hands. And we may now reckon up our gains.

2. I must begin by guarding myself and others. We *have* made an impression on the sanitary state of that vast country, but "impression," so far as this: only to show us the immense work that remains to be done, the immense success that *can* attend it—we cannot yet say the immense work that has been done. But how much this is; what progress since the time we were taught to lament the "hopeless Indian climate"!

The caution is this, as in all epidemic countries, more than in most, the death rates of the Indian Army had shown two characteristics: they fell and they varied according to the nature of the season and the prevailing "epidemic state."

(a) For example, in past and, alas! in present years we can say approximately what districts will be visited by fever or by cholera in "epidemic" times, "if the drainage and water supply and neighbouring ground are left in *that* bad state." When comes the "epidemic," those dwellings may expect it. If air, earth and water continue to be fouled, if foul damp ground be not drained, if the public ways be not better kept, when comes the "fever," when comes the "cholera," those districts will have it.

But why does not cholera come every year to those dwellings? Their state is the same. And why is fever not always in those districts? We do not know. All we can say is, we know into what dwellings cholera and fever will *not* come, however "epidemic" the year; we can put towns and districts into such a state that the *epidemic*, like the medieval witch, is exorcised, so that it cannot come near them. More than this we do not know.

(b) In past years—not so long past—in a great town of England, 47 children out of every 100 used to die before they were five years old. But why those 47? We do know how this infant mortality, or rather massacre of the innocents, can be mitigated or prevented, namely, by cleanliness of house and child, by fresh air, care as to food and clothes, whitewashing, by "minding baby" in short and by avoiding all "soothing syrups" whatever. But we do not know which babies will be taken and which not.

All this is pre-eminently true of India. From the great Sunderbuns, where cholera seems to have had its birthplace and had not been born some centuries ago (great towns, shown in old Portuguese maps, now no longer to be found, seem to attest that the Sunderbuns were not then the home and hearth of epidemics), cholera sets forth on its terrible march over Asia, so reaching Europe, but why in one year and not in another we know not. If the Sunderbuns were drained, cultivated and again rendered fit for human habitations, would cholera disappear?

3. Now, after this caution, to proceed: The results we find, in the last report (Dr Cuningham's Report No. 8) of the Sanitary Commission with the Government of India and in other district reports, have been so striking that they may be fairly accepted as showing, not that India has become "healthy forever" (the year 1871 was a non-epidemic year), but that we can grapple with, that we may one day finally subdue, if we will—spite of the bugbear "climate"—those local conditions which in former days decimated the strength of the army and which, unless preventible and prevented, make up a terrible prospect—that only at such a price could India be held by a British force. And this when man's life was becoming every year more valuable.

In the first part of this century the death rate among British troops serving in India had revolved round 69 per 1000 per annum; that is, 69 men out of every 1000 died on an average every year. The "constantly sick" (on the authority of Mr Annesley) in hospital amounted in old times to 10 percent of the strength; that is, out of every 1000 men 100 were always ill in bed. Or in round numbers, the whole British Army went three times into hospital every year. The royal commission of 1863 gave a table showing, as they state, "that on an average in the stations of Bengal 84 men in a battalion of 1000 were constantly in hospital, where 69 die annually." But men invalided "are a total loss to the service as much as the men who die"; indeed more so, as far as the country is concerned, for they have to be supported. And the loss by invaliding was, as may be supposed, high in proportion—in Bengal as high as between 80 and 90 per 1000 per annum, including all such casualties.

Steps had been taken before (in Bombay sanitary reform began with Sir Robert Grant forty years ago according to *then* lights, and subsequent governors carried the work on, in advance of the *then* Indian ideas; the first scheme for an ample supply of good water to a city was matured in Bombay thirty years ago by Lord Elphinstone and begun five years later—long before any such plans were believed to be possible in any other Indian city), steps were being taken during the inquiries in India of the royal commission for removing some existing sanitary defects, with corresponding improvement of the health of troops.

The report and evidence were printed, with an abstract of evidence from the stations, by Parliament in August 1863. In December, Sir John Lawrence was sent out as governor general (Lord Elgin's death impending) and almost immediately on beginning his vice-reign he formed an organization for grappling with the evils, with this hundred-headed Hydra, in the localities themselves—in the home of the beast.

In this way of late years a vast amount of simple, inexpensive sanitary work has been done in respect of cleansing, draining, improving the water supply. In many of the cities and towns of the North West Provinces this cleansing, the better making and keeping of public ways, the straightening and widening of streets, are now looked after. In the North West Provinces and in Oudh the civil stations have been improving their drainage and the whole subject is marching on. In the Central Provinces, we are told, improvements of various kinds are going on. In Berar the people are thinking about it—thinking how bad is their water supply. One trusts that they will go farther—though thinking is a good thing—and not only think but act. In the Punjab a good deal, we are told, is being quietly done in the towns. In Bengal proper, where most is wanted, least seems to be doing. Many stations all over India—for instance, Barrackpore, Umballa, Muri, Mian Mir—are supplying themselves with better water.

Many have had their barracks improved or reconstructed—not before it was wanted—and sometimes, it must be admitted, not in the most economical way. Still the work has been done, and is being done, very zealously, as is shown by the reports of sanitary commissioners which give as striking instances of results to health from sanitary improvements as could well be imagined, were it even a Hercules who was working for us (these are real miracles of the present day) or as have been realized at home. And this has been done without burning down the city, which, it seems, was the only way of saving London from another great plague.

4. And first, as regards the death rate of the army, for on this subject Dr Cuningham gives some most important facts, especially as regards Bengal, formerly, as we know, the most unhealthy province—if province it can be called—a country of nearly 69,000,000—the most densely populated in the world. Formerly the death rate for all India revolved round 69 per 1000. In 1871 the death rate, including deaths among invalids *after* their arrival in England, was 18.69 per 1000 (the strength was 56,806 non-commissioned officers and men); that is, 18 men died

where 69 died before. Of the invalids sent home to England 16.02 per 1000 on a similar strength were discharged [from] the service.

From these facts we arrive at this result, namely, leaving out the loss from invaliding in the old Indian Army altogether, the total loss to the present Indian Army in 1871 by death *and discharges* was 34.7 per 1000 or just one half of the loss occasioned by the old death rate alone. In other words, we lost, in 1871, 18 men only by death—in India and England both—out of every 1000 of the British Indian Army, and 16 more were discharged as unfit for further service; that is, there was a saving of 51 men in every 1000 in 1871 (a healthy year), or 2858 men in an army of 56,806 were the savings of that year (one year's results) as compared with the average losses of old.

Let us remember, with the mercantile Briton's spirit, that every man costs with his arms £100 set down in India, hence £285,800 was the money saving on recruits in that year. But what is the value of a man otherwise? To *us* these are not figures but men.

Returning to the Bengal presidency, we find in 1871 the deaths 17.83 per 1000, where formerly the Bengal death rate lay between 70 and 80 per 1000, and annual losses from other casualties actually rose to between 80 and 90 per 1000. In other words 17 men only die instead of 70. A few results for 1871, from different groups of formerly most unhealthy Bengal stations, tend to show that the improvement in health is going on thus: in Bengal proper the death rate for the ten years preceding 1870, including a time of sanitary improvement, was 29½ per 1000; and the daily sick nearly 7 percent or 70 per 1000. In 1871 the death rate was 18.72 per 1000 and the daily sick rate 5 percent or 50 per 1000.

Let us here add that in round numbers the whole Indian Army went once-and-a-half times into hospital, and about 5½ percent of the force was always in hospital, during the year 1871 instead of nearly double the number.

We all remember the frightful sickness and mortality of Fort William. Its sick rate continues rather high, but its death rate in 1871 was only 10 per 1000, less than a tenth part of its former death rate, and 2½ per 1000 less than the death rate of 1870.

In Oudh the death rate from 1860 to 1869 was 28½ per 1000. In 1871 it was under 23. The constantly sick had also fallen from 69 to 61 per 1000.

At Kanpur much has been done to improve the site and the station shows a death rate of only 13, while Banaras and Allahabad, in which less has been done, and Dinapore, in which we do not hear of much done, show quite double this rate of death.

Meerut and Rohilcund, in the ten years before 1870, were sick at the rate of 72 per 1000 and sick unto death at the rate of 26½ per 1000. In 1870 these fell to 69 and 18½ respectively, and in 1871 to 65 and 16½. But in this group Roorkee, which has always distinguished itself, and Moradabad died at the rate of only 8 and 5½.

In Agra and Central India, for the ten years before 1870, the sick rate was 74 and the death rate 38½ per 1000. In 1870, though the sick rate was 77, of these there died only 22 per 1000; and in 1871 there were sick only 64 and there died under 18½ per 1000.

In the Punjab there has been apparently some progress in improving the heavy sick list. The ten-year period shows sick at the rate of 56 and dead at 25; but 1870 gives daily sick at 69 and death at under 24½ per 1000; and 1871, sick at 54 and dead at little more than 18 per 1000.

Now the hill stations come in. During the ten years before 1870 the daily sick were 49 and the dead nearly 15 per 1000. In 1870 the sick were 40 and the dead 11. In 1871, 48 and 9. But at one hill station, Raneekhet, the death rate was as high as 24, while at another, Chakrata, it was under 6½, and at Dugshai 5½.

Now for the convalescent depôts. These gave a death rate of nearly 31 per 1000 during the ten-year period; for the men seem to have died rather than convalesced—whereas in 1870 it was little over 22½ and in 1871 under 13 per 1000.

The Army Sanitary Commission concludes its notice of this part of Dr Cuningham's statistics by "congratulation at the improvements already effected in the sanitary condition of stations and troops serving in the Bengal presidency"; especially, it says, when the former history of the old Bengal European Army is considered, with its annual death rate "of from 70 to 80 per 1000"; and "its annual losses from other casualties of between 80 and 90 per 1000." But it warns us not to delay measures for making the statistics of 1871—"an avowedly healthy year"—the real representative statistics of every year in India. For it must not be assumed that the work of improvement is done. Far from it. The general result only indicates progress towards realization, not realization. As yet *what is* BEING *done* is all we have to show.

The royal commission pointed out that the death rate, when we have *prevented preventible* diseases, ought not to be more than ten in the thousand. The importance of the present results consists in showing that India is not necessarily fatal to European lives and that the

Government of India, the India Office at home and the British public have not only a common interest in the results already attained, but that they have a right to expect, and do expect, that their officers' hands shall not be stayed in this good work, that they shall be assisted in every possible way. Expense has been incurred—somewhat more perhaps in certain directions than was necessary—but has there been no gain?

It has been shown that we are in the way of regaining every year a large part of the outlay.

5. Had time permitted, some account should have been given of the success of sanitary work in India in cities and even in country districts. But we must be content with a few illustrations.

Ten years ago I reported to the royal commission that no one of those three large and populous cities—seats of presidencies, Calcutta, Bombay, Madras—had as yet arrived at the degree of civilization in their sanitary arrangements at which the worst parts of our worst towns had arrived before sanitary reform sprang up in England at all. Yet the fault of the inevitable results was laid to the "climate." Bombay, the second city of our empire, had, it is true, a better water supply, but no drainage. Calcutta was being drained, but had no water supply. Two of the seats of government had thus each one half of a sanitary improvement, which halves ought never to be separated. Madras had neither.

This was ten years ago. Now (and I cannot but name the name of the Calcutta municipality engineer, Mr Clark,[14] with this great improvement—let us give him a cheer) Calcutta has its water supply complete; all classes, all castes use it and find, indeed, the fabled virtues of the Ganges in the pure water tap.

Draining has been going on, subsoil and surface, the subsoil water level effectually lowered and not only this but a fine current of water runs through the subsoil from the river on one side to drainage outlets on the other, carrying with it old sewage out of the subsoil. The main drainage of most of the town is complete and native owners of houses are already applying for private drainage—a fact of great importance. Still there remain to be provided for—to make the SEWERAGE perfect—connections between the main sewers and the houses (and especially in large districts of the poorer population and in the

14 William Clark (1821-80), civil engineer in charge of Calcutta drainage.

bustees—"temporary" villages of mat and thatch and mud). Many miles of ditches have been filled up to the great detriment of mosquitoes and great comfort of the inhabitants. Then, also, the sewage is being applied to agriculture.

And what has been the result of all this sanitary engineering? From 1866, when the deaths from cholera in Calcutta were little short of 7000, they have decreased to 800 in 1871, the lowest number of deaths on record. Calcutta in 1871 was more salubrious than Manchester or Liverpool and may be considered soon a sanatarium compared with Vienna or even with Berlin, where the city canals are still fouled with sewage.

Still we must not "sing before we are out of the wood." Much, as Mr Clark and Sir George Campbell would tell us, remains to be done. And before the inhabitants of Calcutta can hope to be free from finding themselves any morning in the claws of some epidemic disease, they must have done a great deal more to the *houses* of the *people*, crowded as they are on small unhealthy space, and to the undrained districts surrounding and especially below Calcutta.

Caste prejudices have been alleged as insuperable stumbling blocks in the way to sanitary improvement, but a curious and cheerful instance of caste prejudice being overcome is this: when the water supply was first introduced into Calcutta, the high-caste Hindus still desired their water carriers to bring them the *sacred* water from the *river*; but these functionaries, finding it much easier to take the water from the new taps, just rubbed in a little (vulgar, not sacred) mud and presented it as Ganges water. When at last the healthy fraud was discovered, public opinion, founded on experience, had already gone too far to return to dirty water. And the new water supply was, at public meetings, adjudged to be theologically as well as physically safe.

Besides its water supply, then, the drainage of Calcutta bids fair to be a wonder of the world, when we remember what has been loudly said, even in this our day, that Calcutta at least was hopeless, because it lies close to the level of the river; and its public health has equally defied the prophets of irremediable evil and will yet improve still further its powers of defiance, while the active—not prophets of evil but performers of good—Mr Clark (unhappily, since this was written, Mr Clark has been obliged to come home invalided) and the energetic lieutenant governor of Bengal and other such authorities live.

Now for Bombay—Bombay, hitherto the pioneer, Bombay the active, not to say restless, the energetic Bombay. Bombay has for years done everything to drain itself, except doing it; it had the best engineer, Major H. Tulloch, to look at it, to plan for it; it has had surveys, plans, reports, paper and print enough to drain all India—writing and talking enough for a thousand years. The only thing it has *not* done is *to do it.*

In the meantime it has had to thank its able Dr Hewlett, the most vigorous of health officers—now alas! no longer at that post—for having, at a quite incredible cost of time and energy, in organizing, personally superintending and being as it were the constantly present head of an immense and most expensive system of hand labour, saved them from cholera epidemics and done that for them, single-handed, or rather single-headed, which should have been better and more cheaply done by the civilized hand of engineering and machinery. He has been a sanitarily engineered city in himself—his own reports are his best witnesses. As for the water supply, much the same may be said. The increased water supply needed by the city is still on paper, some small portion only having been obtained.

And what has Madras done—Madras which had neither—neither water supply nor drainage? Madras has obtained a water supply and has just improved it and is applying part of her sewage to agriculture with success. In other respects she appears to be pretty much as she was, with her filthy Cooum estuary and her foul, undrained area. She has recently had the census taken with the advantage of discovering that Madras is a very unhealthy city.

6. These illustrations would be incomplete if taken only from the large cities. Here, however, are a few experimental results described by the sanitary commissioner for Madras in his report on cholera of 1870. Cuddalore town had forty-two deaths from cholera out of a population of 28,421. Cuddalore jail with 301 prisoners escaped. The jail had those two indispensable requisites—good water and perfect cleanliness—which were absent in the town. Madurai town contains 39,872 people, of whom 376 died of cholera which, on arriving there, found bad conservancy, foul privy arrangements, foul subsoil, contaminated water. There are two jails at Madurai, one old, the other new. The old jail had bad water and other insanitary conditions, and lost four out of fifty prisoners by cholera. The new jail contained 180 prisoners; these were the only persons not exposed to sanitary defects and they all escaped cholera.

Rajahmundry town, where the population live under the usual Indian insanitary conditions, lost 147 people from cholera out of a population of 17,498. The district jail, situated within the town and under similar conditions, lost 16 prisoners out of 89 by cholera. The new central jail, where the sanitary conditions were good, had not a single case of cholera among 845 prisoners, although the disease prevailed "violently in all the country round."

Vellore town lost 67 people out of 30,529 from cholera. It has two jails, one old, the other new. The sanitary condition of the old jail was rigidly attended to and there was no cholera among its 152 prisoners. The new jail had 576 prisoners but no cholera. It occupies a healthy site and its sanitary arrangements were good.

More sanitary experiments of this kind could be cited, but here is one of special interest regarding villages. Mr Kearns, a church missionary in southern India, states that on his arrival at Puthian Puttur, in 1856, few villages had suffered more from cholera and fever. The place was wretched and foul, and had bad water. To remedy this state of things, wells were dug and properly protected; surface drainage was improved, rigid cleanliness enforced, trees planted and other improvements introduced. Similar improvements were carried out in other villages. And they escaped cholera.

It is worthy of remark that the facts were brought out, in reply to a statement made by the Madras government, that this village was exempt from cholera, "cause unknown." Mr Kearns replied to this by showing that he was perfectly well aware of the "cause." Quite recently, improvements of a similar kind, including reconstruction of houses, in the foulest and most unwholesome parts of the city of Madras, have been attended not only by an enormous diminution in the district death rate, but the people have improved in civilization as well as in health.

7. But one more word about country districts. And let us remember that Bengal is the most thickly populated country in the world—a country of villages. Till country drainage is introduced, till agriculture is improved, till irrigation and drainage are combined—both better when together, the first dangerous when apart—no great improvement in health, civilization or vigour of the people can be expected. The "drain" in another sense, the drain upon human life and happiness, of *fever* in India is literally untold. But as far as *can* be told, in 1871, a peculiarly healthy year, about one-and-a-half millions of people died in India from fever, or nearly 12 in every 1000, or twenty-three times as many as cholera destroyed.

But this is a mere trifle compared with the ravage fever commits in sapping the strength and vigour of the country, in making the young old, the healthy infirm for life, the industrious helpless invalids, the rich poor, the thriving country a waste. The deaths must first be multiplied by 50 or 60 to give us the attacks. Then a man who has once had a bad attack of malaria has it for life. And almost all this fever is malarial. Cholera[15] destroys life, but does no more. Fever destroys the life of the country, saps the world in which it is. Look at the Burdwan fever;[16] look at the Dengue fever.[17] "Dengue" is rarely fatal, but in its districts "Dengue" is master and 60 or 70 out of every 100 are "down" with it!

Irrigation is essential in many parts of India, but irrigation with stagnant water is almost as injurious to crops as to health. Irrigation should be accompanied by improving the natural drainages of the country, so as to keep the water moving, however slowly. (As the meagrest discussion of the vital question of irrigation would occupy too much time here, it has been placed in an Appendix.)

Let me tell a curious history told me by one of the members of the first Bengal Sanitary Commission. In 1857 nine miles of country, with twenty-five villages, were laid waste by fever; death came sometimes in three hours; of 600 in a village only a few in the centre houses lived. All the others died or fled. All the other houses were unroofed and tenantless. In the other villages nothing was left but pariah dogs. The crops were uncut. The dead lay about in the hollows, unburied and unburnt, for there was nobody left to bury them. Where the people did live they degenerated mentally and physically.

The cause of all this was a screw turned by a coolie, which flooded the low lands from the Ganges Canal faster than the water could be carried off. The man at the screw (at four rupees a month) ruled the destinies of a large population, not only as to health and life, but as to soul and mind, according as the screw turned to the right or to the left. This, the cause, was found out only a few months before my informant gave me the account, through an inquiry made by Sir John Lawrence. And all the time the people were going on degenerating, except those who were dead.

This melancholy history is given here (merely as an illustration; did time permit, hundreds such might be told), not for our discourage-

---

15 More on cholera and fever in the next section of this volume.

16 "Burdwan fever" refers to an epidemic of malaria that swept central Bengal in the 1860s.

17 "Dengue fever" refers to an infectious epidemic disease transmitted by mosquitoes and characterized by fever and pain in the joints. Also called "breakbone fever."

ment, but for our encouragement; not because it is so hopeless, but because it is so hopeful. If the screw turned too much brings fever, the screw turned just right brings plenty and health.

Let the people only see how much they can do for themselves in improving their surface drainage, in keeping their water supply free from pollution, in cleansing inside and out. Let the government see how much they can do for the people in introducing and stimulating better agriculture, irrigation, combined with drainage works in waterlogged districts; for the two must never be separated there. There is not a country in the world for which so much might be done as for India. There is not a country in the world for which there is so much hope. Only let us do it.

8. Unfortunately there is one disease cause in the British Army quite beyond the influence of engineering works, for every man is his own disease cause and must be his own remedy. And this is drink. The quart of porter and quarter of a pint of spirit per day are still procurable at the canteen and as much more as the men like (and as will destroy them) at the bazaar, and will always send to the graveyard and invaliding depôt a large number of men every year until they are made to understand their own interest and are furnished with employment. (Is there no possibility of checking drunkenness by a system like that of "equivalents" in the navy? so that a man might drink his ration of spirits or have its equivalent in coffee, beer, meat, etc., or in money. Would it not pay government to give men 5 percent compound interest on the price of drams so foregone, either paying in a lump on discharge or, better still, giving an additional pension?)

9. I might have ended here by repeating the caution with which I began: not to stay our hand, because the year 1871 gave a death rate of only 18 per 1000; but the experience of 1872 just coming in justifies, unhappily but too well, all the caution that can be used. The disease death rate of 1872, minus the superadded epidemic death rate, was as low as that of 1871. But cholera intervened and raised the death rate materially in Bengal, though very little in Bombay and Madras.

This is no reason for discouragement but the reverse. It is not a defeat but an attempt of the enemy to turn our flank. We know enough of his strength and his arms to turn the check into a victory, if we are only wise. But is not the following an example of action quite [?] than wise?

The report by the sanitary commissioner with the Government of India on this same cholera of 1872 tells that people have been trusting much to quarantine for safety, and that quarantine has been fully tried with results such as the following: "In a question so intimately connected with the happiness of the human race, it cannot be too widely known that quarantine was tried in the hope of protecting a number of the cantonments of upper India; that in many of them it signally failed and that in no single instance is there the smallest reason to believe that it was productive of any good. The direct evils of quarantine are great enough, but . . . by no means the least indirect evil is this, that so long as men believe that they can escape from cholera by such means, they will never be fully alive to the importance of the greatest safeguard, sanitary improvements."

Forced removals of sick, especially of women, for quarantine purposes, and other restrictions "set the people against everything that is done under the plea of the public health," and the sanitary reformer is regarded "as the greatest destroyer of their domestic comfort and happiness." As a consequence, cholera cases were concealed.

The troops also had to bear their share of this medieval infliction. The evils are described as "very great." "The troops are exposed to form cordons at the very time that exposure, and especially exposure to the night air, is calculated to prove most mischievous." Two stations, Mian Mir and Umballa, appear to have suffered from this. Both supplied complete cordons and both suffered severely from cholera. No better *reductio ad absurdum* [disproof of a proposition by showing the absurdity of its inevitable conclusion] of the whole practice could be given than the fact that the fear of spreading cholera interfered with the more decisive moves of troops which were their best chance of safety from cholera.

And then, to crown the whole, there does not appear to have been a single instance in which quarantine could be rigidly enforced. The government of the Punjab has taken the common-sense course of prohibiting quarantine except by special orders, and in the case of organized bands of pilgrims. Sanitary reformers, like other reformers, have more to fear from their friends than their enemies.

| | |
|---|---|
| Da chi non mi fido, mi guarderò io, | [From whom I do not trust I can protect myself |
| Da chi mi fido, mi guardi Iddio [Dio]. | From whom I trust let God protect me] [Proverb] |

But we must stop, only, however, to bear emphatic witness how great are the sanitary deeds already achieved or in the course of being achieved by the gallant Anglo-Indian, as formerly we bore emphatic witness against the then-existing neglects.

Let the Government of India continue to sustain the energetic efforts of their officers and, at the same time, insist on the municipalities and local authorities prosecuting the good work. This was of importance for the central government to do ten years ago, seeing that there was no local self-government at all; it is, if possible, of still more importance now, when there *is* some local self-government; but it wants guidance, which does not mean that the governor is to *do* municipality himself, even though a very good municipality he would make.

The natives are always ready to be taxed, as far as obtaining, at least, a purer and more plentiful water supply goes. There is never any "discontent" about this. What they do not like is paying the tax and receiving no water, and in this they are not so far wrong.

The lieutenant governor of Bengal has invited, by proclamation, the payers of some of *his* rates (this as regards roads) to claim the benefits (or their share of them) of what they pay for. ("Every taxpayer is encouraged and invited to claim that the tax shall be fairly applied to the village roads or water channels in which he is interested. The government will use every effort to see that such local claims are fairly met and that every taxpayer derives a fair benefit from the tax which he pays." *Proclamation of Bengal Government*, August 1873.)

Thus it will be rendered not only an easy matter to hold the great Indian Empire by a British force, but benefits untold will be conferred on the vast populations of our fellow subjects of whom we have undertaken the charge.

## "Appendix to Life or Death in India"
## How to Make Irrigation Healthy

The cause of irrigation has received a frightful significance from this Bengal famine, irrigation being literally a matter of life and death. Not whether we will have irrigation or not, but how to make it healthy, and how to pay for it, are our questions. Wherever water for irrigation and navigation exists, famine is effectually met.

The paramount necessity of combining drainage with irrigation was never forced upon the attention in southern India as it has of late years been in Bengal and the North West Provinces.

In the great irrigated districts of the Godavari and Kistna in the northern part of Madras, and of the North West Provinces and Punjab, drainage is now being taken in hand on a great scale, as outbreaks of fever have shown the results of its neglect.

In Tanjore, south of Madras, where there are above 1,000,000 acres of irrigated rice, without a weed to be seen, the drainage is said to be of the rudest description, yet the health of the people good. The population is more than 700 per square mile in the Delta. But the climate is a dry one, not moist like that of Bengal. In this part of India the thermometer never falls so low in the cold months as it does farther north, and there appears to be some relation between the range of temperature at that time of the year and the prevalence of fever.

The Hugli drainage investigation was taken up by the able Colonel Haig, then chief engineer of the Irrigation Department, under the orders of the lieutenant governor, Sir G. Campbell, though there are no irrigation works there, in hopes of contributing towards the clearing up of the fever question, which has of late years assumed such enormous importance, or rather its enormous importance has only now come to be known. The fever seems partly owing to entire want of drainage, partly to foul drinking water in the dry season.

Much more information than what Colonel Haig managed, with all his super-eminent ability and energy, to collect in the course of a six months' inquiry, is said to be needed, and there is at least one point, the relative levels of subsoil water, about which we as yet know far too little. Colonel Haig's "Note" embodies certain facts in regard to the rainfall, surface levels and drainage discharges of the district, but, as he states, he has no pretension to having exhausted the subject.

It is not, however, more inquiry that is most needed. Inquiry and investigation are the curse of India, as of any country where we do not act up to the light we have: where evils are investigated and reinvestigated fifty times over, simply as an excuse for *doing* nothing. Everybody has known for half a century that, if the water of Bengal were regulated, the superabundance carried off during the monsoon, and plenty of water, fresh from the rivers, carried through every village in the dry season for irrigation, drinking and carriage, the whole condition of the people would be immeasurably improved. All that is wanted is that the works should be executed, but this is the one thing that will *not* be done.

We shall have the country levelled and surveyed, the works planned and approved, report upon report called for, and commission upon commission appointed: anything that can be done as a reason for *doing nothing.*

1. One question is whether an area of ground, covered to such a depth with water as not to give off malaria from decomposition of

dead organic matter, is necessarily unwholesome. This would be very much the condition of an ordinary tank, or of a lake in which the surface of the water is retained permanently at a fixed, or nearly fixed, level.

In the dry climate of southern India such masses of water are said to be perfectly healthy; but in the warm, moist climate of Bengal the growth of aquatic plants is so prodigious that, unless tanks are periodically cleared of the weeds and mosses, which form in time a dense mat of vegetation on the surface, the water, it is said, becomes unfit to drink and gives out deleterious gases.

But, in point of fact, such cases are extremely rare. As a rule the surface of every tank or collection of water falls several feet during the dry months, and exposes a margin of damp soil more or less saturated with organic matter, which is, of course, unhealthy.

Lower Bengal is one mass of tanks, mostly very small, in which every kind of pollution collects all through the dry season, and from these in many places the people drink. All are natural hollows or formed by excavation—not, as in South and Central India, by damming up the outlets of valleys and hollows. But very few are dug out to such a depth as to leave, during the hot months, a sufficient depth of water to prevent decomposition, and fewer still are properly cleansed and protected from defilement by organic impurities.

Even in Bengal it is the poverty, not the will, of the people that consents to drink bad water. Whenever they have the means, they are glad to fence and line their tanks and wells with masonry. A sure sign of a thriving landowner is masonry tanks and wells on his property. The rich often bring their water from immense distances, in sealed jars, on men's heads, and there is no such popular application of taxation as in improved water supply.

2. Observations of the level of subsoil water are doubtless most important.

The precise relation between the level of subsoil water and the prevalence and intensity of fever has not yet been traced in Lower Bengal. Both irrigation and drainage are there new things. The first irrigation work was not begun until 1862, and that by a private company: the government expended nothing upon works of this class until 1868 or 1869. The Dancienic Drainage Works, in the Hugli district, carried out last year, are the first of their kind.

But in N. W. India—i.e., the N. W. Provinces and Punjab—some important facts have been established. In the districts on the upper part of the Ganges Canal, which were, of course, the first and the most copiously irrigated, there has been for many years a terrible increase of fever. By many it was asserted that the fever owed its origin to the canal, that the Mozuffernuggar District, for example, which is now said to be so unhealthy that it is in general avoided by officials, was formerly one of the healthiest and most popular.

This, however, appears to have been clearly disproved. There is abundant proof of the existence of fever long before the canal was heard of. But this also seems to be certain that, wherever irrigation has been excessive, and stagnant pools and swamps have been formed, by carrying the minor distributary channels (as was formerly frequently done in the hurry of construction or from a faulty system) across the natural drainages, there has been a marked increase in the prevalence and virulence of fever.

Wherever the subsoil levels (which are usually termed the "spring levels" in the N. W. Provinces and Punjab reports) have been raised by supersaturation of soil from their original depth of twenty-five to forty feet to *twelve feet or less*, there has been a terrible increase in the mortality from fever. Though still disputed, this fact is now pretty generally admitted by the best authorities, and in some official "Resolution" of the N. W. Provinces' government, it is distinctly laid down as the basis of remedial measures. Sir W. Muir is a hearty friend to irrigation.

How far this "water-logged" state of the soil in the districts referred to is due to excessive irrigation, and how far to the faulty alignments of distributaries and neglect of drainage above alluded to is not decided. But misuse of water is often made an excuse for not draining. Where the laws of drainage have palpably been violated, of course the remedy is plain and will be certain. And much may be done by selecting new sites for villages on higher ground.

Rice cultivation, which consumes an enormous quantity of water, has greatly increased in the upper part of the Ganges Canal, and no doubt has been one cause of supersaturation. It is said that it has been determined to check this by raising the water rates! In the case of one large town, where the fever had been severe, a committee recommended that the rice cultivation, which had crept right up to one town, should be prohibited within a certain distance of all dwellings.

Scientific sanitary irrigation is in its infancy. The danger is lest the abuse, or ignorant use, of irrigation should lead to its undue restriction, and cause the government to hesitate in carrying out works on the scale required, at least, to secure the food supply of the country.

Possibly, Sir G. Campbell, for one, was unduly influenced in this way, but his government is so imperial that he never had *time* to think properly of the subject.

It is stated, however, that in tracts in Lower Bengal, where the fever has been most deadly, the water level in the dry months is at an unobjectionable depth below the surface, say sixteen feet. But it does not follow from this that, during and immediately after the rains, the subsoil may not give out fatal malaria.

If the water rises too high during the rainy season, the difficulty in a rice-growing district is how to lower it.

The moment you cut a drain the ryots complain of it as injuring their crops by drawing off the water in which they always keep the rice standing to a depth of three to six inches, if they can get enough.

This is, of course, the consequence of partial work. What is wanted is a general *regulation* of the water, so that everywhere water shall be kept at the level required: some inches over the surface for rice, some feet under the surface where irrigation is not needed.

3. The ryots always, and justly, prefer *running* to stagnant water. Irrigation with stagnant water is injurious to health and also to vegetation. Irrigation should be accompanied by improving the natural drainages of the country, so as to keep the water moving, however slowly. But the difficulty is said to be how to supply moving water, and make the works *pay* at the same time, for the whole surface of the country. Everywhere, however, water can be supplied for irrigation at a *cost* enormously below its *value*—the average *cost* of water in works on a large scale being about £2 per acre of rice.

Irrigation works are planned generally to supply one cubic foot per second to every 133 acres, which is the same as one cubic yard per acre per hour, or 1/5 inch in depth on the surface per day. Two thirds of a cubic yard per hour for 100 days are given for wheat or other "dry grain," and two cubic yards per hour for 120 days for rice, including rain—i.e., 1/8 inch per day for dry grains and 3/8 for rice.

To this extent, even if every cultivable acre in the country were irrigated, we can change the water; but, as only a certain proportion of the area commanded by the canals is irrigated, and of this all is not receiving water at the same time, we do, in fact, supply a greater depth, and in that degree renew the water lying on the surface.

In the rice districts in Madras the whole area is irrigated. In the wheat country out of the tropics in the dry-season cultivation a portion only of the area is irrigated.

There is no doubt that the more water that is passed through the rice fields in a running stream, the better the yield, both because stagnant water is more or less injurious, and because more water means more *silt*, which renews and fertilizes the soil, and leaves, together with matter in chemical combination, behind it food for the plant.

It is certain that if the ground were thoroughly and sufficiently intersected by deep drains, and water enough supplied to meet the increased consumption which this would involve, rice cultivation might be a healthy employment. There is rarely fever in a village surrounded by rice swamp as long as the water is moving—"living" as the natives say; the fever time begins when the water falls and stagnates.

*Expense* is the sole thing that stands in the way of all these improvements. As it is, our irrigation works in N. India are said barely to pay the interest on the outlay. Is this because we persist in debiting the works with the cost of all our blunders? Do we make a canal on a bad plan—twice as costly (say) as need be, and only half as useful—excluding navigation and cheap transit; and then, because it only pays 5 percent, do we say, "irrigation won't pay"? If we kept our turnpike road or bridge accounts in the same way, without reckoning consequences, should we not find that road-making and bridge-building was of all things the most fruitless application of public money, and that it was better finance to build houses and let them as gin-shops?

The management of the works may be so wrong that, as in Orissa, the people refuse to use the water, and this is the case in only one out of the seven vast works which the government have executed. The actual results are these: the cost of irrigation on these great works has been from £1 to £3.10*s.* per acre, including the navigation, and the actual increased value of crop[s] is from £1.10*s.* to £2.10*s.* in grain only, besides straw.

Is it not only because we are in such a hurry for results that the people seem slow to take water? Irrigation, unless it come from great rivers in flood season, when it renews the soil requires manure, and manure costs money, and the people have to get a little money or credit before they can use their greatest boon.

Of the value of the canals for transit, the following may give some idea: up the valley of the Ganges at least a million tons a year are carried at present prices, a small quantity by the rail at 1½ d., besides half as much more paid out of taxes, and the main portion at about 1/2d. by the rivers; by the canals this would cost about 1/20d., or £200 a mile for a million tons, against £6000 by rail, or £2000 by river, a perfect steamboat canal, 40 yards broad, on that line costing about £3000 a mile.

The irrigation works in the North West yield an enormous profit in all, about £1.10*s.* in *grain* only, on an expenditure of £2.5*s* per acre, or 60 percent, besides the straw and navigation (on the Ganges Canal).

And the area of irrigation is still extending. About 7 percent net of this now comes into the Treasury. In the Jamna Canals, in the same part of the country, the returns into the Treasury are 25 percent, and in all the Madras districts double and treble that. The question of returns to government, though a point of importance, is of much smaller consequence than that of total benefits to the community. (Official papers are written as though the government were simply a trading company to whom the sole question was: What direct profit can be obtained?) Besides its being a question of life or death, of health or disease, of civilization, comfort and cleanliness, or dirt and barbarism and misery, the average total benefits are at least 100 percent. The Godavari district used to export £60,000 a year; it now exports, by sea only, £800,000 or £900,000 a year, besides the whole population being well fed and well clothed and housed, so that their home consumption is probably doubled. The 560,000 acres irrigated, then, now yield about £1,100,000 a year more in grain, besides straw and navigation, by an expenditure of about £600,000.

The results of the irrigation and navigation works in the Godavari Delta have been so conspicuous that I cannot but give the following short account: in 1843, when the first sketch of them was made by Sir Arthur Cotton, he and Lady Cotton took up their abode in tents and rough sheds on the bank of the river, or rather on the side of the riverbed; for only a narrow thread of water was flowing down the middle of that bed, and on each side of that thread was a mile and half, at least, of hot, deep sand. The want and filth and need of every kind around were a continual, pressing sorrow. The weary faces of the women, toiling through the dry riverbed with their waterpots, creeping out of their huts after the exhausting heat of the day to bring the family supply of water between one and two miles, their naked feet sinking at every step in burning sand, were most distressing; and the thought how insufficient the supply after all the labour, painful to look back upon even now.

Sir Arthur and Lady Cotton remained in that district some years, till the works were fairly set on foot. In 1861, they visited the Godavari Delta again, and describe the happiness of that visit. Instead of dry sand, the riverbed was covered full with abundant water; instead of parched, perishing attempts at cultivation, there were rich crops of many kinds, and trees which seemed to have sprung up as by magic; instead of filthy, *waterless* villages, there were channels, well filled, flowing everywhere; and instead of the weary, overworked women, almost all looked well fed, well washed and comfortable. One great obstacle to religious civilization thus removed, the time and strength of mind and body need no longer be solely taken up with the daily drudgery, which before absorbed every power. But, in this as in other cases, the occurrence of fever has warned us to look to our drainages.

4. No one, nowadays, would think of proposing irrigation without drainage. There is no danger in the one provided the other goes with it. The engineer's problem is to apportion the one to the other, so as to increase production without injuring health.

5. Whether the physical degeneration of the people in and over Bengal is due solely or chiefly to malaria, or to malaria and rack-renting combined, is just the point which a commission might be appointed to investigate. But the drainage and irrigation works should be executed first. About these there is no doubt. This is as well known as St Paul's. And the investigation may be carried on afterwards.

Under the Permanent Settlement the share of the produce of the soil left to the cultivator is often too little for health. A process of slow starvation may thus go on, which so enfeebles the great mass of the people that, when any epidemic sets in, they are swept off wholesale. Land is let and sublet to a degree unknown anywhere else. The zemindar will let his land to a patnidar, the patnidar to a durpatnidar, the durpatnidar again to a seypatnidar, and he again may farm it out to an izaridar.

Under such a system what portion of the produce do we suppose falls to the share of the ryot who tills the soil?

Then, population has increased to a degree that has raised the fear lest it may have outstripped the productive powers of the soil. After at least half a million souls had (in the estimate of the present collector) been swept off by the fever in the Hugli district, the population was still at the rate of 1000 to the square mile. But the productive powers of the soil under irrigation are enormous. *One* crop of rice without any manure at all will produce sufficient to feed a population of 2000 per square mile.

The poor people are glad to go long distances for work and food, if they know where they are to be found. They go readily as coolies to the West Indies and Mauritius. But if Bengal were properly furnished with roads and canals of irrigation, navigation and drainage, might not a population half as large again as the present be maintained in health and comfort? Are not the vast tracts of jungle—fertile land, but without population—quite as striking a feature in Bengal as the dense masses of rural population in the cleared parts?

6. If a complete system of drainage were carried out, periodical inspection by specially appointed officers would be essential to prevent the destruction of the smaller channels and consequent outbursts of fever. It is astonishing how evils are unseen by eyes accustomed to them.

7. Every village should have its pure water supply. The present state of the supply in Bengal is shocking beyond description. The water drunk by a large portion of India is utterly unfit for men's use and is often brought from miles distant. Much might be done by the people themselves, under proper supervision, in the way of clearing out and deepening existing tanks. But this should be combined with a fresh water supply from the great rivers by means of the subsidiary irrigation channels.

Wherever we have irrigation the people have this, and appreciate it highly. But, if we are to have all these things, there *must* be, we are told, some tax of the nature of a water rate (as in towns) to be levied on the whole community.

It is impossible to regulate the drainage and water supply of vast tracts, like those in Bengal, except at an expense which cannot be met, it is said, by the mere receipts from *irrigation,* which (with navigation tolls in the canal) have hitherto been our sole source of profit. There is no question about returns, however, *if the water is used*; and, if it is not, it can only be from mismanagement, as in Orissa. Colonel Haig remarks upon the "far stronger feeling of confidence and security which prevails under a ryotwari settlement" (speaking of the Godavari) "than under a zemindari." When a Cuttack ryot is asked why he does not use the water, which he acknowledges is so profitable, he says, "What is the use of it, when half the profit goes to the zemindar and half to the moneylender?" While the water has been generally refused this year, a considerable extent has been irrigated surreptitiously. And when one of the engineers was reporting about it, a native revenue official told him he had his predecessor turned out, and he would have him turned out too if he reported it. Such is the confusion in these districts. Such the relation between the state and the "creatures of its own creation," the zemindars. Such the difference between the ryotwari and zemindari tenures.

8. It is here, however, that the government hesitate, or rather that they have drawn back. Lord Mayo's government was in favour of a compulsory rate in all irrigated districts. Lord Northbrook [viceroy] and Sir G. Campbell are against it. But, without it, it is said that irrigation and drainage (if the works are to be constructed by government) can never be carried out on a scale commensurate with the wants of the country.

Is there much diversity of opinion, however, where the water is *actually given*? But then no compulsion is needed. Are not the people only too glad to get and pay for the water, as fast as they can prepare their fields and get manure? But are we not always in a hurry? And, after shutting our eyes for years to the truth as to the value of irrigation, always trying to force the poor cultivators to take the water the very instant we ourselves are converted to a sense of its value, and charging them for all the blunders we have made in supplying it?

Nay, do we not even go further and make laws enabling government to charge for the water, even if it is not supplied, if we only intended or promised to supply it? Was not Lord Mayo's proposed law of this character? Had he lived, he would have modified it so as to charge for water only where actually given. But really no *law* is needed. If we only make the works, bring the water and sell it at reasonable rates, the people are only too glad to buy it for their fields.

Was not Lord Mayo misled, for the time, by a policy—better at drawing up symmetrical laws which looked well on paper, than in carrying the people with it to *do* what was needed? The duke of Argyll's final decision against such a rate is said to have stopped two or three immense irrigation schemes (one for five millions of acres in Oudh) in the very part of the country which is either now threatened with famine, or not threatened—the famine is upon us. But was it so much the "duke of Argyll's final decision" as the mistakes of Lord Mayo's unfinished policy which stopped the irrigation schemes?

Did not Lord Mayo fall, for the time, into the hands of the fisherman's wife, who never would make the best of what enchanted fish gave her, but always wanted something better? She, after somewhat violently opposing canalization for years, went far beyond its demands and would do nothing till an act was passed to enable her to tax every ryot in India for water, as soon as she had good intentions for irrigating his fields. And when she was told she must tax only after she had given the water, she sulked and would not amend her act.

So with loans: there was no end of writing and planning, but it never got beyond paper. They never borrowed the money, because they were always following some new butterfly of finance. And so they never had it to spend.

Nothing can be more just than a partial compulsory water rate in the irrigated tracts, because, whether the people irrigate or not, they have the enormous benefits of navigation, drainage, drinking water, forage, etc. Under the Orissa works, at £3.10*s.* per irrigable acre in cost of works, 2¾ rupees an acre would pay 8 percent, leaving the transit free, and the increase of produce 15 rupees an acre at least.

The water rate paid in Godavari on about 500,000 acres, at 4 rupees, is £200,000, but the increase of revenue has been above £300,000. If no water rate at all were levied, it would be impossible to prevent the works paying, from the increased revenue due to the increased wealth of the people. As a native gentleman wisely said, the government of a rich population can never be poor.

But at this moment, including all mistakes in projection from want of experience, and the temporary failure from refusal of water in Orissa, all the new works would show a direct net return of some 20 percent into the treasury, and at least 100 percent in all.

If the canal is completed up the valley of the Ganges, it will carry two million tons a year at 1 1/8d. per mile, and at all speeds, from that of the railway downwards, against 200,000 tons carried by the railway at 1 1/2d. a mile, though supported by half a million a year paid out of the Treasury as interest of its debt.

But railways are wanted as canals. And as matters now stand, must they not be made before canals? Must we not do what comes to our hand to promote communication, without limiting ourselves to what is abstractedly best? It has been truly said that, while "we want wagons to carry hay, we provide phaetons." But, if we want to get across country, do we not take what the country affords—jaunting car or broken-down gig? People here will give their money and labour to make railways and not to make canals. Shall India wait till they get wiser, or let internal improvement, which depends so much on easy intercommunication, stand still till she has made them wiser?

If all the canals which the great artist has devised, and which he could give men to execute, were made, the works would then convert the world. Meantime, we should get all the railroads and common roads made which we could find money or men for, certain that, if not the best and cheapest, they are the next best, next cheapest appliances we can give the country.

Is it not the fact that we want both railway and canal? And must not the canal, which will supersede railways, be very different from any canal we have yet seen? But we may believe in its coming—that is, a canal workable by steam as well as by animal power—and able to carry at 10 miles an hour. That we shall see this in India before it appears in Europe is likely. But will anything save example convert the world? Meantime, even if we give India only railways, the people will neither starve nor stagnate.

9. *There is no great new irrigation work in India that is not paying ample direct net profits,* excepting that of Orissa, and that not at all on account of any real failure in the project, but only from the non-use of the water, which will of course be got over before long, and there is not the least probability of its occurring anywhere else.

Indeed, the so-called failure of the Orissa works is mainly due to the tardy and incomplete execution of the original scheme. Government no sooner saw that the works *must* be a financial success than they bought them—and then starved them—waiting for more plans, estimates and paper, before the money to complete them was given. We saw the "haywagon," in fact, and were charmed with it, and bought it as it stood, half-finished, and have since been doubting whether we can afford to complete the wheels and whether the tires should be broad or narrow.

10. The question will now be *forced* on public attention. It is no longer a question. The famine looms large and terrible upon us, as an awful fact. It must not, however, be supposed that little is being done in the way of irrigation. In Bengal alone we have been spending, for some years past, half a million annually, and that is only one province.

There is said to be a practical limit to the rate at which such extensive works can be carried on, viz., available labour supply. If this is pressed upon unduly, wages rise (Oh, would they should!), and with them the price of all materials of construction. In Southern Bihar and Orissa we are said to have quite reached this limit, for there has been a considerable increase in rates since the works were begun. But is not one of the most important effects of these works that they help to release the labouring population from their bondage to the high castes and wealthy, and in all ways improve their condition and raise wages? (The works in the Godavari essentially altered the condition of the whole body of labourers almost immediately. The employers found that their most energetic men would leave them for the works, if not better treated. And thus the employment of 30,000 people at good wages, with thoroughly good treatment, affected the welfare of a million. The state of the agricultural labourer was low enough in England; it may be supposed what it is under Indian landowners of *high caste.*) Every district could easily provide labourers for an expenditure of £100,000 a year, requiring about 20,000 people, and £30,000,000 could easily be spent in three or four years.

There is said to have been much, too, in our recent experience of irrigation in Bengal—chiefly the unwillingness of the people to take our canal water, except when driven to it by the failure of the rains—to cause the government to pause before beginning new schemes, without some such guarantee for the repayment of the interest on the outlay as a compulsory rate would afford. The works are all carried out with loan funds and the interest must be met from some source. But, as above said, our expenditure has been, and continues to be, £500,000 per annum.

As far as has been seen in India, however, "the unwillingness of the people to take canal water" really means "our own bad management" in some way or another. One can hardly conceive now but that, even had famine been averted, the great drought would not have given a vigorous impulse to this most important class of land improvements.

But famine *has* come.

In Lower Bengal the field for *drainage* is boundless. There, however, the one question which stops the way is whether government will make the zemindars, who are the possessors of the soil, pay for the works or not. Here there is great hesitation. *Are* the zemindars so selfish and worthless a class as to exercise their considerable influence over the government in this way? And *would* they resist, as is said, with all their might?

The drainage, however, of about eighty square miles of swamps on the banks of the Hugli is now being carried out at the expense of the landowners, under a special act, and government would probably have awaited the result of this experiment before extending the act to greater schemes.

But if the famine interrupts everything, it must also urge forward everything. May it not also force the authorities to look in the face the terrible evils of the whole zemindari system? Is not the case something similar to that of the old Bengal Army and, if it is still ignored, may not a similar terrible convulsion ensue? The subject is so vast that it is impossible to do more than just touch upon the principal points here.

## II

1. Irrigation and drainage improve the crop and give crop when and where there would be none. Consequently,

2. These combined works improve the entire value of the land, and the question is, Who is to reap the increase?

3. This must be either the zemindar and his subordinates, who have spent nothing, or the government which finds the money, or the ryot who cultivates. In England we should force the zemindar to bear his part by a Poor Law to compel him to feed the suffering people, in the hope that he would find it cheaper to irrigate and drain than to feed.

Or we should pass a law calling on all proprietors to improve the drainage, irrigation and roads over their property, on pain of being taxed for the support of their people every time that famine comes—something as we did in Ireland, where we charged for famine and where the landlords had to pay over and above what other landlords had to pay, because the people were dying. *Should not the fixed land tax rest only on the basis that the people can live and not die?*

This was, in fact, Lord Cornwallis's[18] principle. People blame his "Permanent Settlement" [in land tenancy], but they forget that the best half of his plan was never carried out by his successors. He clearly intended to make the zemindars maintain a police, make roads and do all other things that a landowner should do. But when he died his successors went to sleep.

4. "*The husbandman that laboureth must be first partaker of the fruits.*"[19] Drainage and irrigation will improve the stamina of the entire working population, but of this improvement the zemindar, if untaxed for the work, will reap the whole profit.

In Godavari there is no comparison between the present condition of the people and that before the works. But the extraordinary effect these works have had in the improvement of the people's bodily strength and spirit is one that is not generally observed. In Godavari the difference between a people underfed and working utterly without hope, and the same people as they now are, is most striking. There is, perhaps, nearly three times the amount of work done by the same population, now that they are well fed and more sure of fair

18 Lord Charles Cornwallis (1738-1805), governor general 1785-93 and 1805.
19 2 Tim 2:6.

treatment than they were before. When we began the works, we used to find, in cutting the canals, that large gangs would average one cubic yard per day; and this rapidly increased to three under exactly the same circumstances. Well-to-do, the people have now no look of poverty.

5. Hence sanitary work, such as this, creates a great surplus value over and above the present value and, when we consider the millions of acres to be improved, the addition will be very great.

6. Would not the best course be in India to take a lesson from the present distress, so as to plan for the future some conjoint liability for the drainage and irrigation works?

The Hugli scheme will afford valuable indications on this point, because the increase can be used as a standard. But the difficulties in the way are said to be enormous, arising from the extremely complicated state of property and innumerable interests in the land in permanently settled Bengal, and from the engagements made with the landholders under existing settlements elsewhere. Some idea of what these are in temporarily settled districts may be gathered from the Orissa irrigation scheme: they are far greater in the permanently settled.

Also, is it right that the revenue for the whole of India should bear the cost of improving the revenue of the Bengal zemindars? Would they wish it themselves? We cannot believe this of a noble body of Indian gentlemen.

Should not the local revenue be augmented to pay for this? Also, if money is borrowed, it must be repaid with interest, although it is applied to the improvement of private estates. Clearly, in some way or other, justice requires that men who own these lands, on which so many thousands die from preventible fevers—and now and then from a famine, which counts its deaths by hundreds of thousands—should either pay, or the government should remove the people (one of our alternatives), in which case the value of land will cease to exist.

7. Should not the landowner be made liable by law to pay for all that is really *done* to improve the land or to save the lives of the people on it? Is not the real practical solution of the financial problem a scheme like that applied to Lancashire after the cotton famine—a fund administered by trustees who lend from it, on security of local revenues, for works of permanent value to the reproductive powers of the locality, the advances to be repaid by instalments from local revenue at such rates as shall extinguish the debt in a reasonable term of

years? Or should not the government do as they did in Ireland—advance money to the landlords, and send to the Encumbered Estates Courts all who could not repay them? Such plans have been often laid before the Government of India and, no doubt, *some time* will be adopted.

One effect of the famine may be predicted, and that is, that it will lead to a revolution in the zemindari system in Bengal, which, in its effects on the mass of the population, can be compared to one thing only, namely, the slavery system as it was in the United States.

8. The wealth of an agricultural country is the result of labour and, in a properly governed country, labour ought always to be producing wealth. Every efficient labourer is a wealth-producing agent, and every efficient labourer, lost by death, is a pecuniary loss to the country. These are truisms.

The people pay 2½ rupees per head in taxes—the interest of 50 rupees, sufficient to irrigate two acres, which would support five people, and in actual famine 10 rupees would certainly provide food per head through the famine.

Scarcity and famine act in two ways: they reduce the wealth-producing power of survivors and destroy the wealth-producing power of those who die. When labourers die by thousands on account of famine and epidemics, because the ground on which they existed was left without irrigation and drainage, it may be affirmed with certainty that the pecuniary loss to the country exceeds what would have been the cost of works.

May not this be safely assumed as a law of the universe, from which there is no escape? We may cry back on account of the cost of doing what Nature says must be done, but this will not prevent her from presenting her bill at the due time, and when presented it must be honoured, whether we will or no. A large part of India is occupied on these conditions, and an awful bill it is.

9. But the people are not the only sufferers. Our noble Indian Army, although it may be saved from famine, is doomed to the inheritance of epidemics which always begin among the people. We know all this now. The sanitary history of the British Army in India begins with the sanitary history of the Indian people.

## III A Few Facts about Canals

Colonel Rundall, the inspector general of irrigation, projected, and for the most part worked out, the plans and estimates for the following schemes: the Son scheme, for the irrigation of the Shahabad, Patna and part of the Gaya districts south of the Ganges, included in the great tract now in danger of being laid waste with this dread famine. This work is in hand.

The canal, from Monghyr to Mirzapur, will be 180 ft. wide at bottom, with a depth of 8 ft. and a length of about 180 miles, of which 30 miles have been excavated to one half of the full section. This canal will be used not only for irrigation, but for connecting the Lower Ganges with the Great Ganges Canal. Its great size renders it well adapted as a relief work, as large numbers can be massed upon it, which has already been done; and the railway, at no great distance, will enable food for the labourers to be supplied at different points along the line.

There are other smaller canals (40 to 50 miles in length each) forming parts of the same scheme. The execution of some of these, it is understood, has been ordered.

The Son works irrigate South Bihar, south of the Ganges. Their value, as part of the grand line of communication up the valley of the Ganges, will be even greater than for irrigation. From Allahabad to Monghyr is 300 miles, and on this part two million tons would be carried per annum, saving, even compared with the river, about 1/2d. ton a mile, or £4,000 a mile or £1,200,000 a year in all. This is besides many hundred miles of branch canals. If the works cost four millions this alone would be 30 percent.

There are two proposed canals on the Gandak, a tributary of the Ganges on the north, to supply the Champarun and Tirhut districts on the one side, and Sarun on the other—through the middle of one district of the famine-stricken country. A fight was certainly made to start one, at least, of these at once.

The Damodar Canal project was brought forward in Lord Mayo's time, and a beginning made, but government afterwards stopped the works, on the ground, it is said, that as coal had been found at Midnapur, it *might* not be necessary to carry the coal from Rannegunj [Raniganj?]. Shortly after, on the convict in charge of the boring at Midnapur being relieved, his successor asked whether any more coal had been found and was told by the native in charge that they had not put any into the bore lately. But on this discovery government did not reorder the Damodar Canal.

Under this pressure of famine, however, it is likely to be resumed, with two or three other stopped works. Two modifications of it, though poor substitutes indeed, were wisely suggested, in hopes of getting some irrigation started, and of them the little canal from the Damodar in the Hugli district has been ordered to be carried out. But the works had not been begun, and we may still rejoice to hear that Colonel Rundall's original scheme has now been accepted by government in its integrity.

There is the great canal, which it is proposed to construct from the Ganges at Rajmahal, and to bring down beside the Bhagirathi (the name given to the upper part of the Hugli) to tide water near Calcutta. This would irrigate Murshidabad, now so cruelly suffering, and Nuddea, and enable boats and steamers to avoid the difficulties of the navigation of the Bhagirathi and the circuitous route through the Sunderbuns.

It would be a magnificent work: was originally proposed by Sir A. Cotton, the most perfect master of the question living (by others, indeed, it is said, before him), and the plans worked out under Colonel Rundall's orders.

The first three schemes, above mentioned, would afford irrigation for at least 2,500,000 acres. If they had now been in operation, the saving of crops, irrespective of the increased yield due to irrigation, would have been half a ton per acre. So that 1,250,000 tons of food would have been *secured*, which has now been lost—enough effectually to have prevented famine and perhaps even scarcity.

In North Bihar and Oudh, the great works projected have all been stopped. Is there one of the many works thus stopped that would not have entirely prevented the famine in its tract?

The Rajmahal Canal has been thoroughly projected and might be begun at once. It will form 200 miles of the main Ganges Valley Canal and can be connected with the Son Canals by a link of about 70 miles. This, with the Sirhind Canal from the Satlej to the Jumna, the Ganges Canal to Kanpur, another lower Ganges Canal to Allahabad, will form 1200 miles of prefect steamboat navigation, the finest navigation in the world, and will save at least £4000 a mile, £5,000,000 a year as compared with *river* transit. On the railway alone there is actually paid £1,600,000 for the carriage of goods only, at 1½d. a ton; on the canal this would cost at 1/10d., £100,000, saving £1,500,000.

Such are the sums India is losing for want of cheap transit. But if a complete system of canals were cut on all the main lines, every part of India would pour food into any distressed tract in any quantities and at a nominal cost of carriage.

A return showing the extent of irrigation in Madras presidency gives 4,800,000 acres, and the real area is above this. This is at the rate of 250,000 acres per district. About 40,000,000 of acres more, besides the works in progress, would give every district in India 250,000 acres, and cost about £100,000,000 producing an additional value of grain of about £200,000,000 a year, besides the transit; the whole benefit being certainly eight or ten times the whole amount of taxation, £40,000,000. That is, it is in our power in this way to do eight or ten times more for enriching India than the abolition of all the taxes.

The total paid into the Treasury in Madras for water is about £3,000,000 a year.

The Son works are now watering more than 130,000 acres—the first year, the water rate of which would be, at 3r., £40,000—on a present expenditure of about £500,000, including all the fundamental works, and the value of crop is estimated at £450,000. Such is the real case of irrigation.

Do not many write as if all irrigation had been a loss to the government, and the one difficulty how to obtain it without overwhelming burdens on the country? The Godavari works alone, in their present unfinished state, pay the interest of £5,000,000.

Is there anything to prevent the government ordering at once the irrigation of from 250,000 to 500,000 acres in every district in India, including a complete network of steamboat canals of 20,000 or 30,000 miles, embracing all India, and to be completed in five years, with an absolute certainty of two or three times the present interest of money in direct returns? The Son works are calculated to irrigate about 2,000,000 acres, paying £500,000 water rate alone, or 12 percent on £4,000,000.

The water rate paid in Godavari is 4rs. per acre of *rice*; on the Ganges Canal 2½rs. an acre of *wheat*. Some of the old irrigation in Madras used to pay 20rs. an acre; some now pay, it is said, 12rs., and much pays 8rs.

Two millions a year are now actually paid for goods transit between Calcutta and the confluence of the Ganges and Brahmaputra, a distance of 130 miles, £15,000 a mile per annum; while £3,000 a mile would make a perfect steamboat canal, carrying at 1/4r. a ton for the whole distance, or £50,000 for the present 2,000,000 tons, producing a saving on the *present traffic* of 500 percent; this is besides about 1,000,000 tons that would be carried along the first 100 miles of the canal for the Upper Ganges. And at this charge the *present traffic* would be soon doubled.

On this little line of 130 miles, a saving would be effected of at least £3,000,000 a year, including the new traffic.

N.B. Seven eighths of the traffic still go by a very bad navigation of 470 miles, three times the distance by rail, and taking six weeks on an average.

Is not the Government of India too much like a dispensary, which does all that man can do to cure when too late to do anything to prevent?

## IV

These facts speak loud: I have no need to add my poor words. He who runs may read. What is the answer given by modern "financial policy" or impolicy? That we must only do what we can pay for out of current revenue, or at least what will pay for itself at once. (Instead of interest enough not being taken in India, too much, it would seem, is taken—an ignorant, unsound interest. So much the worse for India.)

It seems like going back 500 years, to the times when our beds were our banks, and we took out of our old stocking, hid in the mattress or in a hole in the floor, enough for a miserable sustenance day by day, careless of whether we starved or died 100 days hence. Christ himself tells us not to bury our talent in a napkin, but to put it out to interest.[20]

"Sound Indian finance" appears to be what Plato calls "wanting to have money safely kept and not used," or "justice useful" and "money useless." Is it not as though we said: it is "unsound financial policy" to live unless you have money in your stocking; to borrow in order to build, or to trade, or to farm; you must not make railways except you can pay for them out of your income, nor telegraphs, nor any means of communication by steam or water? Is not this reversing the whole principle which has given England her unparallelled success in trade and manufacture—her greatness, as a nation, over the whole globe?

Unless you have money in your stocking to do it, we say in India, don't do it; you must not utilize the money in your neighbour's stocking. You can't eat roads, or railways, or canal banks this year, though they may bring you a hundredfold produce in twenty years. Be not fools who spend their money, unless having £100 in your mattress, you

20 An allusion to Matt 25:24-25.

can see £110 for every £100 in your mattress before Christmas. Eat what you can grow in your garden; you can keep your own money safer than anybody else can use it for you.

Is it "extravagance" to provide for ten years hence, or even, as this famine has but too fatally proved, for one short year hence, what we are to eat then?—or die of starvation—unless we can provide with the money now in hand? Is it "sound finance" to let a man starve a year hence, and live this year by eating up all he has?

Is it cheap to let him die, too dear to make him live, if you have to provide for his next year's food on borrowed capital, even if that capital returns cent percent in future years, and even if—*not* borrowing it—you spend next year millions where you would only have had to spend thousands this year, besides the small item of a few hundreds of thousands of acres of depopulated country? Is it cheaper to let a man "get dead" than to feed him or house him on borrowed capital?

Then comes the drought and costs us tens of millions instead of millions, to say nothing of a million or two of people who "get dead."

To thrust these poor remarks upon those who know it all so much better than I, and can put it so much more forcibly, seems needless.

It will, perhaps, be said that the loan system has now been adopted, and public works are no longer carried on out of current revenue only, that the government is no longer in the position of the old woman with the stocking; that the principle has long since been admitted that the cost of such works should not be borne by the existing generation, which has only a life interest in them, but in the shape of interest upon public loans by succeeding generations, which will equally benefit by them. But this is not true. Loans have been *talked of*, but not raised, nor sanctioned till famine came; and now the money may be spent—not in preventing famine, but in feeding and keeping alive some of its victims.

It will perhaps be said that for years the whole expenditure on irrigation and state railways has been defrayed from special loan funds, but this is not so; that the government is open to blame for not having conceded the first sooner, and also for not having pushed forward such works fast enough, though the immense establishments which it has been necessary to organize could only have been got up by degrees. But this is hardly true. Why did they stop private companies from doing the work?

There has been fatal hesitation for the last three or four years, not so much in carrying on the schemes actually in hand—for some of these have been prosecuted and funds supplied as fast as the engineers could submit estimates and designs—as in starting new schemes. And this has chiefly arisen from the presumed discovery that the promises held out by the advocates of irrigation of high direct returns are illusory (made so indeed by our own mistakes) and that, with the notable exception of some great works in Madras specially conditioned, such schemes do not, and for many years to come will not, pay the current interest on the loan capital invested. This is what is said.

But then why did they abolish the income tax? There is no doubt that such works do vastly enrich the land and add to the general wealth of the community, and it may safely be concluded that, directly or indirectly, they must eventually pay—even in spite of our own mistakes.

In permanently settled Bengal, the government, in laying out money upon irrigation, is always said to be in the position of a man who, having given his property in lease *forever* at a mere quit-rent, proceeds to lay out vast sums upon it. The tenant reaps the whole profit.

From whence, then, are returns to come? Increased wealth will lead to increased consumption, but of what? opium or spirits? God forbid. Let us hope that these two sources of income are to decrease, not increase. Salt? the "poor man's income tax?" God forbid again, we say.

What, then, are we to look to? Should not the government do as they did in Ireland—advancing money to the landlords? or as was done in Lancashire after the cotton famine? But when Lord Mayo's tax was negatived, as above recounted, both he and the members of his government, who had up to that time been staunch irrigators, drew back and refused to advocate any new schemes without such a guarantee. And so matters have stood.

Has not the old woman been to blame, although she had begun a little to mend her ways before the day of retribution came, too late to avert the sad fruits of former error?

This appalling famine speaks louder than any man can do—or woman either. But one must live in order to be a subject for sanitary considerations at all, and one must eat to live. If one is killed off by famine, one certainly need not fear fever or cholera.

## Conclusion

This great essential work of the regulation of the water of India is perhaps at this moment the most important question in the world, or rather not question—action. Nothing can compare with it for the material progress of the people, and their moral progress is greatly dependent upon it; for, till the people are in a measure relieved from their bondage to poverty and want, they cannot attend to other things.

Another very important point, and intimately connected with irrigation in all ways, has to be taken up, and that is the subject of manufacturing in India. There are at this moment at least 100,000 horse water power available and made no use of in the great irrigation canals. The canals will convey the goods to and from manufactories, and the irrigation will set free millions from agricultural labour for such work. With cheap labour, cheap power, cheap carriage and cheap food, India will have the very highest advantages for manufacture, for civilization and also for life and all that makes life worth having to those whom God has created higher than the brutes and only a little "lower than the angels."[21]

**Editor:** The following letters show further efforts by Nightingale to address army and public health in India in the aftermath of her paper, "Life or Death in India."

Source: From a letter/draft/copy to Julius Mohl, Florence Nightingale Museum (LMA) H1/ST/NC1/74/2

Embley
Romsey
14 February 1874

Our general election is almost over and with an overwhelming gain to the Conservatives. As far as my concerns go, I am anything but sorry. In every single respect almost they have gone worse under our own ministry for the last five years than under any other. The three Conservative India ministers I have known, Lord Stanley (now Lord Derby), Lord Salisbury and Sir Stafford Northcote, were literally "angels and ministers of grace" compared with any India minister on our own side. I am in hopes that the Conservatives may still come in time enough to save the remains of wretched Bengal from the famine and

21 An allusion to Heb 2:7.

that Disraeli may give the "surplus" of 4 or 5 millions not to afford us a few more luxuries, but to save a few hundreds of thousands of these Bengalis from being starved to death, all which might have been helped if the duke of Argyll had not stopped our irrigation. . . . Mr Lowe[22] said that this new Parliament would be plutocratic and the next revolutionary. But no man has done more to drag down Mr Gladstone's government than Mr Lowe.

Source: From a letter to Lord Salisbury [at the time secretary of state for India], British Library, Asia, Pacific and Africa Collections, Salisbury Papers, copy Add Mss 45779 f8

25 April 1874

You cannot be so penetrated with my impertinence as I am, and I know will be more ready to excuse me than I am myself for asking you to glance over this little pamphlet which I have just printed ["Life or Death in India"].

One of my reasons is your noble speech about the Indian famine at the Lord Mayor's meeting; another, of course, that we hail the reign at the India Office of one who is a real workman and born ruler of men; a third, that I have now been engaged for fifteen years in Indian sanitary administration and that a great part of its official and private documents passes through my hands.

The first part of my little book has grown out of this, the second out of this dreadful famine. With regard to the first part, Mr [C.C.] Plowden's [India Office clerk] admirable annual digests prepared at the I.O. (his sanitary Blue Books) manage to place every year in small compass before Englishmen what otherwise most of them would know nothing at all about.

With regard to the second part, the *irrigation* facts: there is no one but yourself who could, if you believe in them, turn by their means death into life for India.

**Editor:** Having read "Life or Death in India," Lord Salisbury asked Nightingale "to submit any facts or suggestions to" him on ways to expand measures mentioned in her paper. Nightingale obliged, providing a list of necessary engineering works to first of all improve military stations, then to help peasants by offering them better water supply (canals and irrigation) for agriculture and transportation. In

22 Robert Lowe, then home secretary.

answer Lord Salisbury wrote on 4 November 1874: "I think the best answer I can give you to the details of your letter is to send it out to the viceroy [Lord Northbrook] and ask him to let me have a confidential and unofficial report of his intentions in each of these cases." Lord Northbrook wrote to Lord Salisbury on 11 December 1874 to say:

> I beg you to assure Miss Nightingale that I am not likely so much to forget my training under Sidney Herbert at the War Office as to feel indifferent about the health of the soldier in India. . . . Miss Nightingale is evidently more anxious for the future than dissatisfied with the past. The best thing I can say to reassure her is that in the face of the financial difficulties of last year I left the expenditure upon military public works untouched. . . . I can promise you that, so far as our funds will permit, every attention shall be paid to the health of the British and the native army in India.[23]

In spite of some disagreements, Nightingale thought "Lord Salisbury's worst better than any other secretary of state for India's best. And Lord Salisbury's kindness to me is almost overpowering. I had two letters from him yesterday and day before" (see p 749 below).

Source: From a letter to Lord Salisbury in Cook, *The Life of Florence Nightingale* 2:277-78

Lea Hurst
28 October [1874]

As you were so very good, when you were kind enough to acknowledge my paper on "Life or Death in India," as to *ask* me (where permission was all that I could have expected as most gracious on your part) to submit any facts or suggestions to you, I venture without troubling you with more apology to lay before you the following. . . .

The crown prince of Germany[24] said two months ago . . . that we could add to the strength and numbers of organized armies by sanitary works, and that money well employed in these will as much contribute to military force as money spent on fortifications and on direct military organizations. A great deal has been done already in India, and

23 Northbrook letter, Add Mss 45779 ff16-24.

24 The crown prince of Prussia (1831-88), son of Kaiser Wilhelm I and his wife Augusta. He succeeded to the throne as Frederick III but died only three months later, before he was able to effect liberal changes. He was succeeded by his son Kaiser Wilhelm II. Frederick's wife, the crown princess of Prussia, was Victoria, the princess royal, daughter of Queen Victoria and a correspondent of Nightingale's.

great results to our soldiers' health have followed, but does not much more remain to be done before the results of two or three favourable years (for there was little cholera) can become permanent? . . .

It is the truest economy not to stay your hand in improving the military stations and their surroundings until every station in India has been put in the most healthy state practicable. . . . The improvements required *now* at many stations are the following [a detailed list of ways to improve soldiers' health is included here]. . . .

To you it is needless to say that this relates to one half only of the Indian Army (i.e., that under the direct control of Lord Napier of Magdala), and that Madras and Bombay have (between them) at least an equal proportion of unsupplied wants, for they have not had five years of Lord Napier's wise and humane advocacy.

In India it is always possible to fall into the mistake of spending money uselessly. Fortunately, however, there is a way out of it in the appointment of Mr Clark, the great Calcutta municipality engineer, who has drained and water-supplied Calcutta, to go out and do a similar scheme for Madras.

Source: From a letter to John Sutherland, Add Mss 45757 ff275-76

27 January 1875

Lord Salisbury's statement (about "awakening") seems the very reverse of the real state of the case. In Bengal we have the most industrious peasantry and artisans in the world, in spite of serfdom bowing them to the earth, in spite of the zemindar yoke which we have put (and crushed down) upon their necks, in spite of our having done little or nothing with all our great Western invention to improve or stimulate theirs: see Sir George Campbell in the very same *Times* who says that in 100 years we have introduced no improvement in Eastern agriculture or breeds of cattle. Nothing but indigo has improved by our boasted "enterprise" (although Lord Salisbury draws a disparaging comparison, ending in this most gratuitous assertion that it is no use setting Indian trade free, for they have not British ardour). Nor have we at all done for them what might have justly been expected from Western capital, Western engineering, English public works.

It is doubtful even whether in proportion we have done for them more in some cases than their old rulers. Lord Salisbury says (untruly) that the only remunerative irrigation works are those engrafted on old native works. Yet these people, whom it is said *we* have to "awaken," go on in spite of the heavy burdens our rule lays upon them, in spite of the still heavier atmosphere which our opening *no* career, or a career not much more than a drop in a bucket, for natives of education and intelligence to rise to. . . . In spite of all this these people go on with incredible energy and industry almost unknown to our working classes, who drink or play their three days in the week, husbanding every drop of water for cultivation, keeping up the struggle for life against almost every drawback that can be imposed.

Instead of "awakening" the word should be: lifting off the burdens of an industrious and energetic people, allowing free course to their enterprise, enabling them to work without an incubus, lifting off a system depriving them of the fruits of their labour. Read in the "Progress of India," 1874, just out, of the "extraordinary increase" (this relates to jute) "due solely to the energy of the ryots of Bengal" (this is official testimony), of their "creating the trade" (these are government words), of the "native cotton manufacturing industry" and of the "excellence and durability of the clothes manufactured in India," so superior (it is an I.O. official who writes), of "Manchester goods" so "inferior," of "rapid deterioration" of "Manchester imports" (this is a curious commentary coming out of the I.O. in the same week as the speech of the master of the I.O. at Manchester. Read these things and the jargon talked by the highest quarters about India seems like the nursery song sung by the nurses to their infant, not intended to have other meaning than a jingle to put the baby to sleep. But is Manchester a baby?

With all this, I think like Sir B. Frere, Lord Salisbury's worst better than any other S. of S. for India's best. And Lord Salisbury's kindness to me is almost overpowering. I had two letters from him yesterday and day before.

## Famine Prevention through Irrigation

**Editor:** The recurrence of famines provided Nightingale with a strong argument in favour of developing irrigation works in India, particularly with a view to helping ryots overcome isolation, misery and dependence on the moneylenders. In this cause Nightingale encountered in the 1870s the opposition of the anti-irrigation lobby and the weak support of Lord Salisbury, for whom irrigation could not help prevent famine; on the contrary, he thought irrigation was at the origin of malaria and fever and so contributed to the occurrence of famines. However, Nightingale's ally in the cause, Sir Arthur Cotton, supported her campaign and helped promote important measures.

The appendix to Nightingale's "Life or Death in India," 1873, already dealt with the topic of irrigation, but mainly as a means of preventing disease. There was another aspect to irrigation: it was a way to prevent the return of the scourge that famine was for India. It was Nightingale's hope and that of many experts (such as A. Cotton) that irrigation works and canals, more than railways, were to provide considerable aid in the production and transportation of foodstuffs, thereby making it possible to anticipate periods of crisis, reduce shortages of food and alleviate the suffering of the poor.

Source: From an incomplete letter to Benjamin Jowett, Add Mss 45785 f44

13 June 1874

I thank God, I thank God, who has given irrigation the victory in time, we may trust, to prevent more disastrous periodical famines, yet more to prevent a chronic state of half-starvation. But for this we must yet set our hand to the plough and strike at the root of the zemindari evil. May God hasten His work.

I had had a hint of what was about to happen but had no idea that a great minister [Lord Salisbury] was going thus to nail his colours to the mast or rather pass the Rubicon in such a declaration to the House of Lords.[25] Only let him *wisely* go on with his work, the work for one fifth of the human race and let the House of Commons pass the bill.[26]

Source: From an address to the probationer nurses in the Nightingale Fund School at St Thomas' Hospital, and the nurses who were formerly trained there, Florence Nightingale Museum 1.07562

23 July 1874

Do you know that, in this great Indian famine, every Englishman has worked as if success depended on himself? And in saving a population as large as that of England from death by starvation, do you not think that we have achieved the greatest victory we ever won in India? Suppose we work thus for this home and hospital.

---

25 On 20 March 1874 Salisbury presented papers on the Bengal famine, acknowledging that public works were not satisfactory and that he might in the future ask for a scheme of increased works to provide "remunerative returns" to the famine survivors. Hansard *Parliamentary Debates*, 3rd series (1830-91) 20 March 1874:100.

26 The India Councils Bill allocated moneys for various works in India; it was passed by Parliament in July 1874.

## "Irrigation and Means of Transit in India," 1874

**Editor:** The following letter was prompted by an article in *The Illustrated London News* of 27 June 1874 dealing with the second reading of the India Councils Bill of Lord Salisbury, which was carried in the House of Commons in July, and by an editorial on a meeting of the Executive Committee of the Fund for the Relief of the Sufferers of the Famine in Bengal and Bihar, held on 22 June 1874. Through this letter, Nightingale intended to bend the import of the bill and came up with strong arguments in favour of more substantial investments in irrigation works and communications. Such measures, she felt, would gradually make famine practically impossible. She thought the more funds committed to famine prevention the smaller the famine expenditure would be, for that much less would be required by famine relief.

Source: Florence Nightingale, "Irrigation and Means of Transit in India," a letter (dated 30 July 1874) to the editor of *The Illustrated London News* (1 August 1874) 65:99; also in *The Homeward Mail from India, China and the East, and Official Gazette* (4 August 1874) 20:782-83; and in the *Journal of the National Indian Association* (September 1874) 45:215-19

The second reading of the India Councils Bill of Lord Salisbury—that master workman and born ruler of men—having been carried last night in the House of Commons by a majority of more than three to one, how can we help thanking you for your memorable words: "A great opportunity is before us. An enterprise of surpassing magnitude claims our immediate attention"? For is not this act the first step to carrying out this "enterprise of surpassing magnitude," to laying hold on this "great opportunity"?

"Much has been done already in the way of public works, little, however, as compared with the need of them," you truly say. As an example, take the Punjab: less than one third of that great province (without the holding of which, thanks to Lord Lawrence, during the Mutiny, should we have been enabled to hold India?) has irrigation works, either complete or in progress. More than two thirds are without irrigation and almost without communications. Take the North West Provinces: these are well off comparatively. About five eighths are guaranteed from famine by irrigation; one eighth, though it has no irrigation, has communications. But is not one fourth of this vast district, which equals in size one Ireland and a quarter, wholly destitute both of irrigation and communications?

You say: "Periodical famines ought to be made impossible: will be, we trust." One half of this destitute fourth is the unhappy district of Bundelkund, over and over again desolated by famines, in a most depressed condition, with no means of communication but common roads. Take Bengal. Out of a district—what am I saying?—a kingdom two and a half times the size of Ireland, with more than five times its population, including Patna and all the famine regions of this year, regions which, by this time (but for the Christian heroism of British officials, who have justified our Christianity to the earth, who will never themselves be known by name, but who have created an almost new thing—official heroism in saving, not taking, life), would have been the "abomination of desolation."[27] Take all Jeremiah's strongest epithets and apply them here. Out of this vast country considerably less than one sixth part—about two thirteenths—are all that will be saved from future famines by the only two great irrigation schemes now in progress—viz., the Orissa and the Son works. Of the Patna division—about three fourths the size of Ireland, but with a population twice and a half that of Ireland—less than one third (south of the Ganges) will be protected by the Son scheme, leaving more than two thirds yet to be provided for; and of these a small matter of upwards of 16,000 square miles, or half Ireland, but with a far larger population than all Ireland, less than one third will be protected by the two Gandak schemes, of which the High-Level Canal is to be started. Common roads are at present the only communications of this part (North Bihar).

One of the great advantages of the Son scheme is not only that it protects a country, which, though small, has a population more than that of all Ireland put together, from scarcity, so far as the rice crop is concerned, although storage of the water of minor streams is wanted for the cold-weather crops, of which more anon, but that it secures intercommunication by water. All the Son Canals being connected with the Ganges, South Bihar will become accessible to the river systems of Bengal, the North Western Provinces and Oudh.

But, meanwhile, is anything being done, or proposed to be done, for poor Lower Tirhut? In Darbhanga and N. Bhaugulpur—the centre this year of the severest scarcity, and a pretty large centre, too—is anything being done to utilize a snow-fed river, with always a large volume of water, either for irrigation or navigation? Are there any communi-

27 An allusion to Matt 24:15.

cations but common roads? Has not the first attempt at improving the communications been the railway for transporting the government grain from the Ganges to Darbhanga? Shall I give more than three examples? Are not these three enough to show that, though "much has been done," it is as little compared with what has to be done?

"Periodical famines ought to be made impossible." But, then, the cost, people say. Did not the famine of 1866 cost the government—though one out of three of the starving people died—upwards of two millions? The present famine, where, however, nearly all have been saved, will cost at least five millions. In eight years will not Bengal thus have cost us for only two famines nearly a million a year, with scarcely any return? Would not twice these seven millions insure against future famines, according to estimate, three vast districts of the Punjab, equal to Ireland and one fifth; the wretched Bundelkund, in the North West Provinces; three great tracts of Bengal, the Gandak region, the Damodar and the Nuddea or Lower Ganges? Would not these fourteen millions also complete the Upper Tumbuddra [Tungabhadra?] works in Madras and give tanks to the Central Provinces? This expenditure, and more, Lord Salisbury is advisedly anxious to incur.

Would I not gladly enter here into the question of returns! But I must not presume upon your patience.

"No village in India should be difficult of access: railways, internal roads"—should you not add canal navigation?—"storage of water and well-planned irrigation may be to India trustworthy sources of incalculable wealth." They may indeed. Have we not seen how in every famine food has been more difficult to convey than to procure? Notwithstanding all that has been done, is not the country of India most imperfectly supplied with cheap means of transit? Do not the enormous distances make it imperative to reduce the cost of transit to a minimum? whereas some calculation has been made that "the cost of transit in India is actually eight times what it is in England." Do not, in a poor country, bulky goods of low value form the great mass of traffic? Is not water carriage generally the cheapest, the working expenses being so exceedingly small? The cost of transit generally on canals is 1/8 penny per ton per mile. If an irrigation canal, connected with a Bengal river, be made navigable, does it not become accessible to the whole of the water system, upwards of 3000 miles already?

That the Bengali is not slow to take advantage of this opportunity may be illustrated by the fact that, before the Midnapur Canal had been open six months, native boats were plying on it from such distant places as Banaras, Dacca and Patna. Is not the main feature of Bengal traffic that the boat owners are petty merchants trading on their own account, thus diffusing a wider trade more quickly than where boatmen are carriers only? The moment an article is in demand, is not the whole river plant set in motion to convey it from where it is to be had to where it is wanted? Boats, too, can stop at the exact place where there is a demand for their article, and can serve as warehouses till their cargoes are discharged. As to the additional expense for making irrigation canals navigable, is it not from one third of the whole cost, where there is a steep fall, as in the Midnapur Canal, to one tenth of the whole cost where the slopes are flattish, as in the Punjab and North Western Provinces?

When we find whole kingdoms (as they would be called in Europe) of India with no other means of communication but the common country roads, which mean the worst roads, is it not wonderful that the cost of transit is not eighty times instead of eight what it is in England? For instance, in a doab [tract of land between two converging rivers] almost rainless, between Indus and Chenab, camels are the only carriages, except boats on the Indus. This tract—about two fifths the size of Ireland—stands third on the list of those (of the £14,000,000) most urgently requiring irrigation, the Bundelkund being first and the Gandak second.

If you would give us some of your inimitable sketches of the canal source of plenty, to occupy us during the holidays, we should be halfway to our goal.

I have been too long already for your patience. How take up your time with telling how "storage of water" is generally supposed to be a difficult matter, involving incalculable cost? But is not the case rather the reverse? namely, that there is hardly any other country in the world, which has such admirable sites for storing water in India, at a cost quite insignificant compared with its value? What gold or silver mine equals the value of the water treasure of India?

Then, how compress into few words the explanation that some of the driest regions in the world in India have a fall of ten inches more rain in the year than England, which is a very wet climate? But half the year's supply of rain falls in that region sometimes in two nights, separated by one fortnight. But for a tank system, such a country would be almost uninhabitable.

I hasten to an end. There is no time to spare in India. If only these £14,000,000 were spent on irrigation and navigation, we should be saved from famine expenditure without returns but the sad returns of loss of life; our revenue would be raised by incalculable increase of produce; our intercommunications would supply, as Sir George Campbell says, the millions of one starving province from the abundance of others, at the lowest rates; no extra taxation would be incurred; the traffic would be beyond calculation almost, but for America beyond imagination; and we should be doing our duty to one fifth of the human race—our own fellow countrymen and countrywomen.

Source: From a letter to Lord Salisbury, British Library Asia, Pacific and Africa Collections, Salisbury Papers, copy ADD Mss 45779 ff38-42

5 October 1875

*Irrigation returns India. Private.*In obedience to your most kind letter of 10 May I patiently waited for that irrigation "account" or returns which you said you were "trying to make out for Parliament," "to which" you could "safely give official sanction." Not having seen it appear, I did not like to assault you the moment Parliament was over, nor do I now. But your kindness and the extreme importance of the subject are compulsory.

Your willingness, some months ago, to take steps for securing accurate irrigation statistics from India, and your just complaint that there were none, seem to show you as thinking that there is ample scope for asking for inquiry and make the prayer of me (who have been up to my neck in Indian "returns" for sixteen years) less audacious. You said that you could not be satisfied with the present position of the question. And the irrigation matter is one which [we] cannot drop. Therefore:

1. Might I ask you, would you send me such *irrigation returns* as you have doubtless already procured and "given official sanction" to, since May; I mean of course such as it would not be an impertinence to ask for?

2. And if you are not satisfied with what you have obtained, am I too daring in suggesting that now would be the time to give effect to your desire TO MAKE AN INQUIRY, such as shall secure *results and returns* which *can* be laid before Parliament and the public with confidence?

May I venture to say that the five points or difficulties mentioned in your kind letter of May as standing in the way of obtaining accurate returns suggest the following questions, which are entirely based on your letter? Pardon my troublesomeness and let me go on.

*Irrigation Inquiry*. Might not the inquiry be by a commission (it has been suggested that the commission might be of Sir Andrew Clarke and one good civilian??) if that is the shortest and best way of getting at authenticated *facts*? bearing in mind that what is wanted is *not theory nor opinions*, but *facts and the results of actual experience*. That therefore no special or professional qualifications are required in the inquirer beyond those necessary to enable him to collect and present his facts (great qualifications indeed! perfect independence and impartiality and freedom from bias *as to prevailing or fashionable theories*), with industry and promptitude, so that the inquiry may not (as some of its predecessors have—have they not?) run on for years and official generations.

Might not the inquiry be easily made by means of *printed questions and tables*? (upon a *uniform* basis of course, so as to secure *uniform* data, which *can* be compared and tabulated. As you said, the great difficulty has been that hitherto returns have not been comparable). . . .

I am sure that I need no apology with your kindness and genius and great interest (in a subject so vital to India that I should be impertinent if I were to doubt these). What I do need to make apology for is not in asking for inquiry but perhaps in the length of these notes meant to show the direction inquiry should take, if it is desired to have real results and returns. But these notes can easily be set aside: the inquiry I am sure you will not set aside, since evidence is necessary to show *what is* the duty of the government in promoting irrigation by great works? by small? by wells and tanks? by great and small canals? by private capital? by great national grants and loans?

So many authorities are hopelessly at variance as to facts, or the basis of any theory of government duty (in writing this I am not simply writing as a parrot, if *parrots* write, for I have laboured through and tried to tabulate immense piles of so-called Indian statistics myself), that secretaries of state have almost come to look upon the question perhaps hopelessly too as a mere worrying puzzle; it seems left to Lord Salisbury's genius victoriously to solve it and arrive at real definite results which governments can act upon. Hope deferred makes my heart sick: what must the Indian cultivator's heart be? and the famines?

Source: From a letter to Sir Harry Verney, Wellcome Ms 9007/117

Lea Hurst
14 September 1877

*Private and Confidential.* I think these resolutions are very good, IF they are good. And it is as a mere matter of policy bout which I am no judge that I say as follows: *Proposed Commission* (*second* resolution) would I believe "stink in the nostrils" of both Lord Salisbury and the *duke of Buckingham.*[28] Some time ago I proposed one to Lord Salisbury. I even wrote out in great detail the points (connected with irrigation) *to be inquired into.* Lord Salisbury strongly objected and at last decided that Sir Andrew Clarke and the *duke of Buckingham* should do the work. And my *heads* of *inquiry* were sent out to both *separately.*

Sir A. Clarke has personally proved a complete failure: *the duke of Buckingham's* real interest and (a point of small importance) attention to anything I published has, I supposed, arisen from this. (The story is too long to tell you.) The attention of the public is now strongly directed to India, and *Lord Salisbury* and the duke *might* consent to a *commission.* I know not.

But *who is to form* such a commission? The days when Sidney Herbert worked two royal commissions so as to unite all minds and to produce standing *organizations* which *organized* a complete reform are passed.

Source: From three letters to Edwin Chadwick, ADD Mss 45771 ff158, 159-60 and 161-63

14 September 1877

My mind is full of the dying Indian children, starved by hundreds of thousands from conditions which have been made for them, in this hideous famine. . . . How I wish that someone would now get up an agitation in the country, which shall say to the government, *"You shall,"* as regards Indian famines and the means of preventing them, among which irrigation and water transit must rank foremost. If we had given them water, we should not now have to be giving them bread, as Mr Gladstone did as regards Bulgaria.

16 September 1877

I am glad that you have put in this about India, but I regret that you have not introduced Madras because Madras is the *least* progressive of all the municipalities, because there has been remarkable success in the establishment of *sewage farms,* which intercepted the entire

28 The duke of Buckingham and Chandos (1823-89), governor of Madras.

drainage at certain spots—a system which ought to be adopted generally in Madras—because the whole question of *what* system for the *drainage and sewerage* of Madras shall be adopted is *now* trembling in the balance and because it will be *now or never* if the famine does not stir us up to what we owe to India in irrigation and water transport.

*P 28B:* is there not some misprint at "in developing the sources of epidemics"? Does it not mean "in discovering and *preventing* epidemics at their sources"? Doubtless the India Office's annual sanitary report *just out for "India in 1875-76"* and "*up to June 1877,*" has reached you: read *p 150* on the intolerable talakore (*sweepers and filth carts*) system of Bombay.

With ardent wishes for your best success in *preaching* and *prophecy.*

6 A.M. 16 October 1877

I am afraid I am too busy and too much exhausted to "do" your proof as I ought. Some things no doubt I should have liked to have seen in it done in a different manner. But on the whole it is admirable. The only thing I would really urge is this: pray do not say "Sir Arthur Cotton has *also advocated. . . .* " Sir Arthur Cotton, the master, almost the father in modern times of the art of irrigation, who was twenty-six years or more in charge of irrigation works in Madras presidency (South India), who raised the Godavari district from famine to plenty, who raised its revenue by 150 percent (the three districts of Godavari, Kistna and Tanjore consequently upon works of irrigation now yield £1,850,000 in revenue or £600,000 each, while the average of all India is only about £250,000). You cannot say of such a master, he has "advocated"; and to say of him "also" is like saying: Dr Richardson's[29] sanitary work is. . . . Mr Edwin Chadwick has "also advocated" sanitary measures. (N.B. I am very glad you think well of Dr Richardson.) . . .

I am glad that you are going to do something "at the Society of Arts" on Indian sanitation and irrigation. I was appalled at the ignorance and fallacies of Lord Salisbury's speech at Bradford and Lord G. Hamilton's previous speech in Surrey (the secretary of state and under secretary of state for India!) I am afraid I must say, things were otherwise done in my day.

ever your most faithfully
Florence Nightingale

29 Sir John Richardson (1787-1865), surgeon and naturalist, inspector of hospitals.

P.S. I am afraid the Madras drainage question will be settled against us. I send you a *pamphlet of mine* . . . and a copy of second edition of *Sir A. Cotton's* pamphlet. How I wish he would not write in that style of attack, setting every statesman and newspaper against him, so that one does not like to appear in the same pages. . . .

You know poor Robert Ellis is dead. I saw him this summer just after his return from Madras full of all the Madras questions, drainage, irrigation, hospitals.

Source: Letter, Wellcome (Claydon copy) Ms 5483/10

35 South St.
Park Lane, W.
18 September 1877

*India and Irrigation*
Sir [Rt Hon John Bright, MP[30]]

Pray forgive me for writing to you: your speech at Manchester on the necessity of water to render future famines impossible for the poorest, the most industrious peoples in the world, makes me cry for joy and pity. If we had given them water, we should not now have to be giving them bread and to see the children die by thousands for the want of it.

When I read your noble speech, I knew that God had heard our prayers, that some statesmen, like Mr Gladstone agitating for Bulgaria and Bosnia, might agitate the country for India and irrigation so as to say to the government: *"You shall."*

I venture to send you a poor pamphlet of mine on the subject, and may perhaps take the liberty of sending you something more, which has at least the merit of being short.

Pray believe me, as I rejoice to be,
ever the most faithful of your servants
Florence Nightingale

30 John Bright (1811-89), Liberal MP from 1843. His speech appeared in the *Times* of 14 September 1877. He paid a visit to Nightingale in 1885.

Source: From a letter to Lord Houghton,[31] Trinity College Cambridge, Houghton Collection 18/140, copy ADD MSS 45804 f274

27 November 1877

How sorry I am to hear you give a not good account of your health. I trust that your life may be prolonged for many years. Pray give my dearest love to your children, if they are so good as to remember me. . . .

I have often thought too what you say, how strange that I have lived to see (and take sides with) the Russian entering Turkey. But stranger still to see the Hand bringing good. . . . I earnestly pray against "Turkey becoming a Russian satrapy" as *you* do and meanwhile will not trouble my friends with lucubrations where I can do nothing.

God seems to take things more into His own hands (in history). Perhaps He always did. Only we trace more now the difference between what *we* wanted to do and what is done. Whatever comes out of this cruel war, we may be very sure that both good and evil will be very different from what either side expects. . . .

What interests *me* most at the present moment is the Indian ryot, the irrigation and cheap water transport so urgently needed, the indebtedness to moneylenders, the slavery (in Bengal) to zemindars, worse than any Bulgarian slavery to Turks, the poverty more grinding every year for the last twenty. To take the opportunity, when the famine subscription makes English think, lies heavy at my heart, but my will is greater than my capacity. The care of my mother and other things since my father's death have pressed out my life and prevented me from finishing the most necessary parts, i.e., bringing up to the present moment two papers (two volumes of the same booklet), (1) on the condition of the ryot, (2) on irrigation, etc. (I had beautiful woodcuts and irrigation maps, all cut and engraved, ready—irrigation maps supplied by Indian officials—these have already done service at lectures.)

To my surprise a few days ago, E.I. [East India] Association applied that Reverend James Long[32] (Bengal missionary) should make and read selections from paper No. 1 as a lecture at E.I.A. Rather than let this precious thing go by, I consented. *I wish* somebody would do the same with *paper No. 2*. You see, if people ask: But what works would you recommend now? there is map ready to answer. For eighteen

31 Richard Monckton Milnes (1809-85), made Lord Houghton 1863, poet, friend and unsuccessful suitor; one of the original trustees of the Nightingale Fund.

32 James Long (1814-87), missionary, founder of the Bengal Social Science Association.

years I have done sanitary work for India but, for the last four, have been continually struck with this: what is the good of trying to keep them in health if you can't keep them in life? These ryots are being done to death by floods, by droughts, by zemindars and usurers. You must *live* in order to be well. I wish I could start my facts now, but I too am being done to death.

## "Irrigation and Water Transit in India," 1877

**Editor:** The paper below is substantially based on the *Report* of the Madras Irrigation Company, dated 8 May 1877. Sir Arthur Cotton was, in Nightingale's estimation, "the most perfect master of the [water] question living" (see p 740 above); he carried on an important correspondence with her on problems of irrigation, the neglect of which was a contributory factor in the recent famine.

Source: Florence Nightingale, "Irrigation and Water Transit in India." A letter (dated 29 June 1877) to the Editor of *The Illustrated London News* 71 (7 July 1877): 22-23

Also published as an appendix to "The Madras Famine" with other papers, by Sir A. Cotton (London: Simpkin, Marshall 1877: 25-30)

Also in "Reply to the Report of the Committee of the House of Commons in Indian Public Works and other papers, including a letter by Miss Florence Nightingale," by Sir Arthur Cotton (Dorking: R.J. Clark, Printer 1880: 25-30)

Abridged in "The Great Lesson of the Indian Famine" with appendix, containing letters from Lieutenant General Sir Arthur Cotton, Miss Florence Nightingale, etc., by a journalist (London, Paris and New York: Cassel, Petter & Galpin 1877: vii-x)

Sir, You were so good as to admit a letter from me once [in 1874] on that subject of vital—I should say mortal—importance in India, "Irrigation and Water Carriage." The frightful famine in Madras recalls us all to it. When the government is obliged to feed one million and a half of our fellow subjects—when these have been perishing, in spite of us, at the rate of 930 per 1000 in the relief camps—when nearly half the population of villages have died in a month of "famine cholera"—when men were not put on the relief works till they were too far reduced by starvation to do any real work—when their bullocks were all dead, so that their very means for raising the next crop were gone—we are fain to ask, What has irrigation done for the Madras presidency?

This question a report just issued by the Madras Irrigation and Canal Company, dated 8 May 1877, received at the India Office 19 June, answers for us, at least as to one district.

But first let us observe that there are at this time four districts which ought to have been, like the other twelve, overwhelmed by this terrible calamity, but three of which are not only entirely free from famine themselves, but are in the highest state of prosperity, having a large surplus to supply the famine districts, and the fourth, though not entirely relieved from famine, yet has a very considerable supply of grain.

What has made the difference between these three districts and those which are under the dreadful sufferings of famine? The government irrigation works. The three districts of Tanjore, Godavari and Kistna, instead of adding five millions more to starve, are pouring into the starving districts hundreds of thousands of tons of food. Sir Arthur Cotton, the great master of the irrigation art, twenty-six years in charge of the public works in those very districts, which are, in the heart of famine, supplying food, could tell us more about this.

It was the same in the Bihar famine. The Son works, while they were yet unfit to be opened, were made to water 160,000 acres, producing a crop worth £500,000 in the midst of dearth. The whole cost of the works was actually saved by a single crop and thousands of people saved from death.

But to return to the fourth of the Madras districts referred to: this is Kurnool, N.W. of Madras, in the very depths of the peninsula. This is the district watered by the Madras Irrigation Company, from the Tumbuddra River. The works have cost £1,600,000 and are capable of watering 400,000 acres for two crops, or at the rate of £2 per acre of crop. Then also the navigation would afford carriage at a nominal cost. The main canal alone, from Kurnool to Cuddapah, is 190 miles in length. The officers are to sell the water at the price of twelve shillings an acre, worth to the purchaser £2.

A missionary in the Godavari district told Sir Arthur Cotton that scores of times the people had gratefully said to him: "We never got the Godavari water on our lands till you Christians came here. Truly, the greatest Raj is the English."

In Kurnool last year, however, as indeed before, the water was refused by the people during the main cultivating season, but when the pressure of the famine began to be felt, they forgot all their difficulties and asked urgently for water. By this time the supply was already beginning to be deficient, so that the canal could not be kept full. Nevertheless, let us see what was done by these works. I quote from the report above mentioned:

> The total area that has been supplied with water is 91,000 acres. In addition to the satisfactory revenue thus realized by the company, the food crops raised by the canal have contributed materially to mitigate, in the districts of Kurnool and Cuddapah, the effects of the terrible calamity of drought to which these and other districts of Southern India have been and still are exposed. The money value given in the following statement of the grain grown under the canal is £940,000, none of which could have existed except for the irrigation supplied.

The works having cost £1,600,000, two thirds of the cost have thus been saved by a single partial crop. The report then goes on to complain of their being prevented from using the canal for navigation owing to the delays in the proceedings of government, showing how

> the value of the canal, if it had been used for boats, would have been considerable. The cartage of rice from the Gooty Railway station to Kurnool is 5d. per ton per mile, or £1 6*s.* per ton. But that from Cuddapah to Nundial is 7d. per ton per mile, or £2 3*s.* per ton for the whole distance. The rate by the canal, even at 1½d. a mile, would be 10*s.* (ten shillings). *The want of any better outlet for canal produce has been a bar to the spread of irrigation under the canal.*

Yet this canal produce might have been placed in direct communication with the market of Madras and with all the markets of the world at a nominal cost of internal carriage. The canal now extending to Cuddapah, 190 miles, ends there. The North Coast Canal from Madras extends to Nellore, 110 miles, and the interval between this and Cuddapah is 80 miles. This work has been estimated for, but still remains unexecuted. Had it been executed there would have been a perfect communication between the great irrigated deltas of the Godavari, etc., and the inland districts which are in this terrible condition.

The extension of the North Coast Canal to the Kistna is an immense point gained. The duke of Buckingham is cutting also the short line of canal through Madras to connect the South Coast Canal with the North Coast Canal.

Let us resume our extracts from this important report. "October 1876. Throughout the month not a drop of water has been allowed to run to waste down the Pennair," that is, the whole of it has been used for irrigation. "In another fortnight or so all the accessible dry land for which water is desired will have had a first flooding." Again: "Applications for water have been very numerous, and from all sorts of places, *far beyond the reach of canal water.* . . . We are also much hindered by the quarrelling among the ryots themselves as to who shall first have the water."

In November, it is reported:

> *The most bigoted of the old ryots are now quarrelling and fighting for the water.* The old prejudice is entirely broken down and, as a Curnam expressed it, "They (the ryots) have come to their senses about the water." . . . *The sight of the country commanded by the canal is truly refreshing.* In one village above Canalla I rode through tall cholum fields for a mile or two. There more than three square miles of land were saved from utter drought, and about 300 acres of rice were just ripening. It is very sad to compare this with the rest of the district, where utter failure has occurred, and I regret to say cholera is rapidly increasing.

How we wish that *The Illustrated London News* would give us two of its admirable views—first of the desert, and then of the irrigated land, often seen side by side! Misery and plenty, starvation and comfort.

Again:

> All the crops are reported in good condition, both dry and wet. The former, sown under the canal, are acknowledged by the ryots themselves to be in as fine and healthy condition as any crops they have ever sown. . . . Of the thirteen government tanks commanded by the canal, five were filled before the end of the month, and the remainder will be filled before the middle of next month.

For December, the chief engineer reports in January 1877:

> The result of my calculation is:
> In Cuddapah district, 19,050,000 lbs. food grain.
> In Kurnool district, 65,240,000 lbs. food grain.
> Total 84,290,000 lbs. food grain.
> *Enough to feed the whole district of a million inhabitants for two months,* and probably the straw will be enough to maintain all the cattle not yet perished in the villages under the canal. In this calculation vegetables are not reckoned as being any substitute for food grain, whereas they do, in fact, often save grain—for example, sweet potatoes, crinjals [rice variety], pumpkins, etc.
>
> This grain, at present prices, is worth £700,000; and, if the value of vegetables, indigo, cotton and straw be added, the actual value of the crop created by the canal cannot be more nearly estimated than as one million sterling. But its value in helping the district to tide over the critical month of May, and in supplying village wells with good water, can only be poorly represented by such an estimate.

> The actual saving to government by the provision in the least accessible parts of the district of such a food supply, which would otherwise have had to be bought, is about £500,000. . . .
>
> The government are now feeding at imperial expense a third of the population of Kurnool district. This could scarcely have happened had the ryots not sacrificed the whole of the first crop, which the canal might have matured by irrigating their fields and filling their tanks. This infatuation, fortunately, did not extend to the second crop, about a quarter of which will have been reared *under the already failing water supply of the Tumbuddra.*

Again:

> It is probable that the ryots, under the canal, will save most of their cattle and thus be able to resume their work on the first appearance of rain. Elsewhere in the district, it is probable that much land will be idle, as nearly all the cattle will be dead. The sale of bullocks in Kurnool has been so great that the coolies find it cheaper to buy meat than grain, a bullock selling for three rupees.

Again: "The villagers under the canal may be considered to be in a very prosperous condition, the crops being very good indeed."

In January of this year "the overseer reports that the white cholum sown in Pratakota is magnificent. I have never seen finer fields of this dry crop than those of Banakercherla and Vempeuta [Vempalle?]. The ears were so full and the plants so thickly grown that they were touching one another."

Again: "The average yield per acre of paddy is two putties [cloth bags?], which is above that of the preceding season. This putty has been recently sold at forty-eight rupees. The straw is almost half as valuable as the grain." Thus the whole value of the crop is about 140 rupees, while the charge for water is six rupees, and the total cost of the works is only £3 per acre.

In February it is reported, "The wet crops, more particularly in the Cuddapah and Proddatur taluks [districts, estates], are the finest that have been reaped."

In March it is

> estimated that nearly seventy million pounds of food grain have been grown under the canal in three taluks. This is sufficient to preserve one quarter of the population of the Kurnool district for six months, and to feed more than 8000 pair of bullocks. There can be no doubt that, if the water were properly and timely taken, and with the same eagerness that was displayed this season, when it was too

> late, the grain grown under the canal in the Kurnool district would feed the whole population (amounting to nearly a million) for twelve months, even if no crops were raised except from canal irrigation.

Again, in March:

> There is little doubt that the canal water affects the health of the people considerably. When procurable, canal water is always preferred to well water, some villagers are in the habit of going a distance of two miles for it. While in camp I was unable to find a well in any village containing water fit to drink. In one place, though greatly in need of a draught of water, I was compelled to abstain from drinking any of the water of three wells, as the taste was filthy.

Thus far our quotations. Have these things no bearing upon the famine?

As regards canal transit, grain can be carried by water at one twentieth of the cost of carriage by railway, which, besides, cannot produce one pound of food either for man or beast. Had the millions that this famine will cost been spent in irrigation and navigation, the whole of these provinces would have been secured forever from famine and from ten to twenty millions added to the income of the people.

Further, had the necessary preparations been made when the famine had become certain, the link of the canal might have been cut from Nellore to Cuddapah, and the districts of Bellary, Kurnool and Cuddapah have been put in direct communication with Madras, and with Godavari and Kistna. Thus the famine would have been turned into a blessing and an annual benefit derived to the country far beyond the interest of ten millions.

The extension of the Coast Canal from Nellore to the Kistna has at last been undertaken; by the latest accounts 50,000 people were employed upon it and it was expected to be finished next month. If this is accomplished, putting Madras in communication with those great deltas and with the *coal tracts* of Godavari, it is quite certain that far more will be gained even from this small work than the interest of ten millions. It will complete one line of transit of 550 miles from Madras to the second barrier of the Godavari, and will connect altogether 1200 miles of navigation with that city.

Sir Arthur Cotton has repeatedly pressed upon the authorities, both in India and at home, the necessity of providing for these famines, whenever the failure of the monsoon made such a calamity certain, by marking out an important work of irrigation or navigation, erecting shelter and collecting food and tools beforehand—so that, as soon as the pressure of the famine is felt, well-organized parties may be set to work at once, and before they are reduced to a state unfit for work. Now, their ribs must show the signal for them to be on the relief works.

There is always time for this, but it has never been done. The consequence is, almost the whole of the money expended is lost. Whereas a famine is, in fact, the opportunity of executing in a single season important works to raise India forever out of its present poverty. Hitherto, without exception, not a finger has been moved till the people were actually dying, and then it was too late to organize works effectually. What might not the millions that the last two famines will have cost have done to make famine impossible?

In Mr Monier-Williams's[33] letter to the *Times* from Madurai 28 December, he says:

> All the belts of land reached by the grand system of irrigation which stretches between the Godavari, Kistna and Kaveri rivers—fertilizing the soil wherever it penetrates, and forcing even haters of the English rule to admit that no other raj has ever conferred on India such benefits—present a marvellous contrast to the immense tracts of arid waste which meet the eye of the traveller as he journeys by the Great Indian Peninsula, Madras and South India Railways.

Here are two subjects for *The Illustrated London News.* "Look here upon this picture, and on this."

Had half a million more acres been irrigated in each of these districts, and had they been put in effective communication with the rest of India by steamboat canals, which would have admitted of all India being laid under contribution for food, the famine would have been nothing comparatively. And had the comparative few who would then have had to be fed been employed on further great works, the famine would have been a source of plenty.

General Strachey said, on 18 May, at the Royal Institution:

> We must be content to pass through a condition of periodical suffering of an acute kind, during which . . . ways of escape from these evils will be gradually perfected. These ways of escape are, indeed, already sufficiently evident, and, so far as they have been hitherto applied, have been found to be thoroughly efficacious. They are

33 Sir Monier Monier-Williams (1819-99), India expert, author.

> the provision of artificial irrigation and of improved means of transport. . . .

And he has "passed a large part of his life in seeking for the means of extending those essential material allies in the battle of Indian life."

As regards Bengal, an act is being prepared for a compulsory water rate in Bengal, which, though stopped at present, will be carried through, if possible. It is estimated that the landowners benefit to the extent of two rupees an acre from the irrigation works, even when they do not use the water, through the embanking of the rivers, the drainage of the land, etc. If they pay those two rupees, then they will have the water for nothing.

In the Godavari and Tanjore, where the Tamil and Telugu people had sense enough to know their own interests, it was sufficient to give them the water, and they took and used it. But where the people are as stupid as some people in England who would not have factory laws, there is nothing for it but to make them have them. We see what the famine has done under the Tumbuddra in forcing the poor people there to benefit themselves. Why should we wait for a famine to do this?

It is estimated that the lands in Orissa have actually increased in value three or fourfold since the irrigation works without the water being used, the zemindars thus receiving the whole of the present profits of the works, while the government have had the whole of the expense.

This year, as has been said, a crop in Kurnool is worth 140 rupees, or twenty-four years of their water rate.

If all England could set her face against the Suez Canal we must not be surprised that there are other people almost as stolid. Another nation [France] had to cut the Suez Canal for us, and thus force upon us such an incalculable benefit. In England and Bengal you must take men as you find them, and force blessings upon them.

So we thank God and take courage. We are really gaining ground.

## "The Indian Famine," 1877

**Editor:** The following published letter, addressed to the lord mayor of London, was written in response to an appeal for funds made on behalf of the victims of the Indian famine. In his acknowledgment, the lord mayor declared that "the letter would be worth its weight in gold to the fund." It was an earnest appeal for aid to the ryot, than whom "there is not a more industrious being on the face of the earth." The sum of £78,000 was contributed by Great Britain and the colonies for the relief of the victims of the famine.

Source: Florence Nightingale, "The Indian Famine." A letter, dated 17 August 1877, to the lord mayor, enclosing a cheque for the Mansion House Relief Fund, printed in the *Daily Telegraph*, 19 August 1877 and in the *Times*, 20 August 1877

My Lord

If English people knew what an Indian famine is—worse than a battlefield, worse even than a retreat, and this famine too, in its second year—there is not an English man, woman or child who would not give out of their abundance or out of their economy.

If we do not, we are the Turks who put an end to the wounded—and worse than they, for they put an end to the enemy's wounded, but we neglect our own starving subjects. And there is not a more industrious being on the face of the earth than the Indian ryot. He deserves all we can do.

Having seen your advertisement this morning only, and thanking God that you have initiated this relief, I hasten to enclose what I can—£25—hoping that I may be allowed to repeat the mite again, for all will be wanted. Between this and January our fellow creatures in India will need everybody's mite—given now at once, then repeated again and again. And may God bless the fund!

Pray believe me, my Lord
ever your faithful servant
Florence Nightingale

Source: From a draft letter to Sir Arthur Cotton,[34] Add Mss 45805 ff13-16

16 February 1878

What everyone is calling out is this: "What you tell us is reasonable, but show us the exact facts, show them us on a map and with diagrams and don't irritate the enemy about railways when we want to hear about water and water transit. Show the fact, overcome evil with fact, the fact of water, don't hold out a 'red rag to the bull,' educate us not by invective but by showing us exact plans and what you want to do. Show us on a map. You say we are ignorant and stupid—show us as

34 Against Lord Napier, Sir Arthur Cotton argued for the construction of more canals for transit and irrigation as much cheaper than railways.

stupids and ignorants on a map, e.g., how you propose to deal with the problems of storing water running to waste (e.g., in Bengal, etc.); of extending and feeding the tank system (e.g., in the south); of extending the well system (e.g., as in the Punjab); of extending the inundation canals, system of water transit, steamboat canals, etc. (e.g., as in Bombay, etc.). Show us on a map the other localities where what you have done to save millions on the Godavary, Kistna, etc., can be done elsewhere. But do not irritate our governors." . . .

Victory is not to turn off government but to make them do the right [thing]. . . . This is not time at a public meeting to give details but there is time to give, as you say too, a "scheme" with a map, such a scheme as can be given in the time and don't let the time be wasted in vituperation. . . . Before the House of Commons' committee then more detailed plans should be given by Sir A. Cotton with diagrams as evidence, showing *where* you propose to carry out the respective systems of irrigation and navigation suited to the various locations. He will certainly be asked questions, but Sir A. Cotton is one of the few men who *knows* and can answer questions at once out of the fullness of his personal knowledge whenever he is wanted. . . .

What the "great men" say to me is: let Sir Arthur Cotton show us distinctly work for work, locality for locality, what to do. Practical men *will* take each work on its own merits; according to its own locality each work will and must be taken on its own merits: river deltas on theirs; Madras tanks on theirs; Punjab wells and canals on theirs, etc. . . . Sir A. Cotton is too great an engineer not to tell us this better than anyone else: let him teach us.

Source: From a letter to Mrs Roe, Clendening History of Medicine Library, Kansas University Medical Center

23 March 1878

I am sure that you bid me Godspeed in all my objects: the training of nurses which becomes more and more essential every year; the sanitary reform in our army and country generally; the sanitary development—and above all the "irrigation development" to prevent famines—of India, poor millions of our starving fellow subjects. "I trust that you will do me the favour of accepting a little pamphlet of mine on this subject," which I enclose.

Source: From a letter to (Colonel) James George Fife, Add Mss 45805 ff41-42

5 June 1878

I shall be most happy to see you on Thursday (tomorrow) at 5 P.M., as you kindly propose. When I have the advantage of hearing you talk, I feel so penetrated with the want of knowledge of the real bearings of the irrigation question, under which English people in general and I in particular suffer, that I think I ought not to dare to write a word on the question. What I particularly want to understand is the bearing upon the successful use of the water of the way in which the people are rated for water, whether by paying so much per acre or by paying for the water, whether they take it or not, whether by not being allowed to take any land or any water they like, how it is to be made their *interest* to use the water in the most profitable manner and not to exhaust the land but to cultivate in the best manner.

All this is only to be understood and explained by such men as you are. Also how questions of settlement bear upon the development of irrigation and upon the poverty or well-doing of the people.

I think you are not satisfied with the Sind settlement. I want to understand more why. I wish I could see your evidence. I am very sorry there is no Deccan irrigation map. What is to be done? . . .

A man who can say, "I have completed 3000 miles of beneficent canals" ought to be the happiest man alive.

## "A Water Arrival in India," 1878

**Editor:** The article that follows is based on a report from Mr Buckland, commissioner of Burdwan Division to Bengal government, dated 23 January 1874. Nightingale quotes extensively from that report.

Source: [Florence Nightingale] "A Water Arrival in India" by a Commissioner, *Good Words* (July 1878): 493-96

"The bridegroom cometh."[35]

An Indian famine: the heavens as brass, the earth as brick; men, women and children, as well as cattle, perishing for want of water and food, strength ebbing away, people living, or rather dying, on weeds, on jungle produce perhaps.

A royal progress. Like an epic poem the hero-lover meets his people and his ladye-love; he has delivered his country from the destroyer;

35 Matt 25:6.

the bride's and the people's rejoicings, "with noise of weeping loud,"[36] as they go forth to hail the arrival in triumph of their victorious hero, bringing peace and plenty to his stricken land, the very hour of each meeting is noted.

Such are the contents of this official paper, reporting the opening of some engineering works—opening of the Khana Nuddee (Blind River)—in the Hugli district, one of government's relief measures for a famine not yet here, but hanging over us.

With spade and shovel and at a cost of not more than £1200, the waters of the Damodar are let into their old channel—which had silted up and become "khana," or blind, before the present century—the Khana Nuddee, fifty-seven miles long, joining the Damodar with the Hugli.

"It is easy to imagine," says the commissioner, "the joy and satisfaction of the people in one of the most densely populated parts of Hugli, at seeing a river, five or six feet in depth and from forty to eighty feet in width, suddenly flowing through their villages, especially in such a season as this, when their water supply was in the greatest jeopardy, and they were watching anxiously the few dwindling pools of water that used to lie in the old bed of the river. I venture to say that no such great and appreciable benefit has been so suddenly and so cheaply conferred on such a large number of anxious people during the present century, and this work alone will suffice to make the lieutenant governor's administration memorable in the district of Hugli."

Compare this whole account with the fears often expressed in the highest quarters that the people could not be induced "to use the water" without "compelling" them.

Drinking water collected out of filthy puddles—one must have known a hot country in a time of drought to know what a depth of misery that means—among a people, too, whose only drink is water. But could they afford milk, the milch cattle are dying too for want of water.

> See the conquering hero comes,
> Sound the trumpet, beat the drums.[37]

It is a government report which gives the account: "The works were ready on 27 December; the officials were present, when the waters of

---

36 An allusion to Ezra 3:13.

37 From Nathaniel Lee, *Alexander the Great* iv.2. The quotation was used by Thomas Morell for the libretto of Handel's oratorio "Joshua," then transferred to his "Judas Maccabaeus."

the Damodar were admitted into the bed of the Khana Nuddee, amidst the acclamations of the people who had flocked to the spot." The water arrives eight miles farther. "Great excitement prevails." Again the commissioner's report:

> The villagers taking the greatest interest in its arrival. They turn to watch its progress and, to facilitate its advance, cut the bunds (dams) that held it back. On the evening of the 3rd, the water arrives at Kamalpur. At Kooloot the water arrives during the night of the 4th. At Radhanagar the water arrived at 6 A.M. on the 4th. The greater portion of these and adjoining villages are uncultivated for want of water. At Nundanbatty the water arrived on the 5th at 6 A.M.

Does it not read like a triumphal progress? "The admiration and gratitude" "of the people within reach of the use of the water - -." "In the villages of Nundanbatty" "there are no tanks and the people express great satisfaction at the arrival of the Damodar water."

So comes the conquering hero on, till "at Dukhinkool" the water arrives "on the 6th at 7 A.M." "The people are enthusiastic." (Still the commissioner's report.) "Their tanks were nearly exhausted and would have been quite dry in a month" (think what that means!); "the few tanks they have are extremely foul, and the clean water now brought to them is of immense benefit." And so on, and so on, till "at Bhola the water arrives at 1 P.M. on the 8th." "The people are loud in their gratitude"; "it has saved their lives." It has indeed.

They irrigate "eagerly"; they "commence preparing the land for onions and sugar cane, it being too late for other crops." (These are the "people" who have been accused of immovable want of enterprise. Sugar cane is the crop which requires most labour and care, and is also the most valuable. It takes eleven or twelve months' water to grow sugar.)

"At Anundopore [Anandpur? Anantpur?], thirty-four miles down," "the water has just arrived" (8th, at 9 A.M.). "At this place was a pool of water," "used for steeping jute," "in a filthy condition"; "but the people were using it for drinking and all other purposes." (Does it not seem miraculous that they are alive at all?)

The police, 9 January 1874, report that "the inhabitants are overjoyed," "praising and thanking the English government." "It is a gift from God." "They were 'badly off' (badly indeed) for water, but now they have full and plenty." (See report from Mr Buckland, commissioner of Burdwan Division, to Bengal government, no. 177, dated Burdwan, 23 January 1874. Is not Mr Buckland an epic poet, without knowing it?)

*Normal state of the Burdwan people.* This is not a famine year, though it might easily be mistaken for such. 8*s.* or 10*s.* or 12*s.* *a month,* to maintain themselves and wife and children, and to clothe them against the winter cold. Again it is a medical commissioner who speaks. Daily food, usually one meal a day only. (This is not a district where the people are very particular about cooking for caste reasons, and consequently cannot spare the time to do it more than once a day.) A little rice, with what is called vegetable curry (oil and potherbs) for the whole family, and this the ordinary daily food; extreme poverty; a permanent state of half-starvation; no proper clothing; a whole population of "poor helpless creatures, so impoverished and so enfeebled in constitution" that, when epidemics come, they lie down to die without power to rally. "Dhall (peas) cost too much," they say, "and milk we can never look at."

In 1869, 1870 and 1871 was the fatal, too-notorious Burdwan fever. Of its excessive mortality we have no idea whatever. It is again the government medical commissioner who speaks: "Unless prompt food and careful nursing be given, one half die in the first year, and with the rest it is only a question of time. And the only effectual method of meeting the difficulty is almost impossible as long as the well-to-do people keep aloof and give no help to us."

What is this but a famine fever, assisted by bad or no water supply, bad or no drainage? Yet this is not *called* a famine!

In good times, two or three cooked meals a day of rice (about a pound of rice a day) and dhall (peas). In the best of times they have fish, cured—imperfectly cured, on account of the salt tax making salt too dear—or vegetables.

To sum up: We must "consider the regulation of the water with regard to health. For several years past a great extent of country round Calcutta" (the Burdwan fever is not extinct, it reappears in other places) "has been desolated by fever of such a nature that numbers of villages have been almost emptied by it, tens of thousands having died of it." Its predisposing cause is semi-starvation. Among its immediate causes are, want of drainage in the monsoon, want of good water to drink in the dry season.

This is the state of villages in those dead, alluvial plains: in the monsoon without a foot of dry ground, and surrounded by pools of water; in the dry season, not a drop of wholesome water to drink—nothing but the remains of these pools a few inches deep, in which filth has been accumulating for months. Compare this with an irrigated tract completely pervaded by drainage channels to carry off the waters in the monsoon, and canals of running water, fresh from the river, flowing through every village.

*Irrigation* means: first, water for irrigating land, but also all drainage and other works for complete regulation of water; navigation, and a good water supply for drinking and cooking.

## II. Life or Death on the Godavari

*Death on the Godavari. Before* the irrigation works were begun, from eyewitnesses in tents and rough sheds on the bank of the river, or rather on the side of the riverbed: a narrow thread of water down the middle of that bed, on each side of that thread a mile and a half, at least, of hot, deep sand. Want and filth, and need of every kind around: weary women toiling through the dry riverbed with their waterpots, creeping out of their huts after the exhausting heat of the day to bring the family supply of water between one or two miles, their naked feet sinking at every step in burning sand. How insufficient the supply, after all that labour, need scarcely be told.

Food: in the dry season any kind of vegetable matter that they could get from the jungle to keep themselves alive, cattle reduced to such a state of starvation that when the rains began they were totally unfit for work.

The superintendent of Madras government farms says that we have no idea of the statistics of "*annual* loss by disease amongst Indian livestock, from being kept during two thirds of the year just above starvation point."

"At the commencement of our rule"—it is a government official, a civilian, who speaks—"it" (the Godavari district) "formed a portion of a neglected province, and at one time it was brought to a state of extreme impoverishment and distress. It was desolated by famine and misgoverned by the numerous landlords (under the zemindari system) and their advisors." Happily the ruin was so complete that the government were left free to restore the land in many cases to its real owners or their descendants, some of whom had been robbed in order to transfer the land to people who had no right in it whatever.

If "honesty is the best policy," unjust proceedings are the worst—ruinous to all parties. Irrigation now could take full effect in every way in this district.

*Life on the Godavari.* Eighteen years later, *after* the irrigation works were in full action, from the same eyewitness: instead of dry sand, riverbed covered full with abundant water. Instead of parched, perishing attempts at cultivation, rich crops of many kinds, trees which seemed to have sprung up as if by magic; instead of the wilderness, a garden; instead of filthy waterless villages, channels, well-filled, flowing everywhere; instead of weary, overworked women, all, or almost all, well-fed, well-washed and comfortable; time and strength of mind and body no longer solely taken up with daily drudgery, which before absorbed every power; religious civilization possible.

Cattle strong and healthy, and doing their work. And, best of all, the people are now very generally free from the moneylender.

Now for the official civilian report: "Since the introduction of the admirable system of irrigation" (Sir Arthur Cotton's), "it" (the Godavari district)

> has brightened and revived. Famine is unknown; the people are prosperous and contented; it is the garden of the great Northern Province. The revenue, instead of being reduced, as it once was, to the verge of bankruptcy, is more elastic than it has ever been. Its population has more than doubled; the material prosperity is proved by their being better fed, clothed and educated than formerly; its commerce has flourished and its trade has developed in a marvellous degree; and it may be confidently asserted that it is in as peaceful, happy and prosperous condition as any portion of her imperial majesty's dominions.

Besides water or no water being a question of life or death, of health or disease, of civilization, comfort and cleanliness, or of dirt and barbarism and misery, it is a question of revenue. The Godavari district used to export £60,000 a year; it now exports, by sea only, £800,000 to £900,000 a year. The whole population is well-clothed, well-housed; home consumption doubled. The 560,000 acres, irrigated by an expenditure of about £600,000, yield about £1,100,000 a year more in grain, besides straw, besides navigation. And they can export food to the famine districts, instead of being a famine district—terrible word, but more terrible thing—themselves. A similar change may be seen in the Kistna and Tanjore districts.

In the last Madras famine, not yet over, where among twenty millions three millions have died—where in some places we have lost one fourth of the population—two large districts are exempt: Kistna and Tanjore. Not only this, but their populations have increased, and increased beyond the *estimated* increase of population, while all around have been dying. Why? Because of their irrigation works they have been saved.

No wonder that the ryots of Trichinopoly [Tiruchchirappalli] lately, in November 1877, addressed the governor of Madras, praying that the same benefits might be extended to them. In their memorial they relate how Sir Arthur Cotton "controlled the Coleroon" (in Tanjore) "by means of a gigantic masonry dam, so as to arrest the drying-up of the Kaveri"; how "that great engineer bridled the Godavari, a river five miles broad at the point chosen, in a similar way and with still more magnificent results"; how other such works have been applied to other rivers, "all which works have converted the tracts affected into scenes of matchless fertility and wealth, and have for ever protected them and neighbouring provinces from the disaster of recurring droughts."

The poor ryots of Trichinopoly then mention six particular projects in their own district which they earnestly demand should be executed, amongst these, "a large reservoir at the meeting of the Patchamalai and Kollimatai ranges, the projected Uengar Channel, for part cost of which the ryots have years ago subscribed and paid money." And with picturesque and pathetic simplicity, they pray for these to be carried out.

This is paper and words to us, to them life instead of death. Such are two or three instances of bringing life out of death to our neighbour in India. "Go and do ye likewise."[38]

Note. Even while this is being written new and bad accounts come in from India. In Madras drought has been followed by locusts, famine is not over and the government is preparing to reopen relief works. In part of the Punjab and in extensive tracts in the North West Provinces there is severe suffering, if not actual famine; prices *very* high everywhere. Actual distress anticipated in Shahabad and Patna. In Eastern Bengal complaints that no ploughing can be done for want of rain. The lieutenant governor of Bengal [Ashley Eden] is gallantly giving himself to necessary works: to "good works" in every sense of the word, as understood by *Good Words*. F.N.

## "The People of India," 1878

**Editor:** Fifteen years after the royal commission report, progress in the welfare of the Indian people had been desperately slow. The "state of things" (ravages of famine, poverty of the ryots, social injustice, exploitation by moneylenders, lack of access to clean water) was

38 Luke 10:37.

"hideous" (see p 810 below). One of Nightingale's most vigorous writings on India, "The People of India," constituted a forceful indictment of official apathy and administered a timely shock to British complacency. Following upon the great famine of 1876-78, Nightingale's opening statement was blunt: "We do not care for the people of India"; we have no sympathy for the wretchedness of the Indian peasant.

Faithful to her method, she was keen to collect facts and figures from knowledgeable people on the spot as well as from official sources. She later said: "It was he [Dr Cornish] who gave me the famine statistics which I published . . . and was scolded for my 'exaggeration' as never man was scolded by the India Office. And it turned out that the statistics were *under* the mark" (see p 672 above). Sir Louis Mallet, permanent under secretary at the India Office, came to take the data seriously; he was to say a few months after publication: "I begin to think now that your 'shriek,' " as the article had been called by important men of the office, "was a better expression of the truth than any other utterance."[39] The article prompted the secretary of state, Lord Cranbrook, to write to the viceroy, Lord Lytton: "I shall be truly glad if your legislation can afford a remedy."[40]

Source: Florence Nightingale, "The People of India," *Nineteenth Century* 4,18 (August 1878): 193-221

We do not care for the people of India. This is a heavy indictment: but how else account for the facts about to be given? Do we even care enough to know about their daily lives of lingering death from causes which we could so well remove? We have taken their lands and their rule and their rulers into our charge for state reasons of our own. Nay, the hour is coming, and even now is,[41] when for "state reasons" we are annexing, or preparing to annex, or to reorganize, or to "protect," by whatever name we call it, huge and immeasurable territories because they lie between us and them. But for them themselves—these patient, silent, toiling millions of India, who scarcely but for suffering know their right hand from their left[42] and yet who are so

39 Letter 10 March 1879, in Cook *The Life of Florence Nightingale* 2:292n.

40 Alfred E. Gathorne-Hardy, ed., *Gathorne-Hardy, First Earl of Cranbrook: A Memoir with Extracts from His Diary and Correspondence* 2:80. Edward Robert Bulwer Lytton (1831-91), viceroy of India 1876-80.

41 John 4:23.

42 An allusion to Matt 6:3.

teachable, so ready to abide by law instead of resisting "their enemy the law"— for their daily lives and deaths we do *not* as a nation practically care. Or should we not as a nation practically rise *en masse* to see that the remediable things to which good public servants have so often vainly called attention *shall* be remedied? Have we no voice for these voiceless millions?

What is the saddest sight to be seen in the East, nay, probably, in the world? The saddest sight to be seen is the peasant in our own Eastern Empire. But we do not look at this sight, no, not even those few who travel in India. To speak of India is, however, much as if we were to speak of Europe, since in India there are almost as many races, languages and climates as in Europe; almost as much difference between provinces and presidencies as between Russia, England and Spain. The land tenures are also as different, so large an item in material life. Only debt and usury are much the same all over India. And, alas! a chronic state of semi-starvation.

"The bulk of the people of India are paupers: they can just pay their cesses in a good year and fail altogether when the season is bad. Remissions have to be made perhaps every third year in most districts. There is a bad year in some one district or group of districts every year." Whose striking words are these? Not those of a member of Parliament or advocate making a case or historian or gazetteer writing in his closet. They are those of one of our great English proconsuls ruling in India over a population nearly twice as large as that of France, second only to a viceroy and who has done perhaps more than any in raising the Indian peasant, in giving him a kind of representation, a voice to rate himself, in giving him education, roads and a sort of independence or power to hold his own.

Let us try to take a glimpse of one or two of the various provinces in regard principally to material prosperity or rather adversity; and first of Madras because the famine, not yet over, and the help given by England have tended to fix our eyes just half an hour more than usual upon this presidency as upon India in general. After Madras we will go to the Bombay Deccan (for other provinces this article gives no space).

What we engaged to do was to prevent any from dying of famine. What have we done? In many parts one fourth have died. In Bellary, Kurnool, Cuddapah and Nellore the deaths from famine in one year have been from 21 to 27 percent. At the end of 1876, according to the estimated population, Salem had 2,129,850 souls. On the 14th of

March 1878 she had 1,559,876. More than one fourth were gone. Here, where even yet the famine will not be over for some months, already, therefore, have died considerably over half a million out of some two million souls. In Mysore there has been a waste of life of one fourth. We have lost in one year not less than three millions out of the twenty millions more especially under the famine scourge in Madras presidency, a presidency of 55,000 villages, a population of 35,000,000. In southern India, that is in Mysore, Bombay and Madras, our loss in one year's famine has not been far short of 6,000,000 souls or rather bodies: God takes care of the souls; this has been our care of the bodies, in spite of the unflinching courage and honesty of the government and of every official under it in trying even more than man can do to keep to its purpose of not allowing one famine death, in spite of England and the colonies vying with each other in coming to the rescue by a voluntary subscription of about £800,000, in distributing which all classes in Madras, European and native, worked hard and well and to the best purpose.

What should we say of a war which had killed 6,000,000 in one year in a region not much more than half the size of France, or indeed in all the wars in all Europe of the greatest of conquerors? It has not entered into the imagination of man[43] to conceive of such a destruction. One death from starvation in London fills all the newspapers with reports of the inquest upon the body. There is a machinery which costs us seven millions of money a year to prevent it. Public opinion is now holding—holding, did I say? it is not holding, it ought to hold—a gigantic inquest upon 6,000,000 bodies, dead less indeed by our fault in sparing effort than in spite of every effort to save them from dying of famine, to save them, *not* to *prevent famine.*

Has any effort been made not to prevent deaths from famine but *to prevent famine itself*? Can we show any districts in Madras safe from this thrice fatal scourge? We can. Nay, in four districts we can show, not only that the population has not been decimated or rather *quadrated*—O that we should have in our days to invent such a word to express the suffering!—as in ill-fated Salem, Bellary, Mysore, but that it has increased. In two of them indeed it has increased more than the *estimated* population. (Population in India is estimated to increase at the rate of 1½ percent per annum.)

---

43 A paraphrase of 1 Cor 2:9.

What are these favoured districts? They are those which have been saved by irrigation works: Tanjore and Kistna. In Kistna the increase over the *estimated* population is 5.1 percent, in Tanjore 1.7 percent. In the two other districts the population of 1878 was above that of 1871 (the census year), though not quite equal to the estimated population. One of these districts was within reach of irrigated districts, though not yet thoroughly irrigated itself, and crying out for irrigation: Trichinopoly, in which a decrease of 2.9 percent below the estimated population was found. The other is Tinnevelly, also partially irrigated, with a decrease of 1.9 percent. (See also correspondence in [the] *Times*, 15 May 1878, dated Madras, 20 April.)

The Bengal famine of 1873-74 is past and gone: so short are our memories. But not five years ago we were writing, talking of this, working and working hard at this. The conditions truly of Bengal are different; the land tenures are different; the race and language are different, but the sufferings are the same. Why is this? We shall have to give a separate glance at Bengal.

Between five and six millions have perished then in this Madras famine. These are figures, paper and print to us. How can we realize what the misery is of every one of those figures: a living soul, slowly starving to death? I have had photographs sent me of five or six. An infant with precocious resigned eyes of suffering, a living skeleton in its mother's skeleton arms, a dying boy, a helpless old man, a man stricken down in the prime of life. I could not bear to look at them. I hid them away and would not publish them. But not five or six, but five or six millions lay down thus to die, slowly to die of hunger and thirst, besides the millions who were saved. And when we realize that five or six millions have so died—that we count not by fingers of one hand but by millions, every finger is a million of living, dying people—do we realize what it is to say that many more millions have so lived, been so saved and will so live after the famine, going back to their bare and roofless homes where not a straw remains? All has been taken for famine needs. Without cattle, without seed corn to plough and sow their now-desolated lands, implements wanting, bullocks dead, everything gone; branches to be used instead of ploughs; instead of cattle, men; paupers, unwilling paupers, for years. And this the most industrious, the most frugal, the most thrifty, one might almost say the most heroic, peasantry on the face of the earth.

Let us look at one or two of these moving skeletons in the famine, not because they are uncommon but because they are common specimens, and particularly at the children; for care of the weakest things, of infant life and of diseased life, is certainly in our belief the characteristic of modern Christianity, though we must put in a plea for modern Indian Hinduism and Muhammadanism too. As certainly the sufferings of children, though no whit less patiently borne, are more severe, more agonizing than those of grown-up or old people; for children cannot look forward, cannot understand, can feel nothing but the cruel suffering and weariness of dying, cannot measure the time or see the end. As a child who had fallen into a ditch for one minute said, "I was there for a thousand years."

In the Madras famine children of seven to ten years used to bring poor little naked living skeletons of two and three and four years to the government relief centres, feeding the babies day after day for weeks with the daily dole, asking for nothing for themselves, till the little foster mothers would themselves sink fainting at the gates. These were often of no kin; sometimes even of a different caste or religion. A little kindness "makes the whole world kin." Hundreds of fathers and mothers, going to other parts of the country to get work and food, left children to die in their villages. Little ones who had no little foster mothers wandered about to get a dole of food from any one who would give, then lay down and died with—pass me the word—the heroic agony of childish patience. For example, one missionary from Cuddapah met in one day's journey over one hundred who had no one in this world to care for them. He stopped and helped the oldest, telling them to look after the little ones, but he believed that all, or nearly all, died. This led to himself and his wife opening a "Temporary Home," one only out of many such instances, of course, for children under twelve years. No temptation to idleness was held out and in five weeks many were restored so as to be sent out to work. One orphan boy, nine years old, told as soon as he could speak that he knew of other famine orphans: might he bring them? And he instantly sallied out and brought in first two little Muhammadan boys under six, then carried in from a great distance in his skeleton arms a little girl too far gone to stand or sit up, and who apparently could not live through the night. But with good nursing she was brought round to look like a moving skeleton and eat rice. A tiny Muhammadan of three would call another but a little older who tried to take care of her, her sister. The two could not be parted and both were taken. Both had lost their fathers and mothers of cholera in the relief camps. Mothers often brought in children, breathing their last, to the Temporary Homes. The Famine Fund gave to the Temporary Homes and the missionaries begged "famine orphans" from government and took them into their "boarding schools." The other children uniformly showed kindness to these orphans. The Famine Fund gave bullocks and seed grain to many survivors returning home.

To the Madras famine all this relates. But what is the grinding, chronic semi-starvation of every day in many places where what is called famine does not exist? In 1875-76 Mr Robertson, the superintendent of Madras Government Farms, tells us: He was making an official tour through Coimbatore; and writes his report without any reference to the famine since fallen upon us but not then expected. The condition of the ryots in Coimbatore, he says, was so bad that had they and their families lived in the same "*luxury* as the prisoners in the jail of Coimbatore, they would about eat all their produce and there would be nothing left for rent." These unhappy ryots are landholders under ryotwari tenure; that is, holding land direct from government. There are 215,207 holdings in Coimbatore, the average holding is about twelve acres. Cotton is grown, not because it is profitable but because, as they can't eat cotton, it goes to pay the rent. If they grew grain, which pays better, they would eat it. They have but two meals daily and of the coarsest food. Yet Coimbatore is on a railway, but unirrigated. The ryots are all in the clutch of the moneylender. There are about 100,000 agricultural labourers in the district of Coimbatore; "their condition is a degree worse than that of the small ryots."

We mean to return to Coimbatore, but now let us go north to the Bombay Deccan. Here almost every man has a small holding of land; say, he has a holding of twenty-eight acres and a family of six persons; though they cultivate the land themselves they can scarcely live upon the land; their very salt is heavily taxed; they are bound hand and foot in the grasp of the moneylender. He can sell them up, land and everything they possess, even to the honour of wife and daughter. (Report of Commission on the Deccan Riots.)

We will return to the Deccan, but let us first go northeast to Burdwan. This is in Bengal. What do we find here? They complained in Coimbatore, or rather the Englishman complained for them, of the two coarse meals a day. In Burdwan they had but one—one meal a day only for labourer and wife and children, and that a little rice with what is called vegetable curry. "Milk we can never look at." "Dhall (peas) costs too much." Drinking water in the dry season has to be collected out of filthy puddles. The whole family has to be fed, maintained and clothed against the cold season on 8*s.* or 10*s.* or 12*s.* a month. Here, in Burdwan, the tenure is zemindari—that is, the zemindars, not the state, are landlords; and the ryots hold from the zemindars.

But where is the prosperity of India? This is the adversity.

In Burdwan in 1876-77, the lieutenant governor's reports say that the country was prosperous. Does the "prosperity" then find its way into the pockets, or rather first into the stomachs, of the people? Ought not all such reports to wind up with telling us what constitutes the Bengal labourer's daily food, comparing it not, of course, with the English labourer's, far less with the English navvy's food, but with what is considered necessary to keep a Hindustani sepoy in good condition?

The Hindustani sepoy requires daily to keep him in health *on duty*: 32 oz. of wheat flour, 2 oz. of clarified butter, 4 oz. of peas, 4 oz. of vegetables, ½ oz. of salt and pepper, with an occasional pint of milk. A Bengali labourer requires the same, substituting rice for wheat flour. What does he get? As has been said, usually one meal a day only, of a little rice, with what is called vegetable curry—that is, six or eight ounces of potherbs, cabbage, etc., and half an ounce of oil—for the whole family. And this was the ordinary daily food. Is it any wonder that, when a bad year comes, these poor creatures are struck down in large numbers and that large numbers die? It would be a wonder if it were not so. Prosperity among the Bengalis is believed to mean two or three cooked meals of coarse rice, about a pound a day, and dhall. In the best of times vegetables or fish curry are added. But the salt tax makes salt—a necessary of life to vegetarians even more than to us meat eaters—so dear that imperfectly cured fish is often the cause of disease. And every year tons of fish are wasted for want of cheap salt in the midst of people starving for want of it. Fish, a mere drug in Bengal, is a rare luxury.

In Oudh the cultivators are even worse off than in western Bengal. Eastern Bengal is somewhat better off now. The ryots have found their power. In the irrigated districts of Sind, this is the highest prosperity of the good comfortable Muhammadan ryot: a pound of flour, or the most comfortable may even have two, one for dinner and one for supper, that is luxury: clarified butter, salt, a little chopped onion or chili. He makes a hole in the flour, kneads it all up with his hands, makes a little fire and cooks it. This is not such bad diet; but then he has nothing else. He is not so desperately in the hands of the moneylender as is the Deccan cultivator. This is prosperity, this is.

Now compare these with the English labourer. And first, the Hindus here spoken of use no liquor as a beverage. I could point out a town in England where men can earn wages of 10*s.* a day and drink it all away. Ay, and the women, too. A woman said, "I think no more of my money than of a flea in a churchyard." They are not a penny the better for it, either in clothes, lodging, bedding or any of the decencies, comforts or true interests of life. But we will speak, not of such as these who have no future but the workhouse, the prison, the grave, in this world, as one of their own selves said, and what in the next? and who might have, oh! how good a future if they knew their real interests. We will speak of the sober English labourer, the family man with the gallon of beer a week, the half-pound of tea, sugar, tobacco, untaxed salt, good water and the rest, and the Hindu living on inferior grains for the most part and too little of them, a little vegetable curry, a little salt, too little, and his very salt, as has been said, is taxed. The tax amounts now to £7 a ton, the salt itself being worth 12*s.* 6d. a ton in India. The people make "earth-salt" by washing the earth and boiling the food in the saltwater, and for this miserable product they are punished.

Manufactures are strangled by the tax on salt: such manufactures as bleaching, making of glass, glazing, extraction of metals from ores, salting of provisions; agriculture and the feeding of animals are hindered and livestock die of disease from want of salt. Fish is ruined by being cured with earth-salt. The food of the poor requires more salt than the better diet of the rich, but no man could live without nine pounds of salt per annum. The smuggling of salt was enormous and necessitated a great increase of police. A tower commands the saltworks, occupied by a policeman all day. Moats surround the works, patrolled by policemen all night; workmen are searched to prevent them from carrying off salt in their pockets. (See the Report of the Madras Salt Commission. See also Lord Lawrence's evidence.) The French *gabelle* [salt tax] was "a law of conscription against the well-being of man, a law entailing misery on unborn generations." Can India become prosperous under it?

"The common people who find it hard to live when bread is cheap feel themselves about to die when bread is dear." Can this be wondered at? The drinking water is a fruitful source of misery and disease to the poor in India in the dry season, collected as it is out of filthy pools filled with every impurity. In the dry season, in many districts of India, as in the Godavari districts, before the irrigation works were carried out, any kind of vegetable matter is eaten by the people that they can get from the jungle to keep themselves alive.

So far as to food, but a man must eat to live and it is no bad test of the condition of a people.

His dress is a coarse bit of rag and a scanty sheet. A tumbledown hut of straw and mud, built by himself and not always thatched, a mat for a bed, one or two cooking utensils: this forms absolutely all the house and furniture even of the richer cultivator. And this is commonly shared by the beasts. As a rule he has no money whatever, but in some villages the phenomenon may be seen of a ryot possessing one or even two rupees.

The chief object of this attempt is to ask as well as I can, in so brief a space where only a few questions can be asked or even glanced at, and only in the fewest words, for India is large and time is small, how it is that whole peoples among the most industrious in the world, on perhaps the most fertile soils in the world, are the poorest in the world; how it is that whole peoples always in a state of semi-starvation are from time to time on the brink of famine? and if not actually swept away by famine, it is by their rulers giving food, not water, wholesale. Is there any fatal necessity for this? Is it not due to two or three causes, not only preventible, but which we, their rulers, having ourselves induced, either by doing or by not doing, can ourselves gradually remove? And to come at once to the questions:

1. The great question of moneylending, which overshadows all.

2. Water. (And does the government write as though it were simply a trading company to whom the sole question was: what direct profit can be obtained?) If we had given them water, should we now have to be giving them bread? Water, including *(a)* irrigation; *(b)* cheap canal communications; *(c)* improved methods of agriculture; *(d)* forest plantations.

3. (I reserve for future consideration the great question of land tenure and land assessment. It might be well for the reader to bear in mind that the principal systems of land settlement are: the ryotwari settlement, that is, the revenue settlement made by government with each actual cultivator of the soil for a given term at a stipulated money rent, without the intervention of landlord, zemindar or middleman; this is in the Bombay and Madras presidencies. The zemindari settlement, that is, the Perpetual [Permanent] Settlement made in 1793, creating in the zemindars actual proprietors, enjoying their estates in absolute ownership, out of tax gatherers, who formerly paid to the

government revenue ten elevenths of the fixed net proceeds of the lands, receiving for their trouble but one eleventh of the collections; this is in Bengal. The ryot is the peasant-cultivator. The zemindar is the landlord created out of "collector of revenues on behalf of government" by Lord Cornwallis's Permanent Settlement of 1793. (We might as well create the English collector landholder of his collectorate. He distinguishes himself by all manner of cruel exactions of rent and illegal "abwabs" or cesses levied on his dependent ryots, although expressly forbidden by the Permanent Settlement; and by carrying into effect none of the primary objects of the Permanent Settlement, one of which was to record *all* rights to the land. Sir George Campbell, during his lieutenant governorship of Bengal, made it his aim to restore a record of tenures and rents and rights of ryots, such as has never before been made in Bengal. He did this through the provisions of his Road Cess Act. And already the ryots in many road-cess districts have come forward to take extracts from the returns relating to their holdings and rents. These returns are the first authoritative records ever framed in Bengal of the rents payable by ryots over any large area of country.)

Systems of representation, by which the people may virtually rate themselves according to the surveys of what is wanted and spend the money locally under the elected District Committee's orders; including *(a)* municipalities, *(b)* publicity, or some method of giving the people a voice.

1. The great moneylending question: How to give the ryots, especially in southern India, just and legal help against the moneylender? Otherwise, give the ryot water and the profit will all go into the moneylender's pocket. Into his hands the ancestral lands seem in danger of passing, and the ryot of becoming, not metaphorically, but in some cases literally and legally, the moneylender's slave. We now give the moneylender unjust and legal help to possess himself of the lands of India and to make the ancestral cultivator and the rude tribes his slaves.

Is it not strange that, under a country boasting herself the justest in the world and the abolisher of the slave trade, a poverty, an impecuniosity, an "impropertyness" leading to virtual slavery, should be growing up—actually the *consequence* of our own laws—which outstrips in its miserable results, because it enslaves and renders destitute a land-possessing peasantry (in southern and western India), anything except the worst slave *trades*? And in some respects things are done under us, though not by us, almost as bad as under the tax-farming Turks.

One thing has been much urged: a system of small loans from government at moderate interest to the country ryot (which is now carried out to a very small extent) to be extended to meet the need and supported by British capital. But the ryots, it is said, won't take the loans. We pass over the system of "takavi," that is, money advances made by the government to the cultivators at the time of sowing, especially in the south of India, to be repaid when the crop is gathered, or made in bad seasons—a system which might well be facilitated and extended—and go on to what we can learn of government loan-making. Offering loans to individual ryots is almost given up. For the government sends an officer to see what security the ryot has; then to see whether he is spending the money as he said. This the ryot does not like; he always prefers going to his moneylender, whose interest it used to be *not* to be repaid. And there was this *one* good point in the native moneylending transactions, that the prosperity of the Marwari depended on the prosperity of the ryot. But this is so no longer. (The Marwari represents the moneylending class: most of the sowkars (moneylenders) from Marwar are now colonists of the Deccan.)

Revelations positively astounding have quite recently come home on the chronic state of indebtedness and starvation of the ryot, especially of the poor Deccan ryot; overassessment, his fields sometimes cultivated almost at a loss or "only just repaying cultivation." "Some of this land cannot afford to pay an economic rent at all." The moneylender (and this puts one touch more to the hideous picture) is also the village shop or general dealer and village banker, and not only this, but the valuer also—estimating the advances made *by* him in kind at his own valuation, estimating the repayments also made *to* him in kind at his own valuation.

In the Bombay Deccan, where the ryotwari system prevails—that is, the cultivator holds his land direct from government—the established custom is that the moneylender provides the seed corn and feeds the ryot and his family until the crop is ripe, making also cash advances to pay revenue instalments, buy bullocks, dig wells, etc.

"Grain advanced for seed is repayable at harvest time, bearing 100 percent interest; grain advanced for food carries only 50 percent interest, repayable when the first crop is ripe."

It is said that the Indian case is only the case between capital and labour all over the world; that the only difference is that in Europe it is the rate of wages, while in India it is the rate of interest which is in dispute. But this is "extremely *not* so." For here the ryot is fed beforehand by the moneylender as a regularly established thing. Were the ordinary ryot ever one season beforehand, it would be otherwise. What should we think of the village dealer supporting the whole village to be repaid afterwards?

We have had enough experience in the English Army that the commissariat must never be bankers: this was one of the lessons of the Crimean War. If in a European Army it is found that where the commissariat are also the paymasters the men are almost at its mercy, what must it be with the poor, isolated, defenceless, ignorant Hindu ryot and his moneylender?

The old extinct truck system in England, the old but alas! not extinct, running-tick shop custom here are justice and mercy compared to this.

The mischief is not in the ryot borrowing, but in his being supported beforehand by the village shop and repaying afterwards in kind.

*Co-operative Stores.* Would not the co-operative store, if only possible, be like a new life, a redemption to the Deccan ryot? In an English village, way was opened for a co-operative store thus: a large heap and a small heap of, say, sugar or tea were displayed on the village shop counter side by side. "That, the large heap, you buy by paying ready money; this, the small heap, you buy by running tick."

If these could only be displayed by the general dealer in a Deccan village, how soon he would cease to be moneylender! How infinitesimally small, perhaps hardly visible to the naked eye, would be the small heap, at the moneylender's own valuation! How gigantic would appear to the astonished eyes of the Hindu cultivator the large heap estimated on a system as unknown in India apparently as Arctic voyaging or London commerce—the system of buying and selling with ready money!

Up-country consumers are said to be at the mercy of the retail dealer, "who can create a monopoly and raise prices in proportion to the poverty and isolation of his customers."

The co-operative store would seem to be singularly adapted to the ancient soil of village communities and we hope soon to see a co-operative store in *water*, otherwise called an irrigating community.

"*Debt*" again, it has been said, "is simply working on borrowed capital." It is the system which has created the prosperity of the "Lancashire mill owners" and the Scottish "tenant farmers." But this has nothing to do with the ryot's system of debt. The ryot's system of debt, as has been said, is like, but even worse than, the usurer or pawnbroker feeding and maintaining the whole district and being repaid after long interval at, of course, an enormous and wholly arbitrary rate of interest.

This is quite different from either paying wages or borrowing capital. It is the old truck system: only worse, married to a usury system worse than the worst Jewish usury known in history or poetry—far worse than under the Mosaic law. Well may a government commission say: "When we compare the law of India with that of other countries, we find that not one is so oppressive in this respect, not even the law of Moses, which allowed the debtor a discharge after serving seven years." We shall see what the Deccan debtor has to serve.

"If the moneylender refused to feed the ryot till his crop was ripe, the land would simply go out of cultivation." This is stated as a justification of the system: is it not the worst condemnation?

If, in addition to the mischief of the shop being the bank, a wholly false economic principle—if, in addition to the ryot paying by his *future* labour and *future* property, a wholly different thing to receiving wages for his past week's labour or past week's production; *that* is selling his labour, not borrowing, but what this ryot does is mortgaging it—if, in addition to the rate of interest being 40, 50 or 60 percent or even 100: 50 percent is low, 100 percent is something—if, in addition to all this, *the moneylender, in a land where is no law of insolvency, can bring the ryot into court upon any bond, just or unjust, fictitious or not, which the poor simple ryot subscribed without knowing what it was, and buy up the ryot's land at a tenth or less of its value, nay, may even cause the ryot himself to serve all his life, the general ruin of the ryot is complete.*

A native said: "The English law makes the sale of our land as easy as the sale of a bullock or a turban."

If it is true that a rate of 36, 40, 50, 60 or even 100 or 200 or 300 percent is a not more uncommon rate of interest in the interior of India, as exacted from country ryots by moneylenders, than a rate of 3½, 4, 5, 6 or 10 percent at most is in England, is the greater fear that of the conquest of India by the Russian or of the conquest of India by the moneylender?

Were it possible that England should reconquer India by enabling the indebted country ryot to redeem his lands and pay off his debts, lending him money at 7 or even 10 percent; by introducing factories, perhaps the co-operative store, for which the village community of

India would seem the very soil; by opening cheap village courts, enough to place one within easy reach of every village, so that litigants may be able to go to the court in the morning and return home at night, and be thus subjected to the criticism and public opinion of their fellow villagers; by restoring courts of conciliation, for which also India is the soil, for the settlement of class disputes, as well as courts of arbitration for the cheap and ready disposal of individual suits—panchayats, of these more anon—if England could thus reconquer India from the moneylender, what a glorious conquest that would be! ("A man would often lie in a distant court where nobody knew him, who would not do so in the presence of all his neighbours who knew the real facts." *Report on the Riots in Pune and Ahmadnagar.*)

According to the Hindu law, interest on a loan is never allowed to exceed the principal; that is, however long a term may elapse before the latter be discharged, more than twice the principal could not be exacted. The Bengal and Madras regulations limit the interest of money in those presidencies. The Bombay code does not limit the rate of interest. The banjas or moneychangers evade the Hindu law by obliging their debtors to sign *fresh* bonds for sums made up of the former principal and the interest together; and thus a debt runs on increasing *ad infinitum* through the instrumentality of fresh bonds signed by the ryot who is commonly quite ignorant of what he signs. "A system of registration," says the revenue commissioner of the Northern Division, Bombay presidency, "would check this in some measure by exposing the succession of bonds and showing the sums originally borrowed."

The holder of a decree exacts every year all he can find (little though that be) in the possession of his victim who is scarcely in a condition of solvency. At the end of a few years the poor debtor is shown a large account for interest and to escape being put into jail he is persuaded to sign a new bond for the balance of the old debt with interest thereon since the decree, so that the debt is never cancelled and goes on *ad libitum* unless the patience of the debtor becomes exhausted and he absconds, forsaking the country forever. And of course the moneylender repays himself for this loss by grinding yet more his other unfortunate debtors. The rate of interest is, under the present conditions of the sowkar's trade, in some degree determined by the risk of the worst cases.

The Hindu law favoured credit by making debts payable from generation to generation, but it was a part of that law, as has been said, that the interest demandable should not exceed the principal. But to enable courts to determine the amount of principal actually paid in loan, district registers should be established for the registry of all loans of money to be paid before the District Registering Officer, and the civil courts should only allow the recovery by judicial process of such sums as can be clearly proved to be principal paid and not the accumulated principal and interest of a debt *previously* adjudicated upon.

It is said that *thrift* is what must save the India ryot. We have heard of the horse being made to live (or die) on a straw a day, but we do not know that we ever heard before that the horse ought to exercise "thrift" and save his one straw a day. Yet this is what it appears the country ryot has actually done. (He justified the secretary of state and died.) There is so little danger of pauperization that, in the Madras famine, for one who threw himself without need on the relief measures ten died in silence, almost unknown to our masters (*not* like the wolf, "biting hard"[44]).

There is such an element of endurance and heroism that, quite unknown to our masters, during the greatest starvation and the highest prices, the hoarded grain remained in pits safe in the earth—none betrayed the secret—hoarded, not to sell again at the highest famine prices, but for seed corn against another failure of crop. And not till the present crops were safe has it appeared. This was by the better class of farmers. What thrift, what endurance, have we Westerns compared with this? And we in the West preach thrift to them. The "horse" literally "saved" his one straw a day for his children's sowing. And they call these people not thrifty. It is the very heroism of thrift. Compare the people of some of England's big towns with their drunkenness, their vice and brutal crime, their reckless waste and unthrift, with the industrious peoples of India. Which is highest, even in the scale of civilization? A question not to be asked.

The indebted ryot—indebted, though, except at his children's marriages (and these will be shown not to be so extravagant as is often stated), he is the most frugal of mankind—and the usurious money-lenders are pretty much the same all over India. But I see the "weekly

44 A reference to Thomas Babington Macaulay, "The Prophecy of Capys," in *Lays of Ancient Rome.* Of the she-wolf who nursed Romulus it is said:
"She dies in silence, biting hard,
Amidst the dying hounds."

statement" of the Madras Executive Committee, the 30th of March, reporting: "Within the last few days, the Hindu new year having come, the creditors have closed on their debtors and have sold everything belonging to them." "That will show the intensity of suffering." Indeed it does. Can nothing be done? Government is the first mortgagee on the land. It has all the machinery ready for lending: it would lend at 7 percent. But this is taken advantage of by the ryot in an almost infinitesimal degree. Perhaps in all India only a quarter of a million is out at interest in this way. The question is, why is the indebted ryot unwilling to accept the government loan at 7 percent and why does he prefer going to his own moneylender at five or seven or even ten and fifteen times that rate of interest? Is he afraid of putting himself in the power of minor officials of government? Is he afraid of offending his banker?

It is said, on government authority, in the last India Office Progress Report, that "even when, after floods at Ahmedabad, government sanctioned the advance of £1000 to poor cultivators *without any interest at all*, no one availed himself of the offer." And it is added: "*There are few ryots in a position to offend their banker.* The great object of the moneylender is to evade repayment; if the season is good he lets the debt run on from year to year at 36 percent interest; and this system is preferred by the cultivator *to the tedious formalities and rigid terms of repayment* attached to government advances." It is government which says this. Is there no procedure to obviate it? The same Progress Report speaks of "their" (the moneylenders') "heartless and unscrupulous action towards their debtors," and adds—it is the government who say this: "It is hoped that some amelioration may be effected in the position of the ryots by a modification of the present system of civil procedure."

One echoes the hope that the government is making good their "hope." But the bill now before the Legislature at Simla is not a promising hope. Is it true that the land is passing into the hands of the moneylenders? that three months ago, being the Hindu new year, this process was in great activity? that the ryot is absolutely in the moneylender's power? that the ryot's crops are not his own but the moneylender's? that all over India land is changing hands? that the moneylender sells the ryot up and gets his land for a song? No bidders appear against the Marwari decree holder; a nominal value is put upon the property by the creditor; and, in ninety-nine cases out of a hundred, the property is bought in by him at that nominal price.

What the Marwari is as a landlord may be seen from the Deccan Riots Commission Report, Appendix C. I wish I had room for extracts here. There is no such superiority in intelligence in the ordinary sowkar as would result in improved cultivation. In all that concerns agriculture the Kunbi ryot is superior to the Marwari moneylender and, if the profits of his labour are secured to him, is by no means wanting in industry or enterprise. By converting him into a tenant at a rack rent, these advantages are lost to the land without any compensation whatever. Some of the Marwaris who had accumulated the largest estates were persons who showed open defiance of the law. In civilized countries the lower agricultural class is very much at the mercy of those above it. This evil is intensified in India. And if the Deccan ryot is handed over to such landlords as the Marwaris of Párner, the last state of the ryot will be worse than the first.[45] It is barely a generation in time since government began to divest itself of the powers of an irresponsible landlord for the benefit of the agricultural ryot. To allow these powers to be retransferred to a class with none of the traditions of the hereditary landholder, and probably the least fitted in the whole world to use them, is to sink the ryot into a lower and yet a lower depth.

In the same Progress Report it is stated—it is the financial commissioner who speaks: "That sales and mortgages take place to a large extent is not to be doubted. It is desirable that the landholders should, if possible, retain their lands and should prosper." Probably. It is in relation to the flourishing Punjab that this remark occurs.

In the Bombay ryotwari tenure the independent small landowners, who ought to be the most prosperous, are the most miserable. Is England such a plutocracy that everything naturally runs to favouring money?

But let us favour money in the right way. It is little or not at all considered that whatever money there is in India runs to moneylending and not to manufacture or trade. The tacit encouragement given to usury by our existing law tends to transfer land to the moneylender, a transfer by which, as can be shown, the land does not gain. The landlord is still, of course, the usurer, making the hardest terms possible with his tenant, who is also his debtor and often little better than his slave. But not only this; this same encouragement ties up the capital in

45 A paraphrase of Matt 12:45.

usury instead of letting it flow into commerce, India's great want. In India *capital creates pauperism, not* prosperity through manufacture, trade and commerce or new industries. No one flourishes but the capitalist and *his* flourishing means power of absorbing other people's property. It means reducing to utter misery and slavery a well-to-do and hardworking peasantry. It means that the enormous interest *guaranteed*, one may say, by our own courts to the usurer—with no risk but that of being murdered and this but very seldom, only when the debtor gets desperate—prevents the moneylender or capitalist from doing anything useful with his money, from putting money into honest enterprise, manufacturing, commercial or even agricultural. It means that the use of riches in India is to make the *people poor*, to make them beggars and even to sell them for slaves.

Does the official network of petty administration require improving? In cases where ryots are said to be unwilling to accept the water for irrigation purposes, *why* are ryots unwilling to accept the water? Because it puts them in the power of public works overseers and other minor officials who are all natives. Are bribery, oppression, corruption, bullying the rule, the universal rule with these? They have unlimited power to make themselves disagreeable—almost as much so as the moneylender—and must be bought off with a bribe. In the courts of law, in irrigation works, everywhere, the petty native official steps in and requires a bribe. The cultivator cannot take a single step towards getting justice done him of himself. For instance, our stamp laws meet and baffle him at every turn. He cannot possibly understand them and for every step he has to pay and consult a vakeel (a vakeel is a public authorized pleader in a court of justice), whose dishonesty and cheating is often second only to that of the sowkars. This in itself is almost certain ruin to him. (Deccan Riots Commission: Appendix. See also Mr Pedder's admirable article in *Nineteenth Century* for September 1877. I commend it to the reperusal of those who would see a true picture of this terrible state of things by an eyewitness.)

I come now to individual instances of moneylenders and their victims. The first indication of what led to the Deccan debtors' riots of 1875 is so characteristic that I open with it the saddest series that ever fell to a peaceful periodical to give. It shows that the victims of the Marwari moneylenders are not limited to poor cultivators. It also seems to show that by the arts of peace the Marwaris might be ostracized and ousted, and the villagers might set up their own shops. This occurred in the village of Karde, in the Sirur Taluka of the Pune collectorate. A deshmukh (district hereditary officer) of good family and some influence, a relative of Scindia, who had made a large fortune, in Scindia's service, settled in this village and "fell among thieves,"[46] that is, into the hands of the Marwaris. Two of these, Kalooram and Bhuywadas, got decrees against him and Kalooram took out a warrant of arrest. The deshmukh gave Kalooram personal ornaments and the warrant was not executed. About four months afterwards some ornaments and property belonging to the temple of Vittoba at the deshmukh's house were attached, but at the instance of the villagers Kalooram allowed the attached property to remain in deposit with a third party for two months. It was then taken possession of by Kalooram. A third execution was issued on Kalooram's decree and the deshmukh's houses and lands were sold for a song, there being no bidders against the Marwari decree holder.

The consequences as related here are extracted from a vernacular periodical, which we might call the *Nineteenth Century* of Pune, of January 1875:

> One of the sowkars of Baba Saheb (the deshmukh), by name Kalooram Marwari, obtained decrees against him from the court at Talegaon, put the deshmukh's house up to public auction and purchased it himself for 150 rupees (£15). Kalooram began to pull down the house, though the defendant agreed not only to pay rent for it but to pay his debts. Defendant "took to heart these proceedings" and collected together the village ryots when they came to a unanimous resolution that, as the Marwaris had begun to ruin them, it would be better neither to borrow from them nor to serve them or purchase anything from them in future. [FN:] (How much better!) This unanimous resolution of the villagers put the Marwaris Sachiram, Pratap, Shivram and one or two others to the greatest inconvenience for want of servants, etc. They therefore proposed to remove themselves to Sirur, with the help of the police, by 5 January 1875. When the Marwaris had loaded their carts with their goods and things, the villagers submitted a petition to the sirkar (government) that, as they had given grain to the Marwaris, these should not be allowed to leave the village until the government assessment had been paid by them. "How this application has been disposed of is not known to me."
>
> One of the villagers has opened a grocer's shop at which all purchases are made: "Mr Editor, if the example of these villagers be

46 An allusion to Luke 10:30.

followed everywhere and unanimity of the people secured, the pauperized state of our country will, I think, certainly disappear very soon."

So far the Pune paper, but the story does not, alas! end so well. Besides refusing service as water carriers, barbers, household servants, etc.—in which they were undoubtedly right—the villagers threw dead dogs, etc., into the Marwaris' premises and the moneylenders, retreating to Sirur, the taluka headquarters, petitioned the magistrate, representing themselves as in bodily fear of the villagers.

Five months afterwards, the actual outbreaks occurred in the Pune and Ahmednagar districts. But the remarkable part of these was the absence of serious crime. And in one instance at Damareh, where a Marwari's house was burnt and his leg broken, the rioters themselves saved him by dragging him out of his burning house. The object of the rioters was in every case to obtain and destroy the bonds, decrees, etc., in the possession of their creditors; when these were peaceably given up, nothing more was done. When the moneylender refused or shut himself up, violence was used only to frighten him. In every case inquired into, it appeared that the rioters supposed that the government approved of the proceeding, so deep were their injuries, so strong their trust in us. (The story of this would seem too absurd to be believed even among an Indian peasantry. It was this: that an English *sahib*, having been sold up by a Marwari creditor, had petitioned the queen who had sent out orders that the Marwaris were to give up their bonds. Even the more educated believed that, on a report from India, orders had come from England that the Marwaris were to have their bonds taken from them, that the government officers would connive at the extortion of their bonds from the sowkars. The Mutiny of 1857 affords examples of similar beliefs gaining and holding their ground.) And shall we really not help them by reform, by law, by every means in the power of their law-abiding masters? In most cases the movement was a mere demonstration. It was not so much a rebellion against the oppressor as a attempt to disarm him by taking his weapons (bonds and accounts). The law-abiding spirit of the Kunbi peasantry was shown by their moderation under provocations calculated to produce "dangerous exasperation"—it is the government which says this. And the British authorities themselves allege these disturbances as melancholy proofs how intense were the grievances to drive so patient a people to physical force. (Report on the Pune and Ahmednagar Districts.)

For go to the Bombay Deccan for the deepest tragedies. In Ahmednagar a usurer has, like all the rest, made the helpless ryot sign any bond, having scarcely any knowledge of its contents and powerless to oppose any decree. The civil courts in reality back the fraudulent moneylender by assuming the creditor and debtor to be equals, whereas they are master and slave. A man borrowed of the usurer four maunds of jowari (a sort of Indian corn) worth 6 rupees. Two or three bonds followed and in sixteen months the borrower was sued for 72 rupees, which the lender got with costs—£8 or £9 or £10 for 12*s*. The court considered the thing iniquitous but there was a bond and so they thought they could do nothing. There are thousands of parallel cases. The ryots cannot read or write, the moneylenders forge what documents they please or enter in the bond the most extravagant terms. And these documents are allowed to pass by the courts as "mutual agreements." The borrower has no protection whatever.

Here is a yet deeper depth in the collectorate of Sattara, where the people are the best off, also reported by a government officer (an assistant collector). At Visapur one Appa Rowji owed money on a bond to Hirachand *guzur.* (A guzur is a trader or dealer from Gujarat.) Hirachand threatened to sell him up but promised not to do so if Appa Rowji would get one Appa Malli to go bail for him. The good-natured friend consented and passed a bond for 200 rupees (£20) to the guzur, giving as security for payment his whole house and land. The agreement was that Appa Rowji should at the same time give to Appa Malli a bond of 400 rupees with his land as security. Other money was owing by Appa Rowji to Appa Malli, which made the whole amount up to 400 rupees. This bond, however, was never forthcoming. Time after time Appa Malli was put off. But the guzur was not put off. He lost no time in enforcing *his* bond. He went through all proper proceedings in the civil court. This Shylock[47] was entirely within his bond. And there was no Portia to save poor Appa Malli. His house and lands were seized by the law and given to the moneylender who, adding insult to injury, gave them to Appa Rowji to cultivate. Appa Malli, despairing of all redress by law, waylaid Hirachand guzur and murdered him in open daylight before several witnesses. Appa Malli, so far from concealing anything, courted the fullest inquiry into his money transactions and confessed the murder. He was of course hanged.

---

47 Shakespeare, *The Merchant of Venice*.

Is it thought that this is a solitary instance of this class of maddening wrongs? Extortionate usury, its name is legion.[48] Hear the government officer's remarks: *The ryots learn by bitter experience that they have no chance of obtaining redress in the civil courts, as at present constituted, against the more cunning sowkars* (moneylenders). Without fear for the present or hope for the future, they turn upon their oppressors. Year by year the little independence that is left to the ryots is gradually passing away; and if nothing is done to stop the process, in a few years the whole body of the cultivators will be reduced to the position of mere labourers.

The undue pressure of the land assessment has something to do with this. It is almost out of the question for the cultivators to turn produce into silver without the moneylenders. Some collectors think it would be wise to allow the ryots the option of paying their rents in kind, as in former times. "By no other means, I fear, can the power of the moneylenders be broken." (Deccan Riots Commission Report.) If an administration may have unwittingly brought an ignorant peasantry into such a state as this by requiring an assessment to be paid not in kind but in money, it being utterly impossible for the cultivator to get coin except through the moneylender, it seems rather a sorry jest for an administration to say that it cannot get him out of it—that the results of any fixing of rate of interest by law, of any usurers' act, of any pawnbrokers' act, would be "demoralizing." (See Deccan Riots Commission: Appendix.)

If we have the misfortune to sink a ship with its company of living souls and all its precious freight in deep waters, we do not say that any attempt to prevent similar terrible accidents and to save what can be saved of this would be "demoralizing," that "painful experience" will teach them "prudence," that "the suffering is justified by the results of its teachings upon the sufferers." We hold inquests and inquiries, and we do not rest till we have discovered the causes and how to remove them. Here is a shipwreck, utter, disastrous, of some not hundreds but millions of souls: it is a shipwreck which is repeated every year. *No* hand is stretched out to save. It is a shipwreck which will be repeated, more disastrous, more complete, if that be possible, *every year.* It is not a famine or storm-wave induced by the elements, which comes once in a period. It is the utter demoralization of two races: the

48 An allusion to Mark 5:9.

race that borrows and the race that lends. But no one holds the inquiry. Yes, one commission holds it: the Deccan Riots Commission. But none ask for the report. No one Englishman in Parliament or press has asked the result. There is not a single member of Parliament who has called for it. We do not care for the people of India.

I proceed with the account of the shipwreck. In the collectorate of Dharwad a very large proportion of the cultivators have parted with their occupancy rights: like Esau, they have sold their birthright for a mess of pottage[49] and are now cultivating either as sub-tenants paying high rates, or upon, to them, the most ruinous system of "*kore* tenancy," under which the ryot cultivates the land and hands over to his creditor the bulk of the produce. The moneylender is in fact becoming the small grasping zemindar of the Bombay presidency, so proud of its ryotwari settlement, so contemptuous of the Bengal zemindari settlement. But the moneylender, or in other words the extortionate usurer, is become the occupant and owner not only of the land, but of the ryot. It is not only by rack-renting but by constantly drawing on the debtor-tenant's labour in addition to his rent that the moneylender lives. He is worse and more exacting than the more powerful Bengal zemindar.

Take all the villainies and frauds of the preceding and following instances, multiply *ad libitum* and add to the sum the crowning villainy of all, now to be recounted, and you will have the history of the man the murder of whom is now to be told. In Gujarat a moneylender was murdered on the high road in open day by hired assassins at the instance of his debtors, two of whom were headmen of villages. But besides the quite common villainies he had committed, it was proved in open court (the Sadar court in their criminal capacity) that the price of staving off the creditor's demands had been the dishonour at his hands of the wives and sisters of the peasants who were indebted to him. This is recorded by the court in passing sentence. In the Solapur collectorate, at the other end of the presidency, a moneylender was murdered by some of his debtors, exasperated beyond endurance by the usual grinding oppressions, in the midst of his village, in broad day, among a crowd of his neighbours. All these murderers were of course hanged. The remark of the Revenue Survey commissioner upon these two cases is that they are but aggravated instances of the usual

49 An allusion to Gen 25:29-34.

relations between moneylender and cultivator. The cultivator, proverbially long-suffering, accustomed to ill-usage at all times, yet is goaded at last, having lost all hope of redress from our law or our government, to redress his wrongs by murder and be hanged for it. Even his patient and peaceful nature is roused to desperation by the deeds of such men as these moneylenders. This is the government officer who speaks, not I. (Report of the Deccan Riots Commission.)

What is another and most common means of oppression in certain parts of Bombay presidency? Thousands of instances might be given, resulting from the relations brought about by the action of the courts of civil justice (or injustice) between the moneylending classes and superior holders cultivating by hired labour, and bheels [hired tribal labourers] and members of other rude tribes indebted to the former under various forms of obligation.

Guzur has a bond on stamped paper, purporting to be executed by his servant, acknowledging loan of a sum of money the man can never by any chance repay. Awtya (Awt or aut or aoot is a plough) shows a disposition to leave [the] guzur's service. Instantly his master files a suit against him in the civil court for amount set forth in bond. Awtya, knowing he has no chance of success, does not appear to defend the suit. The court accordingly decrees against him and a distress warrant follows. The poor wretch's few household goods are seized, his wife's little ornaments are taken and he himself is carried off a prisoner to the munsif's court. There his master, having made him utterly helpless, offers him his choice of returning to work or going to the Dhulia jail. He returns to service with his liabilities increased by costs of suit, of his own arrest, etc., and with no proper agreement with his master. It is no part of the court's duty even then to see that his master is bound down to treat him fairly. He serves on for a few more months, or perhaps years, on a pittance of grain and the smallest covering of clothing until, tired out, he again strikes work. Again his master rushes off to the civil court and this time the bheel is not even invited to have his say; another distress warrant is issued without further inquiry. The first the bheel hears of it is from the sepoy come to arrest him. And so it goes on from year to year. What is this man but a slave? He cannot appeal to the judge (not to mention that the judge's court is eighty miles away and months must pass before his complaint can be heard) as, even if his friends did provide the money, he did not defend the suit originally brought in the munsif's court. He is a mere chattel, to be disposed of whenever his master may want money. It is a common occurrence—hundreds of instances could be produced—for one guzur to sell his awtya to another under the pretence of a transfer of the awtya's debts. A well-encumbered bheel, with a decree of the civil court out against him, is a more valuable commodity in the West than one whose liabilities are smaller. (Report of Deccan Riots Commission: Appendix A.)

Here is a very common instance of another and most fatal form of moneylending to bheels. A guzur advances forty rupees to a bheel to buy a bullock, on the understanding that bheel and bullock are to work on the lender's farm, bheel becoming a partner (gowandya) to the extent of half a plough. A bond is made out for the amount advanced, plus 25 percent premium, plus a further amount on account of old debts unjustly claimed. Interest at the rate of 24 percent is charged on the whole amount entered and at the rate of 50 percent on the grain advanced for bheel's food till harvest time. The guzur takes the bheel's labour free for his share of the plough. He keeps the accounts and manages the sales and cheats bheel to his heart's content in the division of the produce. So much so that—it is an assistant collector who reports—this gentleman remembers but two cases in which a gowandya's debt was not *increased* at the end of the year, according to the guzur's accounts, though no one of the bheels ever had more than food and clothes from his partner the guzur.

At the end of the year there is a pretence of adjusting accounts. The first year bheel is put off with the argument that he has to pay for his bullock; next year, too, he gets nothing but clothes and food, and is told he has still something to pay. He asks for a settlement of his account and as a preliminary he is sent for a new stamped paper. His master and two or three "respectable" "*patels*" meet and talk his affairs over. (A patel is the headman of the village who has the general control and management of the village affairs, is head of the police and—this is not ironical—exercises to a limited extent the functions of a magistrate. In some of the cases of fraud I give, the biggest villain was himself a patel. At all events he generally takes care to be "in with" the patels.) A few soft words are said to him. (Of all natives the bheel is the most trusting, the most easy victim. No matter how badly treated, a little present, a promise, puts his neck in the noose again. In former times these same guzurs, after a bheel raid, invited the whole party to a dinner and debauch, as a preface to a settlement, and murdered them all in cold blood when helpless from intoxication.) The bheel is given money to buy his wife a new *sari* and a little liquor for himself. A new bond is made out, the contents of which he does not understand in the least, and he goes back to his work, hoping for a bumper crop and better luck next year. He struggles on for another year or two and then, feeling that the state of things is very unlike partnership—his is all the work and none of the profits—he resolves to leave. Then for the first time he finds out that his partner, or rather his master, has his acceptance for two hundred rupees or more; that the bullock he had toiled for all these years is not his; and that he and all he has are at his master's mercy. The civil court is resorted to and, as in the case of the awtya, all his little goods are seized and sold, and the bheel becomes the guzur's slave.

Are instances of gross oppression of bheels, awtyas and gowandyas by guzurs and others wanted? Again their name is legion. I could fill not only this article but this number and all the numbers of this year of the *Nineteenth Century* and the nineteenth century itself with them. As many labourers, so many oppressions. As many moneylenders, so many frauds, multiplied by an unknown quantity. But room, not subject or inclination, fails me to give more than three typical cases:

HOGA BIN GAYTYA, BHEEL; EERJEE PATEL, GUZUR; PATEL OF MARWAD, TALUKA TALODA

Hoga says he has served for fourteen years and received only ten rupees and his food. Eerjee says that Hoga has worked for him for thirteen years; that he gave him thirty rupees when he first came and nothing since but food and clothes. He now holds his bond executed in 1868 for 175 rupees and has obtained a decree for that amount. The guzur says that his agreement with the bheel was for food only, so he has charged against him every year the cost of his clothes and that these charges, with original advance and interest at 24 percent, mounted up in 1868 to the amount entered in the bond. On its being pointed out to the patel (rather forcibly, I suppose) that slavery is not allowed by the British government and that thirteen years' good work is a very sufficient return for an advance of thirty rupees (£3), he was forced voluntarily to give the bheel an acquittance. This method of compelling voluntary agreement reminds one rather of an English mother who, upon being told that she ought to make her child go to school voluntarily, addressed the infant, stick in hand, thus: "If you don't go to school *woluntally,* I'll bray your brains out." But one very much wishes the method were oftener had recourse to on the money-lenders in the Deccan by government.

The British government does "allow slavery," though not by act of Parliament, nor by act of Legislature of the Government of India, nor of the Viceroy-in-Council, but rather by *want* of act. And the instances where the "slavery is" discovered and "*not* allowed" are the exception, and the instances where it reigns rampant are the rule.

BOODYA BIN KAGRA, BHEEL; RAMDAS PATEL, GUZUR OF NIZUR, IN NANDURBAR

Boodya is now about thirty years old. He has served Ramdas Patel all his life and his father served before him. When he was a boy the patel spent about forty rupees on his marriage. Beyond this amount he cost the patel nothing but food and clothes, and served him for some twenty-five years, first as cattle-herd and later as awtya. Some five years ago the patel agreed to take him as a gowandya and advanced him eighty rupees wherewith to buy a pair of bullocks. At the same time he made him sign a bond for 200 rupees and held a lien on his bullocks and on the whole share of produce that might come to him in the course of his partnership until the amount were paid. Three years ago the patel sold Boodya to Nana Nundram, guzur of the same village, for 200 rupees and next year bought him back for the same amount. Ramdas now holds his bond for 172 rupees with interest at 24 percent, and the same lien on his cattle and share produce; and on his refusing to remain partner longer, seized his bullocks and grain, and threatened him with an action in the munsif's court and imprisonment in the Dhulia jail. Boodya then went to the first assistant collector and on his remonstrating with the patel, Ramdas was obliged to allow that Boodya had been a good and very profitable servant and eventually restored him his bond and his freedom.

To show the extent to which bheels are cheated of their just shares of produce by their guzur partners, the patel's account for the current year as entered in his books (but not paid to the bheel) and the amount as admitted by the patel himself before the assistant collector, are given [in the table below.]

The assistant collector states that "this is by no manner of means the worst case of cheating in account that has come before him, that he rather gives it (query, as an example of the best) because the patel did admit the facts as stated."

My third instance will give the enormous expense to a defendant if, his case being so good that he seems sure of winning, he ventures to meet one of those suits in which we are told the aggrieved party is always sure of finding justice; the account is from the vakeel of one of the parties.

| *Value per Maup* | *As Entered in Ramdas Patel's Account* | | *As Admitted by Patel before Collector* | |
|---|---|---|---|---|
| Rupees | | | | |
| 25 | 15¾ maups | wheat | 21 maups | wheat |
| 32 | 1 " | grain | 2 " | grain |
| 19 | 1 " | linseed | 1 " | linseed |
| 21 | 2 " | toor | 5 " | toor |
| 6½ | 2 " | aniseed | 2 " | aniseed |
| | 60 bundles | tobacco | 80 bundles | tobacco |
| 16 | | | 11 maups | bajri |
| 16 | | | 4 " | rice |
| 12 | | | 1 " | badli |
| | | | 7 maunds | hemp |

NURYA BIN CHAMBARYA, BHEEL, OF SUMSHIRPUR, TALUKA NANDURBAR had executed a bond for forty rupees in favour of gunputsing, sowkar and judoo bin hurjee, patel of the same village. He died some time in August last owning some land. Immediately on his decease his wife (his heir), being unable to cultivate the land, transferred it to Mittya bin Fukera, bheel, a connection of hers. The patel and sowkar brought an action on the bond and the crop (*bajri*—bajri is a smaller Indian corn) growing in Mittya's field was attached in satisfaction of the decree. It was alleged on the other side that the deceased Nurya had sown it and the court eventually decreed that such was the case and sold it for the benefit of the plaintiff, the defendant obtaining nothing from the court for all his labour in tending, weeding, watching, reaping and stacking. And besides he lost his market. The price of bajri during the season was 16 rupees. When the crop was sold the price was but 12½ rupees, and besides he was ruined (see the table below). The unhappy defendant had thus to pay by decree of court nearly £16 on a bond of £4 and we say that we want to induce the bheels to cultivate!

I have given only three instances, taken as three types, but almost at random. There are cases so much worse that "it is perfectly sickening," as the principal bheel agent in Khandeish reports, "to sit and listen to them."

Some few more observations: We are invariably told of the "hopeless" "recklessness," "improvidence" and "extravagance" of the Deccan ryot as constituting a bar to every improvement. His recklessness is necessity, necessity induced by a rack-rent assessment and by the sowkars, backed by our own civil courts, making him forever roll his stone, like Sisyphus, uphill. His extravagance is limited to an occasional marriage festival, said rarely to exceed fifty rupees and never seventy-five. And these occasions occur seldom. His imprudence is no more than that of all uncivilized races who live only in the present. And does the peasant or even the artisan of our civilized race rush spontaneously to lay by in a good year to meet a bad one? And do we consider him "hopeless" or do we multiply government savings' banks, co-operative stores, coffee public houses and the like to save him—though not so much as we ought?

| | Rs. | Annas | Pie |
|---|---|---|---|
| Original claim, principal and interest | 40 | 0 | 0 |
| Costs in the case | 11 | 0 | 6 |
| Durkhast stamp | 0 | 1 | 0 |
| Batta for executing warrant | 1 | 0 | 0 |
| Security stamp | 0 | 8 | 0 |
| Auction notice, first time 4 annas; second time 8 annas | 0 | 12 | 0 |
| Cost of guarding bajri after seizure | 16 | 0 | 0 |
| Revenue assessment (one instalment) | 12 | 4 | 0 |
| Managing Karkun's pay | 8 | 0 | 0 |
| Threshing the bajri | 9 | 0 | 0 |
| Carting bajri to the Court | 9 | 0 | 0 |
| Brokerage 8 annas; cart-hire of bajri from threshing floor | 2 | 0 | 0 |
| Storing of bajri, guards' pay after bajri brought to court | 18 | 0 | 0 |
| Defendant's expenses in defending suit | 28 | 0 | 0 |
| Total | 157 | 9 | 6 |

The results of the commission's inquiries show that undue prominence has been given to the expenditure on marriage and other festivals as a cause of the ryot's indebtedness. . . . In a course of years the total sum spent in this way by any ryot is not larger than he is justified in spending on social and domestic pleasures. . . . The constantly recurring small items of debt for food and other necessaries, for seed, for bullocks, for the government assessment, do more to swell the indebtedness of the ryot than an occasional marriage. . . . *Ancestral* debt is a chief cause of the ryot's indebtedness. (Report of Committee on Pune and Ahmednagar Riots.)

We are told that education will raise the ryot out of this Slough of Despond,[50] out of this Shylock's hands. At the rate at which education is going on now, it will be a long time first, about as long as it takes to create out of a nebula a world. Do we supply the means of education so fast that we expect anything else?

This was already written when important evidence by a collector in the Bombay presidency unhappily confirmed every previous misgiving. He says that in his collectorate:

> The general condition of the people is, as a rule, at the centres of trade, satisfactory. In the agricultural portions the reverse is the case, the cultivators being more or less involved in debt which, with high rate of interest charged—the result, too often, of *fictitious bonds,* combined with the facility with which *civil courts decree against* them—are fast tending to their holdings or land being alienated from them, and they merging into the position of mere serfs; they being permitted by their rapacious creditors still to cultivate their lands, on payment of rental, barely sufficient to support them and their families. The state of these classes of the population was urged some three or four years ago on the attention of higher authority and the adoption of remedial measures suggested for their protection. The question though was stated to be one which *education* alone can in course of time overcome; *when* the remedy may be expected to reach these classes is evidently still a future uncertainty far distant, *if the measures taken to impart education* to these classes be regarded. Unless some other more feasible remedy be adopted, there is little doubt but that the land tenure in the course of years in this district will largely assume that of rack-rentals. (Appendix to Deccan Riots Report.)

"The remedy is education," which is much like saying, education is a sufficient remedy because it is not. We give these people laws and institutions fit only for an educated people; and then we say, they are not educated, therefore, these laws are enough. A feeling of pathetic and sympathetic respect overwhelms one when one sees these collectors and magistrates labouring so hard and so well, often with such an insight (which they alone can have) into the condition of their charges

---

50 An allusion to John Bunyan, *Pilgrim's Progress,* part 1.

and into its causes, and wholly powerless to remove, sometimes even to palliate these causes, while the only remedies urged upon them are those they know to be either none or to be impracticable.

We are told that the ryot has the remedy of English justice; this remedy and that remedy, our courts, and the rest. He has not. A man has not that which he can't use. As one of our noble heroic class of Indian officials well says: "You might as well put a revolver into an Andaman Islander's hand and tell him to take his remedy on a tiger with it. The man doesn't know how to use the remedies he's ironically credited with and if he did, he has no ammunition. What he does is to go with his case to the nearest magistrate, who is obliged with inward rage and shame to tell him he can't help him, and retreats into his tent to shorten the disagreeable interview, while the unlucky petitioner is turned away by the peons, vociferating that there is no justice in the country." (Report of Deccan Riots Commission: Appendix.) And no more there is for him. What is this jargon about "security given by English rule" when there is no security that a man shall not any day be made a slave? The same evidence in this report says that to base a system (in the Bombay presidency) on the principle that "every man can take care of himself" works as would a factory of which the engineers should assume wood to have the properties of steel.

Hear what the government itself says but does not do. Once when a revenue commissioner brought the matter before the Governor-in-Council, the Governor-in-Council recorded the following resolution. He "entertains no doubt of the fact that the labouring classes of the native community suffer enormous injustice from the want of protection by law from the extortionate practice of moneylenders. He believes that our civil courts have become *hateful*" (this is the word of the Governor-in-Council) "to the masses of our Indian subjects from being made the instruments of the almost *incredible* rapacity of usurious capitalists. Nothing can be more calculated to give rise to widespread discontent and disaffection to the British government than the practical working of the present law." Could the greatest orator have opened the matter more forcibly than it is opened by this resolution? "The attention of the Legislative Council on the subject should be requested and"—what is to be done?—"copy of the revenue commissioner's letter forwarded for their consideration." (Report of Committee on Pune and Ahmadnagar Riots.) And so the matter drops.

What are these civil courts which the Governor-in-Council declares "hateful" to the people, and the "instruments of," not the protectors from, "incredible rapacity" and "usurious capitalists"? The civil courts make procedure the whole question, right or wrong is put on one side. As soon as the debtor has acknowledged his signature, it is all over with him. A criminal court investigating the same transaction would discover that the signature was indeed his but obtained by fraud. It is the commonest thing in the world for a bond to promise the payment of money which never has been, and which both parties very well know never will be, paid to the cultivator; for a man to sign as he thinks an acknowledgment of ten rupees and to find himself condemned on his own signature to pay a hundred rupees "with costs," and even for the creditor to avoid by subterfuge the payment of a single pie of the loan for which he holds an acknowledgment conclusive in court. This is the civil court, or rather the law which that court has to administer. The criminal court is cheap; the civil court dear. The criminal, or at any rate the magistrates' courts, where the procedure always begins, are expected to find out the truth by all means in their power. The magistrate is responsible for justice and no excuse is accepted if he, by his own fault, fails to do it. The magisterial courts work under a system of cheap appeals and constant supervision.

> The ruin of the cultivators, the brigandage amounting to open rebellion, the disturbances caused by sheer desperation and almost every difficulty encountered in levying the revenue of government, are caused principally by the sheer inefficiency of our civil courts for the only purpose which gives them a *raison d'être*—the administration of common justice between man and man. (Deccan Riots Commission: Appendix.)

A man said: If an Oxford undergraduate gets into debt, you help him by right of his folly; the courts take his part against the "usurious, grasping moneylender." The court of Chancery, says the report on the Deccan riots, feels itself justified in refusing the help of law to a London moneylender who has taken advantage of the "weakness and necessities of the defendant" by imposing on him terms which would be *moderate* in Ahmadnagar. What are the English young gentleman's "weakness and necessities" compared with those of the poor Indian peasant, guiltless of letters? And how is the ryot served by "English justice"?

In the civil courts the woes of mankind are supposed to be curable by passing decrees. . . . The pressure of work prevents the judges from seeing how those decrees are executed, while their method of conducting business makes them all but inaccessible to poor and ignorant petitioners who find all other officers sitting at the tent door. . . . A return of the percentage of processes served by each peon (a peon is the inferior officer of the court; like all others he may be called not an officer but a bride taker) of all committed to him for service would be a surprising document. (Report of Deccan Riots Commission: Appendix.) On renewal of bonds the creditor bribes the court subordinates *not* to serve the notice on the debtor.

Nay, in two ways we have ourselves been one main cause of the cultivator's miseries, though most unwittingly. The facilities for recovery of debt offered by our civil courts called into existence an inferior class of moneylenders dealing at exorbitant rates of interest with the lower class of agricultural poor. The value of the ryot's title under the Survey Settlements came to be recognized; his own eagerness to extend his cultivation grew; a fresh start was given to the moneylender. Thus a stimulus to borrowing was actually given by our Survey Settlement together with a stimulus to lending by increased facilities for recovery. (Report.)

One more word about the present urgent state of things. The doings of the Marwaris far exceed the limits of fair trading and it is not so much their object to trade with the ryots as to get them by fair means or foul (how often fair?) into their hands, so that they may use them as tools to make their fortunes. (Report of Deccan Riots Commission: Appendix.) This is not I who speak, it is a superintendent of Revenue Survey. "Three fourths of deeds between poor and rich men in this country are false, and the law ... encourages fraud and forgery." Again it is not I who speak, it is a high government officer in the Appendix of the Deccan report.

Is it possible to lay bare a more hideous state of things?.

## Famine Mortality, 1876-79

**Editor:** Questions having been raised as to the exactness of Nightingale's mortality statistics concerning the recent famine, she went into great detail to explain her sources, without losing sight of the huge problem of the unacceptable number of deaths due to famines. There was a special difficulty in determining the actual number of deaths in a famine, not just the "registered deaths"; the latter sometimes amounted to only "22 percent of the real number of deaths" (see p 818 below). In correspondence with Louis Mallet she explained the problem she had encountered, but showed that she was ready to accept his corrections and suggestions; she clarified her statements in a "memorandum" to the India Office (see p 826 below).

Source: Letter, Balliol College, Mallet Papers

35 South St.
Park Lane, W.
10 August 1878

*Article Nineteenth Century. Private and Confidential*
Dear Sir Louis Mallet[51]

I cannot thank you enough for your most kind letter. But the first thing is to try to answer your question, so that all should be at least honestly trying to get at some kind of truth and measure as to the loss in the recent famine.

Your question is: Whence come my "figures" "about the *deaths* from the recent famine"? The "papers from the Government of India" speak only of "*registered*" deaths. And you say "we cannot make up more than about 1,300,000, including Mysore." Now the "famine commissioner" in *Mysore* alone reports "a *decrease in population* of 1,250,000" (scarcely less than the "1,300,000") dealing with such enormous numbers, alas! My unlucky paper ["The People of India," 1878] gives "our LOSS in one year's famine" (*not* "*deaths* FROM famine," still less "*registered* deaths from famine")—the probable *decrease* of population, disappearance of population—"in southern India, that is, in Mysore, Bombay and Madras." Also in the previous sentence, "We have *lost* in one year" "*out of* the 20 millions more especially under the famine scourge in Madras presidency"—meaning *not* the "deaths from famine" but the disappearance (*loss*) of population—what the "famine commissioner" means when he "reports that the results of the partial census" "show a *decrease in population* of" - - Or, as army returns say, "a *loss* of" - - , meaning killed, wounded *and missing.*

2. The only contradiction or explanation of my figures which reached me (and did not reach me till after my paper was out) is this: "At one period there were 200,000 famine refugees in Madras. This would raise the population to say 600,000. Taken over the year 1876-77 the total deaths on this number were 25,000. In 1875-76 the deaths on the normal population were 14,415, so that the famine added 10,585 deaths out of "200,000 refugees." "These 200,000 people all came from deserted villages and would be counted as deaths there, while only 10,585 of them died."

51 Sir Louis Mallet (1823-90), permanent under secretary of state for India 1874-83.

Had this reached me in time, I should have put it in. But it explains so very small (comparatively) a number. And there are not so many "Madras cities." The same authority says, "We have no reliable information about famine *mortality*, except for Madras City." "We cannot get the total mortality without a census."

3. As to "*registered*" deaths, how many were *not* registered? in the deserted villages, in the ditches, by the roadsides, among wanderers into wild places in search of food, deserted children and old people especially: were the dead bodies or the missing "registered," counted or even found? Officially, or unofficially, has it been doubted that those who were *not* may be guessed at but never known? Would not the only way be to take a complete census and compare it with the estimated population from the last census?

4. Would not the "*decrease*/disappearance of population," i.e. (population unaccounted for), as resulting from a census, general or partial, include deaths from famine, cholera, smallpox and fever (indirect consequences of famine), decrease of births, migration, etc.

5. Has the *Bombay* government always declined, and does it decline still, giving any estimate of its famine mortality?

6. The Viceroy-in-Council is said to have stated "that the papers now before the Government of India do *not* furnish means for forming a correct estimate of the famine mortality in southern India during 1876-78." And he is quite right.

7. The "figures" in my "paper" were "taken" from those I saw of the "trial census operations" on 14 March in Madras presidency. Among those I saw were few beyond those I gave. (*Salem* was counted as to its entire population in order to correct error from migration.)

The estimate of "LOSS" (NOT "deaths") "in one year's famine" (*not* FROM famine) "out of the 20 millions more especially under the famine scourge in Madras presidency" and, again, "in Mysore, Bombay and Madras" was appended to this letter. I have sought to point out possible sources of error and discrepancy rather than to justify myself.

N.B. The "papers" give the "*registered deaths*" (how can *all* deaths from famine in a country like India be *registered*? and how can they know the deaths among the migrations?) over a population of *13,765,165* in Madras presidency. Mine gives the probable *loss* over a population of *20 millions* which takes in migration.

Your estimate of "1,300,000" which, may God grant, is the correct one, is it of "*registered* deaths"? and is it of *Bombay*, Madras and Mysore?

I regret more than I can say that I have not been more explicit in my paper as to what "*loss*" means, i.e., population *unaccounted for*, population *disappeared, missing*, and have left out the words "*probably*," "*perhaps*."

And in the first part of the paragraph I have left words in which I cannot justify to myself; but it is *not these* figures which you question, e.g., "deaths from famine," "have died" instead of "were gone" (as I did put in one place) or have *disappeared*, words which, had I known what I do now, I should have modified thus. The alteration of *five words would have done it*. And made it absolutely correct. I waited *two months* for some *con*tradiction and none came—these "figures" appeared in the *Times* of 15 May in a letter from their Madras correspondent of 20 April. And no contradiction, official or unofficial, has appeared.

I would rather say, I *should* regret more than I can say (and God forbid that the estimate in my paper should prove correct even by millions, though I still fear that it may not be much over the mark!)—but that I am sure *you* will not think this "cant"—I should esteem the loss of any (writing) reputation of mine as nothing if only official attention at home could be directed to the broad facts of the condition of the people in India—even by my blunders and stumbles—facts which *are* appreciated by many of the officials out there. But *they* are handcuffed.

And who can appreciate their labours as I do? They need not complain of me. One feels a sort of *agonizing* respect for them.

8. Would you kindly advise me to put in the next No. of the *Nineteenth Century* a sort of fly note explaining what the "figures" in my paper mean: the impossibility of *registering* deaths in a south India famine? Or had I better wait till more perfect information can be had?

9. Would you be so very good as to send me "papers relating to the partial census in the famine-stricken districts of India," including "Extract from Despatch from Government of India to Secretary of State for India about the *North-West Provinces*"? (They have been sent to the *Times*.)

I am glad that you do *not* "defend" me for the cause's sake, which is all we either of us care for: it is "3 millions" times more important that you should not "lose your character" than that I should lose all mine.

As to my paper being "a shriek," we cannot cry without crying, i.e., loud enough to be heard, any more than we can fight without fighting. If a town crier were as old, as worn-out and as cracked as I, his cry *would* be "a shriek." I do not at all quarrel with them for saying that. But what always strikes me as a hypocrisy, worse than that of the "Scribes and Pharisees,"[52] is that, while we prate and gabble as if we were the Apostles of the Gospel of Administration, about our "mission" to govern the "benighted millions" of our "vast Eastern Empire" "for the people's own sakes," etc., scarcely six men can be got together in the House of Commons "for the people's own sakes" when the "millions" of our "vast Indian Empire" are at stake. (Teignmouth Shore[53] said in a sermon, "we talk of the inscrutable dealing of Providence, we had better talk of the inscrutable dealings of Englishmen.")

*I* am amazed at my own moderation (in my paper), e.g., I could have given a list (out of official report) of the principal landholders—Marwari *moneylenders* in Deccan places—against each of whose names figures a list of forgeries, thefts, etc., which Satan himself might have envied. In Madras (but I think I bored you with this before) people say that, if it were once understood *why* the ryot refuses government loans at low interest and prefers paying his moneylender exorbitant rates, the difficulty would soon be overcome, but that officials who wish to know and serve the ryots under their charge rather than please the authorities over them do not as a rule rise high in office.

Had I had time, however, I should have given more coherence, more correctness of expression, less vehemence to my poor little article. But—always, as I am, under severe stress of business and illness—I had to write it between 5 A.M. and 7:30 A.M. in the mornings, as I have written my letters to you. But this, I know, is no excuse for publishing a bad article. *I* judge it more severely than anyone else can, I assure you. But, you will say, this is of little use now.

Do not give me up, that is all I ask. I will never "claim" you. I did not receive your most kind letter of 8 August till this morning (10 August). I am anxious to answer it at once. (I am at Lea Hurst, Cromford,

52 An allusion to Matt 23:13 and many similar passages.

53 John Shore (1751-1834), 1st Baron Teignmouth, governor general of India. He was educated at Harrow and went out to India as a writer in the Bengal Civil Service in 1769. He became a member of the Supreme Council 1787-89, in which capacity he assisted Lord Cornwallis in introducing many reforms, but did not approve his permanent settlement of Bengal. On the retirement of Cornwallis, he became governor general 1793-98. On his return to England he was appointed member of the Board of Control 1807-28 and was for many years president of the British and Foreign Bible Society.

Derby, attending to my mother and have hardly any of my papers here.) I do most cordially echo all you say about Mr Caird's mission and I live in hope of your future "*commission*" *on land tenure* and on the "condition of the people" "to obtain facts."

Pray forgive this letter of unreasonable length and pray believe me, dear Sir Louis Mallet, somewhat penitently but

ever yours faithfully and gratefully
Florence Nightingale

Source: From three letters to Sir Louis Mallet, the first two written on the same day, Balliol College, Mallet Papers

Lea Hurst
Cromford, Derby
13 August 1878

*Article Nineteenth Century.* May I have your permission to send you by *this* afternoon's post a copy of the *Nineteenth Century* article ["The People of India"] with the words *corrected* up to what I *ought* to have said?

You are so kind as to say that you will "have the paper critically examined" at the India Office. Please let it be the *corrected* copy that shall be so "examined." I feel that I can never thank you enough for all your kindness.

13 August 1878

I venture to send you the CORRECTED copy of my paper. . . . It would please me indeed to have this copy "critically examined" as you kindly propose.

After repeated sending to news agents I have at last received the *Pall Mall Gazette* of 25 July and mean at once to study H.'s article.[54]

28-29 August 1878

A man who had been twenty years in India in all kinds of (local) posts says that the intricacy of our procedure in some things, the rigidity of our procedure in others, do so "mystify" the poor ryots that "under the village fig tree"[55] they ascribe all their woes to us. . . .

---

54 Henry Mayers Hyndman (1842-1921), socialist leader, wrote on "The Bankruptcy of India" in *Nineteenth Century* 4 (October 1878): 585-608 and 5 (March 1879): 443-62. The author who signed "H." at the end of an article, "A Famine-Stricken Peasantry" in the *Pall Mall Gazette* of 25 July 1878 seems to be the same Hyndman: he uses the same theme of "bankruptcy."

55 Possibly an allusion to John 1:48, 50.

*Private.* You are so good as to say that you will ask Lord Cranbrook[56] whether he objects to my seeing the papers and reports mentioned in your memo. I had a kind little note from Lord Cranbrook about my poor little paper in the *Nineteenth Century,* but he evidently thinks that the "indebtedness" applies merely to the "Pune and Ahmadnagar" districts and that my paper exaggerates, if not the intensity of the evil there, yet the *extent* of it in India.

Mr Stanhope [Parliamentary under secretary of state for India], in answering a question and presenting the "Deccan Riots" report in the *House of Commons,* said the same thing (I think in answer to Mr Grant-Duff).[57] Surely this can only arise from Lord Cranbrook not yet having had time to examine the subject.

Not only does the "Deccan Riots" report ("Pune and Ahmadnagar") deal with nearly every part of the Bombay presidency, Sind inclusive, but it also deals with the North West Provinces, with the Central Provinces and in some measure with the Punjab and Oudh.

But I have also been "distressed" with letters received from Indian officials and ex-officials in England, directly or indirectly (there has not been time for letters from India), saying, "All this *I* have known in *my district*" or "*I* have had to condemn ryots (according to law) to be bond-slaves without being even allowed (by law) to represent the case to higher authority." As it happened, not one of these men was from the Bombay presidency at all, much less from "Pune" or "Ahmadnagar."

Source: From a letter to William Clark [engineer in Calcutta, then in Madras], Florence Nightingale Museum (LMA) H1/ST/NC1/78/3

6 September 1878

*Private.* About Madras I wish I could give you good and certain news of it. (I had a great correspondence with the governor and the secretary of state for India not quite a year ago about it.) But, I believe, during the famine year the whole municipality resources were engaged in saving life from famine and, except increased expenditure in cleansing

---

56 Né Gathorne Hardy (1814-1906), from 1878 Gathorne-Hardy and 1st Lord Cranbrook, Conservative secretary of state for India.

57 (Sir) Mountstuart Elphinstone Grant-Duff (1829-1906), Parliamentary under secretary of state for India 1868-74 and for colonies 1880-81, governor of Madras 1881-86; speech in Hansard, *Parliamentary Debates,* 3rd series (1830-91) 27 June 1878:321. Lady Grant-Duff helped Nightingale find suitable authors to write health primers in vernacular languages; correspondence with her appears in *Social Change in India.*

for the additional 200,000 people that filled its streets, there was nothing done. The grievances which can only be removed by water supply and house drainage still remain. And the governor, though with an extraordinary knowledge of detail, scarcely seems awake to the necessity of what alone can give efficiency to his details. The India Office has tried to stir him up. I hope you will hear good news on inquiry in London.

And believe me, if you can tell me that your Madras scheme is going to be carried out, I can hear no better news in this world. (But "economy" so-called is all the rage now in India, I fear.)

Source: From a copy of a letter to James Caird, Add Mss 45805 f87

5 October 1878

I cannot thank you enough for all your kindness. I wish you "God-speed" with all my might on your great mission [as member of the Famine Commission]. (You cannot guess how disappointed I am not to be able to see you before you go.) My best wishes will follow your mission everywhere. If I may, I shall perhaps send after you to India any questions that may appear worth suggesting, without of course expecting any answer till your return, which may God prosper with a great freight of important work for India. (If I may, I shall send occasionally to your house in London to know what news of you.)

As you do not leave London till the 9th, I may perhaps venture to send you (in London) on the 7th some questions on the "Printed Questions" of the "Famine Commission." These will of course require no answer; if they are worthless you can but throw them into the Red Sea.

Now God speed your mission and bring you safe home again and bring India safe too.

Source: From a letter to Major General James George Fife, Wayne State University, folder 37 letter (14)

20 December 1878

6. It seems almost too grievous now to recur to the famine, but completed reports are now coming in giving the mortality at actually higher than the estimate I gave and as over 6 millions. Do you remember the papers moved for and presented to Parliament just before it rose in August? These gave the famine deaths at 1,300,000. Now those deaths were the *registered* deaths. I asked at the time what was the estimated proportion of *registered* famine deaths to total actual famine deaths but received no answer.

Shortly after I received from Simla a bundle containing the same papers as those presented to Parliament but it contained one more in which the *registered* deaths were estimated as *22 percent* of the *total deaths* from famine. And the reports now coming in and closely entering into all the deaths, figure by figure, give the total ascertained mortality very much the same as the estimated mortality is given in that Simla paper, *not* presented to Parliament.

These reports are not yet published. The famine is forgotten. People's minds are so taken up with this [Second] Afghan War [1878-80], on one side or the other, that they forget the far deeper tragedy than any that can be acted there, which took place but one short year ago here in southern India, an interest of immeasurably greater magnitude. I have made no use, public or private, of these facts. I was too heartsick.

Source: From four letters to Sir Louis Mallet, Balliol College, Mallet Papers

4 January 1879

*Famine deaths.* People's minds are so taken up with this Afghan War, on one side or the other, that they forget the far deeper tragedy than any that can be acted there, which took place but one short year ago here in southern India, an interest of immeasurably greater weight.

You will have observed the completed reports fast coming in which give the actual ascertained mortality as even higher than the estimated mortality, which was called a "shriek." The papers moved for and presented to Parliament (just before it rose in August last) gave the famine deaths at 1,300,000? And Mr Gladstone, in his paper (*Nineteenth Century* of this month) gives them as 1,400,000? Now the actual ascertained mortality for Madras presidency alone (*not* including "diminished rate of births," etc.) is a little over *2 millions.* The deaths "presented to Parliament" were the *registered* deaths. It was asked at the time what was the probable proportion of *registered* deaths to *actual* famine deaths. But no answer was made. That answer can now be given.

The Famine Commission of Mysore had given the *loss* in that state alone as 1,250,000 for the famine year (see those Parliamentary papers). It is from Mysore that the first accurate intelligence comes to us. Included in those papers but not presented to Parliament (it was sent me from Simla) was an actual statement. It was ascertained for one month (January 1878) by actual enumeration that the *registered* deaths (in Mysore) were *22 percent* of the real number of deaths. "The deaths *registered* in the mortuary returns of the province from January

1877, when famine began to result in increased mortality, up to the end of the year when the test census was taken were 224,813. 1,050,000 represents the actual number of deaths in the famine year, whether due directly to famine and the diseases which follow on it, or to other causes." (This is 22 percent.) This does *not* include the diminished births to be expected, and on the other hand it *allows* for the expected return hereafter of half the emigrants, half of whom are supposed to have died.

In the twenty days between the preliminary and final census in December 1877 and January 1878, "when there was hardly any famine in the country," there was a death rate of 127.8 per 1000 and a birth rate of only 7 per 1000. *The persons who were dead had actually been seen alive by the European officers.* Here then the deaths were actually ascertained (and not registered). "Such a rate of mortality, if continued for 8½ years, would have exterminated the whole population." The death rate and birth rate *thus* taken between preliminary and final census were absolutely correct. The "decrease in population" of Mysore is given, in the papers presented to Parliament, as "one and a quarter millions." The population of Mysore may be taken at 5,200,000 (see chief commissioner). *One fourth of the population* therefore is gone: 24.94 percent. This is what was called a "shriek." (The Madras presidency statements are, if possible, almost more miserable.)

It was ascertained then for one month, by actual counting, that the *registered* deaths (in Mysore) were *22 percent* of the *actual* number of deaths. If the registered deaths in *each* month were 22 percent of the truth, we should have as the *true rate* of mortality a little over a million, or 1,050,000 of actual deaths. If to this be added the mortality among the emigrants in Coory and the Wynaad, it accounts, says the authority (Parliamentary papers), for the million and a quarter lost. ("The mortuary statistics of the province have never made even an approach to accuracy." In ordinary years "in the five years preceding the famine," "about two thirds of the deaths were never recorded.") Thus far quoting from the paper which was one of the packet presented to Parliament but which must have been overlooked.

*Madras Famine.* Now for the complete reports just coming in from Madras presidency and elsewhere, we gather the strangest information as to the methods of registration in Madras presidency, e.g., such famine deaths as were registered being registered under "*All other causes,*" etc., BECAUSE it was announced that "no death was to be allowed by famine."

You know that registration (outside the municipalities) is *not* compulsory, that it is carried out by the village officials, many of whom died or wandered from home like their poor clients; many avoided registering the dead because they received *relief* for the *dead* and many registered only as it would please the European masters. (I should take it as a favour, a distressing favour, if you would direct me to *draw you up a memo of the facts and methods of registration* in the *Madras* presidency, also of the facts and methods of making *lists for famine* relief by *village headmen.* I am tempted to do it here but this letter is already too long. After all, was the famine relief relief or starvation?)

*To return.* In Madras presidency the seventeen months' returns from November 1876 to March 1878 show an *excess* of deaths of 1,140,048 OVER the average of the same months in former years, while the test census shows a decrease of population of at least 3 millions. Such was the disorganization during the famine of village life and communal administration that "not one half of the actual deaths were ever recorded." The losses by DEATH are reckoned by the authorities (roughly) at rather more than *two millions,* the diminished birth rate at one million *besides* or over 3 millions in all.

Much has been made of the famine emigrants who, we hoped, would return. But alas! no more than 100,000 can thus be accounted for. There was no such mystery as was supposed about these emigrations. Whither the various streams *set* from each district was perfectly well known. In most cases, by questioning the survivors at home who had heard from their emigrating relatives (or not heard), accurate information has been obtained as to the deaths. This, family customs in India render easy. I could give such a multitude of facts (and explain methods of enumeration and sources of error) but I will only here sum up this disastrous history. It is stated on the highest authority that the figures given in regard to the famine mortality were *under* the mark, that our probable losses of population in *Madras* are *more than 3 millions* (to wit, over *2* millions *deaths,* 1/3 million diminished births). The loss in *Mysore* has been already estimated at more than *a million* and the losses in *Bombay* and *Hyderabad* "must have been more than two millions." "These facts," it is added, "have come out the more strongly from attempts having been made to explain them away." (In Madras presidency in *ordinary* years about two thirds of the deaths are registered and a little over one half of the births.)

I have made no use, public or private, of these facts. I have not even written to Lord Cranbrook, nor to Mr Stanhope, who presented the false figures in Parliament. I am so heartsick that I do not care to revive the personal question. But you have been so truly kind that I actually venture to appeal to you for advice. *What shall I do?* It did occur to me also that *you* might write some "instruction" to Mr Caird to inquire about these collateral points.

N.B. I have reports speaking of the *money famine* following in the steps of the grain famine and no way of meeting it but by advancing "Takavi" for wells, etc., carrying out public works, etc. It is these after-consequences of famines on the half-starved and ruined survivors that are terrible to think of and in England scarcely thought of. "There are more things 'twixt heaven and earth than are dreamt of"[58] in Simla's "philosophy" or in the India Office's (as I remember you once said). And now here is this Afghan War to drain away the little life there is left—stopping all improvements—as we hear.

10 January 1879

*Famine (Madras).* I am very grateful to you for your most weighty note of yesterday. I will send you *in the course of today* some figures, which I hope will clear up those which you justly say are confused. But the very circumstances of the case are "confusion worse confounded."[59] I too look upon Mr Caird's future report with the very highest hope, as the *only* hope in fact. I mean to live till he comes back, to read it and make much of it. But *you* must tell him that it *must be written in the style of the Deccan Riots Report,*[60] with chapter and verse, *facts* with name and place and individual narratives (and not in the style of the Indian reports with which we are inundated). Then I will venture to say the English public will care and listen.

Would you think well to send him a copy of Mr [Edward] Prinsep's irrigation schedules as far as relates to Madras, etc., by no means as absolute information but as asking *him* for information? Thank you for sending me a copy.

17 January 1879

*Private.* I cannot say how thankful I am that you are looking into this miserable famine mortality, for it is unspeakable. I will answer your last question first.

---

58 Shakespeare, *Hamlet,* Act 1, scene 5.

59 John Milton, *Paradise Lost* ii.995.

60 In 1875 there were agrarian riots in the Deccan, a revolt of peasants overly exploited by moneylenders.

1. "Report on the Test Census in Mysore" by C.A. Elliott dated 10 July 1878 (19 pp) accompanied from Simla (to me) the papers presented by Parliament. But indeed, indeed I did not say or even hint that "Mr Stanhope had suppressed this paper." I do apologize—not only a "Parliamentary" apology—if I used any word that could by possibility be construed into this. I think what I said was (and perhaps I should not have said *that*): Mr Stanhope presented the "false figures" to Parliament. The figures *are* "false," are they not? You yourself, in your letter of yesterday, state the Mysore deaths alone as very nearly the number of the *whole* famine deaths presented to Parliament. But I said the "*figures*" were "false," not that Mr Stanhope was "false." I could not anyhow say or think that they were "falsely" presented, only that they were incorrect.

*Could you be so very kind as to send me a copy of "Mr Elliott's Report" which* you say "reads like Defoe's *History of the Plague*"?[61] I do not think I can have seen it.

2. I will send you, I hope, in the course of tomorrow, the figures which I received from Madras, and which are authoritative, about the Madras mortality. I see you say "the information which has reached us *officially*": I was told that these were sent to me "privately" and that I must not make use of them till they were "issued" by the government officially. (I meant to have sent them you last week as I promised. And I heartily beg your pardon for not doing so. My only excuse is that I am so overworked.)

3. As to Bombay and Hyderabad, those figures also reached me from India, but I have no report and no particulars. (I have today both written and telegraphed for these.) You say truly that Mr Hewlett is an "admirable specimen," I hardly know anyone like him. He is a kind of hero in practice.

I await with the utmost anxiety the "statement of all the information which has reached" you "officially as to famine mortality," which you so kindly mean to send me. I will also send mine, *not* "official." But I would not delay my explanation about the "suppressed paper"—even for my figures—a day. Again saying that you can hardly conceive the relief of knowing that the India Office is fathoming this terrible subject "officially."

---

61 Daniel Defoe was a child during the great plague of London, 1665. He wrote *A Journal of the Plague Year,* 1722, based mainly on his father's and older brother's experiences.

20 January 1879

*Madras famine figures.* I send you the *Madras* famine figures, as promised. I have only dealt with the Madras figures because, as you have Mr Elliott's last report, you probably know as much as or more than I (though I had begun abstracting his figures) for *Mysore.* I have telegraphed and written to India for the *Bombay and Hyderabad* figures in detail. (I have indicated at the bottom of some pages of the enclosed under what headings I could supply you with figures yet more in detail concerning Madras.)

My figures concern only the south India famine. Have you seen a statement of Mr Knight's upon Sir G. Cooper's statement on the "Famine Relief Works" in North West Provinces? (Mr Knight was an under secretary, I believe, of the Government of India and is now, I think, editor of the *Statesman,* Calcutta.) An English official in India sent it to me with a note (I do not know him) containing this "highly treasonable" opinion: "Despotic governments never reform themselves," etc. There would be one hope for India, I mean for interesting the people here in India, if an Indian Dickens could arise or if the *Daily News* would send out a McGahan or a Forbes to travel about the interior of India as "special correspondent," or if the *Times* would think India of almost as much importance as Cyprus, or if your friend *Punch* would go to India.

Source: From a letter to C.B.N. Dunn,[62] Derbyshire Record Office

21 January 1879

The famine mortality figures are coming in from India: they are heart-sickening. Rather more than 2 millions deaths in Madras presidency alone; altogether it will not be short of 3 1/4 millions ascertained deaths in Mysore and Madras alone; and Bombay and Hyderabad figures yet to come in, perhaps 2 millions more.

Source: From a copy of a letter to James Caird, ADD Mss 45805 ff133-35

24 January 1879

*Private.* Once more I come to trouble you, but this time it is only to wish you "Godspeed." We look to your report [Famine Commission report] with the most intense anxiety to arouse the people of England

62 Dr C. Blencowe Noble Dunn (1836-92), physician at Crich, near Lea Hurst, to whom Nightingale referred many patients. See *Public Health Care* (6: 628-57) for correspondence.

to a sense of their duty towards the people of India. We are like children: we have forgotten to learn our lesson (on the state of the people of India) in order to run to the window at the sound of the drums and fifes in the street going—ah me: what devil has done this?—to Kandahar and Jellalabad. The only chance of real reform in India lies in a powerful report such as yours will be, which will interest the people of England. And—if an Indian Dickens could arise? or if the *Times* could think India of as much importance as Cyprus and send out a "special correspondent" to "discover" the interior!! The India Office say in so many words that they hope that Mr Caird will disregard the limitations of the instructions to the commission. And they also hope that you will tell us something about the famine mortality. And so do I.

Another subject: A Mr Digby,[63] whom you will probably see at Madras, says that the Indian government have two courses before them: (1) doing nothing, and a Poor Law will be necessary in a generation; (2) exerting themselves to improve agriculture (active to devise such means as shall increase the food-producing qualities of the soil) "for there is untold wealth a few inches beneath the surface of the soil if an improved plough is used to turn it up." The same Mr Digby says: "With better village government (the enlargement and improvement of the village system), better village statistics and general widening of knowledge, agriculture could be improved, *manufacturing industries* introduced and famine become as impossible in India as it is in France."

No one will know so much about this as you. A leaving of the wretched ryot to his ignorance, his poverty and his plough (which scarcely scratches the soil) is the doctrine which many preach here. I was glad to hear the India Office say that their great hope now of reviving interest in this terrible Madras tragedy was in "Mr Caird's report," but that it will require courage like yours to bring to light damaging facts.

God speed you and God bless you in so divine and Saviour-like a task.

63 Probably William Digby (1849-1904), journalist, editor of the *Madras Times*. See Jharna Gourlay, *Florence Nightingale* 204.

Source: From two letters to Sir Louis Mallet, Balliol College, Mallet Papers

27 January 1879

*Private.* Thank you for your very kind note. I learnt by last mail from India that the reports and papers—from which my memo to you on Madras famine mortality was extracted—are now "published with the government orders on" them, so that its information may, I suppose, be used as you like. But I still think it better that my name should not appear, except, if you please, to Mr Stanhope, who, as you say, "I am sure may be trusted."

I take the liberty of adding a few figures extracted from an official paper sent me from Simla some months ago, if you will be so good as to add these to (No.) *"2" p 1* of my memo, to which heading they belong.

15 February 1879

*Private and Confidential. Mr Caird.* I always feel like a prisoner in extremity appealing to you and as you cannot know why, I rush at once to the point. You have said that you look to Mr Caird as the one "power" that can now awaken attention to India's agricultural condition, to the famine and the state of the people. And so did I. I looked upon him as the "forlorn hope." It is said, upon what appears to be good authority, that he has declared the agriculture of India, taking the climate into consideration, to be on the *best possible footing,* that he is delighted with his reception by the various authorities of India and that he views everything through an enchanted medium or rather through the medium of the authorities.

I cannot and do not believe this. He is too independent-minded and too sound-hearted. You probably have heard from him direct. I hope that he is to write a separate *report,* that is the only way to prevent what *you* would call a "hocus-pocus."

One thing is probable: the *acting* president of the Famine Commission has received instructions from headquarters in India which, being translated into English, mean this: "Go as near to the truth as you can, but don't let it singe you, and above all don't let it singe us." Knowing that this acting president has sent many things to the *Times* which are nothing better than "communiqués," my hopes (IF *Mr Caird* is gone wrong) from the Famine Commission are sunk below zero indeed.

Do you remember the Rhine legend of the archbishop who said: "Let the villagers burn like rats." And a long line of rats swims the Rhine and silently enters his island castle and—nothing is left of the archbishop? Sometimes it seems to me as if we were bringing upon ourselves, in this ignoring of the famine deaths of India, a similar awful ghostly retribution.

Source: From two letters with notes to John Sutherland, Add Mss 45758 ff76-89

15 February 1879

*Private.* You tell me that you are now "doing" the famine figures. I have been in communication with the India Office about this and at their own request furnished them with a *memorandum* of my own, which I enclose. They replied with a *Memorandum* signed by the under secretary, Mr Stanhope (entirely confidential). I also enclose Dr [W. Robert] Cornish's [sanitary commissioner of Madras] statistical paper and Mr Elliott's paper on Mysore with Gordon's covering sheet.

I add the following to the India Office memorandum. . . .

*Epidemic diseases.* This excites my ire. *Epidemic* diseases are one of the worst results of famine. *Therefore* they are not to be considered a result of famine at all; "unusual *epidemics*" are the inevitable consequence of "unusual famine." Therefore they are not to be reckoned to famine at all. Instead of their being added in the awful total, they are to be deducted. (It is like the former fallacy: "*Cholera* is the worst result of insanitary conditions." Therefore deaths from cholera are to be deducted in judging of any increasing mortality due to want of sanitary measures.)

I gave the India Office an abstract of that part of Cornish's report, where he gives the want of accuracy in the (village accountant) registrars, putting down *famine* deaths to fevers, to "bowel complaints" and all "other causes." The orders of the government of India are, as you know, to ignore any deaths but the following six headings: *1. Cholera 2. Smallpox 3. Fevers 4. Bowel Complaints 5. Injuries 6. Other Causes.* But the India Office evidently thinks that *whatever deaths* can be *properly* put down to *fevers*, cholera, *bowel complaints*, etc., *are to be deducted* from *famine deaths* (instead of the reverse).

I cannot say what grief this causes me. It falsifies the whole history and argument from the history (unusual epidemics are a thing quite apart from "unusual famine" in *their* estimation, just as much so, *they* think, as a storm wave or inundation is a thing quite apart from a drought). Sir M. Kennedy, whose famine work in Bombay was prodigiously good, has yet done enormous mischief in this way. *If you could* by *facts* and arguments enable me to dispel the mischievous delusion, it would be an invaluable service.

I cannot conceive how they could present the "registered" deaths as the *actual "famine"* deaths, without any qualification, to an ignorant

House of Commons. (You see too they look the famine mortality only up to *October* 1877, whereas it certainly existed and was severe all over Madras and Mysore even in *January 1878.*)

I asked the question at the time, *what is* the estimated proportion of *registered* deaths to actual famine deaths? No answer was given. Mr Elliott estimates the *registered* deaths for *Mysore* as *22 percent* of the actual famine deaths, Cornish as under *50 percent* for Madras.

19 February 1879

I do not know what estimate of famine mortality has been *officially* presented by Dr Cornish or what estimate *officially* accepted by the Madras government. (The India Office do not dare now to stand up for theirs.) I have read the Bombay reports most carefully and have had but two long interviews with Mr Hewlett (who is yet more of a hero than ever). No reasoning can however be made founded on *Bombay* for *Madras,* e.g., as to what epidemic deaths should be deducted from famine deaths, etc. To show what I mean [concerning famine]:
*Madras:* Population affected 20 millions; population severely affected 17 millions.
*Mysore:* From November 1876 to March 1878 (17 months): death rate still high.
Registered deaths not 50 percent of actual deaths; registered deaths 22 percent of actual deaths according to Mr Elliott. Village accountants (registrars) thought famine deaths at all events not to be recorded.

| | |
|---|---|
| Cholera | = result of famine |
| Smallpox | = result of overcrowding, etc., in relief camps |
| Fever | = famine fever |
| Bowel complaints | = generally (always and nearly always in children) the internal state due to starvation |
| Other | = anemia, innutrition. |

Causes: European supervision neglected or impossible, native petty official corruption hideous, both in the relief works and in distribution of relief, all kinds of bribes taken by the native official. He who could not bribe got nothing. Relief did not reach persons it was intended for, people could not get on relief works even without a bribe.
*Bombay:* Population affected 8 millions; population severely affected 5 millions; famine from January 1877 over in November (10 months).
Registration of deaths better than in ordinary years, more accurate due to increased supervision.
The village headmen (over registrars) were afraid of not having enough deaths on their books and thought their English masters wanted deaths.

| | |
|---|---|
| Cholera | = real cholera |
| Smallpox | = worst where famine was least |
| Fevers | = malarial fevers |
| Bowel complaints | = anemia, innutrition and other direct results of famine classified under these two heads |
| Other Causes | = European supervision made effective by being multiplied through the higher native officials, native gentlemen. Not an anna [1/16 of a rupee] but reached the hand it was meant for. |

If a bribe was taken to get a man put on relief works, it was detected and bribe taker instantly dismissed or punished.

*Madras:* Relief camps and houses models of sanitary defects, overcrowding, want of conservancy, etc. Cholera and smallpox the result.

In Bombay the people on relief works seem to have been actually better off in sanitary things than at home, but it is not denied officially that even in Bombay smallpox and cholera patients succumbed from being half-starved by the famine, who would not otherwise have died.

Peculation immense: almost unchecked or uncheckable. The poor nation had *no* reserves of money or grain, utterly exhausted and in the last stage of emaciation. They were put on relief works and on the insufficient pay or ration. No "special treatment" (including any food judged suitable that could be had) appears to have been given or was perhaps possible. Children's allowance appears to have been neglected or not seen: children wandered away and perished in vast numbers. Villages deserted by the thousand, headmen and village accountants disappeared, perished, wandered away. Registration dropped.

Bombay: *sanitary* supervision of relief camps, relief works, splendid. If a native official neglected the conservancy, European officer was riding up and down the lines and the petty official was instantly dismissed. Grass huts erected every 200 or 300 yards for babies whose mothers were at work on the lines, where the babies were under the care of an old crone.

Even chapathis sold by a trader appointed by European officer that they might not have to cook their own food. Conservancy of relief houses very bad, at first no peculation possible. European or high native official saw the daily pay paid into the people's hands. The poor natives had generally reserves of money or grain. Without these reserves relief works pay would not have been sufficient. Where they had none, they were put on "special treatment" till able to work. Children under seven years had also their allowance and it was *seen to* that they *had it*, also that they *ate* their food in a place where parents could not see them and take it away. No deserted villages, headmen always remained. Registration not suspended. Madras: Europeans have counted ninety corpses by the wayside in a morning's ride. Inquests impossible either on one corpse or on ninety. Three fourths of the deaths in a relief house were from innutrition (starvation). They were so starved when they came in that no food could do them any good.

As a rule women's ornaments all gone (sold): 1 lb. rice not worth, 1 lb. jowari. . . .

Bombay: only five corpses ever seen by wayside by sanitary commissioners. Inquest held upon every such death. . . . They would try and wander home as wild animals to die. . . . 1 lb. jowari much more nutriment [?] than 1 lb. rice.

Sir R. Temple's famine policy very different as governor of Bombay from Sir R. Temple's policy as delegate in Madras. . . .

I have carefully gone over the Bombay reports. I cannot help repeating: Mr Hewlett is as brave a soldier against sanitary evils and famine as the bravest war soldier that ever held a post against overwhelming numbers. The grandeur of his success (and Sir M. Kennedy's too) in the Bombay famine deserves its place in a higher history than ours. Also the Bombay registration of deaths appears to have been more accurate than in ordinary years. Epidemic deaths, at least as far as cholera and smallpox go, appear to have been *epidemic* deaths and not *famine* deaths.

In Madras all this is altered. Still as I look over the Bombay mortality returns, I find my pencil notes on the margins, "But there is no evidence of *famine* deaths in *any* part of this." "The famine might not have been at all. *Famine* deaths might not have been at all, for any evidence there is here." "What are *real* famine deaths then registered under?" "Where are the *famine* deaths?" etc. . . .

It is understood that an authority who is, I believe, accepted by the India Office, does not accept Sir Richard Temple's figures or conclusions. And others, among whom is one great authority at least, considers as quite inadmissible the separation of cholera and smallpox as *unconnected* with famine in Bombay. The first authority also considers that "*ignoring the results of the partial census* makes the Bombay facts unreliable and that they have yet to be subjected to impartial review." . . .

At the same time, it is quite obvious that there was success in overcoming the famine—in registering—in everything in *Bombay* that there was not in Madras. And it has done no little good in softening the bitterness felt by those who knew that the *registered* deaths in Madras were not 50 percent (in Mysore, 22 percent) of the actual deaths. Bitterness felt at what appeared like an official attempt to represent to an ignorant House of Commons *registered* as actual deaths, to know that in Bombay they were more nearly so. But it remains that it is quite impossible to eliminate cholera, smallpox, fever, etc. in Madras from famine deaths. . . . Parliament has entirely obliterated the famine.

I will gladly give these authorities but I have discovered in my old age how Indian ways are like official ways of *Vatican Council* on papal infallibility. The bishops go into the Vatican Council, not only convinced but prophets of the one way of thinking, and come out prophets of the other, a parody of "they that have gone to scoff remain to pray."[64] So is it with official ways of the Government of India.

Source: Excerpts from notes for John Sutherland, ADD Mss 45758 ff90-99

[1879]

Memorandum on South India *famine mortality of 1876-77*, the greatest since 1770, includes nine revenue divisions of Bombay, fourteen districts (out of twenty-one) of Madras, nearly all Mysore, south and east of Nizam's dominions.

1. Money famine, consequence of grain famine.

2. No connection between famine and excessive population.

| Districts with sparse populations as | *Pop. per sq. mile* |
|---|---|
| Kurnool | 130.4 |
| Nellore | 162.7 |
| Cuddapah | 161.5 |
| Bellary | 151.5 |
| suffered the severest famine while | |
| Tanjore | 540.1 saved by Kaveri irrigation |
| Godavari | 255.9 not only grew enough for their own populations but for material help to the famine districts |
| So with Malabar | 376.7 saved by S.W. monsoon |
| Trichinopoly | 341.5 saved wherever there was Kaveri irrigation—saved but crowded with famine-stricken; wanderers from Coimbatore and Salem |

64 Possibly from John Fenimore Cooper, *The Pioneers* 1:11.

3. Defective registration except in municipal towns; in the country no legal power compelling people to register births and deaths. Every village is a commune—more than 50,000 villages—each village has a separate "accountant" who is *ex officio* registrar (the village accountant is the man who keeps the accounts of the government for the lands cultivated by each ryot and the tax due on them). In ordinary times about two thirds of deaths registered, in famine times not one half. Village accountants suffered starvation with the rest and went away in search of food and work. Thousands upon thousands of deaths occurred of people dropping down by the wayside or in desert places, which were of course unregistered. The registration has no absolute but much relative value.

*Non-famine districts:*

*Births* decreased only from 19.9 per 1000 (mean ratio of 5 years) to 19.5 in 1877

*Deaths* increased only from 18.6 (mean ratio of 5 years) to 24.8 in 1877

*Famine districts:*

*Births* decreased from 20.0 (mean ratio of 5 years) to 14.4 in 1877

N.B. decrease of births much greater in 1878

*Deaths* increased from 19.7 (mean ratio of 5 years) to 70.2 in 1877

4. *Madras: the previous famine of 1833-34* practically arrested all development of population *for four years* after famine ended.

In the area now included in the eight districts of Godavary, Kistna (these before irrigation works), Nellore, Cuddapah, Chingleput, N. Arcot, Madurai and Salem, the population in 1838 (next census four years after famine) was *less* in these eight districts by 1,153,000 souls than the ascertained population of 1822 (last census before). (It is not pretended that these numbers are accurate; the ascertained numbers only are given.)

But from 1851 to 1871 (census) the population had increased 35.8 percent in these twenty years. And from 1856-57 to 1871-72 the revenue had increased 58 percent in these fifteen years. . . . There was no material check to the increase and prosperity of the people during these years, except a scarcity in 1853 and 1866; there was none at all between 1871 and 1876.

5. Areas selected for famine census, March 1878: *Salem* (whole district censused, a population of 2 millions):

| *Total pop.* in 1871* | *Total pop. in March 1878* | | |
|---|---|---|---|
| 1,966,995 | 1,559,896 | Decrease | –407,099 |

*Can give the actual number for each of the taluks, if desired.

Salem: Total loss of population thus -20.7 percent (*without* allowing *any* increment for normal growth of population during a prosperous five years)

*Six "selected"* taluks in famine districts, Bellary, Kurnool, Cuddapah, Nellore, Coimbatore, Chingleput; total loss of population 15 percent (these taluks were "selected" as fair averages—neither the best off in the district and certainly by no means the worst).

Four "selected" taluks in non-famine districts, to wit, Kistna, Trichinopoly, Tanjore, Tinnevelly: total *increase* of population: *+6.1 percent* since 1871 or, allowing for villages transferred since 1871 to another boundary; *+8.2 percent*

N.B. (The increase of population was thus *more* than the estimate 7.5 percent in the five years before the beginning of the famine, or the estimated 1.5 percent per annum.)

6. Decrease *not* accounted for by migration: all natural population movements in definite directions to find food and work, e.g., from the districts surrounding Madras to Madras, from Coimbatore to Malabar or Trichinopoly, from Salem to Tanjore (the great irrigated Kaveri delta and Trichinopoly, from Kurnool and N. Nellore to Kistna (irrigated), etc. For example, in Madras, out of some 30,000 in relief camps, not twelve from Salem, the great bulk from Bellore, Chingleput and N. Arcot. (N.B. From Bellary and Cuddapah immigration was encouraged, to "Buckingham Canal," works on Nellore coast. But this was out of the usual (population) course. It was full of disaster to the people and had to be abandoned.) Again Madras famine district, population 20,000,000—they did not go to Mysore, for all Mysore was famine, nor into Bombay, nor into Nizam's dominions for these were worse off than our own. Nizam's and Mysore people came to Bellary for relief. Before end of 1877, the great surplus of emigrants, including even those who went to Ceylon and Travancore, i.e., those who were not dead had returned to their villages. . . .

We have in actual ascertained figures that children under ten years disappeared in double the proportion of persons over ten years. Now these children could not have emigrated: they must have died. This disproves the migration theory as explaining the decrease of population.

7. In the partial famine of 1833-34 upwards of 2 millions of the population disappeared (2,205,578) but for government relief the losses of population in the greater calamity of 1877, extending over fourteen revenue districts, would have been nearer 5 millions than 3.

Decrease of births: they diminish month by month in exact correspondence with the intensity of famine nine months before, but causes of diminished birth rate continue to operate for a long period after famine. . . .

9. Mortality *returns* alone cannot be trusted to show whole absolute mortality. But the seventeen months' RETURNS from November 1876 to March 1878 show an EXCESS of *deaths* of *1,140,048* over average of same months in former years, while test census would indicate a probable decrease of population of at least 3,000,000. Such was the disorganization of village life and communal administration that not one half of the actual deaths were ever recorded. May be reckoned roughly as *deaths* rather more than 2,000,000, accounting for one million (1,000,000) *as* DIMINISHED BIRTHS.

Facts *ascertained* do not account for more than 100,000 of the missing people by *migration*. Famine cuts away population at both ends and it will be well if the census of 1881 does not show the losses to be greater still than are here estimated.

10. Causes of mortality from 1866* to June 1878

*Could furnish the numbers for each year from 1866 to June 1878, if desired.

| Years | Total Deaths | Cholera | Small-pox | Fever | Bowel Complaint | Other Causes |
|---|---|---|---|---|---|---|
| 1876 | 680,384 | 148,193 | 23,469 | 230,092 | 31,876 | 240,454 |
| 1877 | 1,556,312 | 357,430 | 88,321 | 469,241 | 133,366 | 507,934 |
| 1878 | 409,151 | 18,926 | 41,506 | 181,610 | 25,602 | 141,507 |

*Famine* deaths were sometimes registered under "*All other causes*" *because* it was announced that "no death was to be allowed from famine"; sometimes under "*fevers*," yes, but famine fever, although it may have spread among the well-to-do; sometimes under "cholera" or "bowel complaint," affection of the bowels being, especially among children, the very type or characteristic of the famine state.

These methods of registration are to be expected among the village accountants, ex officio registrars, non-professionals, whose only rule of registration often is how to please the English masters.

In camps and relief houses at least *three fourths* of the mortality was the direct result of innutrition (starvation).

11. Madras famine. Food rose to 400 percent above its normal value and under this enormous rise wages were reduced by government 25 percent.

N.B. Roads and railroads and increased facility of communications have very much reduced the practice, before universal, of keeping reserves of grain enough for three or four years. It is obvious that the usual tests of market prices cannot hold here.

Source: From two letters to Sir Louis Mallet, Balliol College, Mallet Papers

18 February 1879

*Private and confidential. Famine deaths.* If you think the enclosed in the least worth showing to Mr Stanhope and if Parliament has not entirely obliterated the famine, pray show it. I may tell *you* what was told me by the *Bombay* authorities themselves, that they had suppressed certain monthly or occasional *famine reports* because they "reflected discredit" and gave statements which they did not wish to have known (I am to see these reports and some have already been communicated to me in "confidence"). . . .

A superior official, who knows the Deccan and the *whole* interior of the Bombay presidency better than any man, and who is a cordial admirer of the Maratha peasantry, told me the other day—of course, in the strictest confidence—that, if there were another mutiny (which, he added, there will be), this fine Maratha peasantry is so disaffected owing to our laws putting "weapons of torture" into the money-lenders' hands—owing to our forcing or administering Western ideas of civilization among these Deccan populations—that they would join a sepoy mutiny against us, IF something were not done in the meantime by our government. [Ed: Famine figures for Bombay and Madras were appended.]

25 February 1879

*Private.* You say, "But surely the facts on which all are agreed are enough: whether this terrible scourge has swept away a few hundred thousands more or less x x scarcely touches the question for practical solution." I do so entirely agree with this that I am quite grateful to you for saying it.

So far as we have gone, we have found that, for *Bombay*, we have a number of *registered* deaths which represents the *maximum* (though I understand it is to be disputed, as not the *maximum possible) excess* of mortality from famine (this results from the extra precautions taken by Mr Hewlett for the registration). So far as we have seen from the

Madras data, all we can get that is trustworthy is the *minimum possible* mortality from famine. And the practical question is, as you say, whether this be not enough and whether to endeavour to come closer to the *actual* mortality is not almost to turn away our eyes from the question? WHAT IS TO BE DONE?

The *minimum* deducible from the *Madras* papers is one of the most awful records of human suffering and destruction the world has ever seen. and if the Government of India and the public are not moved by it to action, the case is hopeless. Much may be done if the government take the case in hand as one of their prime administrative duties. It will not do to judge of it as people might do of an Irish famine or scarcity. The Indian problem is altogether different.

Another problem we have now to solve for practical purposes is the exact relation of *epidemics* to *famine.* If you could order Sir R. Temple's *"Minute on the Famine" of 24 December 1877* to be sent me, I should be the more obliged.

Source: From a letter to Sir Harry Verney, Wellcome (Claydon copy) Ms 9007/183

1 March 1879

*Private. India.* I read Mr Grant-Duff's speech in the House last night[65] with the greatest attention as well as the whole debate. You know how the question interests me. I was glad to see that Mr Grant-Duff attributes so much efficacy "to the action of enlightened English opinion exerted through Parliament upon the great, broad questions of Indian affairs." I am sure that you will bring me home much Indian information (I do not mean political or "policy" information but information about the people of India) from Mr Grant-Duff.

I wonder whether he has any information about the *famine mortality figures* of 1877 with which he would entrust me. As you know, the government gave these figures to the House last August as *1,350,000 deaths* from famine. These were the *registered* deaths, but such was the pressure, which resulted in an amount of human suffering and destruction to which the records of the civilized world scarcely contain a parallel, that the officials altogether failed in counting the dead.

In Madras the registered deaths were not 50 percent of the *actual* famine deaths. In Mysore 22 percent. The government, I believe,

---

65 Hansard, *Parliamentary Debates,* 3rd series (1830-91) 28 February 1879:1991. Grant-Duff opposed Henry Fawcett's views on finance and lack of control over it, discussed in *Social Reform in India.*

themselves now reckon the famine deaths in Madras, Bombay and Mysore alone at *2 millions and a half,* or nearly double what they told the House of Commons. And this does not include the *N. W. Provinces,* where there must have been a famine mortality of something not very far short of half a million; or *Hyderabad,* where the deaths must have been far above a million.

The figures which have reached me bring the loss of population during the famine up to between five and six millions in *southern* India (not reckoning the N. W. Provinces). It is not that we want to substitute an arithmetical dispute, however important, about the number of famine deaths for the far greater questions as to the state of the people and the *prevention* of famines which are, I trust, now forcing themselves to the front. But it is that in India the loss of life by famine is the test, the type of the condition of the people: a test so striking, a type so awful that, if it does not move the Government of India and the people of England to action, the case is indeed hopeless, a test and a culmination, which, thank God, is not to be found in any country of the West, not even Ireland in days gone by. It *is* a *test,* because it is not pretended that there was not food to *be had* in this Indian famine if there had been money to *pay* for it. And the large quantities of grain poured in from the irrigated districts of the Godavari, Kistna and Kaveri (Tanjore) are matters of *official* report.

One other thing which (among *many* others) I should like to know Mr Grant-Duff's opinion about is the controversy which has been going on between Mr Hyndman, Sir Erskine Perry and Mr Morley and others, chiefly in the *Nineteenth Century,* on the so-called "bankruptcy" of India. It would be too much to expect that Mr Grant-Duff should have read my paper on "the people of India"—the part of the subject which interests me—in the August No. of the *Nineteenth Century.* But he has probably made up his mind as to the value of Mr Hyndman's arguments and whether India is getting poorer and poorer, etc. Do you think I ought to make any answer regarding the extraordinary misstatement concerning me and the Indian barracks by *Mr Onslow*[66] in last night's debate, which I should not have seen had I not been reading the whole debate?

---

66 Denzil Roberts Onslow (1839-1908), MP, who argued that Nightingale had caused excessive expenditure on barracks, after seeing them on a visit to India.

Source: From a letter to Sir M.E. Grant-Duff, ADD Mss 45805 ff155-56

1 March 1879

1,350,000 deaths: figures given to the House last August. These were the *registered* deaths, but such was the pressure, which resulted in an amount of human suffering and destruction to which the records of the civilized world scarcely offered a parallel that the officials altogether failed in counting the dead. In Madras the register of deaths was not 50 percent of the actual deaths from famine. In Mysore 22 percent. The government themselves, I believe, now reckon the famine deaths in Madras, Bombay and Mysore at 2½ millions, or nearly double what they told the House of Commons. And this does not include the North West Provinces where there has been a famine mortality of something not very far short of half a million, or Hyderabad where the deaths must have been far above a million. The figures which have reached me bring the loss of population during the famine up to between 5 or 6 millions in southern India, not including the North West Provinces.

It is not that we want to substitute an arithmetic dispute, however important, about the exact number of famine deaths for the far greater questions, as the state of the people and the *prevention* of famine which are, I trust, now forcing themselves to the front.

But it is that in India the loss of life by famine is the test, the type of the condition of people, a test so striking, a type so awful that, if it does not move the Government of India and the people of England to action, the case is indeed hopeless—a test and a culmination which, thank God, can exist in no other country, not even Ireland in days gone by under our rule. It is a test, because it is not precluded that there was not food to be had in this Indian famine, if there had been money to pay for it. And the large quantities of grain poured in from the irrigated districts of the Godavary, Kistna and Kaveri (Tanjore) are matters of official report.

Source: From two letters to Sir Louis Mallet, Balliol College, Mallet Papers

12 March 1879

*Private. Mr Caird's figures.* I am exceedingly obliged to you for your two kind notes and I assure you that I consider your kindness quite "confidential": Mr Caird's figures shall not be betrayed through me.

2. A good Calcutta friend has sent me Mr Elliott's (large) report on the Mysore famine so that I need not now trouble you for that. How much it tells! how much he knows. You may well say that it reads like Defoe's *History of the Plague*.

Thank you for sending me at my request Sir R. Temple's minute on the Bombay famine. I will return it. I suppose I must not say how *little* it tells—it could not well tell less—*not* because he knows little, perhaps because he knows too much. Three times in one page he tells us we "cannot understand it" but he does not help us much to the understanding. . . .

4. People do so very much regret that Mr Caird did not visit the "improving" districts of India, such as the Godavary, Kistna and Tanjore, etc. The list is short.

3 April 1879

*Private and confidential.* Your kind letters are sacred to me, especially sacred what you told me about Mr Caird's figures. (I knew of the "battle raging fierce and strong"[67] between Bombay and Madras, and indeed between everybody and *every*body about famine figures.) But I have seen the statement of North West Provinces' *million* of famine deaths elsewhere and you must not think, if you hear it, that *I* have betrayed confidence.

It is now my turn to ask for confidence again. It is all-important, I believe, that Mr Caird should write the report, that is, if he be not "traitor Scot."[68] As he is to be home this week, we shall soon know "how he looks," as you say.

The intention I have just heard from *Indian* headquarters is that Mr Cunningham and Mr Elliott (I trust the latter more than the former) are "now about to draw up the framework of the report and to throw into form the mass of information which we have collected" *at Simla*, that "the report is to be finally settled in London in the course of the autumn so as to be ready for Parliament next session." Mr Elliott has written by far the most powerful and most incisive and *in-seeing* contribution to the famine history in his "Mysore famine." But I cannot help saying that the value of the report will consist in its being written in England, far from what you call justly "blandishments." No one must be "enguirlandé" [inveighed against]. and it is so difficult to alter a "framework" once put together, is it not?

2. There are the most terrible previsions of scarcity. "The Punjab is in great peril and parts of Bombay are only just, if at all, falling short of scarcity." Oh me! oh me! "a plague of rats is the last misfortune."

---

67 Possible allusion to H.W. Longfellow, "Coplas de Manrique."

68 Possible allusion to Jane Porter, *The Scottish Chiefs* chap 34.

Did I not say that the legendary archbishop, who was in his castle on the Rhine reached by the swimming line of rats, was a prophecy?

F.N.

Mr Gladstone says, in a note to me, that, however bad the means which have brought it about, the time has come when Indian questions *must* "force their way to the front," even in Parliament.

*Burn* please.

## Famine, Retrenchment and Public Works

**Editor:** Nightingale saw a fatal connection between "retrenchment" or curtailments in planned public works announced by the Government of India, especially those linked with irrigation, and the threat of recurrent famines. A list of proposed irrigation works for the next ten years "warms and cheers one's heart. O if they could be carried out!" (in the letter immediately below). But there was serious doubt that they would in fact be realized, which worried her. She had the further evidence that a "money famine" followed "in the steps of the grain famine," adding misery, as the same letter notes, to misery. Retrenchment falls most heavily on the poor of India, "who cannot complain," and least on "the British servant of government" (see p 841 below). There is further material on retrenchment in a section on Indian finance in *Social Change in India.*

Source: From two letters to Major General James George Fife, Wayne State University, folder 37 letters (14) and (16)

20 December 1878

I am very glad to hear from you again and to know you so near.

1. I send the revise of the irrigation map of India with the two proofs from which it was corrected. Please go over it and say whether it is now exactly as it should be before I have some copies made for distribution. Sir Arthur Cotton wishes to have six. How many will you have? It is to *you* we are indebted for this.

2. Thank you very, very much for the Gujarat and Deccan List of Irrigation Works proposed for the next ten years. It warms and cheers one's heart. O if they could be carried out!

I had just been reading a private official report (from Simla) of the latest date, dwelling on the MONEY *famine* among the people, following in the steps of the grain famine, and no way of meeting it but by carrying out public works. . . . And now there comes a telegram—misery twice told—from Bombay saying that no new works are to be undertaken, all public works in progress to be suspended, no applications to be sent in, all expenditure to be retrenched, etc. Do you believe this will be carried out? It is ruin to the people. . . .

I ought to congratulate you on your promotion as major general, but I am so very sorry to hear that there is any difficulty about "compensation."

N.B. 5. I want to ask you to be so very good as to revise something I have written about what you told me as to preparing land for irrigation, etc., in the Deccan and Sind.

4 March 1879

You no doubt saw, some time ago, Sir R. Temple's "Minute on the Famine" of December 1877, acknowledging the immense value of your plans of works for Famine Relief Works. Mr Hewlett, the acting sanitary commissioner for Bombay presidency, who did duty in the famine, told me of a pupil of yours (*Burke?*) who had been of the greatest service by "*following the water*" in procuring a pure water supply.

Source: Notes from an interview with Thomas Gillham Hewlett, Add Mss 45782 f49

2 May 1879

Irrigation. Told Mr Hewlett what Sir Richard Temple has sent me. Sir R.T. does not understand—and few of the high officials in India do—either that none of this gives information such as the mass of the English reading public will care about, nor how important it is to interest the mass of the English reading public *aright* in India, although he says himself (so truly) "acq[uainted] with details." Why are people so much interested in war matters, so little in these far greater interests and disasters of peace? Because the authorities publish the minutest details of a battle—Isandula and Rorke's Drift.[69] The feats of the heroes recommended for Victoria Cross are described even to the hourly doings of Private J.J. [Jones?] who held a hospital

69 During the Zulu War the British were defeated in January 1879 at a hill called Isandhlwana (literally "a little hand"), erroneously called "Isandula," some ten miles from Rorke's Drift astride the Blood River. In the aftermath of Isandlwana, the Zulu reserves mounted a raid on the British border post at Rorke's Drift, but after ten hours of ferocious fighting, the Zulus were driven off by some forty British soldiers. Eleven of the defenders of Rorke's Drift were awarded the Victoria Cross. Defending the post hospital to the last, William and Robert Jones managed to remove six men to safety, the seventh being killed. In July the British finally won the decisive battle of the Anglo-Zulu War of 1879.

ward with the bayonet against so many hundred Zulus. And why will the civil authorities not describe the far greater feats of the far higher heroes who held, not for a night but for a whole year, famine at bay and saved not hundreds but millions from death?

They would so soon find their account in it by seeing how the interest of the people of England would be roused in India. The people who sway the Parliament, which sways the Cabinet, which sways our mighty empire. Possibly the effects in making English capital too flow into India might be momentous. But we know nothing really about India here.

Sir R. Temple's views—efficient sanitary department—satisfactory. Regret your not being sanitary commissioner. But what you have done in Bombay you will do in Sind. God be with you.

Reason why newspaper correspondents mislead on one side by giving only *one side* and partial facts is that the government gives hardly any on the other, at least not with any details that common readers will read. I do not think people say, government gives "inaccurate" "records"; I think they say, government gives *none at all* that we care to read.

Source: Note, Wellcome (Claydon copy) Ms 9007/223

6 May 1879

One thing I must say: the anxiety I feel for the good result of this Famine Commission is so intense that I can only pray for it and for Mr Cunningham on that Famine Commission. There will be a letter from me in each of the two next Nos. of the *Illustrated News.*

Source: From five letters to Lieutenant General James George Fife, Wayne State University, folders 18-22

16 June 1879

I cannot thank you enough for your three letters: the first written in answer to my questions about the effect of the threatened discontinuance of public works, then the two articles in the *Times of India* and still more your commentary on these with regard to whether a water cess were desirable or not. . . . The "one half percent" on all the new works in the Deccan *taken together* "for 1876-77" tells terribly against us. I fear "retrenchment" will fall most heavily on public works because, you see, these chiefly affect the poor people of India, who cannot complain, and not the British servant of government. . . .

I had three letters on "Irrigation and Water Transit," chiefly in Madras, in the *Illustrated News* of 10, 24 and 31 May. If you did not see them and would like to see them, I would send them you. . . .

Alas poor India! Is the *bill* for the "*relief of indebted agriculturists* in the *Deccan*" said, in the *Times* telegram of *today*, to be "introduced" by Mr Hope, *the same* as that of which you have kindly sent me news from time to time?

*How we have broken our promises to these poor people!*

23 June 1879

I am afraid that it is going *against* our irrigation public works in the report of the Public Works Committee (at which you were examined last year) which is now under consideration. They say that none but *old* works, improved by us, are remunerative. And they reckon the Sind works as *old* works (and said this, when I reminded them that the Sind Canals returned 5 percent). This is not the case, is it? that the Sind Canals are, like the Canvery [Kaveri or Godavari?], old works improved.

25 June 1879

Thank you very much for your most important information about Sind Canals. I am appalled by the tide which is running *against* public works now. Public works are sure to be cut down first in the present necessity for retrenchment, because *that* only presses on the natives of India who have no voice. "Hit him hard: he's no friends!"

29 November 1879

God speed the irrigation works! There is no darker cloud [that] hangs over one than the dread that all these retrenchments that are to take place will be death to the public works as to the very things upon which the wealth and welfare of the cultivators most depend. And so *poverty* will come out of economy. I should be anxious to know what *you* think about the retrenchments in the public works, upon which all the economy seems to fall. . . .

*Private and Confidential.* There is some scheme afloat about Punjab irrigation by a combined system of numerous cheap cuts from rivers, supplemented by *wells* irrigation, and on the principle of *lift* as against flow. It is now proposed to work this out, as an auxiliary to a scheme of purchase and colonization of wastelands—the trial sphere of operation to be in the Punjab, colonization to be not European but indigenous—in the form of encouraging emigration from overpeopled tracts to these improvable wastes. Have you been consulted about this? . . .

Would you be so very good *as to write me* a few lines giving your *opinion of the irrigation scheme by lift, etc., in the Punjab*? . . . and let me have them *by tonight.* And please not to say anything about this scheme (which I have no right to mention) until you hear of it publicly.

*Something must* be done in the way of POPULARIZING irrigation, if only they rightly know their way in the *engineering* point of view.

3 January 1880

I should like very much to know what you thought of Mr [Edward] Prinsep's last[70] (Punjab) irrigation scheme and your interview with him.

The Famine Commission is reporting and I understand that their verdict is very much more favourable in the matter of irrigation returns (saving poor Bombay and Madras Irrigation Co) than that of the House of Commons "Public Works" Committee.

I pray for a happy New Year and many of them to you and yours. And oh how I pray, because it seems almost past praying for, for a happy New Year for poor India.

What do you think of the Deccan Ryots Relief Act? O how she suffers. And what do you think, in the other direction, of the stoppage of public works? And what do you think of Afghan affairs? and are steps making [made?] in *your* sense to employ natives?

Source: From a letter to Vaughan Nash,[71] ADD MSS 45795 ff233-34

20 February 1900

I found at an early hour this morning the book we were talking about: [Robert Benton] Buckley's *Irrigation Works of India*, I believe a rare book—at least I never saw but this one copy, which was a present to me. Pray make what use of it you can (it may be you have it already). All success to you on your noble mission. Irrigation is in India, as a Hindu said to me, not food merely but life.

## "Irrigation and Water Transit," 1879

**Editor:** The three published letters below highlight the great benefits derived from irrigation and canals in times of famine. The problem of long-term, underlying poverty is raised, and the possibility of a "money" famine following the initial "grain" famine. These are letters to influence public opinion at home.

70 W. Edward Prinsep, settlement commissioner in the Punjab, brother of Henry T. Prinsep of the India Office.

71 Vaughan Nash (1861-1932), married to Rosalind Shore Smith, then about to leave for India to report on famine for the *Manchester Guardian.*

Source: Florence Nightingale, "Irrigation and Water Transit in India." Three letters to the Editor of *The Illustrated London News*, 10 May (dated 28 April) 1879, 74: 450; 24 May (dated 29 April) 1879, 74: 495; and 31 May (dated 27 May) 1879, 74: 522

28 April 1879

[1]

Sir, You have already been so good as twice to admit observations of mine on irrigation and water transit in India in connection with famine—the last time in July 1877, as regarded the Madras presidency and the late terrible famine. May I offer now a few remarks, correcting also two statements then made by me?

That dreadful scourge of famine is now over, it is supposed. Ah, would it were! But scarcity is returning, which the poverty of the people, not yet recovered from the money famine which followed the grain famine, may convert, but for timely rains, into another disaster.

A magnificent work has been accomplished by the duke of Buckingham, extending the east and north coast canals, or rather connecting the canals north and south of Madras, and thus completing water communication all the way from Kakinada in the north, in the Godavari districts, to Madras in the south and south of Madras—a distance of about 450 miles. There was, it is true, a break of eight miles at Feringhee Dibha, but the canal must now be open all the way. A passenger boat, built at Kakinada, has arrived at Madras. The Buckingham Canal will soon become the main thoroughfare for traffic between Madras and the north coast. When flat-bottomed steamers are placed on the canal, then we shall have speed as well as cheapness. But it seems strange to open the canal without having steamers ready at the same time. Would they treat a railway thus? There will be an immense saving of expense in the movement of troops by the canals.

On 27 January 1879 in the evening a procession of seventy or eighty boats issued from the Junction Canal near the Marine Villa in Madras and passed silently up the Cooum river (a river till lately of most unsavoury and unhealthy reputation), underneath the Government House Bridge, by the General Hospital and away into Cochrane's Canal. They who saw it say that, in the light of the setting sun, it might well have been taken for a scene on the Grand Canal at Venice. Even the top boats gleamed like gondolas and the boatmen, with their long bamboo poles, might have been the gondoliers. The boats carried 1000 souls and their appurtenances, belonging to the 38th Regiment of Native Infantry, on their way from Trichinopoly to Secunderabad—a great part of the journey to be easily travelled by the Buckingham

Canal. (For an account of this see *Madras Mail* of 28 January 1879.) If Canaletti[72] is not here, will not the *Illustrated London News* give us a sketch of this beautiful scene?

And now, not for the picturesque, but for policy. Let us but have the means of moving troops and military stores by water north and south of Madras, and the Coromandel coast becomes almost impregnable, for an enemy could scarcely land his troops without already having a landing place in his possession. In other words, he can land them if he has landed them. The coast canal enables us to send troops and guns to prevent him doing so. For strategy as for commerce, the present water communication is invaluable.

As to expense, it is almost nominal. On the present trip, notwithstanding the small supply of boats available, each sepoy was carried at the rate of seven miles for a penny, each follower at fourteen miles for a penny, while the lowest passenger rate, coolie class, on the railway is four miles for a penny. The canal can now be used where coasting steamers, carts or the railway had to be employed.

It is reckoned that, with steamers similar to those on the upper Godavari, men could be moved at the rate of twenty miles for a penny at ten miles an hour. There is nothing to prevent high speeds on the canals, but we want high speed only for a very few passengers and the mails. As to goods traffic, on the Erie Canal, where they carry two or three million tons a year, the speed is two miles an hour. On the line from Calcutta to the Burhamputra, nine tenths of the traffic go by the river's 400 miles, averaging forty days and, as the direct distance is 130 miles, the average speed is a little over three miles per day. On this coast canal there are only nine locks between the Godavari and Madras, and of these three will be open most of the year, so that there will be no objection to trains of boats drawn by one steamer, which will make the cost at low speeds extremely small. On the Forth and Clyde Canal, at six miles an hour, with twenty locks in forty miles and short trips of only forty miles, the cost of carriage is but a penny for seven miles per ton. On the Coast Canal goods can certainly be carried at the rate of twenty miles for a penny per ton. It offers the cheapest line of communication between the northern parts and the chief port of the presidency, where the shipping of cotton will be greatly facilitated when the harbour is finished. Guntur, in the Kistna

72 Giovanni Antonio Canal (1697-1768), known as Canaletto or Canaletti (form used by Ruskin), Italian painter.

district, is the centre of a large cotton trade; its port is Kakinada, 150 miles off. In the Kistna valley alone are about 100,000 acres of cotton lands; the exports of cotton from Kakinada average about 90,000 cwt a year, besides rice and oil seeds. The trade on the north coast canal was 300,000 tons a year before the Buckingham Canal was opened. What will it be now? Guntur is 250 miles from Madras, the way is now opened by water. A gentleman and his wife arrived at Madras from Guntur, travelling by one of the canal top boats (a clumsy old style of boat worked by men). The journey occupied four or five days and the trip is described as very pleasant with plenty of shooting. The fare for the above journey cost 40 rupees for two persons (of course, with all their servants, goods, etc.).

On cheap water communication depends the vast American trade. Now that Madras has cheap water communication, what the trade will be can scarcely be overestimated. But when the quality and the quantity of the dry crop cotton produced by India is raised by irrigation and improved culture to vie with that of Egypt and America, what may we not hope?

In January of this year, the Buckingham Canal being open from Madras to 200 miles north, where the break of eight miles occurred, three kinds of boats already plied for hire—a small provision of seven or eight cabin boats (budgerows), top boats (that is, with a covered space in the centre) and barges or cargo boats. For the first 200 miles the canal runs within one or two miles of the sea, on the other side a sandy ridge. Pleasant "topes" (groves of mango or cocoa nut or tamarind), good water and supplies for halts, good shooting and fishing (without gamekeepers interfering) for sportsmen and sea bathing in the back waters. But some villages mark "bad water, place feverish" as halts to be avoided. A traveller's bungalow, post office and salt superintendent's cutcherry (court) mark luxury and the great station, as well as the terrible salt tax, alas! And there is the metalled road inland. "Good water *one mile* inland" sounds uninviting. Then comes the Penner River to cross, with its three branches and connecting canal two miles and a half long, and your boat is sailed or poled across. A large village, large bazaars, good tope and camping ground, water good, travellers' bungalow, treasury, post office, police station and sub-magistrate mark civilization. Shallow rivers and deep rivers, 500 to 600 feet wide, you have to cross till you come to Feringhee Dibha, a wild desolate place, where was a Dutch factory 200 years ago. Here comes, or rather came, the break between Feringhee and the canal eight miles to the north.

> Before the work could be completed . . . to the creek near Feringhee Dibha, information was received that his grace the governor wished to proceed from Bezwada to Madras by canal. Obstructions were hastily removed and two temporary locks built, so that in January 1878 the canal was available for navigation. Subsequently, as his grace's visit was postponed, the locks were removed and the canal run dry in order fully to complete the excavation. (Annual Progress Report, P.W. Department, Madras, for 1877-78.)

The canal now completed, the distances onward are: to Bezwada sixty miles, to Rajahmundry on the Godavari ninety miles, to the port Kakinada forty and from Bezwada to Masulipatam forty-eight miles. On the Bezwada and Kakinada canals the passenger boats have general cabins, sometimes for one hundred persons, and fore and aft cabins for well-to-do travellers. They can do fifty miles in twenty-four hours. It reminds one of old days in England or of Nile "tracking."

There are now 1300 miles of navigation in this system between Sironcha at the junction of the Godavari and the Wurdah and including the delta canals, besides 100 miles above Sironcha, with only a transfer at the second barrier near Sironcha. On all these lines it is said that at least two large steamers a day each way might at once be run, making nearly 6000 miles of running per day for passengers alone. What the effect of this line of communication would have been in saving life in the late famine—grain being landed at every point of 700 miles and in any quantities—with employment for hundreds of thousands of people in working the boats, one does not like to think. But there appears little hope that it may not yet be wanted for this use. Had the eighty miles to connect this canal with the Tumbuddra canals been cut, 300 miles more, leading into the very heart of the suffering country, would have been open.

The Government of Madras has been blamed for not making this connection from Cuddapah to Nellore for the purpose of navigation. But the engineering difficulties are such as to have caused the abandonment of the scheme by the company and a careful review of the matter by government has not made it look better. It has to be carried through a high chain of rocky hills, to descend to the plains of the coast by a difficult pass. And if the canal were formed it is doubtful if water enough could be had. When it reaches Nellore, its proposed terminus, it is still some sixteen miles (as the crow flies) from the coast canal navigation, which would have required a canal with several locks, needing a constant supply of water for which there was no source except during the rains.

To return to the coast canal, unfortunately left in abeyance for so long—twenty-five years—shelved and discussed again with every new governor and every new chief engineer; surveyed in 1855, again in 1857, actually begun in 1860, dropped; whole surveying business gone over again, sea level v. fresh water canal; municipality would not help in finding funds; shelved again in 1870. The canal was taken up by the duke of Buckingham's government in the beginning of 1876 with the intention of completing it to the Kistna canals in five years. As the season advanced it appeared probable that labour might be abundant and plans were pushed forward and all necessary organization for supervision of extended works prepared, so that when the failure of the monsoon indicated the need for large works nothing more was wanted than to move the companies of sappers to the place to erect the sheds for hospitals, stores, etc., at the previously selected camping places. And an organization was complete, from the superintending engineer to the hospital attendant, before a man was employed and so much in advance of the wants that for three months the staff was in excess of what the numbers coming to the works required. The expectations were that 30,000 men would come. For months the members were not half that.

The reason of this was that, although the people during the famine forsook their village homes to an enormous extent for the chances of finding food and work, yet all these movements were in definite directions. The people from Bellary, where the famine was intensest, and Cuddapah were encouraged to migrate to the Buckingham Canal works on the sea coast of the Nellore district; but this line of migration being out of the usual course and across a barren hill range, without water communication from Cuddapah to Nellore, though the thing was tried, it failed and the trial was disastrous to the people. But thousands migrated with success to the Kistna and Godavari irrigated districts in the north and to Trichinopoly and Tanjore, the great irrigated delta of the Kaveri in the south and found there food and work.

I propose, by the kindness of *The Illustrated London News,* to tell next week something of the glorious part acted by the Godavari, Kistna and Kaveri irrigation during the famine.

The Buckingham Canal, notwithstanding outbreaks of disease amongst the coolies and damage done by the cyclone of May 1877, was successfully carried on and, owing to the careful previous organization, is now a complete waterway.

To make up for previous scarcity of labour 19,000 coolies arrived almost unexpectedly in July, causing "great difficulty." The work, "for the most part, was carried out on task at little above normal rates."

All hail to the duke of Buckingham who has completed the gift of this wonderful boon—water communication all the way from Madras to Kakinada—the conveyance of troops and stores, of native passengers and of heavy native produce by canal at cheap rates, the one thing needful for native trade—enormous increase of trade in cotton, rice and oil, as well as improvement in the article cotton itself, sure to follow the opening of a navigable canal through.

Coals are now obtained at some of the pits for three rupees a ton, so that when the water transit is opened to the Wurdah the cost of navigating the canal will be greatly reduced.

May we venture to give the duke of Buckingham joy, as we give India and ourselves joy, on the noble results which will be twofold and tenfold every year, especially when steamers have been placed on this grand work? Where, too, so much has been done, more may still be done.

To take up speech and time with *what can't be done* is unworthy of Englishmen. "We can't water from the rivers when there is no water in them and we can't water the steep slopes of the mountains." This is the cry. The slothful man says, "There is a lion in the way." The practical man sees *what can be done.* He sees the full rivers, the hundreds of millions of acres of level land. Instead of lamenting that "Water won't run uphill," he rejoices that it will run downhill and that we can get it at any level the land requires.

[N.B.] Since this was written the glad news has come in from Madras, dated 22 March, that "this last week we have had fine rain over a large area in south India. This will rejoice the hearts of the unfortunate ryots, stimulate them to early culture and ease the tightening markets in regard to food prices."

29 April 1879

[2]

Sir, In India famine does not altogether, alas! cease to darken this year's prospects. The Punjab is in great peril and parts of Bombay are only just, if at all, falling short of scarcity. Orders have most opportunely been given to begin earthworks on the Neera Canal as relief works. But it is much to be feared that the condition of Indian finances will check operations. The Indapur people, too, have been petitioning for the completion of their canal.

A plague of rats is the last misfortune, and a very serious one it is, following upon a plague of locusts. Famine consequences do not disappear for years, even if there be no fresh scarcity. In many parts of Madras you see in village after village from one eighth to one third of the huts a mass of ruined walls, with no sign of anybody belonging to such ruins. Of migration—that is, of corresponding additions to villages in neighbouring districts—not a trace.

Nervously anxious about the safety of our frontier, we lay the burden of a war [the second Afghan war] upon our people at the very time that they are perishing by thousands of hunger. God forbid! but we *may* have another terrible year before us. But for timely rains, already was famine again looming in Madras, over a part of the country stricken in 1877; and in the North West Provinces, Oudh and the Punjab, owing to the deficient rainfall, the crops stand in imminent peril of failure. There will be but scanty harvests, even if famine be averted. And what with the high price of provisions, the extra taxation which this war will render necessary and the impoverished state of the peasantry, a scanty harvest is equivalent to a famine under ordinary circumstances. The people have no money, no grain reserves, no work. It is little known that starvation won its million of deaths in the last famine in the North West Provinces. What a fact that is!

The suffering we have inflicted on our own famished subjects by this costly war is appalling. The general seizure of camels has ruined, it is said, thousands of well-to-do families who, being engaged in trade, depended upon these camels for the conveyance of their merchandise to the proper markets. The price of provisions all over the Bengal presidency has risen to a height which has placed the scantiest means of subsistence beyond the reach of thousands. These die and make no sign. In helplessness, in uncomplaining silence, they lie down to die.

1. But what was the result of the irrigated lands in Madras, when tested by the "great teacher," famine? Was the relief afforded by the irrigated districts estimated? Did it suffice for themselves alone or also for others? Here are some of the results as given officially:

> The irrigation works in the Godavari and Kistna deltas, besides supporting the population of their own districts and a great crowd of hungry immigrants from the surrounding country, and besides exporting over country roads an amount of food grain which the collector of the Godavari estimates at little less than the amount exported by sea, supplied very nearly one fifth of the food grain imported during the worst period of the famine and 44 percent of the food exported from places within the Madras presidency itself

> for the supply of the famine demand during the same time. Tanjore and Trichinopoly, like the Kistna and Godavari, supported their own and all immigrant population, besides exporting by road, as well as by sea and rail, but only supplied by these latter routes 9 percent of the food grains imported and 21 percent of the grain exported from Madras ports between 1 August 1876 and 1 October 1877.

For the Godavari irrigation works, after making all deductions for land revenue, charges for maintenance and collection, etc., "the remainder (£110,000), being net amount left to meet interest charges, gives a clear return of 14.9 percent on the outlay incurred up to the end of the year."

The revenue of the district has actually increased by £240,000 more; £110,000 is added *directly* to the revenue by irrigation. But the fact is that about £300,000 is due directly or indirectly to the irrigation, making 40 percent on the outlay. "In like manner," from the Kistna irrigation works, "10⅓ percent clear interest on the capital outlay to the end of the year" is obtained.

It will be seen farther on that the "clear return" or "net revenue" from Godavari and Kistna irrigation works is put considerably higher by the "Annual Progress Report" "after careful calculation" and "special investigation." But so much the more reliable are the subsequent statements in the official paper, because clearly *within* the mark.

The Godavari returns are given by the "Progress Report" at 21 percent, which on £750,000 would be £150,000 a year. General Strachey's calculation, several years ago, was 28 percent and Mr Thornton, of the India Office, calculated 40 percent on the outlay. But when it is a matter of discussion whether an irrigation work returns 21, 28 or 40 percent, we may rest well content as to its success.

It is given officially that the gross value of the rice raised by means of the Godavari and Kistna canals during a year of famine when, to judge from the condition of neighbouring districts, there would not otherwise have been an acre ripened, "may be taken at 495 lakhs of rupees (£4,950,000) or *four times the whole capital outlay to the end of the year on the canal works of the two deltas* . . . the deduction for dry crops watered being considerably in excess of the reality and no account whatever having been taken of the value of these crops." (The italics are not mine, but those of the government writer.) These official statements of the export of grain and value of the crops raised are of the highest importance.

The united population of the two deltas of the Godavari and Kistna is assumed at about 1,800,000. But that of the Godavari district (not delta) alone was, in 1871, 1,600,000 and then rapidly increasing. And numbers of people during the famine flowed into a district where there was not only plenty of food but also plenty of money, enabling the landowners to make improvements. Overflowing funds and overflowing labour are the strongest inducement to private improvements. And the prosperous Godavari people had before this paid off their moneylenders.

In 1871, the year of the census, the population of Kistna was 1,450,000. That of the whole districts, Kistna and Godavari, cannot now be less than 3,000,000.

If Godavari exported by sea and land together 250,000 tons of grain, it must have saved the lives [of] about three millions of people at a pound a day for 200 days.

2. As to water transit in the deltas of the Godavari and Kistna, by official statement, "In the Godavari delta 425 miles of canal are now navigable and 495 miles will be navigable on the completion of the works. In the Kistna delta 286 miles of canal are now navigable and 320 will be so on completion of the works. . . . The canals of the Godavari and the Kistna are united by the Eluru Canal. . . . A large proportion of the Kistna produce passes down the Godavari canals to the port of Kakinada."

"During 1876-77, 108 passenger and 2093 cargo boats, having a registered tonnage of 45,874 tons, plied on the canals of the two deltas. The ton mileage was equivalent to a goods train carrying about 76 tons net run along the whole length of open canal on each day of the year." . . . "The total cost of carriage would be 4 2.3 [2/3?] pie, or say even 6 pie, per ton per mile." (A pie is less than a halfpenny; 4 pie make an anna, which has a nominal value of 1½d.; 16 annas make a rupee, which has a nominal value of 2*s.*)[73] "The cost by cart on the bad roads of the deltas would certainly not be less than 3 annas, and by pack-bullock 4½ annas per ton per mile, so that the saving effected by the delta canals during 1876-77 on carriage of goods alone must have amounted to at least 30 lakhs of rupees (£300,000)."

---

73 The next letter has a correction on this point: "I have a stupid mistake to correct in my last week's letter. The pie is only a twelfth of an anna; this makes a difference in calculating the cost of carriage, for the "say even six pie per ton per mile" is equivalent to only a half anna—nominally three farthings of our money. Twelve pie go to the anna."

All these are official statements, not mine. No wonder that the official paper adds: "Schemes for extending and developing the Kistna and Godavari works deserve the heartiest support of the Government of India."

3. Again, the government officer says:

> The remissions of the government demand for land revenue form a very correct measure of the condition of a district during a year of drought. In the Godavari district, where the irrigation works are nearly completed, the percentage of remissions on the gross demand of ryotwari revenue during 1876-77 was 1.9; in the Kistna district, of which the irrigation channels are still very incomplete, 15.6; in Chingleput and Bellary, which are dependent upon rain and tanks supplied from local sources, the percentages of remission were 70.4 and 61.4.

Taking famines merely from the financial point of view, it is not only the cost of maintaining the famine-stricken through one or more years of drought—maintaining, did I say maintaining?—when, in spite of all our efforts, public and private, the deaths from starvation are counted, not by ones or by hundreds, but by millions. It is that money is not only going out from the imperial revenues but that money is not coming in. Think what a cutting off of 60 to 70 percent of revenue from the famine districts means! It is docking the revenue at both ends. This is what "remission," necessary, inevitable, means.

4. Still continuing on the financial question, it has been hotly discussed what interest, what profit can be rightly attributed to irrigation works. Secretaries of state and governments of India, as well as the public, have differed upon this and a system of accounting has been ordered, which shall really solve this question. The "Annual Progress Report," Public Works Department, Madras presidency 1878 is the first official document which gives us the result. It says:

> It is only as regards the deltas of the Godavari and Kistna, and that quite recently, that a settlement has been made distinguishing between land assessment and water rate, but even here the principle of the settlement was a consolidated wet rate, of which an arbitrary and uniform portion was called the water rate. . . .

The question, apparently so simple, is really a complicated one, and wends its difficult way through "consolidated wet rates," "land and water gross assessments," "charges against works," etc. The "Progress Report" sums up:

> The necessity for ascertaining with as much accuracy as possible the profits on such enterprises as the irrigation works in the deltas has been long recognized and special investigations have been instituted and are in progress, which have for their object, on the one hand, the summing up of the charges against the works, on the other the determination of the revenue due to the outlay incurred. For five out of the eight systems approximate accounts have been prepared, and the following abstract shows the results which are for the present accepted.

These follow and they give:

| Percentage of net revenue on capital outlay | |
|---|---|
| Godavari delta | 21.25 |
| Kistna delta | 15.48 |
| Kaveri delta | 85.81 |
| Palar Anicut | 1.01 |
| Srivaikuntam | 3.65 |
| | 22.59 |

"*No* credit is allowed on account of land revenue."

The years given are years previous to those of the famine, when Godavari and Kistna works did such twofold and a hundredfold good service. God bless their author!

525,000 acres are under "wet" cultivation in Godavari delta, 246,000 in Kistna delta. 906,000 acres are under "wet" cultivation in the Kaveri delta.

Harking back to the official statement of June 1878, we find:

> while the whole of the works in the Godavari and the Kistna deltas are being carried out at the cost of the British government and aim at the economical distribution of the available supply on the most approved principles, besides providing inland navigation throughout the deltas, the Kaveri irrigation works in the Tanjore and Trichinopoly districts merely regulate, in a more or less imperfect manner, the distribution, broadcast over the surface of the country, of the freshes in the Kaveri river. The water is for the most part turned into spill channels or artificial cuts of such antiquity as to have assumed the appearance of natural channels, while private interests and vested rights of the most virulent type start up on all sides to oppose any but the most cautious attempts to improve on existing arrangements.
>
> The irrigation works in Tanjore and Trichinopoly have cost up to the end of 1876-77, Rs. 13,53,430, and it would be very desirable to spend another fifteen lakhs of rupees on their improvement (£150,000). The remissions in Tanjore amounted to 5.5, and in

Trichinopoly to 3.2 percent of the gross demand of ryotwari revenue during 1876-77.

This official paper discourages "calculations of interest upon outlay" in the case of the "Kaveri works, of which the capital account includes no allowance for the labour expended, in some cases centuries ago, on constructing the various channels of distribution, such as they are."

This, however, need not discourage us from spending another £150,000 on a district where the results have been so admirably large, the remissions so small.

Reverting to the same "Annual Progress Report" previously quoted, we see:

> The Kaveri delta has the largest area of irrigation in Madras. . . . Across the Coleroon (a branch of the Kaveri) a weir called the Upper Anicut was constructed about the year 1834 and was one of the earliest of the great works planned by Sir Arthur Cotton. Its effect on the delta has been very great, and the benefits conferred on the government and on the people of the Tanjore district have more than fulfilled the anticipations of the projector by securing a reliable supply of water and obviating the necessity [FN: (this must never be forgotten)] for collecting annually or, in some seasons several times during the year, several thousands of the cultivators to form temporary works for the diversion of water down the Kaveri. The head of this river is 1950 feet wide and the bed level is regulated by a dam. . . .

For full particulars see the "Progress Report" above mentioned and No. 561, Revenue Department, Madras, dated 9 April 1878. These two papers, if compared together, show the net return on irrigation works fairly chargeable to those works under the loan system, as distinguished from the gross return—that is, gross assessment on land *and* water, "dry" and "wet."

The proportion of revenue fairly attributable to irrigation is given from careful calculation, and the "resulting average rate of water cess per acre" is:

| | Rs. | Annas | Pie |
|---|---|---|---|
| Godavari delta | 3 | 1 | 7 |
| Kistna delta | 3 | 2 | 1 |
| Pennair Anicut | 2 | 10 | 9 |
| Kaveri delta | 3 | 0 | 2 |
| Palar Anicut | 3 | 13 | 8 |
| Srivaikuntam Anicut | 3 | 8 | 7 |

The regular water rate in Godavari is 4 rupees. A great extent of land belonging to the *rich,* it is said, is watered free. We cannot deal, it appears, with a man possessing 5000 acres as we do with a man holding five acres.

Under the old works the tax on irrigated land is from 8 to 12 rupees. It used to be 20 in some places. This includes 1 rupee or 1½ rupee for land tax.

In the last "Report of the Public Works in Bengal" there is an account of the ill-conditioned people they have to deal with in Berar—so different from the sensible, practicable Tamil and Telugu people of Madras presidency. A great portion of the trouble they have had with Berar irrigation arises from this difference of race. But do the worst of them show such perverseness as the English did about the Suez Canal?

5. Shall we not by all means work out the deltas and the river margin where it is to be had? These are *sure.* These will pay. The development of the great deltas, richly, as we see. Shall we not also choose projects of inland storage and channel works, examine them thoroughly and cautiously, to the very bottom, but with the determination to do them justice and even risk those which are much needed, putting up with the temporary loss, if loss there be, for the certain good and future profit, remembering that not only are the people thereby secured from famine, but they also contribute to support famine districts? And not only this, but the government are secured from having to make enormous remissions of revenue. Even were the works slowly done, even did they last twenty years, it were right to do them. Some of the greatest works in the world have been done by the patient cumulative industry of a couple of generations (ten governors).

6. Statesmen will understand that the execution of public works is a perfectly distinct subject from the state of the finances. The finances are one thing, the investment of money is another. These two must not be jumbled together in one account. The more defective the finances the more urgent are public works, which alone can enable the people to pay a higher revenue.

It were impossible to touch upon the famine question without a burst of admiration for the heroes who inch by inch held the famine at bay for long months. Alas! if they were worsted, if it carried off its millions in spite of us, at their door cannot lay the blood of our fellow creatures. But some account of the famine heroes must be given elsewhere. The question is here how to deal with future famines and how to avert them.

The Famine Commission have now concluded their investigation and their report will be presented this year. If the investigation was undertaken, as there can be no doubt it was, not to quiet us by making a show of inquiry, but with a resolution to sift matters to the bottom and then to discover the proper remedies to be applied, and if the Government of India is willing and able, as there can be no doubt it is, to apply the proper remedies, we may confidently expect the greatest strides towards solving this great problem—how to meet, how to prevent famine—famine, not the result *only* of drought from the skies, but, perhaps, in some measure the result also of some drought in wisdom, never in good intentions, wisdom in our legislation and government. Good intentions alone will not pave the way to prosperity. There must be good action too, not hasty and changed viceroy by viceroy, but action steady, continuous, to remedy blunders, if any such there be, in our land laws, in our civil procedure—blunders in aiding and abetting the moneylenders by our own civil courts and hereby the ruin of our cultivators; blunders in keeping up instead of keeping down our too expensive army; blunders in governing India by departments instead of encouraging civil native professions and studying not only to admit the natives more and more into our administration, judicial, financial and professional, but to raise them out of corruption and oppression of their own poorer fellows; blunders in making our government education a training school and nursery for government clerks instead of returning our scholars to their own lives, improved for, and able to improve their agriculture and their trades; blunders in making the land pay all the school cess, so that the ryots pay, the richer classes profit. (In Bombay and Madras the poor agriculturists who can afford neither time nor money to send their children to school pay for those who can afford to pay for their children's schooling.)

We may confidently expect from the Famine Commission not to ignore but to point out abuses and how to remedy them. May God speed the work of the Famine Commission!

But, inverting what Mr Gladstone said last night in the House of Commons, with even more than the fire of his wonted eloquence, as to "what this nation (England) will do in considering its own interests and in making provision for its own fortunes,"[74] let us never forget

74 Hansard, *Parliamentary Debates*, 3rd series (1830-91) 28 April 1879:1294. Gladstone's tough speech generally attacked the Conservative government for its foolhardy military expenditures, its "financial delusions," and defended

that India can neither consider her own interests nor certainly make "provision for her own fortunes." She *must* look to us.

5 May 1879

In today's *Times* a Simla telegram announces the government order that no military charges but all public works are to be stopped or cut down. "No new works, even if already sanctioned are to be commenced without special orders and the outlay on reproductive works is to be largely cut down. Military charges are left untouched for the present but the duty is declared of reducing them to the lowest point compatible with safety. This order is a step in the right direction." (The "duty" and acknowledgment of gravitation is "declared" "a step in the right direction.")

But do people know what the stoppage of government works means? It means throwing 100,000 labourers out of work (in the south of Madras alone) (see *Madras Times Overland Mail* 28 December 1878). It means leaving half a million of souls—those dependent upon the 100,000, including old people and children—to distress and death. It means depriving them of the only work they could get at a time when food grains were still from 50-100 percent higher than usual. It means making recovery from famine impossible.

South of Madras the people are suffering nearly as much as during the worst part of the famine, but then "*officially*" the famine is over and the condition of the people passes unnoticed. In the northern districts the crops were good.

As for public works they were all stopped long ago in order that a surplus might be shown to justify the recent concessions to Manchester.

Not only has nothing been done to help the labourers gradually recovering from famine but the usual public works have this year been stopped.

F.N.

27 May 1879

[3]

Sir, The Indian plot thickens, and a fire is lighted which, God be thanked, all the efforts of all the world will not be able to put out.[75] I

---

his own. He mentioned India only briefly, arguing: "That question has grown to such vast and menacing importance that it must, I think, form the subject of separate, serious and early discussion in this House." He even suggested that Britain might have to assume the debt of India (1290).

75 An allusion to Luke 12:49 or to the burning of Jan Huss.

do not allude to the Pune fires—sad witness of our broken promises to the indebted ryots of the Deccan, when these rose up, four years ago, against the oppression of the moneylenders. God forbid. We are now going to redeem our promises, to fulfill our responsibilities to India. We English have to learn a new language to India. Her day is come. The true friends of India have not only convinced the House of Commons, they have convinced the government also. But government ought not to have wanted convincing. They ought to have known it all before and taken measures to meet and remedy the evils which they now so fairly admit. At last they have spoken out the truth.

But to our business. It is little known that in 1877-78 above four millions of acres less than the ordinary were cultivated, or about 20 percent, in Madras. Agricultural prospects are now there improving, owing to the late good rains. One more instance of life saved by irrigation during the famine. One more instance of returns from irrigation works, not only during the famine, and I have done.

1. Kistna, Trichinopoly, Tanjore and Tinnevelly are composed of irrigated and non-irrigated taluks [districts]. In the *irrigated* taluks the trial census was taken and these areas showed, as was to be expected, an *increase of population,* aggregating about 8 percent in five years. But the *dry* parts of the districts suffered severely from famine, as may be seen from their death rates *registered.* (The *registered* deaths in Madras presidency may be estimated at about one half of the actual deaths in ordinary years and considerably less than that in famine years.) Thus:

| Non-irrigated Taluks | Death Ratios 1877 | Average of Five Years |
|---|---|---|
| Trichinopoly | 66.6 | 19.7 |
| Kistna | 25.2 | 16.9 |
| Tinnevelly | 40.4 | 18.9 |
| Tanjore | 37.4 | 32.3 |
| Mean death rates | 39.7 | 19.7 |

2. Lord Napier and Ettrick, formerly governor of Madras, draws attention particularly to "the Srivaikuntam Anicut (weir) in Tinnevelly, as a representative delta work on a small scale." At present it only

gives 3.65 percentage of net revenue. And people cry, It hardly pays. But see how short-sighted is this cry. It is, on the contrary,

> an example of the profits which may be expected from irrigation works of a very simple character in the present times under present prices. The work is to irrigate about 32,000 acres in an ancient irrigation district on either bank of one of the venerable old Indian rivers, Tambrapani, used from time immemorial as a breadwinner. Acres, 30,000 under cultivation; outlay up to April 1878, 9,19,947 rupees. But there are improvements contemplated. We may assume that the whole work will be perfected and completed within eleven lakhs, perhaps for little more than ten. But let us be *liberal.* Add to this sum a round sum on account of interest due for money borrowed and unprofitable for eight years, in whole or in part, during the construction—say (£10,000) one lakh. Total outlay from loan funds £120,000 (twelve lakhs) proportion of revenue attributable to irrigation 106,297 rupees; knock off 6297 rupees for expense of management, repair, etc., net revenue of return for an outlay of twelve lakhs, one lakh or between 8 and 9 percent. But there are still about 2000 acres to be brought under water. It may be fairly affirmed that, in round numbers, the return on capital expended will be 9 percent. But the capital is borrowed at 4¼ percent; 4¾ are therefore available to extinguish the capital debt.

When this is done "the Srivaikuntam Anicut will therefore pay the Government of India a net increase of revenue of £10,000 a year forever, besides all the indirect revenue accruing on the secured prosperity of the people living on and cultivating 32,000 acres of wet land. There will be very little charge for repairs and no risk of injury, the work being so familiar and simple." (For full particulars see "Annual Progress Report," Public Works Department, Madras Presidency 1878, and No. 61 Revenue Department, Madras, 9 April 1878.)

The moral to be drawn from this is plain. But the day is come when many a new and old moral has to be drawn for India by us English at home—at least by those of us who are neither hard-hearted nor selfish. May we be guided aright.

# Sanitation and the Prevention of Epidemics

Epidemics and infectious diseases, in addition to being recurrent phenomena in India, were, to the eyes of outsiders, endured by the local population with resignation and often with a sense of fatalism. Much work was required of the "sanitarians" to lift the veil of fatalism from over such calamities as cholera, smallpox, malaria and typhoid fever, and to lead people to combat such evils. Moreover, collaborative efforts of scientists and health care providers from everywhere were needed to find adequate diagnostics and cures, and to convince people to do their part in the battle. To Nightingale, sanitary measures were essential in this campaign; she had great motivation for engaging in the campaign as she firmly believed that sanitation not only promised eventual victory over diseases but even brought about civilization.

The fight to prevent epidemics had to begin at the level of elementary hygiene, to which the local population was to be awakened. Basic instruction on means of improving health and withstanding epidemics and infectious diseases was seen as a necessary first step; in this context the preparation of a "practical sanitary primer"[1] to diffuse information received growing attention, with a special emphasis on making sure that such information reached women and girls first of all, particularly those in elementary schools. On that issue Nightingale was led to co-operate with Lady Dufferin, as will be seen in the next volume, *Social Change in India.* After these first steps the right public health officers had to be appointed, which required the utmost care. Nightingale was convinced that "one of the most important functions of the presidency commissions and local authorities was the mitigation or prevention of epidemic disease among the native population. And for this purpose they should have the power of inspection and

1 Letter to Thomas Gillham Hewlett 2 December 1873, in *Social Change in India.*

recommending measures. Or they might be vested temporarily with absolute executive functions" (see p 451 above). Those steps are retraced in the correspondence below.

Nightingale and others also had debated the question as to whether or not the caste system was an impediment to implementing sanitary measures and whether epidemics, in Indians' eyes, were a divine punishment against their lack of resistance to foreign rule and therefore not to be fought.

In the mid-nineteenth century there was little clarity as to the origins of infectious diseases, and even of illness in general.[2] A plethora of theories vied with each other to explain the etiology of disease. The waterborne theory (diseases came from foul water), the zymotic theory (infection was linked to fermentation of matter or blood), the ozonic theory (ozone had an impact on health), the electrical theory, the telluric theory (unhealthy subsoil caused illness) and others were debated, but basically two main theories confronted each other, and their presence is amply found in the material below. First, there was the "miasmatic" (also called atmospheric or environmentalist) theory, which claimed that illness was caused by miasms or effluvia, i.e., by noxious emanations from a polluted source carried through and fouling the air, clinging to walls and inhabiting stagnant water. Conditions in Bengal favoured this view and helped shape the vision of India as a place of pestilence and peril. This theory rejected the role of human agency in the transmission of infectious diseases, and in general the idea that so-called "germs" could cause illness. Opposing the miasmatic theory was the germ theory, which attributed the origin of diseases to germs or micro-organisms of various sorts, bacteria, viruses, parasites, etc., that could be communicated from person to person or that circulated through the air. In the debates surrounding the various theories, political biases and vested interests played a considerable role, as modern scholars have made clear.[3]

2 See David Arnold, "Cholera and Colonialism in British India" 118-51; David Arnold, *Colonizing the Body* and *Science, Technology and Medicine in Colonial India* 57-91; Mark Harrison, *Public Health in British India: Anglo-Indian Preventive Medicine 1859-1914* 99-115; Mariko Ogawa, "Uneasy Bedfellows: Science and Politics in the Refutation of Koch's Bacterial Theory of Cholera" 671-707; and Alan Ramsey Skelley, *The Victorian Army at Home* 31-32.

3 See Mariko Ogawa, "Uneasy Bedfellows."

Nightingale, in agreement with and depending on colleagues in England (Chadwick, Sutherland, Fayrer and D.D. Cunningham; Farr until the 1870s) and in India (J.M. Cuningham, Hewlett, Bryden, various cholera commissioners and most of the Indian Medical Service) preferred the miasmatic theory. Hence Nightingale insisted on ventilation, drainage and the control of filth; conversely she was critical of quarantines, "cordons sanitaires" and other measures preventing physical contact with sick persons. In the eyes of administrators and merchants, quarantine was to be resisted as it endangered the commercial traffic, especially through the Suez Canal, which was opened in 1869 and from 1875 under British control.

The least that can be said is that Nightingale was reluctant to go along with the speculations of germ theory. She preferred the miasmatic or environmental theory for practical and perhaps even moral reasons: germ theory logically led to isolation of the patient at the micro level, and quarantine measures at the macro level. Throughout her life she advocated sturdy measures to remove the causes of infection: dirt, overcrowding, bad ventilation and bad water. She resisted germ theory for its connection with contagion theory—germs being the main disease-causing entities transmitted by contact—although her measures for removing the causes of infection made for good "germ practice." For most of her life she saw the two approaches as mutually exclusive: either germs or filth caused disease. It could not be both. But curiously, in 1858, she had accepted the idea that there was some kind of specific causal agent for a small number of diseases, such as smallpox, cow's pox and syphilis.[4]

Only in the 1880s did she finally accept germ theory as a valid theory—indeed then acknowledging some use for it. Robert Koch's identification of the cholera bacillus in 1883 during a cholera epidemic in Calcutta was the crucial breakthrough (further discussed in the second war volume of this series, for Koch's Calcutta trip followed research in Egypt during an Egyptian campaign). On the publication of Koch's results Dr Sutherland bought a "beautiful Vienna microscope" precisely for the purpose of seeing for himself the comma bacillus (an expression for the comma-shaped cholera bacillus). The task caused him to beg off a meeting with Nightingale that she had needed to prepare material for an interview with Lord Dufferin, who

4 See *Public Health Care* (6:23).

was then about to leave for India as viceroy. Dr Sutherland had explained that "if Dr Koch's cholera bacillus turned out well the discovery would save many more lives than Lord Dufferin, however carefully instructed, was likely to do."[5] Thereafter Nightingale still remained a reluctant germ theorist, grudgingly accepting the theory but continuing to make sarcastic references to it. In 1888 she referred to the "comma bacilli," joking that British rule in India had made things such that there was now "refuse so bad that comma bacilli cannot live in it" (see p 676 above). In 1890 she could still write (facetiously in part) to W.R. Robertson:

> I have found seven nos. of your admirable *Saidapet Journal* of the Agricultural Students Association—*which I trust continues.* It is so profitable to young men to write *exactly*. But I hope that they will not go mad about "bacilli" and "germs" and "bacteriology," which has been the "fad" here. But I think [it] is passing away in its dangerous aspect (Koch's), viz., that of considering the "germs" as the origin, not the product of disease, of which uncleanliness, bad drainage, bad water supply, etc., are the origin.[6]

She was far from alone in her slow acceptance of scientific progress in bacteriology. In England as late as 1894, "the great bacteriological discoveries of Koch and Pasteur were scarcely recognized, or were ridiculed, and Laveran's was almost unheard of."[7]

Nightingale's views of infectious diseases and their causes are related in *Public Health Care* (6:22-23 and 567-68) and in *Hospital Reform.* Readers should beware of secondary sources on this subject, which tend to describe Nightingale as an absolute and blind opponent of germ theory. Certainly she always preferred the miasmatic, environmental approach, which continued to be helpful in guiding preventive measures, but she was gradually attracted by the merits of germ theory and came to understand that bacilli really existed and were harboured and nourished in the right sort of environment. The cholera bacillus thrives in human bowels and is transmitted through

---

5 Cook, *The Life of Florence Nightingale* 2:344; the exchange of material on this in Cook is missing from the appropriate British Library volume.

6 Letter 31 March 1890, Asia, Pacific and Africa Collections Mss Eur B 263 f29.

7 Ronald Ross quoted by Mark Harrison, in *Public Health in British India* 57. Sir Ronald Ross (1857-1929), officer of the Indian Medical Service. In the 1890s he demonstrated a link between malaria and mosquitos. He was awarded the Nobel Prize for Medicine in 1902.

excrement to sewage and water polluted by it, which made plain the need for proper sewer systems. By 1891 she wanted to use the ability to see micro-organisms to stir people to action. She proposed village lectures with "slides" showing germs swimming in polluted water: "Probably the village schoolrooms might be utilized for the lectures, which might be made attractive by object lessons, with the magic lantern showing the noxious living organisms in foul air and water."[8]

When all is said, the two theories are not mutually exclusive; bacteriology and sanitation rather can and do co-exist, as practice since the early twentieth century has demonstrated. To Nightingale and its opponents, germ theory seemed to excuse inaction toward the real causes of disease, the filth or bad water that later science would see as nourishing the growth and spread of germs. But when Nightingale worked at the elimination of filth, inspired as she was by the miasmic vision, she was also killing the germs responsible for the origin and propagation of disease. When firmly applied, sanitary measures knock out undesired micro-organisms.

In the final analysis, Nightingale did not believe that medical doctors had the competence to apply sanitary measures, the only means, in her mind, to fight epidemics; well-trained sanitary engineers and officers had that competence, as she was to state firmly to Lord Dufferin in 1886. To him she explained she held that "sanitation is a speciality; ordinary medical men are all contagionists and would advise quarantine and such things, and not one has studied the question of sanitary construction of buildings, etc." (see p 925 below). Therefore she insisted that more executive power be given to the sanitary officers if progress in public health was to be achieved.

It remains that "British concern with Indian sanitation," in the judgment of T.R. Metcalf, was "obsessive yet ineffectual," and poor at dealing with the problems of a tropical climate. "From Dr Bonavia's hapless endeavour in the 1860s to put an end to public defecation among the citizens of Lucknow to the fierce denunciations, continued up to the present, of 'filthy drains' and 'stagnant cesspools,' India's sanitary shortcomings distinguished it as a land of squalor and of indulgence, of bodies that were out of control."[9]

---

8 Letter to the Poona Sarvajanik Sabha December 1891, in *Quarterly Journal of the Poona Sarvajanik Sabha* 15,1 (July 1892):13-17. The entire text is given in *Social Change in India.*

9 Thomas R. Metcalf, *Ideologies of the Raj* 173.

Cholera, the typical epidemic disease of nineteenth-century India, illustrates the overwhelming difficulties encountered in the fight against illness. The main attacks took place in 1817-21 and variously between 1856 and 1861, 1867 and 1877, and caused millions of deaths. Cholera struck the poor disproportionally and was at its most virulent when it coincided with famine.[10] Pilgrimages were dangerous occasions for spreading the disease due to the multiplied contact with infected people and the practice of "sordid" rituals. Colonial powers were reluctant to criticize such institutions directly, however, since their action would be seen as an attack on Hinduism and risked political backlash. All the same, sanitary measures remained imperative.

The following letters and notes offer a wide conspectus of Nightingale's evolving views of infectious diseases and epidemics, starting in 1860. Included is a small amount of material on the Contagious Diseases Acts, or measures intended to reduce syphilis. Most of the material is on the practical measures required to prevent disease by improving drainage, sewerage and clean water supply, all familiar themes from the royal commission's recommendations.

Source: From fragments of a document, Wiltshire County Record Office, Pembroke Collection 2057/F4/68

[1860-61]

It appears from what Dr Farr said this morning that the chief object he has in view in having a weekly state *printed* is publicity, and the weekly state being accompanied by notes pointing out the most important results of the weekly statistics, as regards the health and efficiency of the troops, he expects, would direct the attention of the commanding officer more pointedly to the sanitary state of his regiment, while the public will be kept fully informed on the sanitary state of the army.

Without giving any opinion either on one side or the other, it may be well to consider how far the Horse Guards would permit this publication. A weekly return is *indispensable* for the working of the sanitary department and *must be had.* Consequently all the forms and books required for this weekly return are indispensable. . . .

The experience of the great loss to the troops from tropical diseases shows the extreme importance of studying carefully the whole subject of army hygiene and tropical epidemics, with special reference to applying such sanitary measures as may remove the local horror of

10 David Arnold, "Cholera" 123-26.

malaria. Whether as regards garrisons, stations, barracks and hospitals—upon which such epidemic outbreaks depend—and diminishing as far as practicable the circumstances of exposure which tend to augment the individual predisposition of the men [breaks off]

Source: From a letter to William Farr, Wellcome Ms 5474/46, typed copy ADD Mss 43399 ff18-19

Hampstead, N.W.
5 October 1861

I do not admit your definition of fanaticism, nor that truth can be fanatical. Either your "contagionists" are in the right and then they are not fanatical; or your "non-contagionists" are in the right and *they* are not fanatical. *Both* cannot be fanatical any more than both can be in the right. Quarantine follows logically and inevitably on "contagion" as sanitary measures on non-contagion.

Farther than this, I do not venture to argue with you, because, as you say, I am not scientific. Neither do I quote the opinion of those men (whom you think I worship) such as Chadwick, for the same reason—he is not scientific—I only modestly and *really* humbly say, I never saw a fact adduced in favour of contagion which would bear scientific inquiry. And I could name to you men whom *you* would acknowledge as scientific who place "contagion" on the same footing as witchcraft and other superstitions.

## Contagious Diseases Acts

**Editor:** Nightingale was involved for many years in the fight against the attempt to reduce syphilis in the army through the compulsory inspection and treatment of suspected (women) prostitutes, and with nothing compulsory for the soldiers (all men). The institution of these Contagious Diseases Acts for Britain is related in detail in *Women* (8:411-515), where only a small portion of the material relates to India. A high rate of syphilis in the British Army in India was, however, a prime factor in prompting recourse to this drastic course (the infection rates were considerably lower among the sepoys, who of course typically were married and able to live with their spouse). Nightingale's view was that prostitution, which the British Army encouraged, was the real problem. The army held to the conventional double sexual standard: men had to have sex, and so required prostitutes when married intercourse was not possible. Prostitutes in turn supplied liquor to soldiers, which further served to undermine their health.

Nightingale rejected the double standard, as did other opponents of the legislation. On the one hand she promoted marriage—but while the army could not stop men from marrying, ensuring limited accommodation for wives was a very effective barrier to normal married life for soldiers. On the other hand, Nightingale consistently advocated military measures to encourage such sublimating activities as exercise, gardening, sports and other decent leisure pursuits as alternatives to bars and brothels (see p 182 above).

She was pleased to keep a recommendation for compulsory inspection and treatment out of the report of the royal commission on India, but the first Contagious Diseases Act was legislated in Britain in 1864 and similar provisions were put in place in India. Both sets of measures were eventually repealed. Nightingale was only peripherally involved in the repeal campaign in Britain, and seems not to have been involved at all in the India debate.

Source: From a letter to Harriet Martineau, Add Mss 45788 ff253-56

14 March 1864

*Private.* You have the two volumes of the India sanitary report. And in Sir A. Tulloch's evidence it is stated that the admissions from syphilis in the army amount to 60 per 1000 per annum—not 400 and 500, as is popularly believed. Mr Acton's table clubs together all kinds of diseases under one denomination.

There is little literature on the subject. What there is relates solely to the *disease*, the mode of treatment. The present movement should be discussed under the head of public morality, public policy, public utility. Proof of all three—overwhelming proof—ought to be produced. Medical *opinion* is absolutely worthless except as to the treatment. As to prevention, that is another thing. About that, they have given us no evidence at all. My evidence is (but all Paris police papers are kept so secret that I cannot produce any) that the Paris police, the only people who know anything about it, state that there the disease among the prostitutes is very small, among the men is very much *increasing*; that, in thousands of cases among *men*, examined and traced at great expense, *not one* was traced to a diseased woman. The act of vice between a man and a prostitute, even not diseased, seems to produce the disease, but not invariably (no more than everybody catches smallpox under bad sanitary conditions) in the man.

Oh that a medical man would observe, as I have observed, in Paris! There, where the perfection of medical police exists, are the worst forms of disease among men—married men. If Paris civil life were to be sent to hospital as our soldiers are, half Paris would be in hospital. The reason is that vice has been made prevalent—there by the fancied immunity from disease, to a degree we have no idea of. . . .

As regards soldiers, until we have provided men with rational means of work and recreation for their spare time, what can we expect but dissipation? and disease?

**Editor:** In the 1880s evidence of rising syphilis in India, i.e., after the repeal of the Contagious Diseases Act, prompted a recommendation to reinstitute the compulsory legislation. There is some correspondence on the issue in the 1880s, but it seems Nightingale took no position on it *(Women* 8:506-07). Then in 1897 she signed a "Women's Memorial," published by the *Times* of 25 May, for "effectual measures" to "be taken to check the spread of contagious diseases among our soldiers, especially in India." Many high-ranking women signed it, including Lady Lawrence, major nursing colleagues and Dr Mary Scharlieb. Nightingale's signature was given subject to the addition of the request that "An independent inquiry be at the same time set on foot at the several stations in India, as recommended by the Governor General of India and Council in the military despatch to the secretary of state for India, No. 184, dated Simla, 4 November 1896, appended to the report of the departmental committee." The memorial was sent to high officials of the government, and its complete text is found in *Women* (8:508-09).

## Disease Prevention and Sanitary Measures

**Editor:** The 1863 royal commission on India recommended, among others, a series of sanitary measures aimed at combatting disease in India. Henceforth Nightingale's correspondence reinforced those recommendations, which she had been instrumental in formulating. We present here an overview of her efforts in the matter from 1863 on.

Among the sanitary measures recommended to prevent disease were drainage, sewerage, water analysis and safe water supply, healthy location of stations and villages, engineering works, proper ventilation, protection against tropical climate, changes in bad habits and the regulation of pilgrimage sites, all measures determined by the current view of the origin of disease. Irrigation also had a role to play in this context, although its major impact was seen in the battle against famine, as shown above.

The diseases that the recommended sanitary measures aimed to reduce included typhus, malaria, cholera, various types of fever and smallpox; these sometimes reached an epidemic magnitude.

Source: From a letter to Robert Rawlinson, Boston University 1/2/32

9 January 1863

We hope to have your views fully stated about the sewering of Indian towns. At present they use a vile system of open cuts in front of the houses, into which all the filth goes and festers there.

As a general principle, and where there is good surface drainage, no doubt the rainfall should mainly sweep over the surface. But in India the great evil in that, after the rains have soaked the ground and as soon as the water level begins to descend below the surface, all kinds of fevers and bowel diseases show themselves; in fact this state of the subsoil is the main cause of army mortality.

The royal commission has recommended drainage for getting rid of this subsoil water. Cuts and water courses do not answer, except during the height of the rainy season. At all other times, they give off malaria, unless very small.

In stating therefore the general principle that flood waters must be allowed to escape in the most natural way, it will be necessary carefully to distinguish between flood waters and subsoil water, the removal of which latter by the most speedy method is the key to the sanitary improvement of stations, so far as draining can have an effect.

In the additions to our paper, which you will kindly make,[11] will you be so good as to keep in view this distinction? If Indian towns are not to be paved, then it is difficult to see how the subsoil can be kept free of water, except by a thorough system of subsoil drainage. And yet the subsoil must be kept dry, if any good is to be done. This is the real engineering work required. There is this difference between English and Indian towns: English towns are paved and surface-drained, by which the water is carried to outlets or underground sewers. Indian towns are not paved and have no surface drains, and the water either evaporates, runs off or, as is the case, it mostly sinks into the subsoil and causes an immense amount of disease. English towns require "sewerage" in your sense. Indian towns in their present state require "sewerage" and "drainage."

---

11 Probably Rawlinson's "Instructions and Suggestions" for the A.S.C.; see letter to Rawlinson 1 January 1864, Boston University 1/3/37.

Source: From a letter to James Pattison Walker, Florence Nightingale Museum (LMA) H1/ST/NC1/64/8

18 June 1864

*Private.* I thank you very heartily for your letter of 7 May and for its enclosure of your minutes. The filter in the Mediterranean report will answer your purpose. It is intended specially for filtering water *before* being tanked for use. If, e.g., you had good tanks for Fort William and if you collected all rainwater from roofs for drinking and cooking, you would pass the whole of it through such a filter before allowing it to enter your tanks. (The War Office commission will recommend it specially for India in the *Suggestions* called for by your president.)

Source: From a letter to Harry Verney, Wellcome (Claydon copy) Ms 9001/48

Hampstead, N.W.

5 August 1864

By the next mail, I shall, without mentioning names, . . . introduce the subject in my letter to Sir John Lawrence. . . . What I shall say to Sir J. Lawrence is this: there is no natural reason why Delhi should not be healthy and, if unhealthy, the cause is removable. With such a rate of sickness, the place is untenable and the disease (Delhi sore) fatal to efficiency. And it must be taken up by the Bengal Sanitary Commission.

The Mediterranean cities suffer from a bad form of carbuncular sore—a tenth part of the cases proving fatal—and inquiry has shown that damp with foul air, by gradually undermining stamina, are predisposing causes.

The Delhi causes can only be understood by careful local inquiry, including not only troops but native population. The following points suggested:

1. Extent to which Delhi sore prevails among natives, especially state of localities where it is most prevalent.

2. Extent to which it has prevailed among troops, comparison between localities they occupy and localities occupied by native population.

3. Minute medical inquiry into nature of diseases, including microscopic examinations into nature of sores—previous symptoms to be very carefully described (whether scorbutic).

4. Minute inquiry and report as to nature of barrack and hospital accommodation in reference to position, drainage, ventilation, cubic space, general construction, state of buildings.

5. Minute chemical analysis of various waters supplied for use, analysis to be both qualitative and quantitative. (Roofwater filtered and stored

would afford sufficient drinking and cooking water.) If the waters are alkaline or contain organic matter, especially animal matter, in any quantity, such waters are unfit for use.

6. Examination of ration, specially as regards pork or bacon, which should be struck off the list of substances used as food.

7. Carefully drawn up report on whole subject to be made, pointing out causes and remedies, immediate steps to be taken to have requisite improvements carried out.

I send to Mr Calvert for you today a copy of *Suggestions* (you will see how particular we are about water supply), sent out to Sir J. Lawrence direct by me, by H.M.'s book post, at his own earnest request (for, of all the slow-going government offices, the India Office is the worst), signed by the said Barrack & Hospital Improvement Commission.

Source: From a letter to Robert Rawlinson, Boston University 1/3/45

22 February 1865

I should be very much obliged to you, if you would be so kind as to give me an opinion, such as I might send to Calcutta, on the enclosed paper regarding disinfectants, sent me from thence. I have just sent Lord Stanley (privately) your opinion regarding the Bombay reference about disinfectants, in the minute by which you replied to Sir C. Wood.

Source: From three letters to James Pattison Walker, Florence Nightingale Museum (LMA) H1/ST/NC1/65/6, 8 and 19

26 February 1865

I am sure you are perfectly right as to taking the conservancy collections out to sea. Proper dung boats, with a small steamer to remove the filth of Calcutta down the river to the sea, is the only plan. This is what we used to do at Balaclava in the Crimea. And *till* we did it, Balaclava was on a small scale what Calcutta is on, alas! too large a one, the hotbed of cholera and typhus, even during the short time we infested it. If, under a very fine climate, a small place like Balaclava became in nine months, i.e., till the dung boats were used, what was very nearly the graveyard of a whole British expedition, what must Calcutta have become in 100 years under a very trying climate?

About the disinfectants: we have had this question referred to us over and over again from the Bombay government and have consulted the Local Government Act Office. I send you an opinion of theirs, though it does not apply precisely to your case.

> It is the old, old story over again—disinfectants in place of removal—and a wish to have things "far sent and dear bought." Wood charcoal dust will do all which the fluids and powders are said to have done. But cleansing and reforming the latrines and drains, with subsequent flushing, washing and regular removal of refuse, at short intervals, will be better. These disinfectants are the right-hand power of ignorance and nothing more. We do not repudiate disinfectants; they have a use, but that use is not to palliate refuse heaps, which ought never to have been allowed to accumulate. A temporary use of disinfectants may be allowed, to enable a safe removal of refuse now existing to be made—the store of poison heaped up by ignorance in past times. But a continuance of poison storing and disinfecting should not be allowed. MacDougall's powder may prevent the heaps of foul refuse killing the men ordered to remove it, or wood charcoal powder, but on the condition that any such heaps and deposits are not to accumulate in future.

I wish such papers as this of the health officer of the municipality of Calcutta could be remitted home for the Barrack and Hospital Improvement Commission (consisting of members of the War and India Offices and Local Government Act Office) to make their suggestions upon. It appears not impossible. At this moment the Bombay engineer [H. Tulloch] is in England, consulting with one engineer of the Local Government Act Office, on the drainage of Bombay.

10 April 1865

I cannot sufficiently thank you for most kind letters, by several mails repeated: for four most valuable and encouraging statistical tables, which we shall make great use of; for a number of printed papers, all more interesting one than the other.

I have consulted several scientific men, both in London and Manchester and at the Army Medical School at Netley, about the water supply analysis question, as to which you did me the honour to write to me.

18 October 1865

*Private.* I am very sorry to hear you are so far from well. But I hope that you have taken holiday in time. John Bull is a conceited ass and thinks the climate ought to take care of him, instead of him taking care of the climate. The French fare much better. Anglo-India has made its capital of a place where the Mughals used to send their state prisoners to die. And people fall ill in Calcutta, and then say, it's the climate. The royal commission never told you all to live in Calcutta.

But you abuse them for not having laid sufficient stress on "climatic influences." *We* are spending just five millions sterling to empty that small gutter, the Thames, of sewage. And this in a temperate climate. What are *you* doing?

It is not that Calcutta might not be made much more healthy than it is, if you were willing to spend several millions. The main question is to keep the subsoil moisture at a certain distance below the ground varying with latitude and local circumstances. This costs money. If it *costs too much*, as perhaps in a place like Calcutta, then the place ought to be abandoned, or never to have been chosen. This is the only real determination of localities, as far as healthy surface of ground is concerned. But people in India, though they are always raving against the "climate," actually tolerate a state of things in their palaces which we here ceased to tolerate in the poorest village in this healthy climate. And yet we have always typhus and sometimes cholera, and at this moment the Poor Law Board is meditating a sweeping bill (for London) for next session, because the vestries are not doing their duty. And the Poor Law Board is quite right. (I tell you this—but it is a secret.)

There are 120 ways of boiling eggs (this *anent* "climatic influences"). Climate is good everywhere. But man and his habits and his manner of selecting places to live in and to build on are as bad as possible (as I say, John Bull's a conceited ass and his conceit is that climates are made to obey him). And hence he confounds climate with his own want of care. He ought to boil his eggs better.

Batavia [Djakarta] was the most deadly place in the world. And now people go there for their health. Can anything be stronger than this?

In the table of mortality for 1859-64, shown in its distribution by months, which you have been good enough to send me, are appended notes as to the climatic elements which are assumed as causing the increasing death rates during certain months. I think this is a pity. They belong to a method of determining causation, which in this country we venture to think we have improved upon. High temperature and moisture are nothing per se. As influencing other causes, they are a great deal—they have immense power. To place them as *causes* is much the same thing logically as it would be to make the perfection or imperfection of roast beef depend on the quantity of coals raised at Newcastle, as if you said, the more fuel the sun puts into his grate, the more unhealthy India becomes.

I have to thank you for your most kind note of 16 August and for its enclosure from Dr Bryden. There is a growing conviction in Europe that, when cholera seizes a population living in bad sanitary conditions, its influence may extend hundreds of miles atmospherically from the centre where it began. And there is a diplomatic proposition to suppress or regulate the Mecca pilgrimage, in order to prevent its becoming the epidemic centre for the West, which it has always been hitherto. The moral is that unless you improve the sanitary condition of the civil populations, you cannot insure immunity for the soldiers from epidemics.

I have to thank you, which I do most cordially, for the valuable draft No. 262 about railway travelling by troops, also for the extract of a letter No. 247 about the jails in the Lower Provinces. How curious and instructive that is, and how terrible. It shows that someone must again set hard to work to reform the management and laws of these jails, like a Howard, and never leave off till he has done. The contrast between the men's and women's health, and between the cubic space for each, startles even me.

But my mind is full of Lord Palmerston's illness. He may be passing away even at this moment. He will be a great loss to us. He made a joke about everything. But, though he made a joke when asked to do the right thing, he always did it. No one else will be able to carry the things through the Cabinet [as] he did. I shall lose in him a powerful protector. Especially in Poor Law and wide sanitary views, he was so much more in earnest than he appeared. He did not do himself justice. His *presumed* successor is so queer-tempered that he cannot manage the Cabinet.

Source: From notes, Add Mss 45836 ff23-26

[1864-65]

Note on relation which should exist between the powers of raising and spending taxes proposed to be granted to local authorities throughout India and the proper execution of sanitary works and measures. Taking for granted that the measures proposed in the *Gazette of India* of 14 September 1864 for the future police administration of towns and districts are the best adapted to meet local circumstances, it is most desirable that every precaution be taken, that the money raised for conservancy purposes is spent in such manner as not only to do no harm to health but to benefit health.

These two principles flow from ascertained experience at home. Much of the work of sanitary improvement in England has consisted in undoing, tearing up, destroying and reconstructing works already existing which had been planned and constructed by local authorities and paid for out of the rates. . . .

It is obviously of the greatest importance to derive all possible benefit from this experience in India and to provide for the following successive steps in the procedure:

1. Some competent sanitary and engineering authority must determine the drainage area and general limits within which sanitary works and improvements are to be carried out by every local authority. The reason of this is obvious: it relates to questions of outfall for drainage, the application of sewage to agricultural purposes, the deposit and utilizing of solid refuse matters, the draining and reclaiming of unhealthy ground near towns, and the prevention or removal of distant sources of nuisance.
2. The same authority should either prepare or sanction a general survey and map of the whole district, laying down the contours, levels, outfall, course of sewers and drains, streets, roads, houses, properties.
3. The same authority should prepare or sanction a general scheme of sanitary improvement, including works of drainage, water supply, paving, cleansing, opening up of streets, laying out new streets and other sanitary measures which are to be carried out in detail and for the execution of which the local authority is to raise the required sums of money.
4. The same authority or some similar authority should inspect works in course of execution to see that they will fulfill the required object.
5. The same authority or some similar authority would have to see that the works were kept in proper and efficient repair and working order.

The royal commission proposed the appointment of the existing presidency sanitary commissions for the express purpose of giving a beneficial direction to all expenditure for sanitary purposes, whether civil or military, and the question has now arrived at this point that it will be necessary to arrange the order in which the various authorities should act.

They [the above proposals] are not put forwards as affording a solution of the difficulty, but solely to show what the difficulty is and how apparently it might be met, in conformity with the inference drawn by the royal commission from past practices in India, viz., constructive works should be executed under the Public Works Department, but you have illustrations of another method of procedure in the cases of Calcutta and Bombay, in both of which places the municipal authority has employed its own engineer as is done in England.

Such a course would be most in conformity with the extended introduction of municipal authorities throughout India. But again it would be very difficult to find a sufficient number of competent sanitary engineers even to make a beginning. The way would be wonderfully smoothed if the capitals were once put into a good sanitary state. A number of engineers would be trained in the process, who might be drafted to other cities. And possibly the chief engineers of the presidency capitals might act as consulting engineers to other municipalities. There are difficulties anyway and the whole case has been stated above, so far as our knowledge here extends, in order that you may have an opportunity of considering in what manner the works (described in the *Suggestions* prepared by the W.O. commission) may be carried out, so far as these works are applicable to Indian cities and towns.

Source: From a draft and three letters to Douglas Galton, ADD Mss 45763 ff83-84, 85-86, 87-89 and 91-93

[before 28 October 1865]

I have had more than one letter from Mr Chadwick about a plan he has for indoctrinating young engineers into the principles of sanitary work. I also saw the draft of a paper he wished [?] to send to Lord de Grey on the subject. He writes me to say that he had sent it in. Now I think the proposal of the greatest importance, and if you can arrange some way [whereby] the men (whose duties on India at least will now to a great extent include sanitary work and great canal and irrigation works) can be brought into contact with the experience acquired at home, you will have done a great good not only to the service but to the country at large. I entirely agree with Mr Chadwick's views on these points and I know Mr Ellis will tell you he thinks the proposed practical instruction is absolutely necessary, for there are scarcely any men in India at the present moment competent to undertake the simplest drainage work. Some time ago I received from Bengal [J.P. Walker's letter of 23 February 1865] an urgent request to supply the commission with the best methods of detecting noxious substances in water.

28 October 1865

*Private.* I am afraid, now that you are come back, you will have a whole pile of "addresses" from me.

No. 1: Mr Chadwick has been perpetually writing to me about his plan for indoctrinating young engineers with the principles of sanitary works. He showed me the draft of his paper to Lord de Grey and asked me for corrections, which I made. I understand from him that Lord de Grey has had it and that Lord de Grey has sent it to you. The proposal is of the greatest importance, as I am sure you will think. And, if you can arrange some way whereby the men (whose duties, in India at least, will now to a great extent include sanitary works and great canal and irrigation works, by Sir J. Lawrence's recent enactment) can be brought into contact with the experience acquired at home, you will do a great good, not only to the service but to the country at large. Mr Ellis (Madras Sanitary Commission's president) thinks the proposed practical instruction is absolutely necessary, for there are scarcely any men in India at the present moment competent to undertake the simplest drainage works.

30 October 1865

Is that unfortunate Christian, Captain Galton, come back? Then here comes No. 2.

Last winter, I received from Bengal an urgent request to supply the Indian commissions with the best methods of finding out how much dirt there is in the water they drink. I consulted your masters and pastors at Netley. But they could make nothing of it. Then I consulted Dr Angus Smith of Manchester (who, I think, is more difficult to manage than the whole Indian government). First, he says one thing, then he says the reverse, then he listens to what his "nephews and nieces in Argyleshire" say (sic) and tears up the paper. (But I had it in type.)

Five mortal months and six mortal times has this paper been through our hands and there is scarcely a word in it which there was in the first revise. But Dr Angus Smith is the only man in Europe who could do it. And this paper is well worth the trouble it has cost us. I have printed this at my own expense, because no mortal office could be required to deal with Dr A. Smith's vagaries. When it has reached the sixtieth revise, I shall make the India Office and the War Office distribute it. *Pray*, make the War Office take copies for the army medical officers, everyone of whom may be placed any time in the position of being obliged to use the methods of testing contained in this paper. (You may do this with perfect safety as it is the best thing of the kind in existence.) But please remember it is quite "private" *at present.* For I must smooth down the ruffled feathers of Messrs Parkes and Hoffmann first. Or they won't recommend it to their pupils.

1 November 1865

*Private and Confidential.* I have not said a word to Dr Sutherland about the subject of your yesterday's note. I would not have you think that I am indifferent as to whether the inhabitants of Malta and Gibraltar have cholera. On the contrary; you will remember that I never left poor Sidney Herbert in peace till he sent you and Dr Sutherland (the last act of his life) to the Mediterranean stations. But Dr Sutherland ought to be *coming back* now, instead of going there *now.* We are full of Indian business, business which must be settled before Parliament meets. Lord Stanley (which I tell you in the closest confidence) has consented to take it up.

*One* item is: Indian jails. And I have pledged myself to have it all ready by the time Parliament meets, a thing I should never have done if I had thought Dr Sutherland would be sent abroad. You are yourself aware that Calcutta water supply has been sent home to us (at my request). And Dr Sutherland told me this morning that *he and I* should have to write the report. (Dr S. is so childish that, if he heard of this Malta and Gibraltar plan, he would instantly declare there was nothing to keep him in England.) *I* do not weigh the importance of the several objects. *That* is for *you* to determine. I merely state to you what is on hand and leave you to judge. *No* one could do the India business but Dr Sutherland. I think there *are* men who could do the Malta and Gibraltar business.

About "ventilation": it was *I* who said to Mr Ellis that Mr Rawlinson knew little about ventilation. I said the War Office knew a great deal. Mr Ellis is terribly bitten (through Mr Chadwick) with French artificial ventilation. And I told him that Dr Sutherland was a dangerous lunatic (and I a harmless lunatic) on the subject of *natural* ventilation. But I think it would be entire loss of time to send Sutherland to Algeria to convert Mr Ellis.

Source: From a letter to James Pattison Walker, Florence Nightingale Museum (LMA) H1/ST/NC1/65/23, typed copy ADD Mss 45781 f307

26 November 1865

*Private. At last* I send you the final revise, which I have just received from the printers, of Dr Angus Smith's paper on water analysis, asked for by you, I am afraid to say, how many months ago. But I can truly say I have not lost a moment. First I applied to our Army Medical School professors, to some of our great government chemists. None were able to satisfy the want. Dr Angus Smith is the only man in Europe who could do it. And this paper is well worth all the trouble.

But what that trouble has been no one who does not know Dr Angus Smith can know. (I think he is more difficult to manage than all the Government of India.) The enclosed paper has been through his hands and mine some fifteen times. And we have had nine revises of it from the printers. The rough proof which I send you, though merely a rough proof, is the final one. It has been seen and approved by the great War Office sanitary authorities. And on Wednesday when they have a meeting, they mean, I believe, to vote the sending it "by authority" to army medical officers abroad and to the school at home as their textbook. But I make haste to send you this copy. And I will send you others, when I have had it printed off. In great haste

yours most gratefully for your many kindnesses
Florence Nightingale

Source: From two letters to Douglas Galton, ADD MSS 45763 ff103-04 and 106-07

28 November 1865

*Private.* I remembered to you the fact of my having been asked from India to obtain a method of water analysis for them, of my having applied to Parkes and others, of their failure, of my applying to Dr Angus Smith, of my printing his paper, which has been fifteen times and ten weary months through our hands, and five months through nine revises through the printers. Here is a rough proof of the final revise. Tomorrow Dr Sutherland presents it at your meeting and proposes a vote for its distribution "by authority" to army medical officers in India and to your school at home. I thought I had better send you a copy first, asking you to consider the number of copies, if you do distribute it "by authority," that you will take, as I have not had it printed off yet and wish to be able to do so. Also to say that I have made up my mind: it is better for me to pretend to know nothing at all about this, instead of making a communication to Dr Parkes to mollify him (for having failed). If it is to become a textbook at the Army Medical School, it is better that Dr Parkes should not know that it has any connection with his failure or with my request. Angus Smith's paper is perfect and (hitherto) unique and well worth all the trouble.

7 December 1865

*Angus Smith's water analysis paper.* I don't know exactly how to answer your note of the 4th. The paper was written at my request, in order to comply with a request from India. The paper will be very useful, but, in order to be useful, it must be circulated. And to be circulated it must be bought, either by you or by me. I shall want 100 copies for myself. Dr Angus Smith (whom I have asked) will want 200. If you can, buy 1500 or 2000 copies --. You may do this any way you like. But don't drag me through the Stationery Office, which I know of old. What thou doest, do quickly.[12] And don't bring me into it. For I would rather pay for it than that. I was in hopes you would have told me how many copies you wanted. And then I should just have had it printed off. It is of the greatest consequence to do it quickly.

The two men in India who originally started the idea and who would have worked it, are both going to resign from ill health. It has been already ten mortal months on hand. And I must have copies to send out (some) by Sunday's (i.e., Monday's) mail. I shall write to Spottiswoode to send me six for this purpose unless I hear from you about the whole number wanted.

Source: From three letters to James Pattison Walker, Florence Nightingale Museum (LMA) H1/ST/NC1/65/27, 66/3 and 6, copy of first letter ADD MSS 45781 ff320-22

18 December 1865

*Private.* I really cannot tell you the grief I felt at your two last letters, which arrived together—both for the account of your health and for the inestimable and irreparable loss which the great sanitary cause in India will sustain from your resignation. I cannot write about it, for I should only intensify my regrets. And that would be of no use. I can only hope that the step you have taken will perfectly and entirely relieve yourself and Mrs Walker of all anxiety about your valuable life. . . .

By last mail but one, I sent to you, directed to Calcutta (I had not then had your fatal news) the first proof of the final revise of Dr Angus Smith's water analysis papers, written at your instigation. By last mail I sent three copies to you at Simla. (I had not strength to write.) I think I told you the ordeal this paper has gone through, in order to excuse its delay. It has been fifteen times through our hands and has gone through nine revises. It is considered now to represent the last and most perfect knowledge on this subject in Europe. I have presented it at the War and India Offices. And they were so much pleased with it that the War Office has asked for 600 copies to distribute "by authority" among its officers, medical and engineering, and at its

12 An allusion to John 13:27.

medical school. The India Office has asked for copies, too. But it takes at least a year for them to do the sum in addition of how many copies it will want. And, as it will be at least another year before it sends them out, I shall send 100 copies (privately) to India for distribution. Could you kindly tell me how this object will be best attained? I send out three more copies by this mail. I give Dr Angus Smith 200 copies. He is a most curious man—do you know him? Nothing but the pressure put upon him would have made him bring this paper to its present point. And yet he is the only man in Europe who could do it. So you see what good you have done. The present paper will circulate through Europe and other parts of the world. And practical scientific men will improve upon it and bring to a farther and still farther progress what Angus Smith has brought to this point only at present.

I have to thank you for the (croquet and archery) photograph, containing yourself and Mrs Walker, which interested me extremely. I wish I could send you some which would interest you as much.

I will not enlarge upon the immense loss to myself of your retirement from the sanitary commission. For indeed I cannot. It is irreparable. But I hope we shall never quite lose sight of each other, while I remain in this world. I cannot thank you for all the kindness you have shown me. But pray believe me,

ever yours and Mrs Walker's gratefully and sincerely
Florence Nightingale

26 March 1866

I have had letters from Sir J. Lawrence and Mr Strachey. As you are aware, the position of the sanitary commissions will be modified in important particulars—I do not pretend to send you Indian news from England. I am at this moment engaged with the Indian secretary of state here about this. In one respect, Lord de Grey is a better Indian secretary of state for us than Sir C. Wood, for Lord de Grey is entirely penetrated with the importance of the sanitary subject as signifying improvement in civilization, more than anything else. . . .

As to Dr Angus Smith's pamphlet, I cannot remember whether I mentioned to you that, after I had finished compiling it and presented it to the Army Sanitary Commission here, which has Indian members, the government was so penetrated with the importance of it that the War Office and India Office each took 600 copies and have distributed these with a printed circular among their medical and some of their engineering officers—abroad—by authority. So you see what good you have done.

I will not write more at present because I scarcely know whether this will reach you. But I hope, when I have your new address, to write about many things more fully. Your letter containing an extract from the engineer's report about the drainage of Calcutta was of the greatest importance to us. Had you been at Calcutta, I should have asked you to ascertain a point for us accurately which arises out of it. But now I know not to whom to apply. I feel as if we had lost our chief friend.

Pray give my most grateful and affectionate regards to Mrs Walker, if she will accept them, and accept the same yourself from

yours ever truly

Florence Nightingale

My birthday, as you are so good as to ask, was on 12 May 1820.

18 May 1866

I know not how to thank you for all your kindnesses to me. I forget whether I told you that I have received your proceedings. They are most valuable. I will send them back as you desire, without making any farther use of them than for myself. They are full of interest, full of the energy of your most energetic men, who have been doing your work in your own way.

We here could not agree with all your methods. But we cannot but agree and rejoice that you are doing all that can be done and that, as you advance, you will improve as we hope even on our procedures in the old country.

I forget whether I mentioned to you that Lord de Grey, at the beginning of this year, sent a commission into Algeria, which has many problems similar to those of India (deep ploughing and draining has made many of their pestilential stations healthy and they can now rear children as well as in any country in Europe). The object of the commission was to inquire into the causes of this decreased mortality. They have already reported in a first rough proof. The first complete proof to be had shall be for me to send to you.

I have received your last kind letter of 4 April with Dr Macnamara's paper on water analysis which I have duly forwarded to Dr Angus Smith with your message.

Source: From four letters to Douglas Galton, ADD Mss 45763 ff181-82, 196-97, 200-01 and 209-11

18 June 1866

*Private.* You know the history of Dr Angus Smith's water analysis pamphlet. Since then, I have had a copy of Dr Macnamara's paper on the same subject forwarded me by the Government of India (quoting Dr Parkes) which is extremely inaccurate and unpractical. Your committee on the aide-mémoire (which of course I need not tell you about) are very desirous that Dr Angus Smith shall supply the water analysis methods, provided you will sanction the expense. It will be well expended; he is undoubtedly the best man (but *he* must see that "Sennacherib" is kept out of the pamphlet, or "Nebuchadnezzar"[13]).

23 June 1866

I transmitted messages, which Dr Sutherland told me he had received from you, to Dr Angus Smith, relative to his writing (for sanitary aide-mémoire) a water analysis chapter and the cost of doing so. He will, I think, undertake it. He wishes not to ask any sum of money until it is seen what he has done. Perhaps the best way will be for your commission to recommend that some remuneration should be given, when you see the work. If this can be managed, we will write out a list of instructions as to what the said water analysis chapter should contain. Please, if you have a moment, tell me the ministerial prospects.

I am furious to that degree at having lost Lord de Grey's five months' ministry at the India Office (mainly owing to that stupid Mr Ellis, consorting and colloquing with Dr Sutherland) that I am fit to blow you all to pieces, with an infernal machine of my own invention, which does me credit.

27 June 1866

*Private.* Now do write to a wretched female (F.N.) about WHO is to come in WHERE.[14] Does General Peel come to the War Office? If so,

---

13 Sennacherib, Assyrian ruler who took the fenced cities of Judah according to 2 Kings 18:13. Nebuchadnezzar, Babylonian king who took Judah and Jerusalem according to 1 Chron 6:15. Perhaps Nightingale meant the avoidance of exotic details.

14 A Tory government under the 14th earl of Derby took office 28 June 1866. General Peel became secretary of state for war and Lord Cranborne secretary of state for India.

will he annihilate our civil sanitary element? Is Sutherland to go all the same to Malta and Gibraltar this autumn? Will General Peel imperil the Army Sanitary Commission? I must know, ye infernal powers. Is Mr Lowe to come in to the India Office? It is all unmitigated disaster to me. For as Lord Stanley is to be [secretary of state for] foreign [affairs] (the only place he can be of *no* use to us), I shall not have a friend in the world. If I were to say any more, I should fall to swearing, I am so indignant.

28 July 1866

*Private and Confidential. Burn.* My situation is this: Lord Cranborne has written to me (urged, of course, by Lord Stanley) that he will do the public health business next—and with me immediately after the officers' claims are settled . . . , that he will bring a metropolitan workhouse infirmary bill before the Cabinet in November, that he will devote the two months after 10 August to preparing it and that he will come to me "to advise and suggest." (About the bill is, I believe, no secret—I think he said so to the deputation on Thursday. It IS, of course, a secret, that I am to have a hand in it.) Now, neither Indian nor Poor Law business should I undertake without Dr Sutherland. (I merely want to know what his course is likely to be.) We let the metropolitan workhouse bill slip through in January, mainly owing to his absence in Algeria. I do not mean to let it slip through now, if I can help it. For myself, I have offered to go and see poor mother (whom we think altered). But I should time my visit home to coincide with Dr Sutherland's visit to the Mediterranean. And I should certainly postpone it to the India and Poor Law business. Indeed, nothing could be easier. Please BURN this.

Source: From a letter to James Pattison Walker, Florence Nightingale Museum (LMA) H1/ST/NC1/66/15

3 September 1866

Could not the Indian authorities try the effect of completely improving the drainage, water supply and sanitary conditions of two or three stations in the manner recommended by the *Suggestions* of the War Office sanitary commission? These are quite in conformity, so far as drainage and water supply are concerned, with what the French have done—of course, independently.

Source: From a letter to Robert Rawlinson, Boston University 1/4/52

6 August 1867

*Private.* Can you tell me what is actually being done about the drainage and sewerage of Bombay? Also, what you think of the civil engineer in charge of the works there? I have a particular reason for asking this question, as I am in communication with Bombay authorities and, therefore, I trust that you will not have wasted your time, if you are so good as to answer.

I communicated immediately with the authorities at Madras as to your kind information about the possibility of having civil sanitary engineers out there and will let you know the result as soon as I hear.

Source: From a letter to Douglas Galton, ADD Mss 45764 f106

13 August 1867

A *Captain [Henry] Tulloch, R.E.* has been sent home by the Madras government, to see drainage, water supply and other sanitary works in England for India. He is an "advanced sanitarian." He is coming to see you. Will you take care that he sees water supply, drainage and irrigation at Aldershot, Herbert Hospital, Woolwich married quarters, *a* new barrack?

Source: From notes for John Sutherland on a meeting with Sir Bartle Frere, ADD Mss 45752 f223

[August-September 1867]

[Sir B. Frere] says that ten years ago there was not a single man in India who would allow that the causes of cholera could be remedied.

He says that from Calcutta to Peshawar is as far as from London to Constantinople and it is positively necessary to have four responsible sanitary centres [in Calcutta and the presidencies] in that line. Your population is increasing every year—the epidemics strike a greater blow at the people and property in a week than the whole cost of the sanitary works.

Source: From a letter to Thomas Gillham Hewlett, Reynolds Historical Library, University of Alabama at Birmingham 5065

3 September 1867

I have to thank you very much for your kindness in sending me your report on the prevention of cholera. I have also received a copy with the municipal commissioner's letter prefixed to it, from the India Office. Let me also thank you very much for your kind letter.

You will perhaps be glad to hear any little hints I can collect from Europe on the sides on the subject of your pamphlet. The best scientific opinion in Europe rather tends now to consider that on which the prevention of cholera is here based as a groundless theory. And we have nothing to do with theories. The system of disposing of house sewage which you mention is essentially the same as has been tried for thirty years at an enormous cost in Paris and which the emperor is now putting an end to by having Paris drained. In a report on Madras drainage by Captain Tulloch, R.E., which he has just brought to England, he shows that the dry system costs more than ten times as much—as much—as the sewer system. But it is not only the cost which is fatal to the dry earth system in towns. Is it not the fact that it is impossible to carry it out with the same safety to health as the sewer system? I know of at least one large institution where an outbreak of cholera was distinctly traced to this. It is always interesting to know what has been said on both sides. In the Madras report, the medical officer recommends the adoption of the dry system and gives an estimate. The engineer shows that it will be ten times as much.

Doubtless I am not telling you anything new. Doubtless you know all that can be said much better than I do. All the Paris sewage is now to be taken away in pipes and applied to agriculture. The Dutch method removes only about a two hundredth part of the sewage of a town.

As to *value,* the latest estimate is just published in the "Rivers Commission" report and shows that *sewer water* gives actual produce equal to £100 per acre. Would it not be at once concentrating and intensifying the energies of each side and preventing waste of power if, as a general rule, the officer of health deals with pointing out *causes of diseases,* the engineer deals with *removal* of those causes and estimate of cost? And though the one report should never be made without being accompanied or closely followed by the other, yet it would save much time and energy if neither were confused with the other. We have grievously erred in this respect in England. And often I have observed (especially since Sidney Herbert's death) that the engineering officer has usurped the medical officer's functions and vice versa. It is probably most easy to avoid this when the two go together.

I hope to send you shortly some reports which our government officers are about to issue on the subjects on which you write so ably. And therefore I will not write at greater length.

Source: From a letter to Dr Shrimpton,[15] ADD Mss 45801 ff117-18

19 September 1868

The Army Sanitary Commission (this is a standing commission for the War and India Offices) is so justly dissatisfied with the state the whole cholera question is in that they are going to carry out a special inquiry all over India simply to arrive at the facts, which have been so bedizened with professional theories that they are like actors in a masquerade. But it is only one manifestation of a mental disease or obliquity or want of philosophical thought, which seems to pervade all subjects of human interest at the present time. You know that the Spaniards *and* Gibraltar have put "British ships" in quarantine under observation for three days!! because we have cholera in London! The wisdom of the quarantine world transcends belief!

Source: From notes to Benjamin Jowett, ADD Mss 45783 ff141-42

[ca. September 1868]

About "contagion," surely the "bad moral" is that of Simon Magus[16] and Co. which teaches there *is* "contagion" (no one is ever able to tell you what it is, where it is, how it is and for a very good reason—because *it is* NOT). There is "contagion" and all you can do is to cut it off, to stamp it out, to kill or to segregate.

Lord R. Montague[17] was strictly logical. And the price of meat is to be doubled for the people, because, for why? for a fancy which has absolutely as little foundation in fact as witchcraft has. Surely the good "moral" is ours (besides having the small advantage that it is founded in fact) there is no such thing as "contagion"—there *is* "infection," but from perfectly well-known causes. Remove the causes and you remove the "infection." There is no such thing as inevitable "infection," quarantine, segregating fever, etc., above all concentrating them in hospitals; these are all means expressly constructed to manufacture the best "infection." Killing the cows is exactly the same as killing the witches. O my professor, are you a doctor in Plato and not know these things![18] Depend upon it, if you can find out the facts in science, edu-

---

15 Dr Charles Shrimpton (1815-?), working at what became the American Hospital in Paris, wrote a pamphlet, *The British Army and Miss Nightingale*, 1864.

16 Nightingale's expression for Sir John Simon, an opponent on sanitary matters.

17 Lord Robert Montague (1825-1902), Conservative MP, speaking of cattle plague.

18 A paraphrase of John 3:10.

cational, physical or sanitary, those *facts* will show a "moral," the best "moral," i.e., show best the perfect God, leading man to perfection. "Contagion" would show God a devil. "Infection" (facts and doctrine) leads man on to social improvement.

Source: From notes to John Sutherland with his comments, Add Mss 45753 ff104, 107-08 and 133

4 November 1868

There is a strong argument of public necessity: it is simply a fact that you cannot keep British troops in health so long as you allow native populations in their vicinity to be decimated by epidemics. In this matter, Providence acts with stern justice. If any government leaves its poor subjects, especially in a tropical climate, a prey to pestilence, the government will have to suffer in men (alas! how many of the noblest governors who ever went to India have died from this cause), in revenue and in all their resources. An epidemic country is always a poor country. It is little short of madness in a country like India for people to fold their hands and to comfort themselves with the idea that it is impossible to raise the mass of the people into health and that health is a blessing Providence intends only for rich Englishmen in England.

[5 November 1868]

During the time that you were taken possession of, by the wiles and graces of Wilbraham,[19] Sir B. Frere came here twice. They have made a paper at the India Office, chiefly embodying our paper, and Sir B. Frere says if we would add in again what they have taken out, he feels almost sure it would be adopted. He has now brought it. [in Dr Sutherland's hand:] This is an admirable paper, and contains quite as much as you should put forth at present. You have included in it all the great principles both sanitary and administrative which the country requires, and now you must keep at these points until they are embodied in local works in India. This will not be in our time, for it takes more than a few years to introduce Christian civilization into a continent. These people are of us and we are of them and in God's good time we shall all of us, I trust, reap the common benefit of obeying all the laws which He has given us for our well-being.

19 Colonel Richard Wilbraham, governor of Woolwich Hospital.

[before 12 December 1868]

[in Dr Sutherland's hand:] In consequence of the loss of nearly a regiment of British troops in India in 1867, besides many thousands of natives, and in consequence of the complete fiasco of medical doctrine and practice in this disease, the Army Sanitary Commission has decided to ask the India Office to join in a great scientific and practical inquiry into the whole subject [Inquiry into Cholera, resulting in "Cholera Instructions" of April 1869]. The Instructions are under consideration and will be sent officially in due time for submission to the secretary of state [for] war and secretary of state [for] India.

One part of the inquiry is altogether special and has been made matter of education of two active young surgeons who were sent to Germany on purpose. One, Dr Cuningham, belongs to the Indian service; the other, Dr Lewis,[20] belongs to the British service in India. Both are going out on the 12th December, and application will be made officially to the India Office.

These specially trained men shall not be sent on general service but shall be kept at their special work until the scientific inquiry is completed. It is no doubt about them now that Dr Maclean[21] wishes to see Sir B. Frere. The object is one of the highest public importance and I would venture to bespeak your kind consideration for the application when it comes.

Source: From an incomplete letter, probably to Parthenope Verney, Wellcome (Claydon copy) Ms 9003/84

31 January 1869

*Peshawar* has been made one of the worst spots in the whole world by bad engineering. The causes of fever and cholera there are perfectly well known. And Lord Napier of Magdala repeated them to me in his peculiarly graphic way (which shows such practical ability) the other day. *Amritsar* has not a single drop of good water to drink. This was well known. But I have quite recently had a report on the subject, which it really is impossible to repeat to "ears polite." As for the *hills*, "your correspondent" is probably not aware that the hills themselves have been repeatedly attacked with cholera from filth, nuisance and bad water, that this subject has been continually before us and that we

20 Timothy Richards Lewis (1841-80), surgeon and pathologist, conducted research on cholera.

21 William Campbell Maclean (1811-98), after serving as the first superintendent of the new medical school in Hyderabad, became professor of military and clinical medicine at Chatham.

have continually had to report thus: improve such and such a hill station; do not occupy it with men till it has been improved; at present it is actually as pestilential as such and such a station in the plains. On all these subjects reports come home to us monthly. Quite latterly I have been engaged in reporting on the very subject "your correspondent" treats of and particularly on the abominable state of the subsoil upon which they have built the new Allahabad barracks, terminating my letter with our strongly expressed opinion that, had this been done in England even, nothing could have saved the inmates from cholera in epidemic years.

Lord Napier of Magdala gave me his own priceless evidence of forty years that we have rather *under*stated than overstated our case. He has sent me (since) confidential printed documents connected with his own command. On one of these I have had to report (confidentially). It contains the account of an outbreak of cholera traced directly to an indecent and abominable neglect which I really cannot transcribe (though I have had to report upon it). Also (but this is by the way) it *has been* repeatedly urged to complete the communications over and under the Indus so as to be able to occupy Attock instead of Peshawar where, if they are making improvements at all, it is at the slowest possible pace. (Peshawar cannot be safely evacuated unless there are means of pouring in troops at the shortest possible notice.)

CONFIDENTIAL. (With regard to sanitary things, it would seem as if the authorities were struck with judicial blindness. Here is a thing which has happened since the New Year at home. After years of representations, complaints and urgencies, followed up since Sidney Herbert's time, we had obtained a water supply for Gibraltar. For the town this was opened by Lady Airey with a formal ceremony. The consequence of the whole new system has been that, for the first time, Gibraltar has been free from cholera or fever at an epidemic time. I reported this to a Cabinet minister at his own desire. £1000 was put on this year's Estimates to extend the water supply to the garrison. *And it was struck off!* We believe that we have succeeded in getting it put on again by a statement that the £1000 would repay itself in three years—not by saving soldiers' lives, that is no matter—but by saving the water carrying and rates. But even of this—its being replaced on the Estimates—we are not quite sure.)

I would gladly enter more fully into the subject (of the letter enclosed). But, as you will, I am sure, see, I who have to report to the authorities have not a moment to spare for non-authorities. I cannot report upon my reports. If you make any use of the above statement, you must not, if you please, mention Lord Napier of Magdala, nor my correspondence with Lord Mayo's government, nor my reporting, nor anything which will point to names. (The Gibraltar story is *quite* confidential, Mr Cardwell does not even know that I know anything about the Estimates.)

Neither should I have written even so much as I have done here, if it had not been that it is proposed (in the letter enclosed) that Sir Harry should "bring on" the "hills" question "in the House," which is simply laying so much in the balance *against* sanitary improvements. I have written amid many interruptions.

Source: From a letter to Douglas Galton, Add Mss 45764 ff131-33

3 February 1869

*Private.* I think *The Lancet* should be answered as we have none so much to boast of in the security of our position. The extract indeed shows nothing more than that the writer is unacquainted with the distinction between administering sanitary regulations, which is the duty of the army medical officer, and the planning of new works and new sanitary procedure of a practical kind. You and I and all of us know what a hopeless confusion the medical officer even in India has made of such questions whenever he has gone beyond his own line, e.g., Dr Goodeve and Dr Farquhar (Sir John Lawrence's physician) in the India Office Blue Book, lately out. And WE have almost weekly experience of the same thing in India. (I have actually a letter from a high authority in India proposing to me that medical officers should positively be *excluded* from all sanitary work on account of their interminable contradictions and theories and fights among each other.)

Half of all our practical work (yours and mine and Dr Sutherland's in this line) consists in neutralizing the evil influence of opinions which, however applicable at the bedside of the sick, are simply injurious when carried into the principles which are to prevent people from being sick. You have, I believe, yourself proposed that, with the view of avoiding all this bringing forward of theory as if it were practice (or practicable), the basis of education of officers of health should be laid not in medicine but in engineering. *I* would do the answer for *The Lancet* but I have so many irons in the fire. And you would do it much better. Dr Farr would put it in for you. But please remember that Dr Goodeve is his friend. And also of course my "high authority in India" must not be mentioned. *Burn.*

Source: From a letter to Lord de Grey, ADD Mss 43546 ff128-31

11 February 1869

*Private and confidential.* I send, according to your kind desire:

1. Letter to the secretary of state from the G.G. No. 7 Sanitary,
2. Report of the Cholera Committee Madras,
3. As to control of pilgrimages, Report Madras,

3a. " " Papers Hardwar.

I am nevertheless almost sorry that I mentioned these to you, because I am afraid it will give you some trouble to listen to my explanation. All these papers are full of the most important facts, but some are *in transitu.* And the "Cholera Committee Report" is something like the Irishman who is always said to make some admission at the end of a most masterly case which nullifies the whole case. For the redeeming point in the Cholera Committee Report (Madras) is that they have inserted (at p 46) the memorial of a large number of good men and true *to the president of the Privy Council* here in March 1868 against itself. Also there is a great deal, in all these reports on cholera and other epidemics, which makes one wish that they had followed the example of the author of the chapter "On Snakes in Iceland": "There are no snakes in Iceland."

More candid or more stupid than English authorities, these Indian authorities produce a number of facts for contagion in cholera which, being interpreted, may be summed up thus: Chapter "On Contagion in Cholera": "There is no contagion in cholera."

The present acting sanitary commissioner with the Government of India writes to me by the last mail thus: "Whatever difference of opinion may exist as to the origin of cholera, and the other theoretical questions which are so difficult to explain, and on which I am afraid we are all still very ignorant, I feel sure we fully agree in the practical part of the matter, viz., the vast importance of all sanitary reforms as the best means of checking the spread of the disease." Yes, but the harm is in putting forward the "theoretical questions" *as if they were* "the practical part of the matter," e.g., cholera is to be prevented by quarantine, being due to contagion. Cholera is to be prevented by "sanitary reforms," being due to unsanitary conditions. Both of these cannot be true. One is. Which?

It is extraordinary that these contradictions, which pertain just as much to all epidemics, whether in man or beast, as they do to cholera, should still exist, that, notwithstanding our free trade, there should still be these quarantine questions. They are not owing to the merchants. Formerly they were. In the twelfth century when the Venetians found out for the first time that epidemic diseases were a good protection "dodge," they worked them to their own advantage, as they have been worked by other states since then. But now no merchant would dream of this.

Yet, in the nineteenth century, we have, in another shape, it is true, the same fallacies renewed. I am sorry to say that that profession which is the least selfish—the medical—has been the sole cause. They bring from the bedside the same sort of reasoning (or un-reasoning), employed in curing disease, into a totally different and much higher region, that of preventing disease. . . .

If you will permit me, I will send you, as soon as it is ready, a copy of proceedings about to be taken on the advice of the Army Sanitary Commission, which you have saved. These proceedings, if fairly carried out, will settle on sure scientific grounds these vexed questions.

Source: From an exchange with John Sutherland, ADD Mss 45753 ff186-87

[ca. 16 February 1869]

I must thank Angus Smith.[22]

[Sutherland] Manufacturing to set up, all is ready made and crying out to be used. Now comes the logic. If all this be true, as Dr Angus Smith has proved it to be, why go about making disinfectants which are not so good and cost money and which after all also require engineering methods to apply them? This is how it strikes an outsider equipped with nothing except a little logical faculty.

[Nightingale] I wonder whether that sort of wild resolutioning does much harm. *I* think it does harm. I have not answered Cuningham of India yet.

Source: From a letter to James M. Cuningham, Johns Hopkins University 3

25 February 1869

As you say, in your kind note to me of 5 January, "whatever difference of opinion may exist as to theoretical questions" (about cholera) we do and shall fully agree "in the practical part of the matter." Yes, but the harm is in putting forward that which is theory, pure theory, as if it were "practical." And, as I am sure you will agree, in some instances, taking two theories, if one is true, the other is *not* true. And the practice which would logically follow from the one (*if we were logical*) would be diametrically opposite to the practice following from the other.

22 Presumably for his book *Disinfectants and Disinfection*, published 1869.

If you will kindly bear with me, I will submit to you one matter, chiefly based on Dr Murray's tables, with regard to the great practical sanitary steps to be taken for mitigating epidemic diseases.

The matter I wish to bring before you is that these hypothetical points, viz., the relation of movement of people to cholera, are fair subjects of discussion, provided due care be taken that views of this class are not made subjects of legislation. Laws are applicable only to proved constant phenomena and the danger is that civilian outsiders, who do not know the grounds of medical discussion, should act as if the views on either side were constant demonstrable facts, and so include them in legislative provisions, as has been done in England uselessly or mischievously.

(You are aware how eminently this was the case in the late cattle plague legislation of this country and the useless destruction which followed. And the last quarantine against cholera in the Mediterranean, which did not in the least stop cholera, cost the Mediterranean trade 4 millions sterling for a mere hypothesis.)

I have studied Dr Murray's report, which you were so kind as to send me, and after examining his curious and interesting tables I find the following results, which do very little indeed, as you will see, towards supporting restrictions on intercourse. Results of Dr Murray's table of the Hardwar *epidemic*:

1. Total number of towns at which pilgrims arrived from Hardwar, 210.

2. In no instance is the date of arrival given, so that it is not possible to judge how far the arrival and subsequent appearance of cholera are related "*in time.*"

3. The evidence is hence summed up as follows: "*Pilgrims arrived and cholera appeared.*"

4. Out of 210 places at which pilgrims arrived cholera appeared in 199.

5. But of these 199 attacked places cholera appeared *among pilgrims only* at eighty-five, so that out of 210 places visited by pilgrims at 199 of which cholera appeared, there were 114 at which the disease showed itself among others than pilgrims.

6. Of these 114 places where pilgrims and residents were attacked the dates of attack and consequently the *relation in time* between the pilgrim cases and those among other residents are given in fifty-one instances only. Hence the only reliable data on which an inquiry could be founded so as to avoid the most obvious fallacies are the following: Pilgrims from Hardwar visited 210 places. At eighty-five of these the

disease appeared among pilgrims and was confined solely to them, affording in these eighty-five cases not even the fundamental fact of communication; in 114 cases cholera appeared among pilgrims and residents but in fifty-one instances only are the dates given and in sixty-three instances there are no dates whatever to show the period of attack. Hence out of 210 places visited by pilgrims there are fifty-one (less than one quarter), in which there is a time relation between the attacks in pilgrims and those among residents.

7. The number of days intervening between attacks among pilgrims and attacks among residents was as follows: in two cases residents were attacked before pilgrims (one [in] two days, one [in] nearly a month); in ten cases residents and pilgrims were attacked the same day; in one case pilgrims were attacked two days before residents; in nine cases three days; in seven cases four days; in seven cases five days; in seven cases six days; in two cases seven days; in two cases nine days; in one case ten days; in one case eleven days; in one case fifteen days; in one case eighteen days.

8. The tables include only the towns to which pilgrims went and take no cognizance of the multitude of localities in which cholera appeared and to which no pilgrims went.

9. The tables do not include many places to which pilgrims went and where there was no cholera.

What is wanted for legal purposes are constant uniform facts. Out of any given number of epidemic facts some must always be on one side, some on another, and it is of course only by the most careful inquiries, many times repeated and many times sifted, that we can arrive at real practical truth. We shall want you to help us. And that very much and very often.

Source: Note for John Sutherland, Add Mss 45753 f201

[ca. 1 March 1869]

Sir B. Frere talked to me especially about the Bombay drainage. He says Aitken's[23] pamphlet has never been sent home to the India Office, that he believes Bombay will settle the drainage question itself and settle it in the right way and that he doubts it's being referred home at all, which he says is very good. Sir B. Frere says, if they had meant to take Aitken's scheme, they would have referred it home. They have not. He infers they don't mean.

---

23 Sir William Aitken (1825-92), professor of pathology in Edinburgh.

Source: From a note and an undated note to John Sutherland, ADD Mss 45753 ff238 and 216

13 April 1869

I beg leave to remark that I found a letter of yours this morning dated early in December (which I mean to show you), in which, with the strongest objurgations of me, you told me that you could not come because you intended to get the cholera instructions [for the special Cholera Inquiry] through by 12 *December* 1868.

My dear soul, really Sir Bartle Frere could not have known the fatal, the exhausting labour he has put you all to: to produce that in four months must prove fatal to all your constitutions! I really cannot take upon myself to go farther, to tell you what he asks. He is an ogre.

Source: Letter, University Library, Cambridge, Mayo Collection, ADD Ms 7490/132/1

7 May 1869

*Private*

Dear Lord Mayo

You were so kind in inviting me to address myself directly to you, in the event, which was sure to happen, of your all-powerful hand being wanted to right the sanitary ship in India, that I consider the best mode of service is to take you at your word and without farther apologies (which waste your time) to write the following petition to you.

You will have heard from the India Office—probably from Sir Bartle Frere also—about an inquiry, long desired and becoming every day more essential, into cholera in India. Something of the kind was proposed by the "Conference" at Constantinople. The present inquiry will however include all that they wanted and much more. It arose out of India's own reports of the 1867 epidemic, which were referred to the Army Sanitary Commission here. As you will see, if you could spare an instant to glance at their memorandum (which I enclose), the only lesson taught by this latest experience was that a searching inquiry should be instituted. A code of "Instructions" was drawn up here (of which I also beg to enclose a copy), which not only covers the whole ground of this terrible cholera but will, it is hoped, point the direction for similar inquiries elsewhere.

People here are warmly in favour of this inquiry and great things are expected from it in time. But with you in India will rest the honour of doing that most difficult thing, viz., ascertaining what is true, what is problematical and what is untrue about the causes of cholera and the means of preventing it.

The hopes of scientific men both in England and Europe have been greatly excited by the prospect of this inquiry. And a German of high repute declared it a most worthy act in the British government to undertake it. Of course everything will depend upon its being carried out heartily and carefully.

The "Instructions" are more difficult in appearance than in reality—chiefly on account of their technical nature. But as they are to be complied with by men who understand the subject more or less, this apparent objection matters but little. The real question involved in them is the sanitary improvement of India, because, if you succeed in telling us what cholera is and what are the best means of limiting its ravages, the very discovery will limit it and, if this is done, other diseases, especially these terrible fevers and dysenteries, which afflict the country, will be at the same time limited.

I will not say: May I bespeak your kind consideration and support for this great work—no greater has occupied the attention of the Government of India—because I know that you will further it, if you think it important. Epidemics always mean not only loss of life, but loss of productive power, loss of stamina, loss of prosperity, waste of national resources in fact. And they have consequently at all times attracted the painful attention of governments. But the present object is to do more. It is to bring them, please God, within the domain of science that they may be practically dealt with. You have now in India examined and analyzed the principal water sources all the way North Westward from Calcutta to Peshawar, including those of thirty-eight cities and stations, and nearly 400 sources of water supply. This opens up quite a new field of work. Your wells are deplorable and must be seen to with the least possible delay. You will perhaps find cholera, dysentery and fever at the bottom of not a few of them. As the cholera season is approaching, indeed already here, might I ask you, if you think well, not to let the subject of the "Instructions" be either smothered or neglected? (It is indeed unfortunate that copies were sent out so late.)

We heard with delight of your triumph at the Umballa Durbar, where I have no doubt we should much have liked to have been to see what kind of a rascal he was whom you had to subdue. But I must not abuse your kindness by taking up your time. I look forward to the period with great hope when, long after Afghanistan dynasties are things of the past, these poor Indian races will have cause to bless the civilization which your reign has brought them.

May I ask, if Lady Mayo is so kind as to remember me, to be respectfully recommended to her? I beg that you will believe me, dear Lord Mayo,

ever your faithful servant
Florence Nightingale

Source: From a letter to John Strachey, Columbia University, Presbyterian Hospital School of Nursing C94

14 May 1869

Let me mention to you the proposed inquiry into cholera. I write to you, who did so much in the former inquiry, to ask your kind aid and co-operation in giving effect to the present one. The question of these epidemics has assumed a high degree of importance in Europe, both scientifically and practically, since your former report, so much so that we are no longer as it were standing on the same ground. And, as the Constantinople [Sanitary] Conference [1866] has failed to give light either to scientific or to practical men, we now look to you in India for a final settlement of the question.

The matter has been so complicated by medical theories and other similar impracticabilities that nobody believes anything. And what we now want is an exhaustive statement of *fact—no opinions.* We here are adept in forming opinions and theories containing any amount of contradictions. And we leave governments and merchants to find their way through our darkness as best they can. If you can tell us one real *fact* about cholera—and I am sure you will tell us many—this will be a great gain. A set of pointed questions has been sent out (800 copies) to practised scientific observers. And we are looking forward eagerly and with confidence to this that, before long, you will send us not one but a great many facts and that eventually you will be able to supply the means of solving all the difficulties of Indian, therefore of Asiatic and European, epidemics. We look to you.

If India cannot furnish the reply we want, then we must rest satisfied with merely negative knowledge. However, we would earnestly bespeak your best assistance in this great work—a work not for India alone but for all humanity.

Source: Note on Bombay sanitation for John Sutherland, Add Mss 45753 ff253-54

8 October 1869

The discussions respecting drainage plans for Bombay are not as yet satisfactorily concluded. Two methods of dealing with the question have been advocated, one for providing sewers of large dimensions for carrying off the tropical rainfall of Bombay, together with the sewage of the city, the whole to be discharged into the sea, leaving the sewers nearly empty during the dry season. The other, proposed by Mr Rawlinson and adopted by Captain Tulloch, R.E., who was specially sent to England by the Madras government to study the various questions regarding town drainage and the utilization of sewage: this latter project provides for draining and sewering the city by conduits large enough only to convey away the sewage and for applying the sewage to agriculture at a distance from the city. It is objected to the first proposal that the large sewers being left almost empty during the dry season will become generators of foul air and tend to deteriorate the health of the city, while it is objected to the second plan that there must of necessity be partial flooding of the surface during heavy rains when the tide is unusually high.

It appears to be an important element in the discussion to bear in mind that town sewers and drains are primarily intended for removing the foul water of the population, and not for removing rainfall, while any attempt in such a climate as that of India to provide for rainfall by sewers must entail an enormous outlay for an occasional and temporary purpose. It might be well in any further discussions which take place on this subject to consider the two questions as separate problems, so that, while foul water only is removed in underground sewers, the point of surface drainage may be settled, and the proper outfalls for this water into the sea provided for.

Source: From a draft memorandum (not in Nightingale's hand) for the India Office, Add Mss 45780 ff150-57

[1869]

The abstract of Indian reports up to "General Conclusions" page 30 [of "Memorandum on Measures . . . "] gives a correct picture of the facts as they presented themselves to the Indian medical officers. But it is well known that of late years the medical profession has been declining in its powers of accurate observation, and has either supplemented this deficiency by theory or has observed from a theory as a centre. The older and abler race of Indian medical officers now extinct avoided this error and hence the earlier Indian reports on cholera are still standard works of reference. . . .

There are but two ways of dealing with the 1867 reports, either to criticize them or merely to give the facts without comment. . . .

Now it will be stated to you that the result of the examination of the reports has been to show that it would be most desirable to undertake a special inquiry into the whole subject of epidemic cholera in the East. . . .

*Deficiency in information regarding the cholera of 1867:* As the abstract stands, it places the whole, or almost the whole, causation of cholera in contagion. There is nothing said on the sanitary state of attacked towns and villages. There is nothing said about the water supply, while the analyses now about to be reported on by the Army Sanitary Commission to the India Office show that there is scarcely a town or station over the whole region attacked by cholera in which the water is not dangerous during epidemic seasons. Peshawar is specially distinguished in this respect.

There is no account of the sanitary state of any attacked barrack, station or hospital or of any prison. This defect in the reports sent to you from India should be noticed. None of them are properly speaking sanitary reports. They are medico-statistical reports, based on contagion.

You ought to require a sanitary report year by year from every Indian station.

Source: From a letter to Sir Harry Verney, Wellcome (Claydon copy) Ms 9004/5

11 January 1870

*Private.* I am sure that you will not make any motion in the House on the subject of the "*Hills*" without fully consulting first with Sir Bartle Frere and also, if possible, with Lord Napier of Magdala. It is a policy entirely reversing that of the royal commission, presided over (1) by Sidney Herbert, (2) by Lord Stanley, which was based on the fullest and largest evidence ever taken in the world, which every year's evidence and every year's experience has more and more firmly corroborated, as well as every successive ruler of India. It would be stultifying all our strenuous efforts of eleven years and without any evidence, except that of the R.E. and commanding officers whose own almost guilty neglect has been the cause of many of the outbreaks of cholera. No doubt you know about the Hugli fever. It is the old story. But Lord Mayo's government (as one of its members who is in correspondence with me about it tells me) are going to pass an act to enable us to deal with the proprietors on whose lands the fever is bred, which no one even pretends is *not preventible.* Some hundreds of thousands will probably die first.

Source: Note for John Sutherland on a meeting with James M. Cuningham, Add Mss 45754 ff79-84

February 1870

He [Dr Cuningham] is a man brimming with information, very candid, without prejudice or prepossession, quite without affectation or pretension of any kind, and exceedingly full of our work and of getting all kinds of instruction here. But—he is about 7 ft. 2 inches high.

First of all, he says that he has been all over the presidency [Bengal] during the last year (during which cholera has been more fatal than we have any idea of) and can find *no proof whatever* of cholera being communicated *by contagion*. He says you cannot tell except by the monthly gazettes how many new barracks are finished, that they know nothing of Bombay and Madras presidencies, that Colonel Crommelin is the man who gives, in the monthly report, how many barracks are finished for his presidency, that Jullundur, Allahabad and Agra have new barracks but not all their new barracks finished, that complaints have come in from all these three—and also from Peshawar—principally from the commanding officers (Rawalpindi), that he, Cuningham, has gone into all these complaints himself, those from Jullundur he thinks not substantiated. All the complaints from all five places are of the same nature—very hot sun beats on the walls, no overhanging roofs or penthouses. Cuningham says it is quite true and a horrible defect; the *immense block of masonry* in these new barracks strikes one at once as most incongruous and improper because, he says, even huts with great verandahs would be so much better—they really are "palatial."

He was asked, just before he came away, whether he was prepared to advocate double-storeyed barracks for *all* stations. He reported, Certainly not; he held by what the Army Sanitary Commission here had said; he says, where double-storeyed barracks *are* necessary, it is not necessary to make a great palace, without any kind of shelter from the sun.

He says you have no idea how costly and absurd they are—very hot, even at night, very cold in the hills in winter. He says he saw the men quite shivering and ill with cold. They [barracks] leak. That is of course a building stupidity. The men say, We can't drag our cots out on hot nights, it takes two men to drag them downstairs; we used to drag them out into the verandahs or even out of doors; the verandahs, even where there are verandahs, are so hot they are no good and we don't like the trouble of the stairs. The upper rooms *are* ceiled. In only one instance had he complaints of radiant heat from the ceilings.

The upper storeys are hot through the day and night. Thermometrical observations have been made at Allahabad, Lucknow, Jullundur between the old and new barracks. *He* says, very imperfectly. *They* assert that, at Jullundur, there is 10° difference between old and new. He says that the men leave their sleeping rooms at 4 A.M. but return to them at 7 A.M., that it is impossible to lock them up, that the men spend eighteen hours in them as a general rule, that nothing but a commanding officer, such as they have not, could prevent this, that government won't and can't supply a punkah [fan] and tattie [screen] establishment for upper and lower floors; therefore there is only one for the upper. He says that the recreation and workrooms are there, but nothing but forms and tables in them—no books; that only a commanding officer who would invent occupation to interest the men and drag them off their beds would do any good, that the men have no motive to leave their beds. And they lie there, thinking about the cholera, for eighteen hours a day. He says the recreation and workrooms are only *nominally* used—only a very small number are put to any real use.

He says Rawalpindi is a very healthy station. So is Jullundur. But the cholera at Rawalpindi has been frightful. And that *typhoid fever* has nearly taken a quarter of the garrison at Jullundur. The regiment (92nd Highlanders) at Jullundur was so frightfully mismanaged, brought up the Indus in overcrowded boats, very young Irish recruits in the hot season, that they brought typhoid fever with them. It is *not* attributable to the station. The commanding officer is a grumbler. He says there *is* a great difference between the protection from the sun to the walls in the old and new barracks. That, he says, is their great mistake. You know, Lord Napier of Magdala told me that Colonel Crommelin was only a third-class man. This man did not dare to say as much. But it was easy to see it. And now he says Colonel Crommelin is to be head of a commission to tell Lord Mayo what to do.

Cholera has appeared in the new barracks of Allahabad, Peshawar, Lucknow, Morar, but also in the old. Not *all* the new barracks at these stations are finished. He cannot say that any troops with cholera have been moved into the new barracks. He told me a hideous story where he found that dirty coolie families with diseases (he himself saw a case of smallpox) had been allowed to inhabit the new barracks before they were occupied.

He told me a most interesting story of Peshawar: cholera appeared (say) on 11 September; they moved out one wing (104th regiment) on the 13th outside the cantonment, but two men died out of three attacks

[in] another wing on the 17th. They lost sixty-two [sixty-seven?][24] men (out of sixty-eight attacks). In another [wing] of the 36th regiment, on the 19th they lost eighty-six [171] men out of 180 attacks. He says there has been cholera in the vicinity of all the barracks at the time, except *Sabathu* (which is a healthy hill station!!!). At Sabathu our troops have been ravaged with cholera in 1867 and 1869. And a very dirty bazaar close by has had none. He does not believe in hill stations. Some of our most frightful choleras have been at hill stations.

He says Beatson and Murray are quite mad about hill stations. He says, the British Army might as well be kept at Suez. But, he says, what *does* do the troops good is to send them to *work* on roads in the hills. He says the 55th working at Chakrata (where our friend Dr Walker is) is perfectly healthy and all their sick men recovered. He says that nothing has really been done to improve any native towns; that the Government of India says cantonments must be near native towns, because the cutcherries and civil boards of magistrature must be in the towns and cantonments must be near to protect them; that at Allahabad the new barracks are close to the city; that Amritsar is a vast dirty native city, as dirty as when it was born—without improvements; that just now a plan and estimate (for 20 lakhs of rupees) was made for improving it; that Mr Strachey has taken off the octroi [municipal levy], upon which all municipal improvements depended for funds, and that now they have no funds and there is a furious outcry.

The water supply at Amritsar has not been improved and is as bad as possible. The water supply has not been improved in any of the native towns. The stations' water supply has been improved merely as far as this: the best wells have been selected and great care has been taken by roofing in, etc., to protect them from pollution, but there are no pumps, no means of distribution. And that is all. He says the jails are really their only success, that not one jail except Larikpur in Upper India has had cholera. He says they have actually built vast, costly, palatial buildings for the native regiments' sick and that the sick got well in the huts and don't get well in the palatial buildings. He says the C.O. is really the doctor of his regiment; the health of the regiment depends on the commanding officer. If the commanding officers would devise something sufficiently interesting to pull the men out of bed, *that* is their best hope of health.

---

24 Those numbers are hard to decipher.

Married quarters—*not* at Jullundur—a success. But, he says, it was mainly the commanding officer's fault. He says, Durand is for going on just with the same vast expense as before, Mansfield is for stopping every kind of expenditure. And it appears that Crommelin is to decide, except that Lord Mayo will wait for my letter. And Strachey told him he was very much impressed by the letter he had received from me. He says that the native town of Kanpur *has* been improved, but there is still cholera, that they are now borrowing 5 lakhs rupees at 5 percent from government to carry out their farther scheme.

He asked particularly what we thought of Bryden's[25] report. He says cholera does not follow the area of bad drainage and stops where drainage has been improved. It follows a certain area, outside that it will stop even where there is bad drainage, bad water supply. But certainly good drainage will prevent. He says there will certainly be cholera this year in India.

Source: Letter, University Library, Cambridge, Mayo Collection ADD Ms 7490/132/8

24 March 1870

Dear Lord Mayo

I am exceedingly obliged to you for your kind letter of 11 January. I waited to answer it till after I had talked over the whole matter with Dr Cuningham. I have had great pleasure in making his acquaintance. He is brimming with information, without prepossession and full of his work, which I hope I may also call ours.

Not to take up your hardly pressed time, I had better at once proceed "to business," viz., the present aspect of the public health question in India, including the supposed "partial failures" in barrack construction, and submit the practical points to you. (Possibly there may be too great a tendency in India to "invent first principles." And the crisis arrived at from want of money might have come, even had there been plenty of money.)

An immense deal however has been done in India. We must never forget that, nor cease to be grateful to those who have worked so hard—and so well—ever remembering what an enormous, what a colossal field India is. It is like working at a continent instead of a country.

---

25 Dr J.L. Bryden (1833-80), civil surgeon of the Bengal presidency; he believed in the airborne theory of cholera spread and wrote several cholera reports.

I will take the barracks first, if you will allow me, and then the administrative points and will try to be as short as I can.

I. *Barracks.*

1. The new barracks certainly seem to have been built after a too costly fashion. But might not the complaints of their being "too hot" be easily modified? (a) *Plaster and whitewash* outside to protect the walls from sun radiation, (b) *Fill the tall verandah arches with venetians* to protect the room walls. The lofty arches are right enough but the upper part of the arch of the verandah should be filled up with broad wooden jalousies admitting of adjustment to let in light and keep out sun, or the space between the pillars even should be filled up thus. These two remedies can easily be tried at any station and a comparison made of the effect in temperature, ventilation and comfort with other blocks.

2. New barrack building *alone* will not cure the sick, lower the death rate or guarantee from epidemics. So much (as I need hardly say) enters into the improvement of a station besides the actual putting up of a new house! The four things which are essential to the health of troops—on which their health depends—are: (a) a thorough drainage of ground occupied by stations; (b) an abundant supply of pure water distributed over stations; (c) healthy principles of barrack and hospital construction, *including means of employment,* exercise and recreation; (d) improved sanitary police of stations, bazaars and adjacent native towns. These four things are, as is well known to you, in reality *one* as regards health. To omit the three and build the one is to spend much money with little hope of money's worth. For on (a) the condition of the surrounding native population and (b) the water supply, drainage, etc., depends very much whether we shall have epidemics or not.

Whether it is necessary to construct new barracks and what their construction shall be must be determined on the spot after competent inquiry into the general sanitary condition of the station where it is proposed to build. The *construction* of the new barracks does not appear to have had anything to do with cholera, fever or other diseases in these buildings. The construction may even have lessened the sick rate, for there are plenty, unfortunately, of causes of sickness undealt with, which lie outside the rooms altogether, e.g., Allahabad.

May I suggest to you to inquire what is the condition of the neighbourhood of these barracks? You can easily command a more graphic account than any I can give you of the filthy towns where cholera flourishes almost perennially, where there is neither drainage nor wholesome water, and this close to the new barracks. All the barrack building in the world would make but little difference in the epidemic susceptibility (to use a grand word) of troops exposed to malaria day and night, more especially during sleep. Is Allahabad a solitary example, an exception? Are there not instances of new barracks suffering from foul ground covered with filth by work people and others? (One instance we knew of at Nusserabad, where the nuisance directly produced cholera among the troops. But I spare you this instance. You must be saturated with such cases.) In India improved construction, sufficient space and ventilation, upper floor sleeping rooms, where necessary, have no other object than to remove the depressing constitutional influences of foul air and to enable the men to resist other disease causes, not themselves connected with the barracks.

3. Such causes require to be attacked always outside the barracks, sometimes outside the cantonment, and it may be at a considerable distance from its boundary. Filthy towns and bazaars, or foul native houses and inhabitants *inside cantonment* boundaries, or too close to them, are constant sources of danger. Of course the only real safeguard is to keep such population out of cantonments and at a safe distance to leeward. This, we are told, is not always possible. Also we are told that, for civil purposes, troops must be near the civil population. Then either the native population must be put under efficient sanitary police or the troops (and natives too and civilians too) must suffer.

4. I will not weary you with repeating what has been said by the royal India sanitary commission, presided over by Sidney Herbert and then by Lord Stanley (Lord Derby), and by the present Army Sanitary Commission. There is no difference of opinion as to men sleeping as far as necessary above the level of the ground. The principle is applicable to all climates and countries. The only question as regards India is the amount of elevation. This has been fully discussed in the reports referred to and must be determined by local and climatic inquiry on the spot.

5. But whatever the height of the sleeping room as raised above the ground, the great principle must never be overlooked that, in Indian climates, men cannot be always in the same rooms, inhabiting the same rooms day and night, with safety. (If they are, the floors and walls get impregnated with "men," as in European climates is the case with hospitals constantly inhabited.) Their day and dining rooms must be separate from their sleeping rooms. (This is a "*must*," not

"may"—as I am sure you agree.) And there must be means of occupying the men at trades, remunerative work, or reading, or exercises, instead of lying on their beds, thinking of cholera for perhaps eighteen hours out of the twenty-four. And there must be commanding officers who will devise, support and encourage such remunerative employment, such active industry and recreation among the men as will *pull* them out of bed by force of interest.

Such things have been done and may be done again and done more extensively although of course there is much talk about "impossibility" and "difficulty." "Si c'est possible, c'est fait: si c'est impossible, cela se fera" [if it is possible, it is done: if it is impossible, it will be done], as I well know, under you. Road making in India, as is acknowledged, has cured the troops, engaged in it, of sickness. But, besides this, every commanding officer is learning in India the elementary principle in physiology that men eat and sleep solely to lay in a store of force to be expended under the action of the will. If this force is not expended in healthy production, it will be expended in unhealthy or diseased products. Half the diseased predisposition in India among the men arises from "lolling" on their beds. But men can't *will* themselves active. They must have the necessary room and appliances, the necessary means and inducements for work and recreation, in order to find the requisite means of cure. If the lower floors of barracks are furnished only with a bench or two, if they have neither fittings nor punkahs nor anything to do (in them), of course the men won't go into them, of course the men won't do anything in them. Either these appliances are necessary or not, and if they are, they must be had or, if not had, the men must suffer. Any way there is no saving, for men in India cost more than tables, tools or punkahs. But all the workshops and appliances in the world will be of no use, unless the officers see to their use. And officers nowadays will soon acknowledge that their men's health is of more importance to the state than their own "difficulties." Also you have a commander-in-chief coming out who has been as successful in these matters as he has been in war and engineering.

6. There seem to be matters of barrack detail requiring improvement, e.g., the men complain they can't move their beds easily into the verandahs and don't like the stairs, etc. Points of this kind can only be dealt with in India. One thing seems essential to their comfort: every man should have his bed space, whether on or off duty, whether in barracks or in hospital. Our principle here has been to

give by regulation *every bed*, occupied or not, its quota of space. A soldier's bed is his home, the only home he has. He ornaments it with his little pictures and things. And no good was ever done to a Briton by destroying his notion of home. (In England attempts have frequently been made to alter this. We have always resisted. The secretary of state alone can grant a dispensation in special cases for sufficient cause shown.) At cool hill stations or at damp changeable other stations the barrack room should always have its fireplace for use and comfort.

7. Then, there are the gardens. We have not heard so much lately about extending these, though the government is certainly not less solicitous about usefully occupying its men year by year. These gardens used to be worked with success and only want encouragement. Almost every regiment should supply itself with vegetables, one of the prime elements of healthy diet in India. (But England can't preach to India on these scores. England is the land of "parochial" jobbing. And when I think of our workhouses, workhouse contractors—*kinsmen* to guardians—and the palming off of their last week's stock of vegetables and meat, etc., which they couldn't sell, of workhouse inmates and workhouse sick, I am dumb.)

8. I am afraid India is rather short of that (not unknown) article: a pump. I think I shall make India a present of a pump—provided you will have it engraved on my tomb, as on that of the ex-maire: "Il a doué [doté] sa commune d'une pompe," and provided you will guarantee me from being thrown into my own well by the bheesties or coolies, whose trade I shall have damaged. But, seriously, would not steam pumps, forcing pumps, might not they answer as well in Indian as in European latitudes? We do not here depend upon "natural head-works" nor upon water carriers. You will soon have at your elbow the first of engineers—in your commander-in-chief.

II. *Administrative points*

As to the present state of the public health question in India compared with what it was before the report of the royal Indian sanitary commission, there is

A. 1. A much greater and more intelligent acknowledgment of the importance of discovering sanitary laws on the part of persons in high places. But I am afraid you will retort, as a great personage once did, that that is no more than if I said that government had acknowledged the law of gravitation.

2. Much more is known of disease causes than formerly. But:

3. There is still a great amount of preventible disease and mortality in the army, although the death rates have been lowered.

4. The civil health question is in much the same position practically as it was, although there has been some legislation about it.

5. Conservancy arrangements for cantonments and bazaars depend for their efficiency, but too much, on the efficiency of commanding officers or cantonment magistrates.

6. A number of new barracks and hospitals have been built but water supply and drainage of barracks, cantonments and native towns are much in the same state as they were.

7. There is practically *no executive* for public health works.

8. There is too little money.

9. Improvements have been initiated at the three presidency capitals and the results have been even greater than was anticipated by those who knew Bombay and Calcutta five years ago, showing that Indian climate is *not* the inexorable enemy to health and life, if only the common measures to secure health and life elsewhere are adopted in India, as elsewhere.

10. An admirable amount of reporting and discussing and theorizing on public health questions has been done but not much in dealing with them. There has not been much of real practical grasp. This raises the question of improved administrative arrangements.

B. The "reports" and "suggestions" (of the English Indian commissions), too often referred to above, have anticipated almost all I have to say. Perhaps a greater advance in sanitary work might have been made if the arrangements therein recommended had been persistently carried out. Clearly enough, dwellings, towns and even areas of country may become diseased just like human bodies and, being so, may lower or destroy vitality in human beings living in them. No specific remedy is applicable to all cases, for there are no specifics in public health any more than in private patients. Each case must be taken by itself, its symptoms examined by competent persons and remedies, surgical or other, pointed out. It was with this view that the royal commission recommended presidency commissions of health so constituted as to represent all the elements of health problems throughout India, i.e., the engineering as well as the sanitary and medical elements, the civil as well as the military element. But when they were appointed, men were put on, especially the members who represented the engineering and military elements, who were already so overworked that they had not even time to attend more than two or three meetings, much less to go upon inspections of stations (without which inspections the thing is as absurd as prescribing for your patient without seeing him). So the commissions cost too much money for too little work. They were transformed into one (generally medical) commissioner for each presidency. These men were very good. India is quite as well supplied with men of this class as our municipal and parochial authorities are in England, though, in both countries, some of them are too much given to theorizing and trusting to books rather than to observation. All will improve by practice.

C. But then how is their work given effect to? Where is the executive to carry it out? Is the reporting the be-all and the end-all? What is the machinery to follow it up with measures? For instance, all that a medical health officer can do for us is to tell us how many people have been sick or have died, to what extent epidemics have prevailed, their nature and probable causes. This being done, someone conversant with other problems altogether is wanted, who can trace the causes to their source, draw up estimates for these and see that the works are carried out, i.e., advise, survey and superintend the required works of water supply, drainage, etc. (An instance occurred the other day—one out of many—when a medical officer and an English engineer went to an unhealthy station to select a site for barracks. The engineer pointed out that the real remedy wanted for the station was not so much new buildings as drainage of a water-logged subsoil, which could be done at a small comparative cost. This illustrates the kind of talent and experience which India wants and has not, and yet could have.) But then it must be paid, as is other valuable labour.

The whole matter is summed up in the following list of duties of the proposed presidency health commissions which is in the "recommendations" of the royal Indian sanitary commission:

> To give advice and assistance in all matters relating to the public health, such as the selection of new stations and the sanitary improvement of existing stations and bazaars, to examine new plans for barracks and hospitals, to advise in the laying out of stations and bazaars, the sanitary improvement of native towns, prevention and mitigation of epidemic diseases, and generally to exercise a constant oversight of the sanitary condition of the population, European and native, to report on the prevalence, causes of and means of preventing sickness and disease.

*But*, the royal commission adds: "*and, further, that administrative measures be adopted to give effect to the advice of the presidency commissions.*" (Of course it is no use to make a regulation that your chimney shall not smoke or that water shall not lie, or even to ascertain the cause of the chimney smoking or the water lying, unless there is an executive to take measures and unless the measures *are* taken to carry off the water, to prevent the chimney smoking, etc.)

D. Also it is quite clear that no medical officer can undertake all this, unless indeed he were especially educated in sanitary engineering and other departments of knowledge—just like a sanitary engineer. It is also quite clear that the work is so special that it cannot be taken up merely as *part of other* work. It must be made a *specially responsible* proceeding. In all inquiries of the kind two things have to be discovered: (1) the diseases to be diminished, (2) the causes of these traced to their fountainhead and the *practical remedies and cost laid before you.*

E. Probably there is no idea of reconstituting the original commissions. Then, would not the best step be for your commander-in-chief, whose own special sanitary engineering knowledge is of the first order, to select a few good royal engineers, to direct them to make sanitary work their specialty (if he judges it necessary, to let them come home to study the great European sanitary works) and to set them, with your medical commissioner, to make inspections of stations, inquiries, examinations, reports and estimates? Funds and means of execution would then have to be provided. Much of the preventible disease among troops and civil population may be "stamped out" by drainage and water supply (not by quarantine). The Indian problem is so vast that it can only be solved in details. Sick India cannot be cured in a year or two (people in England are rather too apt to forget that).

An admirable beginning has been made in Bombay and Calcutta. The first Indian sewage farm (at Madras) augurs a great success in India. (£58 per acre per annum of grass produce is a better return for money than building costly hospitals for sick.) This Madras experiment is perhaps the key to the improvement of Indian cities. China is far before us in this aspect.

F. As regards water, it is stated, on the first authority, that there is scarcely a station in India which might not be supplied with water enough by good engineering, e.g., steam-pumping, etc. (There is scarcely an out-of-the-way railway station in the United Kingdom not supplied with water in this way, also with gas made by portable apparatus to be had to any extent in England.) Hardly anything needs *inventing* in India, except indeed "How to do it?"

G. One current remedy is applicable everywhere, and that is *cleanliness.* Much of the native ill-health can be destroyed, as at Bombay, by vigorous cleansing measures carried out by an energetic commissioner, aided by his health officer.

H. We have no cause to sing our sanitary triumphs in England. But at least the standing commission (Barrack and Hospital Improvement Commission, now Army Sanitary Commission), initiated by Sidney Herbert and presided over by himself till his death, has done its work well. This is its method of proceeding at home and Mediterranean stations: (1) A careful examination of the past history of the station was made, particularly as regarded the prevailing diseases and their proportionate importance. (2) An equally careful examination was next made of the station and its surroundings, including the native population, their diseases and mortality, the sanitary defects to which these were due, the state of the barrack, hospital and married quarters, stables, etc., and the general sanitary police of the station. (3) A statement of requirements was then made out, estimates were framed and submitted to the government authorities, money was provided, the improvements were carried out gradually as regarded the military buildings and defects among the civil population were brought under the notice of the local authorities. (4) The death rate has become one half of what it was. We did not trust to building new barracks for improving the health of the army but brought experience in sanitary questions to bear practically on disease causes with the view of removing them at as little cost as possible. And this proceeding is the key to sanitary work everywhere. In India the populations are so vast that sanitary progress cannot be rapid. Should you not begin (as we did here) with the worst cases: cleanse first subsoil drain; where necessary, pump up and supply water and drain buildings? A single station completed, a single village or town cured of its epidemics, will do more to forward improvement than any amount of discussion. Improved agriculture has often been introduced in a backward country by simply showing that a single farm could be well cultivated and would yield a larger profit. The "solvitur ambulando" [it is solved by walking, i.e., by doing] argument has more influence in the progress of improvement than any amount of paper work.

Lastly permit me one word as to what you say about the "localities" in India being made "to do more for themselves" in this work. This is most important. I believe that what they want is not so much interest, or even knowledge, as encouragement and a "grant" of—*powers.* A few good terse instructions in the vernacular (much as already been done in this way, and done well), pointing out the causes of the high death rates, such as filthy customs, bad water and the like, and urging constant cleanliness would be (and have been) well received and do good. (Indian native gentlemen, on their travels, have written to and called upon me and advocated the introduction of sanitary reform into their native cities and villages.) Would not the best way of creating an effectual interest be, in sending such instructions, to grant powers of doing simple work, cleansing, well-digging, etc. for themselves? You can always have their work inspected. Nothing gives men so much interest in any work as *letting them do it,* after showing them how necessary it is for their own welfare. (I am told by great authority that the native Indian will always gladly *pay* for what he *sees,* i.e., for what he *sees* is *doing him good.*)

I do not apologize for this immensely long letter, though much for its stupidity, believing that I have but obeyed your instructions in writing it, which I have done as well as I could, though, I fear, my "could" is but small in its wisdom. Pray believe me, dear Lord Mayo,

ever your faithful servant
Florence Nightingale

Source: From a letter to Lord Mayo, University Library, Cambridge, Mayo Collection Add Ms 7490/132/9

31 March 1870

*Private and Confidential.* I cannot thank you enough for the true kindness of your letter of 11 January and for your wishing to bring us into direct communication with Dr Cuningham's work. You ask me to tell you what I "think of Dr C.'s ideas and opinions." I think him a most intelligent man, a very "full" man, ready to receive any amount of experience, immensely interested in his work, excellent as a reporting and inspecting officer, not perhaps so good as an executive officer—not having any very special ideas or opinions on sanitary matters.

To illustrate the difference of the talents in this work: Dr Hewlett, the Bombay officer of health, has cleansed Bombay almost by his own personal exertions. His practical energy in his special dirty work is something extraordinary. Dr Lumsdaine[26] (whom I do not know), who has succeeded Dr Hewlett, is, I am told, a still better man. And the practical result of their work has been that Bombay is now a comparatively

26 John Lumsdaine (1826-1906), sanitary commissioner for Bombay 1878-83.

healthy city. Either would make shorter work of your dirty native towns at Allahabad and elsewhere than Dr Cuningham. But so far as one can judge by the work done by all of them, Dr Cuningham has more power of sifting and abstracting reports, and tracing disease causes. But this kind of talent, though indispensable, is not all you want. Dr Cuningham very properly keeps clear of engineering questions (of which he knows nothing). But sanitary engineering questions are amongst the most important and frequent with which you will have to deal. Nevertheless, if you were to put the best sanitary engineer in Dr Cuningham's place, the engineer would be lacking in Dr C.'s special knowledge, talent and experience of disease causes. It comes round to the original point that no one man and no number of men "of one class" can improve India. You must have able and experienced engineering work as well as medical opinion.

Pardon me this long sentence. I was anxious to answer as accurately as I can the question you did me the honour to put to me. Nothing but this anxiety would make me venture on the impertinence of saying a word upon financial matters in their bearing on the important sanitary subject. We here are trying to fill our purse by sewing up the hole in the bottom of it. It is a simple operation, but neither satisfactory nor lasting, for in the course of things the hole is worn again. In India the government has spent more than it has gathered. But I am sure that you will not stop every improvement until your purse is filled. With so vast an empire of taxpayers, it is a *good investment* to render the payers more able to pay. This argument is far stronger with troops for, as we have found bitterly and to our cost at home, if we save with them by cutting off expenditure necessary for health, there comes in a dreadful bill afterwards, a bill which always has to be paid. The sickliness, the cholera of this last year in India, is but too terrible a proof of this.

I am sure that you will rather pause before letting people finally act in a way which may be a great cause of subsequent regret. To save this mail I send this unfinished note. But I am ashamed to say that I have still something to answer to your letter, which I am afraid I shall trouble you with by a subsequent mail.

Source: From a letter to Emily Verney, Wellcome (Claydon copy) Ms 9004/45

12 June 1870

N.B. Behold the miraculous effects of *Bride-cake*! As some of Mrs Fred Verney's had been kindly sent me for the orthodox purpose, as I supposed. I place a crumb under my pillow *and dreamt*. And I dreamt that

I was under secretary for India with a balance of 10 millions on the right side of my sheet and that I was irrigating Orissa and draining the deltas of Hugli and Brahmaputra, and famine was vanishing away and cholera almost extinct. Tell Mrs F. Verney.

## "Letter to *The Lancet*," 1870

**Editor:** Nightingale's reply to Dr Maclean's criticisms of her fear of pure theory was accompanied by Dr Maclean's second, brief letter which said:

> Miss Nightingale has been so good as to send me the enclosed letter, written, you will observe, for publication in your journal, in reply to what Miss Nightingale is good enough to call my "kind and gentle criticism." I am glad to find that this very influential writer had no intention or desire to throw cold water on the [cholera] inquiry in defence of which I wrote. I wish, however, to state that I was not singular in thinking such was likely to be the effect of Miss Nightingale's observations. In conclusion, I wish your readers to understand that the inquiry in defence of which I took up my pen was not the one instituted by the sanitary committee of the War Office, of which Miss Nightingale "was one of the first and strongest advocates," but that more special inquiry suggested by the senate of the Army Medical School, and now being carried on by Drs Cuningham and Lewis.

Source: Florence Nightingale, "To the Editor of *The Lancet*" (dated 14 November 1870), *The Lancet* (19 November 1870) 96:725

Sir, In your number of 29 October you inserted a kind and gentle criticism from Professor Maclean on certain parts of my "few words" appended to the last annual India Office report on sanitary measures.

Since the outbreak of this most terrible of all earth's wars [the Franco-Prussian War], I have had a hard time of it in defending others, and I have not had the least little moment to defend myself. Still, Sir, if you will allow me, I should wish to say that Professor Maclean seems to have read from a point of view opposite to that which was in my mind when writing these "few words." And I am glad that he has given me an opportunity, with your permission, to explain them.

My object was, as I need scarcely say, purely practical. It was to deprecate a tendency complained of by all of late years (this very complaint came to me from India), viz., the tendency to base sanitary proceedings on theory. Dr Maclean appears to think that I question the propriety of the cholera inquiry now proceeding in India. I was one of its first and strongest advocates. I strenuously urged the granting of necessary funds to carry it out, and I consider it one of the most important public Indian inquiries which has been ever undertaken on our subject. The very importance of it lies in this: if a fact is proved, it ceases to be theory. The inquiry in question is to ascertain, as far as may be, what *is* fact. This was the meaning of the passage which Dr Maclean interprets as implying "ridicule" on my part.

What I said about the present state of the fungoid theory I learnt from the published report of Drs Cuningham and Lewis, about the ground water from Dr Townsend's Report on Cholera in the Central Provinces. These statements are not theories, but facts. If they are facts, they cease to be theories. The theories remain just where they were. Of course, if the theories were found on longer inquiry to be true, they too would be no longer theories, but facts and as such would afford good ground for expending public money in applying the *facts* to save life.

The case of Jenner,[27] cited by Dr Maclean, is in reality my case. Jenner first started a theory, but the Vaccination Acts, with the costs and penalties, were not enacted until Jenner's theory had become a fact by long experience.

We all have the same object in view, viz., saving human life. This cannot be done without expenditure. And as theories are many and uncertain, all we ask is that the public should know what we are spending their money for. This the said cholera inquiry will, perhaps more than anything else, help to tell us.

Also, in what I said about cholera excreta, I simply dealt again with the facts. Dr Bryden has shown in his report on cholera, p 214, that the dry-earth system, which, in its application, would prevent the dangers of putrid cholera excreta, had not stayed the ravages of cholera. Hence Dr Bryden himself calls in question the theory. And I have done no more.

At p 59, para 170 of the report for 1869 by the "sanitary commissioner with the Government of India," just received, the results of dealing with cholera excreta are stated as follows: "With regard to the effect of the careful disinfection and safe disposal of evacuations which seem to have been generally practised, there is no evidence to show that any results can be professedly attributed to them."

27 Sir William Jenner (1815-98), physician to Queen Victoria, distinguished typhus from typhoid fever.

Since Professor Maclean's letter appeared in *The Lancet* of 29 October, I have received Dr Lewis's able and most interesting report, the first instalment of the scientific inquiry into cholera which Dr Maclean fears my remarks may injure. It confirms the former joint reports of Drs Lewis and Cuningham by a host of microscopic examinations and drawings, from which the following conclusion (No. 3, p 164, sanitary commissioner's report) is deduced by Dr Lewis: "3. That no special fungus has been developed in cholera stools, the fungus described by [Ernst] Hallier[28] being certainly not confined to such stools." But these are the theories which have hitherto occupied the attention of the observers.

Even this information, though most important, we shall not, however, receive as final. We must inquire into objections and ask further questions. The real inquiry is only about to begin. Mere controversy is here useless.

With many apologies for writing so long a letter, which, had I had more time, I could have made shorter. Pray believe me, Sir,

your faithful servant
Florence Nightingale

Source: From two letters to William Clark [civil engineer to the municipality of Calcutta], University of North Carolina 5/7/61

Evening 5 October 1872

In Mr Chadwick's paper in the India Office Blue Book, to which you refer, this [that no engineering principle is applicable to all cases] is overlooked. And when the Government of India printed it for circulation in India, they actually appended a note to the effect that Mr Chadwick's paper was useful but he had quite misunderstood the Kanpur case. An engineer should of course deal with every separate town just as a doctor deals with every separate patient, applying the principles of his art to the particular case.

Much controversy would have been spared had you explained the facts about the sewers of your Calcutta system, which you have been so kind as to tell me. In telling me you have clearly described your case, you have replied completely to Mr Chadwick and to all people who hold by a principle and not by an application.

May I repeat what I said this morning about the desirableness of your giving to the world this your new chapter on sanitary engineering? A principle which would certainly not apply in many cases can scarcely be laid down as an infallible law, like a law of nature. Here was how the

---

28 Ernst Hallier (1831-1904), botanist.

Metropolitan Sanitary Commission and Mr Chadwick arrived at their views about sewers: London was sewered by great sewers; they had these sewers gauged after heavy rains and then they calculated what size of drainpipe would carry away the sewage; they found that quite small tubes would do; and then they laid down the same principle as of universal application. The Calcutta problem was quite different than the London one. You had to free continuously a town subsoil not only charged by rainfall but by river water. (I suppose that, though the sizes of your sewers are somewhat overcalculated for the existing flow, if the entire city were drained into your outlets, they would not be too large.)

2 December 1873

*Major* Tulloch says that it did not occur to him, when he saw you to recommend (as your successor) "a *Mr Hart*, who has been in the *Bombay* Public Works Department for some years and who is a very scientific engineer with at the same time a good deal of practical experience. He would be a capital man for the post, if the Bombay government would spare him. Mr Hart is a man of about thirty-five or forty, no doubt knows the vernacular, a great advantage." You may know something of *him, Mr Hart.*

Source: From a letter to Julius Mohl, Florence Nightingale Museum (LMA) H1/ST/NC1/73/5

30 December 1873

In India all tree vegetation is considered healthy in epidemic times. But as malaria exists notwithstanding trees, we must insist (not on eucalyptus but) on drainage works.

The famine, instead of making us redouble our efforts to prevent such horrors, seems likely to shrivel up all our small attempts, by sanitary engineering, draining and irrigation, to render such calamities less possible. Gulliver (Campbell [lieutenant governor] of Bengal) is doing excellently well. So is Lord Northbrook [viceroy], but he has as yet hardly realized the tremendous extent of the calamity which looms in the distance. And the zemindars and their foolish English advisors are still trying to mislead Gulliver by will-o'-the-wisps.

Source: From a letter to William Clark, University of North Carolina 5/7/61

25 June 1875

I thank you very much for the copy of your invaluable report on the Madras drainage and for your kind note. I was very glad to hear that you are come back and I shall be still more glad to hear that you are going out again *to do it.*

When your principles are carried out and the houses drained, we shall hear little of high Madras death rates. The principles are so sound that the question reduces itself to one simply of engineering detail. . . .

There is small doubt that Lord Hobart[29] died of delay, i.e., in carrying out drainage. Europeans are under the scourge of typhoid fever in India for not acting up to our lights in sanitarily doing our duty. Some years ago we did not know that the fatal Indian fever *is typhoid.* In 1874, 101 soldiers died of it in India. And you must seize it by the throat, please God.

Source: From notes, Royal Holloway, University of London 2

16 March 1878

Believe myself that the great rivers coming down from Himalayas bring malaria. . . . Deltas are malarious; have never been able to learn why Indus Delta is not used as Godavari Delta for irrigation.

Dr Thornton, representative of Punjab in viceroy's council (but that council packed), says Punjabi fever on Bari Duab [?] and western Jumna canal and talks of that "fashionable panacea" irrigation; in greater part of Punjab crops can no more be grown without water as without land.

Sind ditto, well irrigated.

Burdwan fever goes always as it comes, we don't know how: we drained, it did not subside; where we did not drain, it did. Hugli drainage scheme at expense of landowners; they behaved very well; it succeeded very well, great encouragement to go on.

Source: From a draft letter to Sir George Campbell, Add Mss 45805 f32

30 March 1878

Food supply: river water for potable and culinary, guarding from impurities avoidable and unavoidable where no proper supply, would remove one of the worst causes of fever [of the] poor Bengal peasant as also [giving] power to clear his land of surplus water when rice crop sufficiently advanced and yet to be able to claim water from an artificial source when he wants to put a second crop into the ground. Burdwan fever a famine fever; now regulation of water, i.e., combining drainage with irrigation and a good water supply; exciting cause in poor creatures whose normal state is semi-starvation.

---

29 Vere Henry Hampden Hobart (1818-75), governor of Madras 1872-75.

Source: From a letter to Thomas Gillham Hewlett, Columbia University, Presbyterian Hospital School of Nursing C155

27 July 1883

Alas! I wish I could say that we are making progress in Europe in sanitary things. It seems rather as if we were making retrogression (since twenty years ago). The insanity of our doctrines about "germs" and proceedings about cholera is so virulent. Our whole Indian experience tends to, nay actually proves, that cholera is not communicable from person to person, that it is a local disease depending on pollution of buildings, earth, air and water, that quarantines, cordons, medical inspection and the like are all fatal aggravations of the disease, that the only preventives are, first, to remove healthy troops, healthy people, from the locality, to put earth, air and water and buildings into a healthy state by scavenging, limewashing and all sanitary work. (Had we done what you did in Bombay city as officers of health, when we decided to stay in Egypt, cholera would never have come, or but a slight epidemic.) Is this not so ? . . . That attendants do *not* "catch" the disease from the sick, anymore than they do from poisoned cases. Is not all this so? Yet look at Egypt and Europe now. It is this doctrine of "germs" which has "poisoned" us. Our only reason now against enforcing quarantine is *not* that it is an efficient mode of breeding disease, but that it *cannot* be enforced; "if it could be, all would be well." As I heard one of the few good men and true say: People will soon believe that you can take a railway ticket for cholera. Pray help us.

Source: From a letter to John Sutherland, ADD Mss 45758 ff170-71

30 July 1883

I know not whether you know what has been passing in your absence about "Precautions against Cholera." Before he left England Dr Cuningham attended a meeting at the Local Government Board, in which Buchanan and Jenner[30] carried all before them, and Dr Cuningham and Sir Joseph Fayrer were left absolutely alone in protesting against "germ" measures and "isolation" measures and *for* sanitary measures. Dr Cuningham, whom I saw twice, was positively broken-hearted. He left with me a letter which I got into the *Times*. And you see his excellent epidemiological lecture is in full in the *Medical Times* of 21 July.

30 Probable reference to Andrew Buchanan (1798-1882) and Edward Jenner (1749-1823), both physicians linked with cholera research and, in the present context, apparent precursors of the germ theory; the latter developed a vaccine against smallpox.

Source: From a letter to James M. Cuningham, Johns Hopkins University 5

9 October 1884

*Private.* As regards works of drainage these will at first, we suppose, be confined to large cities. And where the populations are small, may not much be done by simple inexpensive surface drainage? Besides, do we not still require more experience of house drainage in India? We *must* agree with all our mights with you as to the dangers arising from sanitary ignorance among M.D.s. This can scarcely be overrated. Would we could see a remedy in Netley! But "who shall guard the guardians"[31] there? The chief enemies of Indian progress are disease theorists. As the local councils gain practical knowledge, one hopes that they will disregard these disease theorists. Dr Koch[32] will not do much mischief except through such men. Was not his "discovery" made thirty years ago in London, and then estimated at *nil*? All that he has done has been to found a theory on it. What is the result of the work of the I.O.'s scientific commission? And has Dr Koch's "discovery" gone the way of all such "discoveries"? . . .

What is wanted here is that a tight hand should be kept on all the Indian people doing sanitary work. Dr Sutherland warned Colonel Yule some time ago that if Dr Koch merely stated what he had seen in the East there would be an outcry; and his return to Berlin was followed by a declaration of Virchow[33] that the English Government of India was a perpetual menace to the world. Is not this becoming more and more true, because men are now learning what we told them long ago that cholera was not spread by contagion but by overflow from India?

Source: From two letters to Douglas Galton, ADD Mss 45765 ff248-49 and 250

4 February 1885

Have you seen Dr Cuningham's small book, "Cholera, What Can the State Do to Prevent It?" intended as the introduction to his *last* annual report but instead published separate. It seems to me very good. He wants to get the book reviewed "by suitable hands." "If it falls into the hands of the ordinary theoretical reviewer," "the experience of India may be lost." "The public remain blinded to the real facts regarding

---

31 "Quis custodiet ipsos custodes?" is from Juvenal, *Satires* VI.347.

32 Robert Koch (1843-1910), bacteriologist, demonstrated the germ theory in 1884, awarded the Nobel Prize for medicine in 1905 for his work on tuberculosis.

33 Rudolf Ludwig Karl Virchow (1821-1902), pathologist, anthropologist and politician.

cholera and the real nature of the protection required." He sends home (purposely not till next mail) copies to *Times, Standard, Daily News, Morning Post, Spectator, Saturday R[eview], Pall Mall G[azette]*, *St James G[azette]*, medical papers. *Could you be so very good as to help in getting it properly reviewed?* The aim is a good one.

5 February 1885

Dr Cuningham sent a copy of his book to "Sir Joseph Fayrer" with, I have no doubt, the same request as he did to me. Also to Dr Sutherland. I do not know about "Klein."[34] Could you be so very kind as to look up somebody to review it properly in some of the papers he, Dr C., mentions? I wish I had more copies, I would give one to Lord Reay and to some others.

Source: From a letter to James M. Cuningham, Johns Hopkins University letter 6

13 February 1885

Very many thanks for your kind note and for the copy of your invaluable book on cholera and how it is to be prevented by the state. Would that all our state authorities, all our military and medical authorities, would lay it to heart and learn it not by heart but in practice!

The mania of tracing any disease not to some glaring obvious sanitary defect, but to insects, bacteria, bacilli, protoplasms—what can I call them?—is becoming an incurable lunacy, so much so that an outbreak of diarrhea, seizing eighteen nurses at once—in an institution that shall be nameless [St Thomas' Hospital]—we were quite afraid would be considered due to some of these delusions and not to sewer air from a wastepipe going direct into a drain with a cistern supplying both W.C.s, sinks and drinking water, and a choked up W.C.

I regret more than I can say that you are leaving India. You will not thank me for this regret but you seemed the main bulwark against all this madness with the Government of India. Who will be your successor? and what will he do? If you could tell me before you leave what are the prospects of the local self-government working with regard to sanitary things, I should be deeply obliged. (You were so good as to write me a summary of the powers and sanitary duties of a local self-

34 Dr Edward Emanuel Klein (1844-1925), physician and microbiologist. He was sent to India with Dr Heneage Gibbes to investigate the causes of cholera; they were chosen because of their opposition to Koch's bacteriological theory on the source of cholera.

government act.) Is the village sanitary work likely to be done well by the new boards and likely to be well supervised by our officials without, as you will say, needless worrying and interfering with the people's domestic happiness by forcible removal of sick and other contagious theory? May we hope to see "judicious guiding" by our officials? How I wish we could have had you to "guide" the work at least for the first year or two!

I have done what I could, and I am sure others will also, to have your book properly reviewed. But, as you may suppose, attention here is concentrated on the fall of Khartoum, Gordon's death and the prosecuting of General Wolseley's expedition. But we will try again. I will write again before you leave India.

**Editor:** Mainly in order to reduce expenditures, a proposal was made in Bombay in 1886 to amalgamate the office of sanitary commissioner with that of the surgeon general. The news gave Nightingale the occasion to express her passionate disapproval of the proposal and the reasons for her opposition to similar proposals: sanitary knowledge was a specialty and ordinary medical men did not have it. The proposal would slow down the steps being taken to control epidemics. Epidemics could best be combatted by sanitary engineers and officers who possess concrete knowledge of local circumstances and enjoy administrative and executive power; Hewlett was their model. No medical officer had such competence (see p 928 below). That is why, in the following letter to Lord Dufferin, Nightingale insisted on the dangers of accepting the proposed amalgamation. Effective prevention of epidemics belonged to sanitary measures applied to towns and villages, enforced and monitored by officers trained in that kind of work.

Source: Letter, British Library, Asia, Pacific and Africa Collections, Dufferin papers, Eur Mss fol 130-24, No. 228

10 South Street
Park Lane, W.
4 November 1886

*Private and Confidential*
Dear Lord Dufferin

May I avail myself of your kind leave to write to you on what seems a very pressing matter. And may I claim credit for not having troubled you before, even about pressing matters, knowing the enormous weight of responsibility and work which rests upon you?

My "matter" is that the Finance Committee is said to be threatening our sanitary commissionerships, to abolish them or rather to amalgamate them with the surgeon generalships (this at least as far as regards Bombay). In some respects our best authorities think that the latter proposal, the amalgamation of the sanitary office with that of the surgeon general, the worse of the two.

As to Bombay, it was stated on high sanitary authorities—what we, here, concur in—that in very, "very rare instances would the surgeon general be fit to be sanitary commissioner, that any such amalgamation would be fatal to the Sanitary Department." It would be manifestly unjust to the deputy sanitary commissioners who have had held out to them by the secretary of state for India repeated hopes that the sanitary commissioners would be chosen from their ranks.

"If this proposition is carried into effect," it was added,

> good-bye to all hopes of sanitary reform in India. Sanitation is a speciality; ordinary medical men are all contagionists and would advise quarantine and such things. And not one has studied the question of sanitary construction of buildings, etc.
>
> The Finance Committee appeals, anxious to reduce the deputy sanitary commissioners' salaries, so that it will be impossible to retain good men in the department. All this is most unsettling and does great harm, as it takes all life out of men.

So far as to Bombay.

But it is not only for saving our sanitary commissioners that we wish to plead, it is because we need a sanitary executive as advised in the royal commission "on the sanitary state of the Indian Army," of which Sidney Herbert and Lord Derby were presidents and which reported in 1863.

*Where* are we now in sanitary work (after twenty-three years)? Disease and death-reporting have done their work, but practical proceedings on the results have still to be taken. They *have* been taken in the British and native armies, and are being taken in the jails. But in these cases the means of execution and of carrying out improvements existed on the spot, and death rates in all these cases have gone down (in European troops to one sixth). There has been some improvement in the general cities' death rates. Some with more or less effective work show best. But generally the cities show want of intelligent execution of measures. The results show mainly what *might* be done.

The country population, living in some 3/4 of a million of villages—for is not India a land of villages?—shows no improvement, but rather increasing death rates, especially from epidemics, which are the real touchstones of sanitary conditions. No provision has hitherto been made for executive sanitary work in the villages, except that at Bombay Lord Reay, with Mr Hewlett, sanitary commissioner, and Mr Crawford, revenue commissioner, is making a noble effort to initiate or restore some villages' cleaning organization, which effort is made much more difficult by our blunder in dispersing the Mhars and Mangs (the sweeper people). The *towns*, which are supposed to have some municipal government, have a population of about twelve millions, while the unprotected *villages* have a population of above 185½ millions.

Pardon me a very few figures. I will not give many. Our latest total mortality returns for the civil population show:

| *Deaths from epidemics* | |
|---|---|
| In 1883 | 3,618,021 |
| In 1884 | 4,201,032 |

| | |
|---|---|
| To wit: *Fevers* which carry off *every* year ten times as many as cholera | 3,306,285 |
| *Cholera* | 287,609 |
| Other like complaints | 274,234 |
| Smallpox | 332,904 |
| Total | 4,201,032 |

[They] show an increase of epidemic deaths in 1884 of 583,011 and, so far as we have the 1885 returns, the increase is still in progress. This is our case, for which must there not be found a remedy?

It is the fashion to say that the natives do not care and that they make a grievance of sanitary measures. If so, more shame for the sanitary officers, who ought to be sanitary missionaries. Where they have been so, as Mr Hewlett, sanitary commissioner of Bombay, has been, things are very different. Formerly if there were 200 or 300 deaths from cholera a day, the people remained passive or accused the goddess of - - ? Now if there are one or two cholera deaths, they hurry to Mr Hewlett: "Bestir yourselves, gentlemen; don't you see we're all dead?"

In a district very near you at Calcutta, [in] the twenty-four pergunnas, a high-caste Brahmin was the sanitary missionary. (He is now here, in charge of a section of the Indo-Colonial Exhibition and gave me the account himself.) His whole family perished of fever. Every year for two months, the whole population is entirely laid up *and unproductive* from fever. The causes are perfectly well known: fouled tanks, growths under the large trees, allowed to rot, muddy roads. All these could be removed with a little organization on the part of government by the people themselves. In many places, are not the people themselves crying out to do this?

India finances are at this moment an enormous difficulty. But this is a thing which could be done with so little money—only a little organization. And think of the money saved, the productiveness of the population restored. In fever districts the people are half alive and the next generation deteriorates from the present.

It is an exaggeration to say that, next to the protection of life and property from criminals, is the protection of life and property from epidemics—if indeed it ought not as a department of government to take the lead. For is it not doubtful if, since the world began, criminals have destroyed more life and property on the earth than are destroyed year after year in India annually by preventible epidemics?

People must *live* in order to plough. They must live and be in health in order to work. It seems strange that thirty years after Sidney Herbert began his great sanitary operations in the army and in India, and after the immense reduction in death rates in some directions (not by medicine but by sanitary work), such propositions as these about the sanitary commissionerships should be possible, and by way of economy!! The saving of money is surely as conspicuous, is it not? as the saving of life by sanitary measures.

But we humbly look to Lord Dufferin to do vast good and signalize his government by initiating real sanitary works, as Lady Dufferin is doing in forwarding sanitary education.

The sanitary commissioners have shown statistically that, for nearly 200 millions of our fellow subjects, nothing of much consequence has been done and that India suffers enormous death and property losses from epidemics. But the executive is wanting and the real function of the present sanitary commissioners is to tell us how many people die of preventible diseases. Better it would be if the government would discuss whether a sanitary executive might not be, to do the administrative and executive engineering work on steadily ascertained sanitary lines. The recommendation of the royal commission was this course: to examine local causes, prescribe local remedies, institute the necessary local means of execution and keep a firm hold over the work. (In Bombay presidency an able sanitary engineering officer has been appointed for the towns.) These are the duties of the sanitary engineer and sanitary officer properly so-called. No medical officer that we know of has any competence for such duties, and they can only be discharged economically by trained and experienced officers.

Would not the change advised of uniting or amalgamating the two offices, *medical* and *sanitary*, be the first step downwards to non-entity? The step downwards being that there would be no necessary sanitary knowledge among the successive principal medical officers appointed, and there would be no continuity of sanitary knowledge. Every new man would have to learn not only sanitary work, but its peculiarities in his district. And then all the while but little money is being saved, while the people would be swept away. There would be an increase of epidemics among the troops. And every life lost costs India £100. The only effect would be to put it into the surgeon general's hands and *do nothing*.

But would not the effect upon the natives be that of our not deeming to care about sanitary improvement after all among themselves? Ought not sanitary commissioner to be, as *e.g.*, Mr Hewlett and Dr [H.W.] Belew [Punjab] are, missionaries or prophets of sanitation to the natives, propagandists, teachers or preachers of sanitary knowledge? Where such are, the people who used to think the most destructive epidemic was fate or the fault of the goddess of smallpox or the "mother" of something else, now think it is *our* fault. What an improvement that is!

Local agencies must be provided by which the work may be done! And a few competent sanitary engineering officers to superintend and inspect on all local works and measures required for towns and villages, in communication with the sanitary officer. Probably 90 percent of the total sanitary work required for India lies in the villages and this work ought to be done directly or indirectly by the people themselves. (Village rules for Bombay presidency *are* being, or are to be, issued under Lord Reay's authority.)

In the cities the matter is not proceeding so well and Madras after twenty years' work returned in 1884 a death rate of 50 per 1000. Up to the present time then, only the statistical reporting work has been attended to. Can any method be devised in India whereby the two necessities can be met without material increase of cost?

In the present state of things the giving up these sanitary officers is really giving up the sanitary executive, because we should not have the instruments with which to work it. Are there not great political objections in the natives' discontent if what affects *them* is the thing cut down, if cheese-paring by governments of things which appear to do the natives directly some good (while the army, the great expense, is left untouched or increased) is carried on? if it is thought worthwhile, for the sake of some very small reduction, to destroy works the people are very much interested in? Is not public opinion becoming a greatly increased power, not to be disregarded? At home a much greater interest is taken in India than formerly.

Sanitary things in India can never be carried out without a sanitary executive all over India. That sounds like large sums. But large sums in a great country, are they not small sums really? Small indeed compared with the vast loss of life and productiveness which takes place year after year, which the natives themselves begin to see might be prevented by very simple measures and may be clearly traced to the absence of a proper sanitary executive to deal with, above all, *village* problems.

I can make no excuse for this long and tiresome letter, except by not lengthening it with my excuses. Pardon me and let me be, dear Lord Dufferin,

ever your excellency's faithful servant, wishing a Godspeed to all your measures for the people

Florence Nightingale

Source: From two letters to Douglas Galton, ADD Mss 45765 f318 and 45766 ff1-2

7 December 1886

He [Hewlett] says that the very high proportion of death to attacks of cholera in Bombay harbour is owing to the long distances they have to be carried to hospital. Government contradicts him and he persists, saying what we all of us know to be true, that a cholera patient had better be let alone at home than moved a long distance to the best hospital. Surely this should be noticed so as to be understood.

19 January 1887

Are you there? We want an example—it is for a presidency in India—of the working of the Local Government Act Office and the country board or authority here when, e.g., typhoid fever has broken out and defect in the drinking water is suspected. I have been asked for a real case here—it is for the Bombay presidency. This is, *if a real case*, what would be useful, viz., that (as at Bangor) on the breaking out of typhoid fever the inhabitants, acting through their own board or representatives (or individuals can apply direct), should write up to the Local Government Act Office to send down an inspector who comes down, inspects and reports. The country board sits upon the report, adopts the suggestions, the cause being discovered to be fouled drinking water. The works are sanctioned, carried out, inspected (the inhabitants taxing themselves by direct rate or raising money from government [?]). The cause is removed, the disease ceases (but the dead cannot be recalled to life).

Could you farther tell us what happens in an *entirely rural* place, whether *they* will report themselves to the Local Government Act Office and get themselves put to rights? . . . Please, I ought, if possible, to have this information ready today. I could see you this afternoon, if you would be so good.

Source: Notes on a meeting with James M. Cuningham, ADD Mss 45827 ff165-66

30 September 1887

Here are these poor people, these millions for whom we are responsible. We who know all the secrets of life or death and health or disease, of which they know hardly anything, we can give them life and health, and we won't. We could stamp out cholera in two years. They are longing for it, they don't like being ill or dying any more than we do. They appreciate a pure water supply, even more than we do; they will sacrifice even caste for it; they *are* clean in their bodies and, wherever they can be, they are beginning to appreciate sanitation. It's the landlord interest, the rich man interest in Calcutta which keeps sanitation down (as it is in London). The poor man *would* pay; he is rated for the drainage and sewerage which he does not get, and then he is rated for removing the filth because it has not been removed by the process he *has* paid for. Is it not a government's business to give its knowledge to save its people's lives? Criminal epidemics.

**Editor:** The following letter to Lord Cross, secretary of state for India, was requested from Nightingale by Lord Cross himself to help clarify the staffing, functions and powers of the proposed executive sanitary boards to be introduced in each presidency; they were expected to become a more adequate instrument in the battle against epidemics than the presidency commissions had been since 1864.

Source: From a letter/draft/copy to Lord Cross, ADD Mss 45807 ff281-90

September 1887

*Private and Confidential.* You were so good as to desire me to write to you on the sanitary evils persistent in India owing to the want of a sanitary executive which you intended, you kindly told me, to make the subject of a despatch to the Government of India. These evils are undoubtedly, we fear, increasing evils, for the epidemic death rate is undoubtedly increasing, in the villages especially which form 19/20ths of the whole population of India. The increase of epidemic deaths in 1884 over 1883 was nearly 600,000 and they were still increasing up to our last reports.

And as far as we yet know it would seem as if this year 1887 would bring us the highest epidemic death rate of all. We *now know that, if every town were put in the best sanitary state possible, the outside villages would go on supplying the epidemics.* We have lost in ten years 38 millions of our fellow subjects in India from epidemics, in addition to all other disease losses, owing to the government having no executive and apparently thinking that the terrible and practical information, with which the best of the sanitary commissioners have never ceased to supply us, is an end and not a mere means. Does not the protection of life and property from preventible epidemics rank next to protection of life and property from criminals, as a responsibility of government, if indeed it is not even higher in importance? For since the world began, criminals have apparently not destroyed more life and property than do epidemics *every year* in India. Yet we certainly should not think crimes to be merely a subject for statistics, without taking any executive action.

But while the sanitary evils have been increasing, the sanitary intelligence of the people has also been increasing, though at present its good influence is perhaps but little felt beyond the larger towns. But *where* the English district officer or sanitary commissioner or British Raj *has taken them into his confidence,* has brought them into consultation with him, they have begun, most salutary change! not only to cease helplessly to "submit to fate," because "the goddess of cholera" or of "smallpox" has done it, and even to cry aloud upon the "sirkar" or to the sanitary commissioner to "bestir themselves: Don't you see we are all dead?" Some have gone farther still, even Brahmins of high caste and, in places where notoriously nothing has been done by us, have put their own (sacred) hands to the plough and bestirred themselves to do their part in the matter of cleanliness and pure water.

The last five years have seen a notable change in the temper of some of the peoples of India, fruit of the education you have given them and perhaps of their ill temper too, and of their attention having been turned to local self-government. And if there is still resistance and great reluctance to tax themselves for their own health, it is not so very long since the same thing has been exhibited in England, not so long since sanitation, now so popular and "fashionable," was a bugbear to the people. And they would have nothing to do "with they fou' things," meaning drains and sewers. You who have done so much for the housing of the working classes must remember this.

But anyhow, whether we like self-government or not, we *must* carry the people with us in any sanitary action. Or whatever act we may pass will remain a dead letter. Engage the educated natives on your side, as has been so well done, especially where you have native associations. Money is not the only or even the chief thing wanted in the state of the villages. Enforcing the ordinary rules of cleanliness is the chief thing, "simple cleanliness is all we want."

The Central Provinces, outstripping Bombay, have already their Village Conservancy Act, providing for the removal of all sweepings and all night soil to appointed places outside, insisting on the conservation of water and on other good sanitary rules. Bombay, making friends of its native associations, is bringing out a Village Conservancy Bill and is prepared to give pecuniary aid towards a wholesome water supply and for providing manure yards outside villages. But daily scavenging and removal of street sweepings, etc., must also be enforced.

And this brings us, though our facts are so terrible as to appear almost hopeless, and things seem going from bad to worse, to the "talents"[?] of the hereditary scavengers. The more hopeful view: work, more than money, and though work means money, yet it is or if it is the money for a wholesome water supply it may be met partly or wholly from local funds, and does not need an enormous loan to be repaid by a heavy rate. It means the careful maintenance of village sanitation, and this most especially in the large towns where the most costly works have failed in usefulness from want of maintenance, not being kept in an efficient state. And it means a technical executive to overlook on the part of government and consolidation of present law as regards nuisances and offences in the villages. This is what it means, rather than a large outlay: a clean surface water supply, reform of wells. There is nothing the native understands better than the necessity of a pure water supply. Then when he sees that, through this, fever is diminishing, ask him for the rest. It means probably the appointment of an advising sanitary engineer (we know of only one).

If other arguments were wanting to show the urgency of the case, the truly vital urgency, for it is a matter of the life and death of millions of our fellow creatures under our own government, there is one with which the secretary of state for India is too familiar: are we not a byword to the nations for our management of India, where epidemics begin, or our no-management? They say: You, England, at once resist quarantine; one is glad to hear the recent Vienna decision against the utility of quarantine and you keep us in constant terror, under a perennial threat of disease and danger, by keeping India as a pest or a nest of epidemic pestilence, which justifies and more than justifies us and our Constantinople Board in putting on quarantine against your endemic cholera ports of India. Is not Europe against us, to put hindrances on our trade and commerce, because of the way we behave ourselves in India?

But more, far more than all these considerations is humanity compelling us, our responsibility as a government which holds, far more than any European government does, the lives and health and happiness of its subjects, our 200 millions of fellow subjects, in its hands, a fifth part of the human race.

A high epidemic death rate means feeble health to those who survive, lays up the whole population for weeks or months *every year* with the corresponding loss of productiveness and degeneration of the race, for its want of power to cultivate the land so as to give more than a bare sustenance. And so they go on *more* deteriorating. A Brahmin of high caste in a fertile district neighbouring the district of the capital of Bengal and the seat of government said to me: Well, you see me I have lost my whole family from fever; for two months in every year the whole population of my district is laid up with fever and incapacitated from doing anything. We know quite well what it arises from. It arises from (1) foul water supply; the tanks for drinking water are used for every purpose; (2) rank and rotting undergrowths remaining uncleared and stagnating the air, growths which in some cases might be articles of trade with England; (3) muddy bad roads. Well, you see me: you know that in my country we Brahmins are next to God (forgive this outburst of pride; it is often said that Hindus will say anything they think will please the ruling race. I do not find this. I like their incivility). We Brahmins must not lay our hands to manual work. Well, such was the need that I with my people set to work (and he then detailed what they had done with their own hands). And why, he said with the natural dignity of an Oriental, why does the government do nothing? If there were only a short act about tanks, *we* would see it carried out. Enlist the Brahmins and you enlist the people.

This is not a solitary instance. Many such could be given from other presidencies where the people are more advanced. Anglo-Indians rave against the resistance of the people (of Bengal especially), the danger of unpopularity if an executive were to put compulsion on them, at the same time acknowledging that little or nothing has been done by the government to bring the people into our counsels. Possibly the danger may soon be the other way, the danger of unpopularity *because* we do *nothing*.

Finance. Always of course the finance question, the revenue problem must come in: "India is such a poor country." An epidemic country is *always* a poor country. Nothing is so expensive as an epidemic country. If the health of the people could be improved, enabling them to work the land, in a country where 90 percent, or is it more? of the population are agricultural, if they were not a hotbed of fever and cholera (fever is always with them and besides following famine and cholera. If they are down with fever, how can they—they cannot—cultivate the land properly), would not the revenue be raised?

That sad instance has just occurred of a most valuable man, the man you most value, Sir M. Melville, losing his life from cholera directly from his own disbelief and neglect of sanitation. I had the whole sad story from his friend.

Source: From notes, Add Mss 45836 f211

7 May 1888

Sir R. Rawlinson says a million of lives lost in Crimean War. F.N. a million of lives lost every year from fever and epidemics in India.

Source: From a postscript to a letter to Thomas Gillham Hewlett, Reynolds Historical Library, University of Alabama at Birmingham 5080, copy Wellcome 9090/214

27 November 1888

Could you kindly tell me what chair of hygiene and sanitary science and practice there is at *Bombay*. I mean a professor (such as Dr Parkes was) with two laboratories under his control, one for chemical (water, food and air analysis), one for practical physiological instruction *and work*, including bacteriology? And are these laboratories more than little rooms? And could you tell me whether medical officers are instructed how to do the analysis of water supply *in the field*, I don't mean quantitative analysis, but enough to prevent troops being poisoned with bad water?

## "Letter on Sanitation," 1888

**Editor:** The publication of this letter on "sanitation in India" is thus prefaced by W.J. Simmons: "The Council are sure the following letter from Miss Nightingale will be read with the very greatest interest."

Source: Letter from Miss Nightingale to W.J. Simmons, Esq., Honorary Secretary, Public Health Society, 6 Hastings Street, Calcutta, in *Journal of the Public Health Society* 4,2 (October 1888):63-65

27 July 1888

Sir

Allow me to thank you most gratefully for your kindness in sending me from time to time the various papers and documents which interest me so deeply, and especially for your society's journal, and the suggestions of your committee on the then pending municipal bill, now carried.

It is remarkable how the memorandum of the Army Sanitary Commission in this country on the municipal reports for 1884 and 1885 confirms the conclusions which it is the object of your society to establish and make popular. It must be a matter of great satisfaction and encouragement to you and your good fellow workers in the cause of Indian sanitation to find that your views are so completely in accordance with those of a body so experienced and authoritative in the things of Indian sanitation as the Army Sanitary Committee.

Having thus received the highest official sanction in this country, they cannot fail, we trust, to influence the future policy of the government in respect of this most important subject. And you may, with reasonable confidence, we may hope, expect that neither indifference, prejudice, nor short-sighted economy, nor any other of the well-known obstacles to improvement, will be allowed in the future to stand in the way of reforms which you have shown to be so necessary, and which are advocated by the Army Sanitary Commission with no less urgency than by yourselves.

Of the vast additions to human happiness which these reforms are calculated to produce, of the deplorable amount of human suffering and sorrow which they would obviate, of the enormous money loss which such a mass of preventible disease and death entails on the community in which it is permitted, it is unnecessary now to speak.

Your reports have made these truths emphatic with results which are startling only to those who are too careless to study the subject. It appears to be demonstrated that sanitary improvements are fully as effective in diminishing disease in India as they are in England. The success which has attended the introduction of proper drainage and water supply into parts of Calcutta is itself a striking example. Where the sanitation has been complete, your mortality is as low as in the healthiest of English cities. Where it has been incomplete, where the water supply is inadequate or impure, where the drains have been allowed to be encumbered with deposit, or to remain untrapped, where dwellings are huddled together without reference to the requirements of the inhabitants in the way of air, water, purity of soil or prompt and effectual removal of filth, there I find that the mortality of Calcutta rises to a level which is happily now unknown in England, and that epidemics, against which we trust the English population is now effectually safeguarded, rage with as much violence as ever. We were much struck by the fact that, in the severe outburst which occurred in the last quarter of 1886, and which cost Calcutta more than 900 lives, the Park Street ward (with the exception of four deaths in October) enjoyed absolute immunity—a circumstance which seems to illustrate very forcibly the fact that, even when cholera is epidemic, systematic sanitation will prove, in India as it does [in] England, an effectual safeguard.

It now remains for those who like yourself appreciate at their true worth the blessings of health to the community, to see that the invaluable advantages which have been secured for the richer portions of Calcutta shall be enjoyed equally by the poorer and by the inhabitants of the suburbs whose mortality is now so greatly in excess of that of the city. Your health officer has clearly indicated the causes of the evil and the means by which it can be obviated.

Calcutta and its suburbs must not go on losing, as they did in 1886, 3500 lives annually (Calcutta: 1741; suburbs: 1845 = 3586) from an epidemic which your statistics show to be to so large an extent amenable to human control, and which in England, we have good reason to hope, has been effectually kept at bay by efficient sanitation. The same result it is doubtless within human competence in other parts of the world to attain by the means which science indicates. I feel the deepest sympathy with the inestimable labours of the Health Society to promote this result in India.

The Army Sanitary Commission reckon, I observe, that 38 millions of deaths have occurred in India within the last decade from epidemics which in other parts of the world have been either wholly obviated or curtailed within narrow limits.

But this is not the worst. If we reckon, as I believe is the correct estimate, twenty cases of severe disease for each death, the mind really sinks oppressed under the idea of the pecuniary loss, the laying aside of cultivators from their daily labour for weeks, if not months, every year, the deterioration in the physical powers of the races, the bodily sufferings, mental sorrow, family bereavement which such a death rate indicates. And all this, or the greater part, might be spared.

I can only wish you and your fellow workers Godspeed in what we must all regard as a most important and benevolent project. It must cost you I know much labour. Such things are not achieved without effort, patience, long delays and frequent disappointment. But you will succeed. And your success will brighten the lives and lessen the sufferings of millions who, but for sanitary reforms, would fall victims to preventible disease. I have written at length, but you will forgive me. The subject is near my heart. Pray believe me,

ever the faithful servant of the cause and yourselves

Florence Nightingale

# SUGGESTIONS ON A SYSTEM OF NURSING FOR HOSPITALS IN INDIA.

To the Secretary of the Sanitary Commission for Bengal.

Sir,

In reply to your letter of November 21, 1864, requesting me to send to you any suggestions which might occur to me regarding the organization of a system of Female Nursing in Indian Hospitals, I beg herewith to transmit a paper of suggestions which I hope may assist you in considering the subject.

In order to supply the requisite number of Nurses for the Hospitals of India, you must have schools for their instruction and training, either in England or in India, or in both. For these schools there must be competent teachers to instruct and train the untaught, and if such teachers cannot at present be found in India, they must be sent from England. Unless it is assumed that the development of excellence in all that relates to nursing will be as rapid and the teaching as good in India as in England, it would be necessary to provide for a continued supply of teachers, that is, of Matrons and Head Nurses, trained at home. No one, probably, who is acquainted with European life in India will doubt that such a continuous stream of fresh blood and advanced knowledge will be necessary to prevent progressive deterioration.

Then, if this be so, you will require a sort of normal school in England at which Matrons and Head Nurses may be thoroughly trained for service in India, not merely as Nurses but as teachers of nursing. A great part of the training must be conducted by the Head Nurses, even where there is a Training Matron. There does not appear to be any other practicable mode of adequately supplying what is required. Whether you train in India or not, the Government of India ought to make arrangements for the training, in England, of Matrons and Head Nurses for service in India, on such a footing as may reasonably be expected to supply annually the number required to keep up, to its full amount, the establishment of Matrons and Head Nurses, trained in Europe, which may be considered desirable.

The inducements which the Government of India would no doubt be prepared to hold out, would probably attract to their service a very competent and trustworthy class of persons, more especially if it were, as it probably ought to be, a "covenanted service"—a service in which employers and employed entered into a formal contract or covenant. In that case what the Government undertook to do would be fixed by regulations which the persons entering the service would engage to observe and the Government would be bound to act up to.

One of the advantages of making it a regular service would be that you might then, to a limited extent, hold out a prospect of promotion, not of course by seniority but by selection for superior merit and distinguished service, in which length of service would be considered. This need not exclude recruiting in India, especially for the ranks. It is probable that in some parts of India persons, either born in this country or of English or Anglo-Indian parentage, and of suitable character and education, might desire to enter such a service, and some of them might rise in it. Such persons might be very useful from their knowledge of the native languages and of local circumstances of which persons arriving from England would necessarily be ignorant.

One of the most obvious difficulties, in the way of carrying out any such systematic organization as is above suggested, would arise from the inducements to marry, which

11623. A

The first page of "Suggestions on a System of Nursing for Hospitals in India," as printed by Eyre and Spottiswoode 1865.

# Nursing in India

By 1864 Nightingale had become a recognized authority in matters of nursing and in the training of nurses. She had acquired much experience in the Crimean War (1854-56), written on nursing in military hospitals, written on hospitals (military and civil), opened a nurses' training school at St Thomas' Hospital, published *Notes on Nursing* (1860), which saw numerous editions, and had been a major force in two royal commissions that examined the state of hospitals and nursing. Her total work on nursing and nursing education will be related in volumes 12 and 13 of the present series.

Prior to 1864 the employment of female nurses in Indian hospitals had been timidly initiated by the vicereine, Lady Canning, and limited to some institutions in Calcutta and Allahabad. Service in military hospitals was mainly provided by untrained male coolies. With the setting up of the Bengal Sanitary Commission in 1864, immediately it appeared that something had to be done to improve the staffing of Indian hospitals. The commission, prompted by Sir John Lawrence, decided to seek advice from Nightingale. She had long been committed to providing care for the poor and was then getting workhouse infirmary nursing started. Nursing for the poor in India fitted in perfectly with these objectives.

Nursing in India then became a concrete issue in 1864 with Lawrence's request for guidance in the use of matrons and nurses in military hospitals and the training of nurses in India (see p 949 below). Nightingale was formally invited to submit her recommendations in a letter from the secretary of the Bengal Sanitary Commission, Dr James Pattison Walker. She obliged with "Suggestions on a System of Nursing for Hospitals in India." As was her custom she first consulted with experts such as Sir John McNeill and Mary Jones. The introductory part was actually written by McNeill, reflecting both his and Nightingale's views. The "Suggestions" were largely based on her experience and practice in England. They were sent to Walker and also soon thereafter to John Strachey.

However, upon receiving the paper, John Lawrence referred the matter to his medical advisors, who so vastly expanded the project that it became no longer recognizable. Nightingale had proposed starting in a limited number of places (first of all in Calcutta where, being the capital, the chances of success were greatest), but instead of the "small, well-considered beginning" (see p 974 below) she had recommended, officials in India opted for a wide and comprehensive scheme that was to be applied to seven hospitals at once. It would cost too much and be difficult to monitor. The Government of India indeed shuddered at the cost and in 1867 vetoed the whole proposal.[1] At that time, disappointed, Nightingale set out the whole sorry story for John Lawrence, ending with the sad point that what she had proposed, "in obedience to the government's desire," had "never been considered at all by the government on its own merits" (see p 970 below).

Furthermore, the employment of female nurses in military hospitals at that time appeared somewhat risky as no one could vouch for the good behaviour of convalescent soldiers. Nightingale wanted nurses in general or acute-care hospitals, not regimental or convalescent hospitals, where "discipline" could pose a problem. She was also concerned with the kind of woman the government seemed to be considering for staffing the hospitals. She felt strongly that only well-trained nurses should be appointed, the equivalent of "head nurses" in England. That the Indian government was considering women of lower qualifications was evident in the idea that "stopping" their beer might be used as a punishment! This would prevent "good and respectable women" from joining: "if you treat nurses like female convicts you will have female convicts for your nurses" (see pp 967-68 below).

With government in India having failed to establish nursing, Nightingale looked for other options and received requests from Indian nationals to take up the work. She hoped to train nurses and matrons for India (with the understanding that head nurses would be Europeans or at least Eurasians, Indian nationals then not having the status for those roles), with financing provided by the Nightingale Fund. She wrote to Robert S. Ellis in 1867: "There ought to be a continuous stream of trained nurses coming out of England to India. You cannot depend on recruiting *in* the country, though you must do all in your power to promote it" (see p 961 below). As for John Lawrence,

---

1 See Cook, *The Life of Florence Nightingale* 2:55 and 156-57.

always the heroic reformer for Nightingale, he failed to deliver on this matter. Female nursing in Indian military hospitals was instead "introduced on a limited scale shortly afterwards in the Madras presidency by its governor, Lord Napier,"[2] and Ettrick, whom Nightingale had known from the Crimean War. He visited her to be briefed on sanitary work before he left to take office.[3] It was only in 1887 that female nurses were generally accepted in military hospitals and the first nurses were sent to India; Indian women began working in military hospitals only during the First World War.[4] Further, later material on the subject appears in *Social Change in India.*

Letters constituting the background to "Suggestions" are given here first.

Source: From notes on Indian hospitals, ADD Mss 45751 ff147-48

[ca. 6 February 1860]

Dr Hunter *of Bombay*. I saw him, I liked him the best of all the Indian hospital men who have been sent me. . . . Dr Hunter was short, not sweet and to the point. He says he wants a trained matron for the Jamsetjee Hospital (one fourth women), which consists of 500 beds for general cases, about 250 lying-in and children, about 250 eye cases. He is the head of the college; he likes the Hindu students better than the Parsi. . . .

Dr Hunter proposes a married Englishwoman, the wife of a sergeant major who eloped with the daughter of his *colonel*, to be trained at St Thomas' as matron of the Jamsetjee. He says that Eurasian women and European women born in India, if trained at St Thomas', would do very well for a year and then fall into fine lady habits.

Source: From a letter probably to Parthenope Verney, Wellcome (Claydon copy) Ms 9000/9

20 February 1862

I would have answered Lady Cranworth's[5] kind letter yesterday. But it was quite impossible. I have heard of Lady Canning's Memorial Fund before. Some weeks ago, a lady wrote to me, desiring me to draw up a plan. But (and Lady Cranworth shares my feeling entirely) they give

---

2 Jharna Gourlay, *Florence Nightingale* 73.

3 Cook, *The Life of Florence Nightingale* 2:112.

4 See Jharna Gourlay, *Florence Nightingale* 66-74.

5 Laura Rolfe Cranworth (1807-68), member of the Harley St Hospital committee.

no definite statement, they have no definite idea of how the thing is to be done. They have not considered what is meant by "training nurses" nor the funds required.

I enclose all the papers relating to St Thomas' for Lady Cranworth, and the only one printed relating to King's College, less as an illustration (which is little use in India) than because she has been so kindly interested about the subject. The whole of the income of the Fund (called by my name) is now appropriated to these two objects. It is something above £1400 a year. The accounts of St Thomas' (one year, also enclosed) will show the number of nurses who can have a *thorough* training even in so large a hospital on so large a sum.

But this is not the main thing. There are no means of training nurses at Calcutta. There is, it is true, a large and bad general hospital. But who the matron is we do not know. It seems to me that the first thing is to ascertain what are the capabilities for training at Calcutta and to show them to be satisfactory. They will probably have to get a matron from England, or what would be much better to send one home from Calcutta, chosen there, to be trained in England. Then they should make some *kind of* guess at what kind of sum they want and what they are likely to raise. Also what kind of subjects for training they are likely to find. (The poor flighty woman who wrote to me had not an idea on any one of these subjects and actually wanted to take soldiers' wives for training.)

How difficult it has been to find good subjects, even with all England to choose out of—Lady Canning's "Home" is a useful comprehensible scheme. But in its present state the training establishment proposed cannot be said to be comprehensible. And I cannot see how any good would come of it with any number of names. First get a good workable scheme, then an estimate of the cost and *probable* income. People will be sure to support it. At present there is nothing to support.

You may depend upon it that Lady Cranworth thinks all this herself and that she is the person who will carry it through to a useful well-digested scheme, if it can be carried through.

I shall be most glad to give any little help in my power (for the sake of so good an object) when it has assumed the form of an object. But Lady Cranworth knows how little that power is. And she kindly says that I should not be expected to collect subscriptions or anything of that kind.

Source: From a letter to Mary Jones, Florence Nightingale Museum (LMA) H1/ST/NC1/65/3

24 January 1865

*Confidential*

My dearest friend

For some time I have been expecting, rather than hoping, that Sir J. Lawrence would lay upon me the formation of a nursing staff for the East. And I am afraid the same fear will possess you (when you see my letter) that does me.

His letter is most liberal: he says that "whatever expense" is required must be met for such an object. The idea is to nurse the military *general* hospitals by European trained women, and *all* the female regimental hospitals which, as you know, means the soldiers' wives and children (many of the cases being lying-in cases) by European trained women. This for a beginning. But of course they must establish one or more training schools in each presidency, for how can we supply them with so many nurses, who cannot supply ourselves?

Here comes the difficulty. The material to be trained is almost *nil.* Every decent woman they get marries directly. There are nothing but soldiers' wives and widows, and they candidly say that, besides the losing them directly, they are a wretched set, worse than their husbands. A religious society would be the only thing. And I am sure I would help them to a religious society, if I could. But there is but one person to do it, and that is you. And I am quite sure the danger in India would be far greater than it is in England of what we have seen nevertheless too often here, viz., the absurdities religious (nursing?) orders have fallen into: if not really losing their hands to the work in hospitals and under a good discipline. (I have been quite afraid of writing to you upon Sir John Lawrence's letter, because I thought you would either volunteer yourself or volunteer Sister Laura.[6] Now I do think that, unless a higher voice directs you, it is far more important to keep the kernel together at home and send out branches to India.)

I enclose you a printed paper, which has been sent to me from India for my guidance. But, at the same time, the private information which accompanies it, almost negatives it:

1. They laugh at Dr Beatson's [principal medical officer of the British troops in India] admiration of the nurses at Allahabad, who,

6 Laura Girdlestone (1831-?), widow of Major Girdlestone, went to India much later as a trained sister.

they say, were soldiers' wives, picked up anywhere, and that Dr Beatson liked them, because he was their matron and superintendent. (All our medical officers in the Crimea, of whom he was one, always wanted to be matrons themselves. What an odd taste!) Of course where there are *two* nurses, one must be matron.

2. The Medical College Hospital at Calcutta is such an abominable place that they are now urging us to say (which we shall do) that it must be pulled down and reconstructed elsewhere.

3. The General Hospital at Calcutta is half military, half civil, half under the military authorities, half under the lieutenant governor of Bengal. This occasions many difficulties if it were to be used as a real training school for nurses.

4. The ladies of the committee, of whom Mrs Williams[7] is the head (who, in fact, wrote the paper I enclose), though very useful and zealous, are not really qualified by knowledge to govern a training school or to judge of nurses.

It seems that they have no such thing as a matron who would really take charge of a real training school. Such a person, if we sent one out, must be quite above the possibility of marrying, such as Mrs Girdlestone or Mrs Shaw Stewart.[8] (You see even Mrs Polehampton, who offered herself both to you and to me, was not.)

Now, what is to be done? I shall send out to Sir John Lawrence all our experience as to training schools, military hospital nursing, etc. But what is the good of that? The thing would be to be able to tell him: we have 1, 2, 3, etc., who would do to send out as matrons, whose health would stand the climate, or we shall have within -- months. And we have 4, 5, 6, etc., who would do to send out as nurses for military hospitals, and 7, 8, 9, etc., for female regimental hospitals, whose health would stand the climate, or we shall have within -- months.

I am quite sure India deserves from us all she can get from us. And if you could train persons for India here, you would be doing a greater deed than by going out yourself, which would be abandoning the root. (How I wish I could go! Do you know I have received a most pressing invitation to go out, invalid as I am, everything to be provided for me as for an invalid? But it is nonsense to wish! It would be quite madness!) The difficulty of finding working persons is to me

7 Rachel Williams, later Norris (1840-1908), trained at St Thomas' Hospital.

8 Jane Elizabeth Shaw Stewart (d. 1905), nursed in the Crimea, superintendent general at Netley Hospital.

inconceivable. It seems to me to increase in the proportion that the outcry for women's "fields" increases. Manchester writes to me for a superintendent. And I answer: a place like Manchester must find one for themselves and send her up to us to train.

I know Mrs Shaw Stewart can't help us, though she ought to be the training school for all military British hospitals, at home and abroad. But she will have the utmost difficulty in taking on Woolwich, which is nearly ready.

Sir John Lawrence's application could not have come at a worse time for Mrs Wardroper.[9] For, as you know, we have been drained by Liverpool. And not only Manchester but several other places have engaged every vacancy we have.

And what are fifteen among so many?[10] It really goes to my heart to write you such a letter, if, as I am afraid, the beginning of the year is with you, as it is with us, a particularly busy time. But I think you would be as sorry as I should be, if such an opening as Sir John Lawrence affords the cause, should be allowed to fall through. God bless you.

ever yours

F.N.

I have been writing this before the morning light, not really having time in the course of the day.

Source: From a letter to Mary Jones, Florence Nightingale Museum (LMA) H1/ST/NC1/65/4

6 February 1865

*Private.* I venture to send you the first rough draft of a paper I am obliged to draw up for Sir John Lawrence. Please do remember that in India they print everything, that if I did not print for them what I don't mind being printed they would print for me what I should not like to be printed. But I have said, I shall say, in private letters to Sir John Lawrence, a great deal about this nursing matter I cannot put in a printed paper.

If you don't like the tone of this printed paper, no more do I—probably less than you do. But what I want to add to it principally (though many other things will have to be added, of course) is some account of your system, your society, your sisterhood. . . .

9 Sarah Elizabeth Wardroper (c1813-92), matron and superintendent of the Nightingale school at St Thomas' Hospital.

10 A paraphrase of John 6:9.

And this is what I principally write about now. But I will ask you to criticize everything.

I have never thanked you for your most encouraging letter. I fully expect that Sir John Lawrence will call upon us for more than we can do for him and for all we can do. There is plenty of room to spare in India for every kind of nursing effort. Would we were as ready for him as he is for us.

Source: From a letter to Sir John McNeill, Florence Nightingale Museum (LMA) H1/ST/NC3/SU156, typed copy Add Mss 45768 ff190-92

7 February 1865

I always fly to you when in difficulty. I have had the most enormous order from Sir John Lawrence for matrons and nurses for India, of which a trifling item is: sixty-six head nurses, 112 assistants for female regimental hospitals. These are already "sanctioned." [He] wishes, besides, to nurse all military general hospitals, of which ten are named, and to establish training schools in all civil hospitals. He does not, like a wise man as he is, positively engage for or desire any particular specified thing. But he asks for advice on the largest scale and "the Governor-General-in-Council" states that "whatever expense is requisite must be met."

(There is a private and most pressing invitation to me myself to go out. If the doctors would give me six months there, I would go. There is nothing in the whole world I should like better.) Of course I lost no time in consulting our training schools as to what we could do. Of this more hereafter.

But they in India ask for a printed paper. And I venture to submit to you the first rough draft of one, knowing that you, if you have time to glance at it, will help me more than anyone. Of course conclusions and some other things must be added to the paper. All the rest I think had better be written privately to Sir John Lawrence, not the "Governor-General-in-Council." . . .

The more chattering and noise there is about "Woman's Mission," the less of efficient women we can find. It makes me mad to hear people talk about unemployed women. If they are unemployed, it is because they won't work. The highest salaries given to women at all, we can secure to women trained by us. But we can't find the women. They won't come. Both our training schools are most anxious to help. The superintendent of King's College Hospital would take another hospital to train women for us, but she cannot admit more in King's College.

If we send women out to India, we should of course engage them expressly for this purpose.

Source: From a letter to Henry Bonham Carter,[11] ADD MSS 47714 ff88-93

10 February 1865

*Private.* I have an order from Sir John Lawrence, of which a trifling item is: sixty-six head midwifery nurses, 112 assistant midwifery nurses (these are already "sanctioned"); nurses for ten military general hospitals; training matrons and head nurses for civil presidency hospitals to form training schools for nurses. . . .

Of course it is vain for us to think of sending out nurses by the hundred. What I wish we *could* think of is to send out trained training matrons, wherever we are asked. . . .

The only matron they ever had in India was paid £360 a year (and everything "found," as the servants say). The highest salaries women receive at all (queens and actresses excepted) might be secured by women trained by us. . . .

Supposing we train for India—if the committee agree. (I do not exactly know on what terms to expense.) Of course if we train for India, we must advertise and engage women expressly for that purpose, as health and other circumstances must be taken into account. Terms must also be offered, and this I cannot do, without a reply from Sir John Lawrence.

A great difficulty will be that women will accept our terms, on purpose to be sent out to India on very advantageous conditions for marrying well. . . .

I send you the first rough draft of a sketch for Sir John Lawrence. Please NOT to show it to Mrs Wardroper, but to return it to me, if with any suggestions of your own, I shall be much obliged. It is to accompany some "Conclusions" and a private letter to Sir John Lawrence from me.

Source: Notes on nursing in India for John Sutherland, ADD MSS 45752 ff4-5

[January-February 1865]

1. Where were the Allahabad women nurses got? soldiers' wives, Eurasians, widows, women of English parents born in India? . . . Widows, yes; I hate wives.

11 Henry Bonham Carter (1827-1921), secretary of the Nightingale Fund 1861-1914.

How the linen can be taken care of in India and what sort of accommodation required for it? Subsidiary orderly service, in carrying and piling of linen, etc., to be done by orderlies or native servants?

Where the nursing material is to come from? what it is? Matron must be not only a linen keeper but a trainer of nurses. Who trains?

2. The superintendent general must be herself a trained nurse. Ask particulars about system of government possible.

3. Wherever there are two nurses, there must be a matron; she must be supreme and have power over discipline, just as Beatson claimed for himself; same matron might do for female hospital. At regimental female hospitals, one should be matron again. All nurses at any given station under one matron. Position of native nurses and midwives with regard to English nurses? Pay of matrons *must* be liberal; she must have the power to select and take on probationers.

4. Who must be the court of appeal over the matron? as the secretary of state for war is here. What commanding officer? to whom must she be responsible?

5. Should there not be a superintendent general for each presidency? Can single ladies travel in the way she would be required to travel?

6. How far would English method of governors for general hospitals do in India? what relation should the governor have to nurses and superintendents?

## "Suggestions on a System of Nursing for Hospitals in India," 1865

**Editor:** The "Suggestions" were sent in the form of a letter to Dr James Pattison Walker on 24 February 1865. They constitute no less than a short treatise on a "system of nursing" for India. The Army Medical Department spoke approvingly of Nightingale's paper; its report for 1867[12] fully endorsed its contents.

Since the regulations given as an appendix in the paper were lifted from those of St Thomas', they are omitted here (they appear in the first volume on nursing). Letters to colleagues Walker and Strachey accompanying the final paper are given immediately below, then the paper itself and finally the letters relating the unhappy aftermath.

12 *British Parliamentary Papers* 1868-69, vol. 37:391-93.

Source: From a draft letter to James Pattison Walker, Add Mss 45781 ff272-73

10 March 1865

I have the honour to acknowledge the receipt of your letter of 21 November 1864, in which you request me to send any suggestions that might occur to me regarding the organization of a system of female nursing for Indian hospitals. I have much pleasure in complying with your request and beg to enclose a few copies of a paper, which I have drawn up on the subject. I have thought it better to have it printed for greater facility of reference.

In preparing this paper, I have laboured under the disadvantage of personal unacquaintance with many facts and circumstances essential for me to know in order to give you that precise advice and information which I should otherwise have considered desirable.

It has been my endeavour, as far as possible, to attempt to realize the conditions under which you have to introduce this great improvement. And having done the best I could I must leave the case in your hands and in the hands of the Government of India, in the hope that the experience I have described may enable you to draw up an independent scheme suitable to the country. When you have done this I would like it as a favour if you would send it to me, in order that I might have the opportunity of going very carefully over it in the hope that in this way we might among us be able to do the best possible in assisting the Indian government in carrying out this great and benevolent scheme.

Source: From a letter to John Strachey, Columbia University, Presbyterian Hospital School of Nursing C83

26 April 1865

*Private.* With regard to your kind question about the nursing, I thought it best, on the whole, to send out, as Dr Walker will tell you, such a (private) paper as I could write on the information I had. It may possibly enable you, which would be much the best course, to draw up a scheme suitable for *your* circumstances. And I need hardly say that, should you then think well to send it to me, I will carefully go over it, with all the experience in details of nurse training which I may have, and give you all the light I can.

Source: Florence Nightingale, "Suggestions on a System of Nursing for Hospitals in India," a letter to the secretary of the Sanitary Commission for Bengal (London: Eyre and Spottiswoode)

Sir 24 February 1865

In reply to your letter of 21 November 1864 requesting me to send to you any suggestions which might occur to me regarding the organization of a system of female nursing in Indian hospitals, I beg herewith to transmit a paper of suggestions which I hope may assist you in considering the subject.

In order to supply the requisite number of nurses for the hospitals of India you must have schools for their instruction and training, either in England or in India, or in both. For these schools there must be competent teachers to instruct and train the untaught, and if such teachers cannot at present be found in India, they must be sent from England. Unless it is assumed that the development of excellence in all that relates to nursing will be as rapid and the teaching as good in India as in England, it would be necessary to provide for a continued supply of teachers, that is, of matrons and head nurses, trained at home. No one, probably, who is acquainted with European life in India, will doubt that such a continuous stream of fresh blood and advanced knowledge will be necessary to prevent progressive deterioration.

Then, if this be so, you will require a sort of normal school in England at which matrons and head nurses may be thoroughly trained for service in India, not merely as nurses but as teachers of nursing. A great part of the training must be conducted by the head nurses, even where there is a training matron. There does not appear to be any other practicable mode of adequately supplying what is required. Whether you train in India or not, the Government of India ought to make arrangements for the training, in England, of matrons and head nurses for service in India, on such a footing as may reasonably be expected to supply annually the number required to keep up, to its full amount, the establishment of matrons and head nurses, trained in Europe, which may be considered desirable.

The inducements, which the Government of India would no doubt be prepared to hold out, would probably attract to their service a very competent and trustworthy class of persons, more especially if it were, as it probably ought to be, a "covenanted service," a service in which employers and employed entered into a formal contract or covenant. In that case what the government undertook to do would be fixed by regulations, which the persons entering the service would engage to observe and the government would be bound to act up to.

One of the advantages of making it a regular service would be that you might then, to a limited extent, hold out a prospect of promotion, not of course by seniority but by selection for superior merit and distinguished service, in which length of service would be considered. This need not exclude recruiting in India, especially for the ranks. It is probable that in some parts of India persons, either born in this country or of English or Anglo-Indian parentage, and of suitable character and education, might desire to enter such a service, and some of them might rise in it. Such persons might be very useful from their knowledge of the native languages and of local circumstances, of which persons arriving from England would necessarily be ignorant.

One of the most obvious difficulties in the way of carrying out any such systematic organization, as is above suggested, would arise from the inducements to marry, which would beset nurses of all grades in India, and the consequent danger that the government might thus lose the services of persons who had been trained and conveyed thither at great cost. A certain term of service in India might be made a condition of employment, but if this condition were violated by marriage, dismissal from the service would be no punishment and would not even involve any sacrifice which the nurse had not predetermined to make. A breach of the contract might no doubt involve certain penalties, which might be enforced by legal proceedings, but there would probably be a disinclination to prosecute or, in case of prosecution, to convict or to give adequate damages.

Perhaps the best course might be to annex a specified pecuniary penalty to breach of the contract, by marriage or otherwise, the amount to diminish with each year of service actually performed in India. This might go far to reimburse the government for the loss of service and might incline both the nurse and her suitor to postpone their nuptials until the stipulated term of service should have been completed, for I presume that the husband, on his marriage, would become liable for the amount of the penalty, being a debt due by his wife.

If the attempt to supply the hospitals of India with female nurses is not to be a failure, it is plain that it must be made on some organized plan, which, being based on a stable foundation, may be expected to give permanence and efficiency to the system. Were it as easy to find competent matrons and head nurses as it is to find female mill workers, it may be questioned whether it would be advisable to send out a shipload of them at once, to be scattered over the country from Cape Comorin to Peshawar. To place the majority thus beyond the control and guidance of the heads of their own very special department would be not only to exclude all hope of efficient and uniform organization, but almost to ensure the failure of the majority of them and, with it, a discreditable breakdown of the whole system. But this is a danger that cannot be incurred, for the nurses do not exist, and years must elapse before a sufficient number can be "made" to supply the hospitals of India. There is therefore ample time and opportunity to devise a suitable scheme and to pursue it in a tentative manner, correcting and adjusting it as the experiments are being worked out.

At how many stations in India it would be desirable to institute such tentative trials of nursing would depend not only on the local circumstances, but also on the number of competent and suitable persons who could be selected in this country to carry out the scheme. It would be better to begin with one well-selected establishment, sufficient only for one hospital, than to attempt more than one with more doubtful materials. Much—no one can foresee how much—will depend upon the success of the first attempt. The value of the whole will, in public estimation, be determined by the quality of the first sample that is exhibited.

Then the question arises if there is, at starting, to be only one hospital nursed, which hospital ought it to be? There can be no doubt that it ought to be where it will be under the fostering care of the governor general. Success at Calcutta would probably carry with it public opinion all over India and would therefore be of greater value than success anywhere else. But assuming that the government is satisfied that female nursing ought to be provided for the hospitals of India, and considering that the government must be the ultimate judges of success or failure, there is no necessity or good reason why *éclat* should be desired; and, on the other hand, in carrying out such an experiment it is but just and right, seeing how many difficulties must in any circumstances be encountered, that it should be tried in the circumstances most favourable to success. If it succeeds, the experience acquired there will enable you to extend it, under less favourable circumstances, with a better prospect of success. In beginning new things we commence with the easier and, having mastered these, proceed to the more difficult. But this is a question the ultimate decision of which must rest with the governor general.

On a consideration of the whole circumstances, then, it appears that there are two things which may be set about immediately. First—to put in operation means of training matrons and head nurses for service in the general hospitals and the civil and female hospitals of India, to be employed on such terms and under such conditions as the Government of India may be disposed or induced to offer. Second—to find a matron fitted to be the leading pioneer in such a field, and to provide her with a well-selected staff of head nurses and nurses capable of showing what nursing really is, to be employed in such hospital as the governor general may determine after due consideration. Whatever aid I can give in obtaining suitable matrons and nurses shall gladly be given.

The exclusion of all interference with the department of nurses, so far as relates to discipline, as hereinafter stated, is obviously indispensable.

The regulations given in the appendix may, with trifling modifications, be adopted for India.

If suitable persons can be found, matrons and nurses for more than one hospital might be sent out, and the governor general would determine to what hospitals the different matrons, with their respective establishments, should be sent.

If several matrons, with nursing establishments, are sent out, then a general superintendent of nurses should go out at the same time, so that she may hold the reins from the moment of starting. Looking to the extent and population of the Bengal presidency (including therein the Upper Provinces and the Punjab) and to the presence of the governor general, it might be expedient that the three or four matrons and establishments first formed should be employed there under a general superintendent for that presidency. Madras and Bombay could wait for a time.

In case you may consider it advisable to train nurses in India, I have, in the following suggestions, given such an account of our method of training in England as might enable you to organize a system of training in India.

## SUGGESTIONS

1. The evidence obtained by the Royal Commission on the Sanitary State of the Indian Army and the information contained in the minute No. 151 of the Sanitary Commission for Bengal show that the systematic introduction of female nursing into civil, military general and regimental female hospitals would be of great service for the sick in India.

2. The evidence shows that the class of women hitherto employed in this work has been of a comparatively humble character and without due training, while the nursing has been at the same time highly appreciated by the sick.

3. The desirableness of introducing an organized system of nursing is certainly undoubted, and it cannot but excite great satisfaction that the Governor-General-in-Council has decided that this improvement shall take place.

4. At the beginning of so important a measure, it is to be feared that nothing but difficulties have to be encountered. But there is no reason why these should not be eventually overcome. It is necessary to state this at the commencement, lest any apparent want of success at first should lead to discontinuance of effort.

5. So far as can be seen the difficulties in India will be of the same kind as, but greater in degree than, those we have had to encounter at home.

We have had to introduce an entirely new system, to which the older systems of nursing bear but slight resemblance. Our constant feeling has been that the need is universal and that our means are limited, mainly because the study and practice of nursing as a profession, second only in importance to medicine itself, dates only a few years back in England. It exists neither in Scotland nor in Ireland at the present time. And we, out of our limited means, have to supply a trained nurse or matron here and there, in the hope that each may become a centre of improvement, however small, until the growing conviction of the importance of the vast field of usefulness which we have opened for women shall supply us with agents sufficient in number and of such character as will enable us to meet the all but overwhelming demands for help which we receive from all quarters.

6. It will be seen that our means of assisting India directly are at present very limited, and yet we are most anxious to send some seed. Good nursing does not grow of itself; it is the result of study, teaching, training, practice, ending in sound tradition which can be transferred elsewhere.

7. The great difficulty to begin with is obtaining suitable material for training. Even in England, where there is such a constant outcry of want of women's work, comparatively few apply even as candidates for instruction, although we pay all the costs of training, including payments in the name of wages to probationers.

Of those admitted for training, a proportion are found on trial to be unfit. But all our nurses to whom we grant certificates are taken up at once by different institutions. (We have just sent twelve and a matron to Liverpool, and are besides training nineteen for Manchester.) And every woman at all competent is at once appointed matron to a hospital.

It is necessary that at the very beginning the difficulties which have to be met in organizing a system of nursing for India should be known. It is taken for granted that the difficulties in India, to say the very least of it, will not be fewer than ours at home.

8. Supposing, for the sake of argument, that you have the means of training, viz., a capable matron, medical officers willing to help and suitable material, probably you could not do better than frame your procedure upon a model which has hitherto been found to answer very well, viz., the rules for admission and training nurses at St Thomas' and King's College Hospitals, London, under the "Nightingale Fund." The probationer nurses at St Thomas' are trained in general nursing duties, those at King's College Hospital specially in midwifery and midwifery nursing. (The nursing of King's College Hospital is carried on by the Society of St John's House, which is a Protestant religious house, a sisterhood having for its main object the care and nursing of the sick in hospitals, among the poor in their own dwellings and in private families of the higher classes, besides the training and education of nurses for this work. The sisters are gentlewomen, trained—for two years or more—in all that relates to the nursing of the sick, the routine management of hospitals, wards, etc. Some of these sisters have charge of wards in hospital, and the training and instruction of probationers, the oversight and direction of nurses, etc., both in wards and when off duty. Each sister has *definite* duty, either in wards or teaching probationers otherwise, attending the sick poor, or control of housekeeping matters, and oversight of domestic servants—the system being to guide and encourage those engaged in the paid labour of the society by the aid of others—the sisters—who are unpaid, more intelligent, educated, with a view to raising the whole tone and character of the nursing attendants of the sick.

Each probationer passes one year in special training for her future duties, by instruction in the manual work of a nurse, attending classes for various instruction by sisters, lectures given by the medical men on physiology, etc., before ranking as nurse, being then drafted off for either hospital work, nursing in private families or among the poor, but continuing in the service of St John's House.)

Source: Notes on a meeting with Mary Carpenter for Dr Sutherland, Add Mss 45752 ff177-78

[7 June 1867]

Well—Miss Carpenter came here yesterday on very serious business. She began by telling me what everyone knows best which seemed to have struck her as something new, the awful state of the India native women. I won't dwell upon this. She has got some enlightened Parsis [Furdoonji,[13] etc.] who have followed her to London. She enlarged upon the horrible Parsi observances, the women defiling themselves with the priests as an act of worship. At Bombay, at Calcutta, the Bengali women mewed up in dark, close out of the way cells, while the men enjoyed the drawing rooms (but that's the way of men all over the world—Editor's [F.N.] Note).

Now for the business she came to me about: she says the hospitals are in the most awful condition. She gave me the most curious account of the Memorial Nursing School founded in memory of Lady Canning. It is *entirely broken up. The Englishwomen all drank.*

But in the Medical College Hospital at Calcutta, where it was founded, the Eurasian women who before would not lay their hands to anything, when they saw the Englishwomen doing it, began to do it too. And the Eurasian matron and Eurasian nurses make a very tidy staff now at Calcutta Medical College Hospital. She says the material *is* there, if it were trained, that there are many Eurasians, many natives and even many Englishwomen out there who could be trained, Englishwomen who don't marry because they are too poor to marry educated men and too well educated to marry soldiers.

She describes the state of the nursing in Bombay and Madras hospitals as something inconceivable both by the native men and native women, worse than anything you can possibly describe. She says, if I wait for the action of government I shall wait forever. She wants to put me into communication with diverse people at Madras and Bombay and she says, if *I* don't do it, she shall ask Miss Edwards of Bristol.

She says, Lord Napier would do anything and she would advise me to write to him, as I know him. She also says, there is a Dr Hunter, of the eye and general hospitals at Bombay, who is now in London (he came over with her) who would do anything. Also she says there is a Parsi of Bombay, now in London for a month, whom she would like to put me in communication with.

13 Naoroji Furdoonji (1817-85), social reformer.

This is on another subject. Miss Carpenter says she finds Sir S. Northcote [secretary of state for India] very amenable indeed both on the subject of her model training schools and of jails. He actually wrote to her to come up and see him.[14]

Source: From a draft letter to John Lawrence in Dr Sutherland's hand, ADD Mss 45777 f97

10 June 1867

I do not wish to hurry you, and the reason of my writing at present is to say that events nowadays appear to move so rapidly that established forms of procedure do not keep pace with them and I fear that, unless we put the whole matter in train, it will practically be taken out of our hands. I have just had such accounts of the nursing or rather nursing pretence of your Indian hospitals as have shocked me greatly. I had no idea that things were in such a state. But they are described to me as they have been seen by intelligent and discerning eyes. . . .

The short and the long of it is that I have had a formal request made to me to place myself at the head of a nursing movement for India on the plea that it is no use to wait for the action of government and with a threat that if I don't act other parties will be found who will. It appears that not only Europeans but native Indians would take the work up. Of course all I could do would be to offer them the same assistance that I have offered to you. That is, they to find the money and administer the funds and I to help in providing trained matrons and head nurses to train natives in India.

I have stated that at present I am in communication with you on the subject and I am now very desirous that the work should be started as soon as possible, because it will take some time after I get your decision to prepare and send out the persons who are to take charge of the training.

14 Carpenter wrote to Nightingale 30 July 1867 to express her intention of establishing female normal schools in India (ADD Mss 45789 ff110-11).

Source: From a letter to William Rathbone,[15] Liverpool Record Office, Rathbone Collection 610 RAT 1/8

22 June 1867

*Private.* I sincerely hope and trust that, even beyond the sphere of our Christian religion, your example will spread and take root. Lately I have had from Parsi merchants in Bombay a desire expressed that I should found a training school for nurses there. As the government has been in correspondence with me for founding such training schools in India, I must, of course, be careful that such efforts should work into one another, not clash with each other, also not to speak of them prematurely.

Source: Notes on a meeting with Dr Porteous for John Sutherland, ADD MSS 45752 ff204-08

31 July 1867

Porteous [deputy inspector general, Madras?]: Well, he came evidently intent on proving to me that no matron was wanted, that the doctor ought to be matron and that wretched coolie women under the doctor were the best nurses. But, luckily for me, he was drunk. And before he went (he was here 2½ hours) he had admitted everything.

The general hospital is half military (3rd Battalion) and half civil. The military (sixty patients) have the same amount of room as the civil (290 patients). The civil have 250 beds male, forty female. The female is so bad that Porteous recommends the government incessantly to pull it down. He says, *nothing* else will do. (By the way, he says that no respectable woman goes into hospital. They are all prostitutes.)

He says that these (which is made such a fuss about) "hospital nurses" are only for the small infirmary (ten beds, all scabies and sore eyes) of the asylum itself, that the "passed hospital nurses" know nothing whatever and are *never* "passed" into any other hospital and are no use. They only have a few lectures from the doctor. And this (he said) after having said that there was no need to send out any trained nurses to Madras, that their nurses were perfect. However, he came to. And he said that in that general hospital our training school must begin, that it was no use connecting it with that. Well, he said, first of all, that they had nurses and to spare at Madras, then that we

15 William Rathbone (1819-1902), Unitarian, Liberal MP, trustee, then chair of the Nightingale Fund. See the biographical sketch in *Public Health Care* (6:677).

could get *no* material at all to train at Madras, then that we might get a few Eurasians and natives to train.

He gave a most deplorable account of the prospect of European life. He said, why you can't get your drummer boys out of soldiers' children and you won't get your nurses out of soldiers' girls. You are obliged to have your lady's maids out from Europe. And they won't stay with you. They get sick and either have to be sent back or marry. He said he was afraid our nurses would not be able to keep their health there. He is strongly of opinion (I don't agree) only to send out a matron, that she should be supreme in the hospital, that she should train Eurasians and natives (I think she *must,* but which was the one built by Sir C. Trevelyan, which he says is capital and have two head nurses *at least* to support her). He says we must ask *not* less than £20 to £25 a month *and a house,* that no woman could keep her health for less and that her position ought to be *supreme.* He says the Eurasians and natives are most untrustworthy, that they never can command the respect of the soldier patients who always rebel against them and call them "blackie." He says he doesn't believe we can find more pupils (and *no* European pupils) than will do for Madras alone in Madras, nor for Bangalore alone in Bangalore. He says it's no use looking for supply to soldiers' widows or daughters.

Monthly salary of teachers of college, of medical college and high school? government teachers? normal school? . . .

Eurasians at the lying-in hospital. He repeated over and over again. We are so proud of this: 200 beds—no puerperal fever. All Eurasian patients (half-caste). Midwives here trained but no permanent midwife. The matron, of whom he spoke enthusiastically, only housekeeper. The pupils deliver *all* the ordinary cases without a midwife and without a doctor. (No native patients, all Eurasians.) The doctor comes in for the extraordinary cases and the doctor gives lectures. I said, and they are by to see the extraordinary cases delivered. Here he got so drunk that he spent at least half an hour in explaining to me that there was nothing to be "seen," that everything was under the bedclothes. But, he says, these midwives (who are paid by government) are employed exclusively among the rich.

He gives the most deplorable account of the medical subordinates. He says the money we have spent too in sending natives to be educated as doctors here is lost, that they pass their examinations splendidly, but that they don't live like gentlemen afterwards, are not respected and sink into contempt.

He says that all these "dispensaries" have twenty-forty beds, chiefly alas! prostitutes, that they are waited upon by native women who know *nothing*, that they ought to be abolished.

The native infirmary is large and he would like to unite the female part of the general hospital with it. They have eighty leper beds, always full. He says the lying-in patients always have their food brought in to them at the hospital by their friends. The hospital neither feeds nor cooks for them. All the women, except the Europeans, are naked in bed. He says it answers very well. (I can't understand it.)

He says the hospital patients *never* stay in bed. They pull off the bedclothes (the moment the doctor is gone) and lie about the floor, the same in the asylums.

He says that Lord and Lady Napier have devoted themselves entirely to the hospitals, and would do anything. He gave me a most interesting account of Lord Napier's famine tour. Lord Napier used to work sixteen hours a day and would actually go to see the sick put up (on the tour) after the day's work.

Source: From two letters to Henry Bonham Carter, ADD Mss 47715 ff22 and 39

12 August 1867

I think we might quite well begin to try to catch someone for the India service. Bombay is certain to employ us. Until or unless the India Office founds a school, if it does, under us, I think we ought to train the first nurses and matrons at the expense of the Nightingale Fund, because India contributed so largely to it, as it always has done to every such kind of charitable fund.

20 August 1867

I have just had Sir S. Northcote here about the Public Health Service business and am rather done. But I took the opportunity of saying to him how all this nurse school affair for India hung fire and showed him the correspondence with the Governor-General-in-Council. Also I have heard from the Parsi [Naoroji Furdoonji] again and it is evident to me that he does not think the Parsis at Bombay can raise the money without government money.

I question whether he (Furdoonji) will have time to call upon you. Would you think it well to write me a letter for him saying exactly what our fund can and cannot do?

Source: From a copy of a letter (mostly in Nightingale's hand) to Robert S. Ellis [president of the Madras Sanitary Commission], Add Mss 45782 ff93-99

August 1867

I have thought over your proposition about the nurses and lady superintendent in every possible way. I have had a long interview with Mr Porteous, at Lady Napier's desire, in order to collect local particulars. And, as you are aware, the nursing subject, even as regards India, is not new to me, for I was applied to officially more than two years ago from the Governor-General-in-Council about sending out or training nurses for India, since which time there has been much written and little done.

I fully hope that we shall be able to answer your call [for sending out matrons and nurses], not at once, not without frequent references backwards and forwards, of course, but still that we shall be able to do what you wish ultimately. But I must ask you to let me explain a little of the nature of the case and our difficulties in order that you may not think our scruples and our conditions extravagant.

When in December 1864 the Government of India first consulted me on this subject of sending out matrons and nurses, I, of course, consulted men conversant both with India and hospital organizations. We all came to the same conclusions:

1. There ought to be a continuous stream of trained nurses coming out from England to India. You cannot depend on recruiting *in* the country, though you must do all in your power to promote it. You ought, therefore, as you have your civil school, as you have your military school—expressly for India in England—so you ought to have your nurse school. The India Office ought to do this (in concert of course, with the governor general) finding the funds. And we, if they please, will find the organization. Our training school cannot give a sufficient supply; our matrons and nurses are taken up for at least a year beforehand and we have been called upon to supply one of our colonies [New South Wales, Australia]. Besides this, the home market will probably be more attractive to good Englishwomen (i.e., to Englishwomen who don't go out to "get married") for a long time to come than the Indian market. They are now well paid at home, they are near their own friends, and they have not the dreaded India climate before them. Therefore, all our experience tells us that, if India is to have good nursing from England, it must be done as a special service, by contract, by women who engage expressly for India and are trained with that view.

2. People rarely look at the enormous difference there is between organizing a woman service and a man service for India. If we send you

out an engineer, you have not to look after his private life. If he drinks or goes to the bad, so long as it does not interfere with his public service, the public need not make it their business to keep him in order. But it is quite different, I need hardly say, with women. If they drink or go to the bad, their usefulness is over, the thing is a failure, you *must* have a woman as high in character as in efficiency for her to do any good.

3. This, of course, includes the important question of discipline. And the consideration of discipline includes the fact that it can only be exercised over women by a woman. (Hitherto, in India, the discipline of a hospital has been exclusively in the hands of a doctor.) A peccadillo which a lady superintendent would and ought to dismiss a woman for, a commanding officer will think nothing of—a *medical officer still less.* It is vain to think of sending out women to be under men.

If nursing is to be ever efficiently introduced into India, there ought to be four superintendents: one for Madras, one for Bombay, one for Calcutta, one for the Upper Provinces, trained, of high character and position, in direct communication with the local government, who, in connection with that government, should manage all nursing affairs: dismiss, appoint, remove, etc., and take charge of the continuous stream of nurses coming out from England, but coming out on the superintendence's requisition, only at the desire of the local government. (The complete failure of the Calcutta scheme, made in memory of poor Lady Canning, has but confirmed these views.)

4. Had we plenty of women, *on whom we could entirely depend,* ready to our hands, there would be no need of all this "embarras" [trouble]. We could send out what India wants (for already we have a similar request from another part of India) as soon as an agreement could be made. But we have not. Also if one or two nurses were sent out to India who—either from not being selected and trained with due care, or from not being put under a discipline out in India such as to ensure due care—were unhappily to prove a failure -- then the whole thing would be ruined for a generation to come. You know what the vulgar mind is all over the world. The one individual instance under the eye tells, the experience of a dozen countries does not tell. The one individual instance becomes the law.

Therefore we must ask India to take into consideration the conditions which alone can give a fair chance of success to the experiment, which she herself has proposed to make (if I could go out myself, as I fain would do, that would be different. Then we should not have to worry *you).*

Now to come to the particular question put by you and Lady Napier:

1. If Lady Napier will take the thing under her own special protection, I think that what you propose might be done, viz., that a lady superintendent and "two or three head nurses" might be found and trained and sent out to you. (But would "two or three" be enough to make the nucleus of a training school?)

2. Of what hospital do you propose to put the superintendent in nursing charge? To train nurses you must have a hospital (with both sexes, medical and surgical cases) to train in. It is always better to take the whole nursing charge of any one hospital at once, but if this cannot be done, then to limit the nurses from England to a part of the hospital, while putting the superintendent in nursing charge of the whole. (You see, in India the thing must be begun from the beginning because there is nothing that we call nursing in India now at all. And, in some respects, this is an advantage.) I have gone over on paper all the Madras hospitals with Mr Porteous. The General Hospital would be, of course, the least bad for the purpose. I had hoped that the "passed hospital nurses" of the Military Female Asylum might have afforded us material. But the number and character of cases (principally scabies and sore eyes) is much too limited to give the nurses any right to their name.

3. To the superintendent must be given a complete and well-defined position, as one who has undisputed charge of the nursing of the hospital, the responsibility of having the orders of the medical officers carried out, undisputed charge of the discipline of her nurses and training school.

4. Now about the pay of superintendent and nurses (it is the interest of the government, if it has out nurses at all at such an expense, to do what will secure and retain the best women). After much inquiry, I should advise the salary of such a trained superintendent as you want to be not under 300 rupees (£30) a month, rising to (say) 350 rupees in four years, 400 rupees in four years more and a house or good healthy quarters immediately adjoining her duties, to contain the nurses also, that is to say, if it is the custom in Madras for a woman to board herself (we prefer giving board), *plus* provision in the event of sickness and provision on ultimate retirement either by grant or pension, free first-class passage out and home if she returns home sick on medical certificate, to return to India on recovery, then some maintenance while at home. For the head nurses a rising scale, similar provisions for sickness and retirement. It would not be desirable for these

women to board themselves. They ought of course to live with the superintendent in her quarters immediately attached to the hospital. And she ought to be allowed a sum to board them and herself (in which case some small deduction might be made on her pay). What the rising scale for the nurses ought to be I think I must leave to your consideration. As a guide, the nurses whom we are sending out to N.S. Wales are for a three years' engagement to have £50 the first year, £60 the second, £70 the third, *and* board and lodging.

[not in FN's hand] There is also a condition that the cost of the passage out shall be repaid, e.g., in case of breach of engagement. This however cannot be considered as regards the nurses as likely to be of much practical effect. [FN resumes] The chances of ill-health and also of marriage are, of course, far greater in India than in the colonies. But I must leave the calculations of these to your greater knowledge. . . .

Mr Porteous desired me to ask you, as guide to the superintendent's salary, what was the monthly salary of teachers of colleges, of medical college and high school, of government teachers of normal schools? And he said that sufficient pay and a supreme position as matron were indispensable for a superintendent.

I should hope that a branch training school for nurses might ultimately be founded at Bangalore.

When it comes to the point of making agreements, Henry Bonham Carter, the secretary to our committee, of which Sir Harry Verney, whom I think you know, is the chairman, would be the person to address. I am the more anxious to put this on a right footing because permanency in India and life in me are so precarious. You might leave Madras, leaving no sufficient minute behind you. Then where are our poor women to go? The agreements ought to be made between some permanent body in Madras on the one hand and our committee on the other. Ultimately I should trust that the India Office will be your *agent* in London. But to make it so now would be simply to shelve the whole thing. It must be borne in mind that to find suitable women and to train them will require time. Our period of training is a year; we cannot hold out any prospect of finding a suitable matron among those who have already been trained, nor that she could be prepared in less than a year.

Source: From a letter to Sir John McNeill, Florence Nightingale Museum (LMA) H1/ST/NC3/SU157, ADD Mss 45768 ff202-09

10 September 1867

*Private.* The matter (on which I want to consult you as to what my answer should be to the India government) is that of trained nurses, upon which you were so very good as to help me before. You will see by the papers which will accompany this that I adopted your suggestions in full. If you will be so very good as to help me again, I shall esteem it as I always do, the greatest favour I can receive.

I enclose a letter from Major Malleson, who is now sole sanitary commissioner for Bengal, and the papers which accompanied it. You will see that they have constructed an immense scheme upon mine, or rather ours. And then they condemn this scheme, which is in some respects the opposite of mine, and call it mine, e.g., they propose to put nurses in all regimental hospitals, which is what we never would consent to. . . .

Our paper ["Suggestions on a System of Nursing . . . ," 1865, above] (of which yours was the best part) was a reply to the letter of the secretary of the Bengal Sanitary Commission of 21 November 1864. . . . Our paper, while doing the best we could at a distance, and without local knowledge to furnish the desired information, at the same time advised that a small tentative experiment should in the first instance be made. And we offered to help in this. The cost would not have been very great. And I must say that, after reading over all the papers, I still adhere to that opinion.

I cannot but feel how unwisely they have begun by rearing up in the first instance (on paper) an extensive superstructure of nursing for all the military hospitals. . . . *Nurses* among *convalescent* soldiers in the wards are quite out of place and always will be. They would become playthings and very improper ones. There are not half a dozen military hospitals in India to which female nursing would be applicable. Certainly not at first. The object would be to induce India to begin as New South Wales is beginning and many other places, viz., to send to us for a small trained efficient staff to take charge of one hospital and to try the work of nursing and training nurses. . . .

Now why cannot the Bengal people do the same, instead of making gigantic cut and dry systems on paper and then condemning them, whereas of all things nursing in military hospitals requires painful, careful trial, because it must always be an experiment, and a new experiment every time you try it, to put down a few women among a parcel of men, this being the only occupation where a woman is really in actual charge and control of grown-up men. So much depends on the discretion of the superintendent, on the character of the medical and military officers, etc.

As to the proposal concerning Protestant nuns in Major Malleson's manuscript letter, enclosed, he falls into the common mistake, viz., of believing that if he would but lay aside religious prejudices, we should have 15,000 Protestant Sisters of Charity as the French have 15,000 Roman Catholic Sisters of Charity. Now, this is not a matter to theorize about. It is already a matter of fact and experience. I should have *more* difficulty in sending him an efficient nursing staff, composed of "sisters," whether R.C. or Protestant, than in sending him a staff out of our ordinary materials at St Thomas', great as that difficulty is.

In these "orders" the material is always doubtful, and the number are far too few. And the best women do not choose to enter "orders." Also it is found that women who had really entered the service of God in hospitals (e.g., Miss Agnes Jones[16] of Liverpool Workhouse) are just as little likely to marry out of "orders" as in them. (Miss A. Jones is remarkably pretty and attractive.)

There are now four London hospitals nursed by Protestant "orders." Of these, the nursing of two is beneath contempt, and therefore shall not be mentioned here, other than to show that so far from the prejudice supposed by Major M. being in active existence, every facility is given to the rising up of nursing "orders" in hospitals. The other two, King's College and Charing Cross, are nursed by St John's House, of which my dear friend and "pupil" Miss [Mary] Jones is superintendent. . . .

I have consulted her and Mrs Wardroper equally about the India nursing. I cannot therefore be supposed to speak as an enemy. But her system of nursing, which is first rate, has taken even less extension than ours has. The fact is that orders in England (and this is quite as much the case with the R.C.s who are exactly in the same difficulty as we are) do not extend for this reason: the best women fit to be heads do *not* enter orders in England, which generally consist of one good head and a number of fools, or rather a very few fools. Add to which: women who wish to marry will marry (and have married) from our "orders" because we can't take the same "vows" as R.C.s and women who don't wish to marry won't marry, even if not in "orders."

---

16 Agnes Elizabeth Jones (1832-68), nurse, superintendent, Liverpool Workhouse Infirmary. See the biographical sketch in *Public Health Care* (6:677).

I should wish to be guided entirely by your opinion as to what reply I should make to the Government of India, if you will be so very good as to take it into consideration. My impression is what they want in India is a well-considered small beginning, and that we should advise them still to try this, and again offer our help in training.

Would you advise me to say that the scheme to which Dr Farquhar takes objection is not mine, that I have no scheme, that if the Government of India wish for my advice regarding a scheme (vide Major Malleson) it is for them and not for me to propose one; that I consider (and experience has always led me to advocate) female nursing as applicable only in general hospitals in the army, and not in either convalescent depots or in regimental hospitals; that as to have "assistant nurses" in military hospitals, the thing is totally and entirely out of the question, whether in Europe or in India, and as far as one can see, always will be so. (The place of assistant nurses in civil hospitals must always be filled in military hospitals by men.) And no women below the class and education and position of a head nurse in a civil hospital should ever be suffered in military hospital.

As to that stuff about the "enthusiasm" of the nursing in the "Crimean Campaign," that is all bosh. We had, unfortunately for us, scarcely one woman sent out to us who was even up to the level of a head nurse, and we suffered for it, and even now, when I look back, I cannot think how we dragged through. But instead of taking that time as an "enthusiasm" which cannot now or again be equalled, we have learnt from it a great deal as to what ought to be the principle and routine of female nursing in the ordinary general military hospitals and as to what ought to be avoided and sought.

I am throwing a great burden upon you to read through all these papers. I have read many tons of papers in the last eleven years. But I don't think I have ever seen such a farrago as this. They send our nursing scheme to a captain of engineers and to a major in the army to discuss. I hope when next they have a war in Bhotan, they will send the proposed artillery to Mrs Wardroper to criticize. Perhaps I need hardly say that such rules as are here proposed, e.g., that as a punishment the nurses' beer should be "stopped," would completely and always "stop" (not the "beer" but) any chance of raising the service to that of good and respectable women.

It shows how wise we were to insist upon, at first and as a *sine qua non,* that the nurses should be under a superintendent of their sex, and not under the medical officers. If you treat nurses like female convicts, you will have female convicts for your nurses. The only idea these papers appear to have of business is to print my paper over and over again. To mount upon it schemes which have nothing to do with it, and then to renounce them as too expensive.

Source: From a letter or a copy of a letter to Sir John Lawrence, Add Mss 45777 ff149-55

18 September 1867

I hope that you will forgive me for addressing you directly on the subject of female nursing in India.

I take the liberty of doing so because, having received at various times from the president of the Bengal Sanitary Commission printed papers relating to the employment of female nurses in hospitals in India, I see that the last contains the decision of the Government of India (Mil. Dep. No. 232, 10 June 1867). It appears to me to call for a direct reply addressed to yourself personally, which I will make as short as I can. But I fear I shall be obliged to trouble you in this with stating the facts of the case, in order to show that there is really no connection between the humble proposal I made at the request of the India government and the scheme which was condemned without even having been referred to me. But had it been referred to me, I, being *entirely* de l'avis de monsieur pour la raison contraire [I agree with the gentleman, but for the opposite reason], should without doubt or hesitation have condemned it quite as emphatically as H.E. the Governor-General-of-India-in-Council, not only on the score of its cost, but because I never could have meant my aid or sanction in any way, humble as they are, to giving effect to any such system, which the experience of my whole life tells me contains proposals which would swamp every principle of good nursing. I would recur to this.

From the voluminous Indian documents which have been sent me, I gather that female nursing in general hospitals in India, so far as it has yet been tried under very unfavourable circumstances, has been found to be of inestimable advantage to the patients. On this point the evidence of Dr Beatson,[17] P.M.O. of the British troops in India and of Dr Bruce, principal inspector general of the Indian Medical Department, is conclusive. Both consider a trained department of nurses essential and feel confident that the very greatest benefits to the sick will result from its adoption, if properly carried out. No one, in short,

17 George Stewart Beatson (1814-87), inspector general of hospitals.

from the governor general and commandant-in-chief to the heads of the medical department and the sanitary commission, seems to have expressed or entertained any doubt on this subject, until Colonel Broome's estimate of the cost of the "complete scheme" which the government had called for and the sanitary commission had submitted, startled the Government of India by its extravagance.

But the scheme on which Colonel Broome founded his estimate is totally inconsistent with the course of proceeding which at the request of the Government of India I had suggested and for which that government had stated its readiness to provide the requisite funds. The scheme on which Colonel Broome's estimate is based proposes the immediate introduction of a complete nursing establishment in *seven* general hospitals in Bengal, *five* of which are convalescent hospitals. In my letter of 24 February 1865 (the only communication of mine that is referred to) I recommend that the experiment should be tried in only one hospital and that it should be regarded merely as an experimental or tentative measure. . . .

It thus appears that the estimated expenditure, which so much alarmed the Indian government as to cause it to renounce in toto its intention of extending to any portion of the army in India the acknowledged advantages of female nursing, was founded upon a scheme devised in India and has no relation to or connection with the course of proceeding which I, when consulted, recommended as the best.

The most singular part of the story is that the Government of India, having done me the honour to ask my advice with a view to be guided (it is a false humility and an incivility to the government for me to disparage this step of theirs), having no experience of their own to guide them, should have set aside my recommendation to begin with only one hospital as a tentative measure in order to obtain the experience and knowledge required for future guidance in a new and peculiar country; that it should have altogether disregarded my distinct intimation that it was not only inexpedient but absolutely impracticable to carry out at once an extended scheme; and that it should have called upon some of its own military officers, who could not have the required practical knowledge or experience (not being matrons, any more than matrons would have the power of advising them on engineering or artillery points) to submit for consideration a "complete scheme for the employment of female nurses in military hospitals," which was understood to mean, and no doubt did mean, all the military hospitals in the Bengal presidency. Thus called upon to submit "a complete scheme" for the Bengal presidency, the sanitary commission submitted such a scheme prepared by Captain Williams of the Royal Engineers and approved by Major Malleson; and the government, considering that scheme too expensive, thereupon resolved not to fall back upon the comparatively inexpensive tentative course which I had recommended, but that no attempt should be made to afford to the sick of the Army in India what the evidence before them from the highest medical authorities represented as an inestimable advantage.

It is not for me or for anyone to doubt the duty of the Government of India to avoid and to prevent undue expenditure, and there is a limit to the burden that can be justly imposed on the people of India, even for the purpose of promoting the welfare and efficiency of the British Army in that country. Summarily to reject as inadmissible and useless any attempt to introduce, even as a tentative measure, in India the trained female nursing which has been adopted in almost every civilized community—and an application has now been made to me by a portion of the native community even in India to introduce it there—and to reject and disparage it merely because a specially extravagant and impracticable scheme, submitted by persons necessarily imperfectly informed on the subject, was considered too expensive, is a course of which the advantage might perhaps be doubted, while there was the alternative of adopting the more safe, judicious and inexpensive course which I had from the first ventured to recommend.

The only account we have of the grounds on which the government may be supposed to have acted is that contained in Dr Farquhar's memorandum. That paper, while it contains the extravagant scheme (as I should do) hardly attempts to deal either one way or the other with the course which I, when I was asked, took the liberty to recommend. The chief objection urged against it is that it might interfere with the Ladies Committee at Calcutta. I do not read the resolution of the Governor-General-in-Council, para 2, as holding out any prospect of the employment of any other description of nurses than those who have hitherto been employed; it only contemplates putting "existing establishments" on a better footing.

So far as I am aware, the course I ventured to suggest, in obedience to the government's desire, as the best, has never been considered at all by the government on its own merits.

Source: From a draft letter to Sir Bartle Frere in Dr Sutherland's hand, ADD Mss 45780 ff71-72

[20 September 1867]

Under these circumstances I feel myself functioning [ex] officio in this matter, at the very time when we are sending to New South Wales a superintendent and staff of nurses trained here at the request of the colonial government, and which staff might have been landed at Calcutta. And at the very time when applications are coming to me from natives in India for help in improving the hospital nursing there.

Source: From a letter to Sir John McNeill, Florence Nightingale Museum (LMA) H1/ST/NC3/SU158, copy ADD Mss 45768 ff216-18

21 September 1867

*Private.* I had received your first letter, on the subject of female nursing in India which, as everything you always do, puts "the situation" clearly before me. And I had written, according to your advice, a simple protest, without proposing anything anew, to Sir John Lawrence himself. But, rather luckily for me, I think, I could not get my letter ready for the mail of the 18th, because by desire of some members of the India Office, I had to write him a long letter and paper on the introduction of a Public Health Service by that mail.

Then came your second most clear and emphatic letter. And I somewhat recast mine to Sir J. Lawrence, to go by *next* mail, when yesterday arrives this letter from him, enclosing the paper from Dr Farquhar, which I also enclose.

I am quite ashamed of troubling you again, when I had already received so lucid and comprehensive a sketch from you of the view I ought to take. But I will only ask you now to be so very good as to look over the enclosures in the light of the previous correspondence and to tell me whether they in any way alter your opinion, as expressed on the whole question in your last letters, or your view of the answer I ought to make. The matter is certainly quite hopeless at present.

I believe you hit on the right solution of the extraordinary proceeding, as it seems, of a government taking and giving all this trouble, not only to me but to a number of its own officers, for the pure pleasure of doing a great deal of utterly useless writing. But you can have no idea of the degree to which this has gone in every department of the India government. What we have gone through in writing on the Public Health Service no one can tell, during these last 3½ years. I should think myself impatient and restless (though I am not much of a novice) did I not hear what Sir B. Frere says, which is much stronger than what I say. He thinks that this very kind of administration or no-administration is bringing all government in India to a deadlock.

I could give you the most extraordinary instances derived from our own branch of administration alone. Our foolscap is sent all over India to see how many fools' heads it will fit. Of course if fits a good many. Then there comes home to us a mass of papers, incredible to any who did not see them. And we have to answer them all seriously. Then answers come back from India. It is so easy to answer, if you don't want to act. Latterly, a proposition about doors versus windows in barracks was sent round to every British department, 6 (six) in every British province in India, only one of which departments knew anything about it at all, and then came home to us with all the opinions of all the *cooks* printed. With Sir B. Frere's assistance, however, I hope now that we shall have a regular department organized for ourselves at the India Office, and in each administrative division of India for itself, to save some of this fearful waste of time.

Before Sir B. Frere came home, I was getting quite desperate. He is to us what you are or would be if we had you here. I have often intended to trouble you about these Indian public health affairs, but it was entailing such an immense amount of "papers" upon you.

Pray remember me most heartily to Lady McNeill and believe me,
ever most gratefully and sincerely yours
Florence Nightingale

*Please burn.*

Source: From a draft letter to Sir John Lawrence, ADD Mss 45777 ff156-58

26 September 1867

I have received your kind letter of 16 August with the manuscript note by Dr Farquhar enclosed, and I have also received from Major Malleson the voluminous printed papers, appended to the resolution of government of 10 June, deciding on not employing female nursing in the military hospitals in India.

I will now venture to remind you that I only gave my opinion when it was sought, that I gave it gladly, hoping that a great benefit, as it was described to be by the evidence of Dr Beatson, principal medical officer of the British troops in India, and of Dr Bruce, principal inspector general of the Indian Medical Department, was about to be conferred on the British Army in India. The method proposed for giving effect to my recommendation, and which the Government of India has rejected, was not mine—and indeed contained proposals to which I never could have agreed.

Having carefully perused the papers, manuscript and printed, which have been sent to me, I have not found in them anything that could lead me to change my opinion as to the benefits to be derived from trained nursing in India, and as to the manner in which it should have been introduced.

But it is for you who are primarily responsible for the welfare of the British Army in India, and not for me, to determine what ought to be done with a view to improve the condition of the sick of that army. If I can, at any future time, contribute to the promotion of so desirable an object, I shall be glad to have an opportunity of rendering such assistance as I may be able to give, believing, as I still do, that much progress in the right direction might be made at a cost so moderate that the Government of New South Wales have not hesitated to undertake it and the Parsis of Bombay are desirous to pursue a similar course. Pray believe me, dear Sir John Lawrence,

ever your faithful servant
Florence Nightingale

Source: From a letter to G.B. Malleson, ADD Mss 45782 ff255-57

26 September 1867

*Private.* Since I received your letter . . . with its printed enclosures, I have received a letter from Sir John Lawrence on the same subject (the rejection by the Government of India of female nursing in the military hospitals). And I have replied to him. It is unnecessary therefore that I should trouble you with any farther reply. And it is only in acknowledgment of your courtesy that I hazard the following remarks in obedience to your desire.

1. I do not read the resolution of the Governor-General-in-Council, para 2, as holding out any prospect of the employment of any other description of nurses then those who have hitherto been employed; it only contemplates putting "existing establishments" on a better footing. I do not therefore see how I can follow the suggestion in your kind letter and aid you in this as I would so gladly do.

2. The extensive and (as I venture to believe) impracticable scheme drawn up at the request of and rejected by the Government of India, is not mine. In fact, the experience of my whole life would lead me to reject it even more positively than the Government of India has done. I will mention a few of the propositions, to which, as I have never consented, so I never could consent to, in any establishments for which I was responsible. E.g., (1) the employment of female nurses in *regimental* hospitals or (2) in *convalescent* depots or (3) the employment of

*assistant* nurses or of any below the class of *head* nurses in *military* hospitals. Also (4) women of such a class could never be found who would submit to such a degrading rule as being deprived of their "beer" as a "punishment." And it would be useless to attempt the governing them except under a lady superintendent of their own. Of course if women are to be treated as female convicts none but women of the class of female convicts would be found to come. But it is useless for me to trouble you with any more than these few examples since the scheme is not now in hand.

N.B. It is implied in one of the printed papers that I successfully employed female nurses in *regimental* hospitals in the Crimean War. Never. I never employed nurses in any but *general* (military) hospitals either in war or in peace.

3. The chief objection urged in two papers is that the scheme might interfere with the "Ladies' Committee at Calcutta." Again, in one of two papers by the same hand, the unfitness of the "raw material" to be procured in India is insisted upon as an insuperable objection to the introduction of female trained nursing in military hospitals in that country, unless at the inadmissible cost of importing a whole establishment of such nurses from England. And it is urged that, even if that great expense were incurred, the attempt must fail because the services of such nurses could not be retained, that therefore the attempt to introduce female trained nursing must inevitably fail in whatever way it might be tried, and therefore ought not to be made.

But, in the second paper, we are assured with equal confidence that the nurses procured and trained in India "do sufficiently well," that they are not only spoken of "with almost uniform approbation by the medical men for the way in which the work is done in the hospital" but are largely employed in remunerative private nursing, that "they combine with hospital work the nursing of sick officers" and that "it may well be conceived how welcome to the sick a well-trained nurse must be who understands what is said and can help them in their helplessness." This in justification of a resolution—not to employ, not even to entertain the idea of employing female trained nurses, of any class or description, in any military hospital.

4. I have never dissembled the difficulties (on the contrary, I have always urged even to pertinacity that a small, well-considered beginning should alone be made, tentative to be treated merely as an experiment at first) but a restatement of difficulties with which everyone has long been familiar and which it is certainly much easier to

succumb to than to combat and overcome is hardly "the way to win." I should not have troubled you even with these few remarks, were it not that your (private) letter seemed to desire it and to ask for suggestions. But the only one which my life's experience can justify me in making is what I have made before, viz., a small tentative beginning with trained nurses from England.

Source: From a note to Henry Bonham Carter, Add Mss 47715 f87

[after 6 November 1867]

*Private. Madras and Bombay.*

*Madras.* I have heard from Lord Napier. We shall have call for a superintendent and a few head nurses in about a year. Nothing official as yet, but I am sure we may be looking out for probationers—it is none so easy to find such a lady.

*Bombay.* I have had a new Parsi here. And he wants to found a midwifery school for nurses, and offered to take trainers temporarily into his house, until they could be established, to train midwives to attend upon ladies and poor. Loss of life not so much now as to the custom of leaving mother and child for forty days in dirt, owing to the prejudice as to "impurity."

Nothing definite as yet.

Source: From a letter to Henry Bonham Carter, Add Mss 47714 ff256-57

[1867]

I am so completely worn out with seeing a Parsi gentleman from Bombay by Sir B. Frere's desire, and a deputy inspector general from Madras by Lady Napier's desire, that I am almost incoherent.

We are pushing the Public Health Service in India very much now by Sir B. Frere with Sir S. Northcote. We may *quite well* begin *to train* for Madras and Bombay both—matron and nurses—though as yet it is only semi-official—the invitation. I was going to write to you all about it.

Source: From a letter to Lucy Leighton,[18] "A Florence Nightingale Letter," *Celebrate the Century 1898-1998* 101-02, Toronto Western Hospital; copy ADD MSS 45803 ff63-66

35 South St.
2 May 1873

I am sure that you well know the interest I feel in the career and prospects of success or failure, in the highest as well as the ordinary sense, of every one of our flock and will not doubt that any delay in answering yours has only risen from the always almost overwhelming pressure of business and illness upon me, and also—must I say it?—from the great difficulty of saying anything which will be at once true to experience and to God—and not what will seem cold to you—and the almost impossibility of giving you advice personally, as you ask, because, while these Indian missions are almost one of the highest interests I have, I cannot think but that the Female Medical Missions will prove a failure if undertaken as they are now proposed.

Let me say at once, as you seem to wish it, that I do not think you break any engagement to *us*. I quite understood that on Dr Peacock's report we not only considered you free to but wished you to seek other employment better suited to your health. . . .

You will be sure how sincerely I pray that your proposed employment in India may be good for both body and soul, and also that I am very glad things are so arranged that you may leave St Thomas' immediately, as the time will be all too short for you to prepare yourself, by even the most elementary training, for India "by October." Indeed I was most anxious that you should be set free immediately.

I will say nothing about the absolute self-abnegation, the severe mental training, the acquiring the languages of Hindustan (I have been now working for India for fourteen years and know something of these things, though my work has been principally in sanitary administration) that are required for the work you propose. But I will limit myself to the learning and qualifying yourself in midwifery, diseases of women and children, dispensing, which, I understand from your note, you expect to do "by October." I should think *two years* all too short for a training in these things.

We had, as you are perhaps aware, a training school for women in midwifery for some years. We gave a *six months'* training, much more

18 Lucy Leighton (1840-74), trained at St Thomas', looked for alternative work, died at sea en route to India.

complete both in length of time under instruction, in scientific and practical training than any midwifery instruction which could then be had in London. Yet we would not allow our women to be certified as midwives or as other than midwifery *nurses*, i.e., qualified to conduct normal lying-in and to detect when anything abnormal was going on, so as to call in a doctor. I have known a much shorter and more incomplete training in London obtain a woman the certificate of "midwife," "accoucheuse" and even "physician accoucheuse." Over and over again we have been asked to admit ladies going out as you are to India (to practise as "*physician accoucheuses*") for one month, three months, six months' training, and have always steadily declined. If we would not do this for England, where a midwife can always have a doctor at hand or within reach, how could we do this for India, where this is so far from being the case that the very circumstance that it is not is made the reason for having lady doctors—and a very good reason too.

But I will not detain you, my dear Miss Leighton, with these considerations, which probably will not commend themselves to you now, if they have not already. I will only commend you to our Father who will work out all things for good,[19] if only we go to Him humbly, sincerely and lovingly, as I am sure you do. . . .

May I send you a copy of a little book of mine on "Lying-in Institutions" for your kind acceptance? You will find some remarks in the appendix on "physician accoucheuses."

Source: From a letter to Henry Cunningham (written in the third person), in Margaret M. Verney, *Sir Henry Stewart Cunningham* 71

29 October 1873

Florence Nightingale is informed by her sister Lady Verney that Mr Cunningham wishes to see her before he leaves England, with regard to nursing affairs in Madras. She is afraid this information must be incorrect as her Indian correspondence for the last ten years on the subject of nursing alone would fill this house, and with Madras a room of this house. And its fruitlessness can only be matched by its size. Nevertheless, if Mr Cunningham takes it up, possibly the impossible may be done.

19 An allusion to Rom 8:28.

Source: From two letter to Henry Bonham Carter, Add Mss 47719 ff35-36 and 37-38

25 May 1874

*Madras Matron.* Dr Mackenzie clamours for an answer, and as he is *in London* you see it is *very impossible to* put him off.

I am not sure that you do not mean your "remark" that you have "no remark" to be a final answer: and if so I am not sure that it is not the best. I am as unwilling as unable to resume all these Indian nursing correspondences; it is impossible for me to waste more months (I have literally wasted *months*) like a squirrel in a cage in going round and round with these Madras people. I saw Henry Cunningham about it too. The plan proposed is one we could never consent to: one matron, one nurse for two years, to be under the medical officer, to train native men and (I understand) to be over several hospitals.

I conceive that, if we entertain the application at all, we must send one matron, one assistant, three or four head nurses, stipulate for her being an officer of the *government* (to be responsible for carrying out medical orders), ascertain and define her position in the "several hospitals," if to undertake the training of "native men" at all, this can only be as it is done (or not done) at Netley by the head nurses training the orderlies *in* the wards. For one matron (and one nurse) to undertake the "training of native men" even in one hospital is unmitigated folly. Also, we cannot possibly consent to have our women judged of by one doctor out of Great Northern, and one out of King's College Hospitals. Any dealing must be between us and the Madras authorities. Also, we must have a full year's notice.

(Mrs Wardroper has seen Dr Mackenzie twice and without entering into the least condition, has asked Miss Hincks if she would go as matron. Mrs W. thinks that we might send by and bye Miss Hincks, Miss Crossland and some nurses. I have piles of letters from Lord Napier, Mr Ellis, etc., from Madras on the subject in past years. I do not feel at all equal to the task of converting Dr Mackenzie) or even of selecting from my papers for him (and yet am very unwilling to quash the thing). Please return me *this* with your answer.

25 May 1874

*Madras No. 2.* Since I wrote to you this morning, I have received these papers (by Indian post) with letter *from Henry Cunningham.* I do *not* think the "matron's salary" offered "conclusive against the scheme." But any woman *must* be *crazy* who accepts such a position as this. (Mrs Wardroper asked Miss Hincks without giving *me* any idea that she was doing so.) I feel quite unable to combat "*Lady Hobart*" and the *doctors* too.

F.N.

I have merely *glanced* over the printed papers and made a few hasty pencil comments, not wishing to give you the trouble of reading the packet sent this morning, *except* with this packet, received since. *Accommodation, everything,* seems to make the position untenable, and for *one* (woman) lady to teach *coolies*!!!!

Source: From notes, ADD Mss 47751 f65

12 April 1876

Miss [Frances] Elizabeth Spencer (Sister Alexandra) came in November 1872; January 1874 wished to go to India in the zenanas.

Source: From notes on an interview with Mary Carpenter, ADD Mss 45789 ff164-65

15 May 1876

*Nursing in India. . . . Madras:* Eurasian women only poor sick women; before no nursing; so delighted with Miss Marter's kindness. . . . Miss Carpenter would write to her to ask if she will send one to St Thomas' to be trained. . . . In Madras workhouse no matron. Train Eurasian women from without for six months . . . ; then they have six months in lying-in hospital, also no matron; then certificated and go out as nurses. . . .

[In] *Bombay* Dr Hunter trains Eurasian women.

Begum of Bhopal founds a *female* hospital [in] memory of prince of Wales's visit; asked an American medical woman to be doctress but she asked 700 a month and was bumptious. . . .

Jails everywhere better than hospitals, but at Dacca very bad. . . . W.C.s mere cesspits in women's apartments, smell atrocious; European officials' ladies made ill by it, husbands won't let them visit.

Source: From a letter to Henry Bonham Carter, ADD Mss 47719 ff203-04

27 July 1877

Mrs Furnell. Madras Hospital Nursing. Her note reached me THE DAY I LEFT LONDON. Since then as you know my difficulty has been rather how to live at all, and make others live, than how to answer letters (which I have entirely given up). Would you say this to her? and say that now I would gladly "answer her few questions"? forwarded through you.

To *you* I say that I had meanwhile seen Lady Anna Gore-Langton,[20] (who, I was told, knew more about the matter than all the Furnells put together), had made copious notes of her information and through her received a paper of answers from the fountainhead herself, the Madras lady superintendent who is *returned*, and also had seen Mr Ellis, my old Madras correspondent, now member of India Council here.

The matter is perfectly clear, though there have been faults of judgment and temper in the superintendent it was madness to try to work it—*no one* could work it—under such conditions, as you will see, as were given. The question is *can we do anything to help?*

**Editor:** It is interesting to note in closing how much Nightingale's early Crimean War contacts played a role in the India work. Lord Napier and Ettrick, governor of Madras, had met Nightingale the day of her arrival at Scutari—he was then a diplomat at the Constantinople Embassy. He later recounted to her that he remembered Scutari and was "one of the few original faithful left." Cook observed that Napier indeed carried a nursing measure through (in Madras) when John Lawrence was "unfaithful."[21] Letters from Napier reporting progress on nursing and public health issues generally are warm and full. One recounts reading "the beautiful account of 'Una' . . . driving along the melancholy shore," signing himself "ever your faithful, grateful and devoted servant, Napier."[22]

Nightingale later sent him a copy of her *Introductory Notes on Lying-in Institutions*, with a dedication:

> To His Excellency the Lord Napier, Madras, this little book, though on a most unsavoury subject, yet one which, entering into His Excellency's plans for the good of those under his enlightened rule, is not foreign to his thoughts—is offered by Florence Nightingale. London 10 October 1871. (Cook, *The Life of Florence Nightingale* 2:171)

## A Few Last Words on Public Health in India

**Editor:** Nightingale's efforts to introduce female nursing in India were aborted. Thereafter she turned to other issues, although the question of nursing kept occupying her and others' minds. The results of her

20 Anna Gore-Langton (1820-79), supporter of medical education for women, then in Madras with her brother, the duke of Buckingham, who was governor.
21 Cook, *The Life of Florence Nightingale* 2:170.
22 Letter 3 September 1869, Add Mss 45779 f222.

India work up to the mid-1870s can be seen in other fields, and more will be said on her overall contribution at the end of *Social Change in India.* Certainly the royal commission, which she did so much to instigate and promote and whose results she assiduously monitored, had many highly positive outcomes. The infrastructure for the next decades of actual public health work was established as recommended. The presidency sanitary commissions in fact became the mechanism for practical reforms. In 1871, according to Nightingale's paper of 1873, "Life or Death in India," the death rate in the Indian Army had been lowered in a remarkable way to one half of what it was (from 6.9 to 3.47 percent), in the whole Bengal presidency from between 7 and 8 to 1.7 percent. The city of Calcutta was said to be more salubrious than Manchester and Liverpool, all progress due to sanitary work. Obviously, however, epidemics and famines raised the death rates unacceptably and pointed to the huge task to be tackled if both were to be controlled.

Much that was recommended by the royal commission was implemented, but much as well did not happen, thanks to inertia, mixed agendas if not motives, and sometimes bureaucratic blundering. Some reforms took an inordinate amount of energy, either to get the problem properly understood or to dissuade officials from taking the wrong approach and to get them moving. An example of a typically rough ride was the proposal for introducing female nursing just related, which was botched, then dropped.

In the wake of epidemics, famines and general malnutrition new problems emerged and more attention had to be given to the Indian population at large. The sources of those phenomena had to be investigated and, if possible, eliminated. British policy on taxation of Indians and the removal of that money from productive uses to pay for military forays continued, despite the protests of Nightingale and a very few others. Exploitation of cultivators rendered many measures for sanitary improvement dictated from above impracticable. Parliamentary interest in India remained minimal—something neither Nightingale nor anybody, it seems, could do anything about. In short the limits of top-down reforms, however well researched and planned, became increasingly more evident. Support for measures of self-government and work with Indian nationals already emerged as a strategy in this volume. We will see the focus shifting much more to those tactics in the next volume, *Social Change in India.*

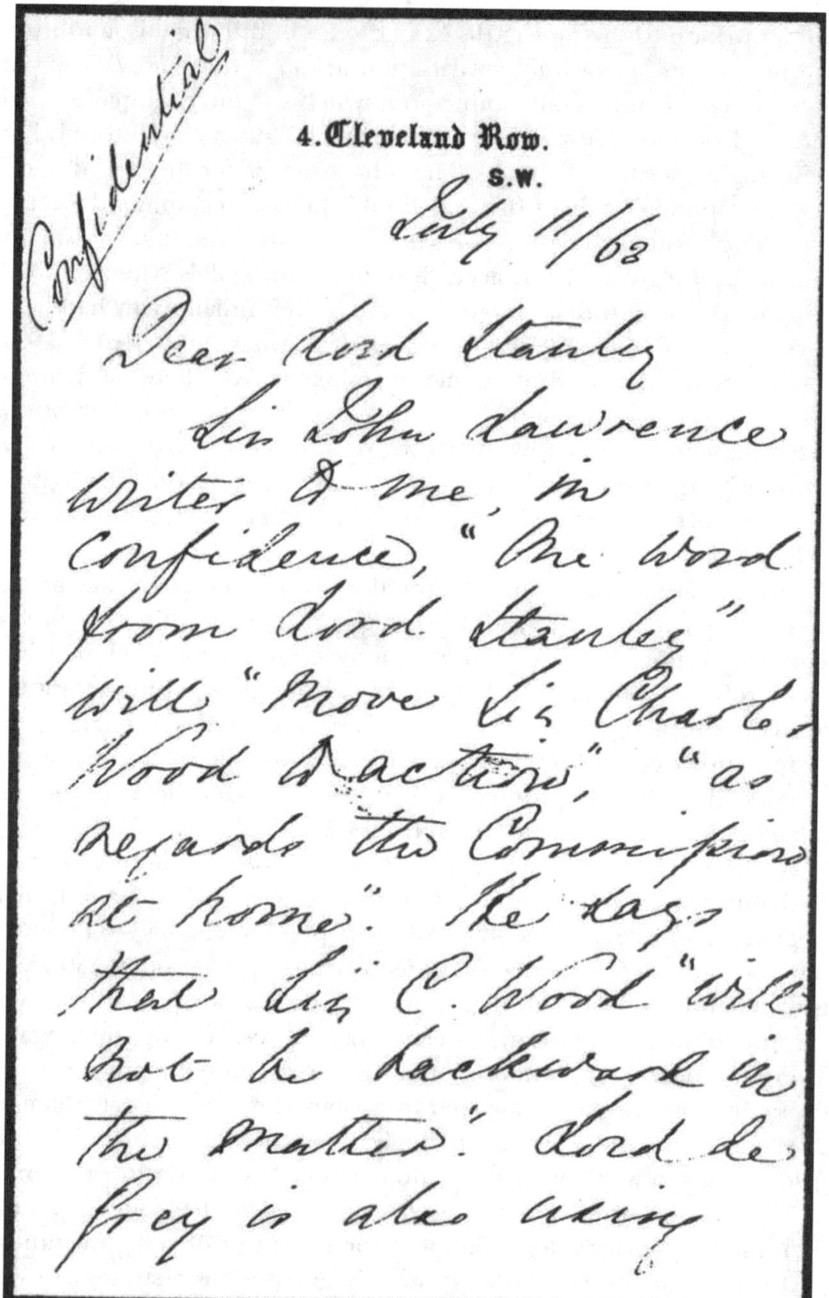

Confidential

4. Cleveland Row.
S.W.

July 11/63

Dear Lord Stanley

Sir John Lawrence writes to me, in confidence, "One word from Lord Stanley" will "move Sir Charles Wood to action", "as regards the Commission at home". He says that Sir C. Wood "will not be backward in the matter". Lord de Grey is also using

Nightingale letter, Derby Collection, Liverpool Record Office. Reproduced courtesy of the earl of Derby.

# Appendix A: Biographical Sketches

## Lord Stanley, 15th Earl of Derby (1826-93)

Edward Henry Stanley[1] received his degree from Cambridge University and travelled in 1848 to the West Indies, Canada and the United States. During his absence he was elected (Conservative) member of Parliament for King's Lynn, which he represented until 1869. This was the beginning of a long career as a British statesman. In 1852 he went to India and, while there, was appointed under secretary for foreign affairs in his father's first administration. His liberal tendencies led the Liberal Lord Palmerston to offer him the post of secretary of state for the colonies. On his father's advice he refused the offer but accepted the post in his father's second administration (1858). In the House of Commons he had charge of the India Bill of 1858 that ended the rule of the East India Company and marked the beginning of crown rule, the raj. Soon (May 1858) he was transferred to the India Office as secretary of state for India, a post which he held for a short time only as the Conservative government fell. He was then called upon to replace Sidney Herbert as president of the Royal Commission on the Sanitary State of the Army in India (1859-63). It was in that function that his close relationship with Nightingale developed, attested to by an extensive correspondence. Once the report of the commission was completed, he remained active in its implementation and worked in connection with the Council of India. Throughout his career he was committed to the respect of Indian religions and established rights.

Nightingale sometimes expressed impatience with Stanley's slow pace in conducting business, mainly due to the ineluctable fact that

1 On Lord Stanley, the eldest son of the 14th earl of Derby, see the *Oxford Dictionary of National Biography* (2004) 52:191-98.

he was not Sidney Herbert, but on the whole she was appreciative of his work and commitment to India, and respected his political wisdom and generosity. He assisted her also by smoothing the way for her with Conservative politicians. She knew how to spur him, especially at the time of the implementation of the commission's recommendations, and he regularly followed her advice. The abundant correspondence that has been preserved gives evidence of a real reciprocity. Her letters to him were generally marked "Answered" with the date.

In 1866-68 Lord Stanley became secretary of state for foreign affairs in his father's third administration, and again in 1874-78 in Disraeli's government. By 1879 he was already showing that he had thrown his lot with the Liberal Party and in 1880 he publicly announced his change of allegiance. From 1882-85 he held the post of colonial secretary in Gladstone's second government. When in 1886 the old Liberal party split over home rule, Lord Stanley/Lord Derby became a Liberal Unionist, taking an active part in the general management of the party and leading it in the House of Lords until 1891. He died in April 1893.

Lord Stanley's moderate liberalism was similar to Nightingale's, although hers was the politics of her family, while his was a departure from his. There never was a close friendship between the two but their working relationship was solid and effective.

## Sir John Lawrence (1811-79)

John Laird Mair Lawrence,[2] descendent of a famous Whig family and controversial civil servant, went to India in 1829 along with his older brother, Sir Henry Lawrence, to serve with the East India Company. He soon became a magistrate and tax collector in Delhi, where he was known for his interest in the plight of the peasantry. During the First Sikh War, 1845-46, Lawrence organized the provision of supplies to the British Army in the Punjab and became commissioner of the Jullundur district, serving under his brother, who was then governor of the province. In that role he was known for his administrative reforms, for subduing the hill tribes and for his attempts to end the custom of suttee.

In 1849, following the Second Sikh War, he became a member of the Punjab Board of Administration, again under his brother. In that

2 On John Lawrence see Charles U. Aitchison, *Lord Lawrence*; Reginald Bosworth Smith, *Life of Lord Lawrence*; and Dharm Pal, *The Administration of Sir John Lawrence in India 1864-1869*.

function he was responsible for numerous reforms of the province, including the abolition of internal duties and the establishment of a common currency and a postal system. His efforts to limit the power of local elites brought him into conflict with his brother and ultimately led to the abolition of the Administrative Board. He then became chief commissioner in the executive branch of the province. In that role Lawrence was partly responsible for preventing the spread of the Mutiny to the Punjab in 1857. He negotiated a treaty with the Afghan ruler Dost Muhammad Khan and later led the troops which recaptured Delhi from the rebellious sepoys. For that he was called the "saviour of the Punjab," that is, for the British Empire.

Lawrence returned to England in 1859. Nightingale met him in 1860 at the time he was serving on the Council of India. He gave evidence to the royal commission on India. Correspondence with him was exchanged in 1862 on her *Observations.* Then in 1863 Lord Elgin, the governor general, fell ill. Late in life (1898-99) she recalled that Lord Stanley had come to her "on Lord Elgin's sudden prostration to consult whether he should name Sir John Lawrence as his successor." He was to go out taking temporary office if Lord Elgin were better, permanent if he was dead, which in fact he was when Lawrence arrived: "I gave Lord Stanley all the information I could, showed how he had saved India to us in Mutiny. Sir J. Lawrence was, I believe, the first instance of an Indian serviceman taking high office from England." Lord Stanley then asked her to see Sir John Lawrence—he "would send him. And Lord Stanley actually came like a footman to the door afterwards to ask if I had seen him. I had" (in *Social Change in India*).

As viceroy Lawrence pursued a cautious policy, avoiding entanglement in Afghanistan and the Persian Gulf. In domestic affairs he increased educational opportunities for Indians, but at the same time limited the use of native Indians in high civil service posts. For her part, Nightingale praised his achievements with unbounded enthusiasm and considered him a close friend, while criticizing his tendency to "caesarism."

Lawrence was raised to the peerage as Baron Lawrence of the Punjab on his return to England in 1869. He died ten years later and was buried in Westminster Abbey following a funeral service at which the sermon, "An Indian Statesman," was given by the dean of Westminster, Arthur Penrhyn Stanley. Nightingale kept a portrait of him in her room, and after his death Lady Lawrence paid her visits: the two women had been friends for a long time.

For Nightingale Lawrence brought no less than civilization to India by instituting sanitary measures. She singled out the establishment of the sanitary commissions for the Bengal, Bombay and Madras presidencies as a historical development. Lawrence himself, though, was more modest about his achievements: "I think that . . . you attribute a great deal too much in the way of sanitary reform to me. . . . Few things are more difficult to accomplish in India than real sanitary improvements, and their expense is very large and almost beyond our means. We must therefore of necessity progress but slowly."[3] Nightingale felt let down by Lord Lawrence on the failure to introduce female nursing in India. And she later realized that Lord Ripon was able to do a lot more in many respects. For his part, Dharm Pal hit a moderate tone in evaluating Lawrence's India work: "Several plans of post-Mutiny reconstruction were laid or fructified during his regime. Such were for example the prison reforms, improvements in the organization and administration of the departments of health, sanitation, railways, canals, forests and elementary education."[4] He certainly cared for Indians and knew them well, but he never could overcome a sense of religious and cultural superiority that limited his effectiveness.

## Sir Bartle Frere (1815-84)

Henry Bartle Edward Frere[5] was one of the leading statesmen of the Victorian era. Most of his career was spent in work on behalf of India, where altogether he spent thirty-three years. He was governor of Bombay 1862-67. In 1875 he accompanied the prince of Wales to India, and was made baronet in 1876.

Frere held the (paternalistic) view that it was Britain's duty to rule it to the best advantage of the people until such time that they could rule themselves. To this end he promoted economic development—the cities of Bombay and Karachi owe much to him. He encouraged education and worked to preserve the religion and culture of India against those who wished to see the country Christianized and anglicized.

---

3 Letter of 6 February 1865, ADD Mss 45777 f62.

4 Dharm Pal, *Administration of Sir John Lawrence* iv. See also 95-107 on public health and prison reform.

5 On Bartle Frere see John Martineau, ed., *The Life and Correspondence of the Rt Hon Sir Bartle Frere*, and Damian O'Connor, *The Zulu and the Raj: The Life and Times of Sir Bartle Frere 1815-84.*

He first met Nightingale in 1867 upon his return to London and his appointment to the India Council (1866-77) and the India Office Sanitary Committee (1867-73). He immediately made a strong and lasting impression on her for his competence and keenness, power and loyalty. She could declare emphatically in 1867: "I have seen Sir Bartle Frere. He came on Friday [13 June] by his own appointment. And we had a great talk. He impressed me wonderfully—more than any Indian I have ever seen except Sir John Lawrence, and I seemed to learn more in an hour from him upon Indian administration and the way it is going than I did from Ellis in six months, or from Strachey in two days, or from Indian councils (secretaries of state and royal commissions and all) in six years."[6] He was able to provide her with the best information not only on Indian administration but also on the concrete conditions of soldiers and citizens in India. From then on and for years he was her consultant and advisor, and his input was large; she knew how to use his expertise and he her influence. Friendship ensued as well as an abundant correspondence.

Frere was a strong opponent of slavery. In 1873 he was sent by the Foreign Office to Zanzibar to work out a treaty for the suppression of the slave trade. By means of gunboat diplomacy he forced the sultan to give in. He was named high commissioner for South Africa and governor of Cape Town, serving 1877-80. He was among those who were concerned about defending the British Empire from threats, real or apparent, posed by the emergence of France, Russia, Germany and the United States as rising powers. The ports of the empire, notably Cape Town, were overly exposed to attacks by naval forces, he believed. Fearing a Russian march on South Africa during the 1878 Balkan crisis he made a pre-emptive strike against the Zulus. As a result of what appeared to be reckless acts he incurred the opposition of W.E. Gladstone, whom he had somewhat upstaged. Frere criticized Gladstone in his writings, and Gladstone retaliated when he came into office again in 1880. He dismissed him without giving him a chance to justify himself. He lost his post as high commissioner for South Africa under the pretext of having started the Anglo-Zulu War of 1879.

For our purposes, Frere remains one of the most helpful collaborators of Nightingale in the central period of her Indian work, and one she particularly admired for his knowledge of India.

---

6 Letter to Douglas Galton 16 June 1867, Add Mss 45764 ff76-77.

## Sir Charles Edward Trevelyan (1807-86)

Charles Trevelyan entered the East India Company's Bengal service as a writer in 1826. A year later he was appointed assistant to the commissioner at Delhi, where he worked at improving the living conditions of the local Indian population and eliminating duties on internal trade. He went to Calcutta in 1831 as deputy secretary to the government, where he devoted his efforts to the cause of education. He married the sister of Lord Macaulay in 1834 and returned to London in 1838. (The Macaulays were friends of the Nightingale family.) He became assistant secretary to the Treasury in 1840, a post which he held for nineteen years and transformed into the function of watchdog of the entire civil service. In fact he is now regarded as the father of the modern civil service.

Nightingale's acquaintance with him dates to 1854, when at the Treasury he was responsible for her arrangements to go to the Crimean War. In 1859 Sir Charles Trevelyan became governor of Madras, where he organized a new police system and established land rights. In 1860 he opposed the plan of severe retrenchment and taxation issued by Calcutta, authored a minute of dissent which he published in the newspapers, was censured and recalled to England for an action deemed "subversive to all authority." His disgrace was softened by the praise he received for his character and independence. In 1862 his views were vindicated and he was sent back to India as finance minister. For three years he opened the coffers of the government for increased public expenditure, especially on public works, which gained him Nightingale's respect and admiration. Upon his return to London in 1865 he authored *The British Army in 1868* and was involved in a variety of social and charitable activities. Nightingale found in him a trusted friend and a congenial supporter.

## Sir James Ranald Martin (1793-1874)

James Ranald Martin[7] was one of the most knowledgeable persons on army and public health in India, and one of the leading British authorities on tropical diseases and medicine. Appointed surgeon in the Bengal Medical Service in 1817, he practised in Calcutta. He retired from the army in 1826 but remained in private practice until

7 On his life see Joseph Fayrer, *Inspector General Sir James Ranald Martin.*

1840. In 1837 he published *Medical Topography of Calcutta* on the diseases of Bengal and their remedies. After having been a believer in the importance of the environment in the genesis of diseases, he turned his attention to the sanitary condition of Indian towns, which he thought could be improved by Western medicine.

Back in London he was made fellow of the Royal College of Surgeons and of the Royal Society in 1845. He was a member of the first royal commission on the reform of the army. As an "old India hand," he gave evidence to the second royal commission, of which he was also a member, and became a friend of Nightingale. He was appointed inspector general of army hospitals and member of the Army Sanitary Commission, and helped set up the military hospital at Netley. In 1841 he revised James Johnson's *The Influence of Tropical Climates on European Constitutions,* which was updated in 1856 and saw its eighth edition in 1861. His *Brief Topographical and Historical Notice of Calcutta* augmented his reputation in medical and Indian circles. In opposition to Western practitioners interested in an encounter with Indian medicine, he insisted on the study of the influence of climate and landscape on people's health. He was knighted in 1860.

Nightingale was aware of Martin's remarkable expertise and sought him out as a collaborator. She had a copy of *Notes on Nursing* sent to him in 1859, and invited him to breakfast with delegates to the International Statistical Congress in 1860. She made large use of his expertise, which was aided by the deep friendship that developed between the two. She had no trouble in agreeing with him when, after 1856, he called for a system of state medicine in India that would promote increased security of life and the study of factors jeopardizing public health. The two could lament together the reluctance of the colonial government to move in that direction. When he died Nightingale lost "the last of my royal commission," except Dr Sutherland.

## Sir John Strachey (1823-1907)

Administrator in India for four decades, he occupied various important positions and willingly provided Nightingale with detailed information on Indian conditions through minutes, proceedings, papers and letters. After qualifying for the Bengal civil service in 1842 he served as district officer in the North West Provinces. He married in 1856 and was on leave in England when the Mutiny broke out. Back in India he chaired the Cholera Commission of 1861, was appointed chief judge in the Central Provinces in 1862 and became president of the newly formed Bengal Sanitary Commission in 1864; in that capacity he was close to John Lawrence and in regular contact with Nightingale. In 1866 he was appointed chief commissioner of Oudh and in 1874 became lieutenant governor of the North West Provinces. Then, as finance minister for the Government of India in Calcutta 1876-80, his popularity suffered due to the abolition of import duties on British goods and the escalating expenses of the Afghan campaign. After 1880 he travelled to Italy, wrote *The Finances and Public Works of India* (1882) with his brother Richard, lectured and published *India: Its Administration and Progress* (1888) in justification of the raj. He was a member of the Council of India 1885-95. Throughout his career he worked at removing prejudices against Muslims. Nightingale praised his "immense energy, practical ability and determination."

## Dr James Pattison Walker (1823-1906)

Soon after completing his studies in medicine at Aberdeen in 1845, James Pattison Walker was appointed assistant surgeon in the Bengal Medical Service. There he remained for thirty-two years until his retirement, thus amassing a rich experience in Indian health conditions. He lived through the Second Sikh War of 1845-46 and the Mutiny of 1857-58. In 1851 he was appointed superintendent of a new penal colony established at Port Blair on the Andaman Islands to incarcerate political prisoners. After almost three hundred inmates escaped within weeks of their arrival, some eighty of them returned, fleeing the island aborigines. Walker had them all hanged within one day and, although he was not officially censured, he was relieved of his port in 1859, returning to his medical career on mainland India. He was made secretary of the Bengal Sanitary Commission from its inception in 1864 and retired in 1877.

For many years Nightingale corresponded with Walker, who provided her with fresh and concrete information, especially on the conditions in jails. She was particularly touched when Walker and his wife invited her to come to India and stay with them. This was not to happen, but she kept the memory of the generous friends who had made the offer.

## Dr Thomas Gillham Hewlett (1832-89)

Thomas Gillham Hewlett[8] was one of the people Nightingale most admired. She repeatedly called him a "hero," for his day-and-night relief work in the great Bombay famine, also a "missionary" for his willingness to die in the cause. She consulted him frequently on matters of sanitary science, as seen throughout this volume, and recommended him to others. There are further instances of both in *Social Change in India.* Nightingale considered his written reports exemplary, not only instructive and sound in judgment, but persuasively illustrated. He did not follow other officials in making things out to look more pleasant than they were, for which, Nightingale thought, somebody else would pay later. He was practical and got things done.

Hewlett started his long Indian career as assistant surgeon of the Bombay Army in 1854 and served during the Mutiny. When the Bombay Sanitary Commission was organized in 1864 he was appointed one of its five members. He became sanitary commissioner upon its reduction to two members. He was given the honour of a C.I.E. (commander of the Indian Empire) in 1878. Hewlett next became deputy surgeon general in Bombay 1879 and then sanitary commissioner again in 1883-87. Nightingale also had an early connection with him through the treasurer of St Thomas' Hospital, his uncle, Dr Whitfield.

Throughout his activities in Bombay, Hewlett provided Nightingale with crucial information on the army and public health in the form of official reports and private correspondence. She in turn sought to promote his career, in 1885 recommending him (albeit without success) to Sir Richard Temple for the post of surgeon general. Nightingale wanted Hewlett to be Dr Sutherland's replacement on his retirement from the Army Sanitary Commission. She started consulting officials as early as 1885 on how to achieve this. She was pleased when Dr Sutherland himself recommended Hewlett, without qualification, to be his successor. Hewlett returned to England in June 1888 but soon fell ill.

Nightingale met with him on his return and advised him step-by-step on the delicate appointment process, and possible intermediate

---

8 Sue Goldie's *Calendar of Letters* lists thirty-five surviving letters by Nightingale to him, mainly in the Reynolds Library, University of Alabama at Birmingham; the Woodward Biomedical Library, University of British Columbia, and much about him with Douglas Galton in ADD Mss 45767; correspondence about him with Lord Rosebery is in the National Library of Scotland Ms 10088.

posts, the whole matter being complicated by a reorganization of the commission. She wrote the new viceroy, Lord Lansdowne, urging Hewlett's appointment.

In 1889 Nightingale wrote a letter of introduction for Hewlett to Lord Rosebery, chair of the London County Council, to arrange a meeting. Hewlett's illness, however, required a postponement and eventually nothing came of the matter. There is much other correspondence with Hewlett, and later his widow, on such personal matters as his failing health, visits and their daughter's engagement. Hewlett died suddenly in October 1889.

After his death Nightingale wrote and organized other letters on behalf of Mrs Hewlett, whose income had been cut in half, and still had two sons to raise (there are letters to this end into 1896). In 1893 she tried to get a cadetship for a Hewlett son. All this correspondence with and on behalf of Hewlett shows a warm relationship, appreciation of his work and even what was considered his "bad temper," for he, like Nightingale, did not mince words.

Her comments to Galton just after Hewlett's death, including a comparison with General Gordon (of Khartoum), are a tribute indeed:

> In him we have lost the last and perhaps the first man in India on whose practical knowledge and information we could absolutely depend. . . . he cannot be replaced. He was one whose knowledge of sanitary details was so far ahead of all his compeers that he could be consulted with absolute confidence on every point by the native leaders. . . . Though intemperate in speech, it was always on the right side—never for self—but for righteous indignation, like Gordon, of whom he often reminded me. He was absolutely disinterested . . . making the sacrifice, which to him was no sacrifice, of himself for India. (Letter 15 October 1889, ADD MSS 45766 ff273-74)

# Appendix B: The War and India Offices

## The War Office

The War Office was established in 1661 to impose civilian control over military affairs. Until 1855 it was run by a "secretary at war," a junior minister, under a "secretary for war," the senior minister. Duties were variously distributed between the army and civilians. The commander-in-chief and his staff were known as the Horse Guards, named after the mounted troops who guarded the queen. The War Office was located on Horse Guards Avenue. The secretary at war was the army's spokesman in Parliament. The War Office's thirteen departments were staffed by civilians responsible to Parliament. All this made for a complicated machine, difficult to mobilize for a unified operation.

In view of the inefficiencies particularly revealed in the years 1854-56 of the Crimean War, the Whig Lord Panmure, secretary of state for war, perceptively declared: "The lamentable results which have attended our present expedition . . . [are] solely to be attributed to the want of proper control by a single minister over every department of the army."[1] Henceforth all administrative duties were consolidated under a single minister, the (civilian) secretary of state for war, now a Cabinet post, at the head of the departments. The War Office now had two permanent under secretaries of state, one military and one civilian. While this reform did somewhat streamline the chaotic administrative structure and strengthen Parliamentary control, it did not eliminate the tensions between the secretary of state and the military men, nor did the further series of reforms between 1858 and 1905 mean much amelioration in that respect. Relations between the army and its civilian minister were further complicated by the fact that

1 Memorandum of February 1855, quoted by John Sweetman, *War and Administration: The Significance of the Crimean War for the British Army* 107.

for much of this period the commander-in-chief was a high-ranking royal, the duke of Cambridge, but the minister a mere Mr or peer. As well, the commander-in-chief had the advantage of long service (the duke of Cambridge served thirty-nine years), while ministers lasted only a few years, or even months.

In 1870 the Horse Guards and the War Office combined into a single department under the control of the secretary of state for war. Tensions with Parliament remained, as with the India Office, when both offices were called upon to co-operate, for instance, on sanitary measures to be implemented in the army. The secretary of state and the commander-in-chief continued to operate quite independently, underscoring the uneasy relations between the civil and the military. Some progress was made in 1906 when the office of the commander-in-chief was abolished and a general staff was established as co-ordinating body. Finally in 1964 a ministry of defence emerged, with a secretary of state for war at its head.

The Crimean War had created a national emergency that allowed those eager to see reforms in the army to rally support for their cause. Administrative changes were made during the war but the postwar period was characterized by apathy. However, a certain momentum for the betterment of the health conditions of the troops was evidenced after the appalling reports that had reached the public from abroad. The Mutiny of 1857-58 added to the conviction that reforms of the army in general, and of its sanitary conditions in particular, were imperative. This is the point at which Nightingale and Sidney Herbert began to orchestrate their actions. Their collaboration on administrative reform, begun in 1854, continued untill his death in 1861, embodied in the two royal commissions on sanitary measures for the army (1857-58 and 1859-63). Thereafter Nightingale continued to have influence through various collaborators and friends.

Meanwhile, the Barrack and Hospital Improvement Commission, one of the four subcommissions struck by the first royal commission, produced reports on improving the sanitary conditions of the army (1861, 1863, etc.). In 1865 it was renamed the "Army Sanitary Commission/Committee," and kept working toward the same goals. Along with the Army Medical Department, this is the committee which Nightingale deployed her energies to move; it was her point of entry into the army establishment for her campaign of furthering health reforms for the troops. She had here the co-operation of such people as John Sutherland, Douglas Galton, J.J. Frederick, Robert Rawlinson, Thomas Longmore and, in his several capacities, Lord de Grey (later marquess of Ripon), all people we often meet in her writings. Her concerns were effective to the extent that they corresponded to efforts already made in the army to improve sanitary conditions,[2] as well as to general trends noticeable in society at large toward reforms of public health.

## The India Office

The India Office was created in the aftermath of the Mutiny by the Queen's Proclamation of 1858 and the transfer of authority, at least formally, from the East India Company to the crown. The spectre of the Company, "which had hovered over the India Office well into the 1870s and dominated it in terms of procedures and personnel," did not disappear until the 1880s.[3] For example, in 1858 nine (according to Williams) or eleven (according to Kaminsky) out of the fifteen members of the Council of India were drawn from the Company; fourteen, however, had been in India. At any rate, a secretary of state for India was appointed and a new office created, the India Office, responsible to Parliament through its minister. First housed in the headquarters of the Company, the office was moved to the Westminster Palace Hotel in 1860, then to a new building adjacent to the Foreign Office in 1867.

While including an army of technical "sub-departments," secretaries, assistant secretaries, clerks and writers, the new office was essentially structured as follows:[4]

1. The secretary of state for India, member of the Cabinet, changing with changes of the governing party; he was expected to act corporately with the Council of India.

2. The Council of India; it had fifteen members in 1858, including the secretary of state, but was reduced to as few as four at one point of its existence when it became "more of a consultative and less of a controlling body."[5]

---

2 On the "health of the rank and file" during the period that concerns us, see Alan Ramsay Skelley, *The Victorian Army at Home* 21-84. Skelley is careful to note Nightingale's impact on the reform measures taken through that period.

3 Arnold P. Kaminsky, *The India Office 1880-1910* 6.

4 See Donovan Williams, *The India Office 1858-1869*. Unfortunately Williams's study does not include the activities of the military department nor the influence of pressure groups on the office (xvi).

5 Williams, *India Office* 473.

3. The departments (of the India Office): seven in 1858 (financial; revenue; judicial and legislative; public, educational and ecclesiastical; political and secret; railway and telegraph; public works); the departments drafted despatches for discussion by the committees.

4. The committees (of the Council): three in 1858 (finance, home and public works; political and military; revenue, judicial and legislative), reshuffled into six in 1860 after Charles Wood's reform of the India Office in November 1859, and into eight in 1867 (the sanitary committee was added in 1867); they lost importance in the 1870s and 1880s; the committees conveyed the despatches to the secretary of state and to the council.

5. The under secretaries of state:

a. The Parliamentary under secretary, who looked after the preparation of Parliamentary returns (there was a succession of ten such officers between 1858 and 1869, and eighteen between 1883-1909);

b. The permanent under secretary, central to the work of the office and the formulation of Indian policy; he reviewed the despatches before they reached the committees and supervised the departments. There were four permanent under secretaries between 1858 and 1909:

1858-60 Sir George Russell Clerk,
1860-74 Herman Merivale,
1874-83 Sir Louis Mallet,
1883-1909 Arthur Godley.

The secretary of state was free to appoint separate or ad hoc committees for the consideration of special business, e.g., the "Commission on the Sanitary State of the Army in India" in 1859. A Medical Board was added in 1864.

The India Office was a complex organization; it was rendered still more complex by its being exposed to influences from the crown, Cabinet, Parliament, other departments of state and the Government of India.

Nightingale's work had close connection with the military and the political departments and committees, and some connection with the Public Works Department and committee. She was in direct communication with the secretary of state for India and with members of the India Office, and in indirect communication with Parliament through such persons as Sir Harry Verney. But because her first interest was the well-being of the army, her contacts with the War Office were crucial and at least as important as her contacts with the India Office.

# Bibliography

Abbott, Evelyn, and Lewis Campbell, eds. *Life and Letters of Benjamin Jowett.* 2 vols. London: John Murray 1897.

Aitchison, Charles U. *Lord Lawrence.* Oxford: Clarendon Press 1892.

Allen, Charles. *The Search for the Buddha: The Men who Discovered India's Lost Religion.* New York: Carroll & Graf 2003.

Arnold, David. "Cholera and Colonialism in British India." *Past and Present* 113 (1986): 118-51.

_______. *Famine: Social Crisis and Historical Change.* Oxford: Basil Blackwell 1988.

_______. *Colonizing the Body: State Medicine and Epidemic Disease in Nineteenth-Century India.* Berkeley: University of California Press 1993.

_______. *Science, Technology and Medicine in Colonial India.* Vol. III.5 of *The New Cambridge History of India.* Cambridge: Cambridge University Press 2000.

Ballhatchet, Kenneth. *Race, Sex and Class under the Raj: Imperial Attitudes and Policies and their Critics 1793-1905.* London: Weidenfeld & Nicolson 1980.

Bartlett, John. *Familiar Quotations.* Boston: Little, Brown 1863.

Bayly, Christopher Alan. *Indian Society and the Making of the British Empire.* Vol. II.1 of *The New Cambridge History of India.* Cambridge: Cambridge University Press 1988.

_______. *Empire and Information: Intelligence Gathering and Social Communication in India 1780-1870.* Cambridge: Cambridge University Press 1996.

_______, ed. *The Raj: India and the British 1600-1947.* London: National Portrait Gallery Publications 1990.

Bhatia, B.M. *Famines in India: A Study in some Aspects of the Economic History of India 1860- 1965.* Bombay: Asia Publishing House 1963.

Bishop, William John, and Sue Goldie. *A Bio-Bibliography of Florence Nightingale.* London: Dawsons of Pall Mall for the International Council of Nurses 1962.

Blakeley, Brian L. *The Colonial Office 1868-1892.* Durham NC: Duke University Press 1972.

Buckland, Charles E. *Dictionary of Indian Biography.* London: Sonnenschein 1906.

Buckley, Robert Burton. *Irrigation Works of India and Their Financial Results.* London: W.H. Allen 1880.

Burke, Edmund. *The Works of the Rt Hon Edmund Burke.* 3 vols. London: J. Dodsley 1792. New ed. 6 vols. London: F.C. & J. Rivington 1808.

Campbell, George. *Memoirs of My Indian Career,* ed. Sir Charles E. Bernard. 2 vols. London: Macmillan 1893.

Cell, John W. *British Colonial Administration in the Mid-Nineteenth Century: The Policy-Making Process.* New Haven: Yale University Press 1970.

Clifford, Edward. *Father Damien: A Journey from Cashmere to His Home in Hawaii.* London: Macmillan 1889.

Cook, Chris, and Brendan Keith. *British Historical Facts 1830-1900.* London: Macmillan 1975.

Cook, E.T. *The Life of Florence Nightingale.* 2 vols. London: Macmillan 1913.

Cotton, Arthur. *Public Works in India.* London: Allen 1854.

———. *The Madras Famine.* London: Simpkin, Marshall 1877.

Cuningham, James M. *Cholera: What Can the State Do to Prevent it?* Calcutta: Superintendent of Government Printing 1864.

David, Saul. *The Indian Mutiny: 1857.* London: Viking 2003.

Dossey, Barbara M. *Florence Nightingale: Mystic, Visionary and Healer.* Philadelphia: Springhouse 1999.

Edwardes, Sir Herbert B. *Prospect of the Triumph of Christianity in India.* London: Church Missionary Society 1866.

Ewart, Sir Joseph. *A Digest of the Vital Statistics of the European and Native Armies in India.* London: Smith, Elder 1859.

———. *The Sanitary Condition and Discipline of Indian Jails.* London: Smith, Elder 1861.

Fayrer, Joseph. *Inspector-General Sir James Ranald Martin.* London: A.D. Innes 1897.

———. *Recollections of my Life.* London: William Blackwood 1900.

Gathorne-Hardy, Alfred E., ed. *Gathorne-Hardy, First Earl of Cranbrook: A Memoir with Extracts from His Diary and Correspondence.* 2 vols. London: Longmans 1910.

Gopal, Sarvepalli. *British Policy in India 1858-1905.* Cambridge: Cambridge University Press 1965.

Gordon, Charles A. *Army Hygiene.* London: Churchill 1866.

Gourlay, Jharna. *Florence Nightingale and the Health of the Raj.* Aldershot, Hants: Ashgate 2003.

Hall, Henry L. *The Colonial Office: A History.* London: Longmans, Green 1937.

Harrison, Mark. *Public Health in British India: Anglo-Indian Preventive Medicine 1859-1914.* Cambridge: Cambridge University Press 1994.

Hawkins, R.E., ed. *Common Indian Words in English.* Delhi: Oxford University Press 1984.

Hewlett, Thomas Gillham. *Report on Enteric Fever.* Bombay: Presidency Sanitary Department 1883.

Hopkirk, Peter. *The Great Game: On Secret Service in High Asia.* London: J. Murray 1990.

Hunter, William W. *The Old Missionary.* London: Froude 1897.

Isaacs, Jeremy D. "D.D. Cunningham and the Aetiology of Cholera in British India 1869-1897." *Medical History* 42 (1998):279-305.

James, Lawrence. *Raj: The Making and Unmaking of British India.* London: Little, Brown 1997.

Jones, Kenneth W. *Socio-Religious Reform Movements in British India.* Vol. III.1 of *The New Cambridge History of India.* Cambridge: Cambridge University Press 1989.

Jones, Ray. *The Nineteenth-Century Foreign Office: An Administrative History.* London: Weidenfeld & Nicolson 1971.

Kaminsky, Arnold P. *The India Office 1880-1910.* New York: Greenwood Press 1986.

Keay, John. *India Discovered: The Achievement of the British Raj.* London: Harper Collins 1992.

________. *The Honourable Company: A History of the English East India Company.* New York: Macmillan 1994.

________. *India: A History.* London: Harper Collins 1999.

Kumar, Anil. *Medicine and the Raj: British Medical Policy in India 1835-1911.* Walnut Creek CA: Altamira 1998.

Leith, A.H. *Report on the General Sanitary Condition of the Bombay Army.* Bombay: Education Society's Press 1864.

Logan, Deborah, ed. *Harriet Martineau's Writing on the British Empire.* Vol. 5: *The India Question.* 5 vols. London: Pickering & Chatto 2004.

Macaulay, Thomas Babington. *Lays of Ancient Rome.* 1842.

———. *History of England.* 4 vols. London: Longman, Brown, Green & Longmans 1849-61.

Maclagan, Michael. *"Clemency" Canning.* London: Macmillan 1962.

MacPherson, Duncan. *Antiquities of Kertch and Researches in the Cimmerian Bosphorus: With Remarks on the Ethnological and Physical History of the Crimea.* London: Smith, Elder 1857.

Maharatna, Arup. *The Demography of Famines.* Oxford: Clarendon Press 1996.

Martin, Sir James Ranald. *Notes on the Medical Topography of Calcutta.* Calcutta: Huttmann 1837.

———. "Suggestions for Promoting the Health and Efficiency of the British Troops Serving in the East Indies." *The Lancet* 13 February 1858.

Martineau, John, ed. *The Life and Correspondence of the Rt Hon Sir Bartle Frere.* 2 vols. London: J. Murray 1895.

Masselos, J. "The Discourse from the Other Side; Perceptions of Science and Technology in Western India in the Nineteenth Century," in N.K. Wagle, ed., *Writers, Editors and Reformers: Social and Political Transformations of Maharashtra 1830-1930.* New Delhi: Manohar 1999:114-29.

Matthew, Henry C.G., and Brian H. Harrison, eds., *Oxford Dictionary of National Biography.* Oxford: Oxford University Press 2004.

McAlpin, Michelle Burge. *Subject to Famine: Food Crises and Economic Change in Western India 1860-1920.* Princeton: Princeton University Press 1983.

Metcalf, Barbara Daly, and Thomas R. Metcalf. *A Concise History of India.* Cambridge: Cambridge University Press 2002.

Metcalf, Thomas R. *The Aftermath of Revolt: India 1857-1870.* Princeton: Princeton University Press 1964.

———. *Ideologies of the Raj.* Vol. III.4 of *The New Cambridge History of India.* Cambridge: Cambridge University Press 1994.

Mill, James. *History of British India.* 5th ed. 6 vols. London: Madden 1858.

Misra, Bankey Bihari. *The Administrative History of India 1834-1947.* Bombay: Oxford University Press 1970.

Mohanty, Bidyut. "Orissa Famine of 1866: Demographic and Economic Consequences." *Economic and Political Weekly* 28 (1993):55-66.

Moore, Robin James. *Sir Charles Wood's Indian Policy 1853-1866.* Manchester: Manchester University Press 1966.

Morley, John. *The Life of William Ewart Gladstone.* 3 vols. London: Macmillan 1903, 1912.

Murdoch, John. *India's Needs: Material, Political, Social, Moral and Religious.* Madras: SPCK 1886.

O'Connor, Damian. *The Zulu and the Raj: The Life and Times of Sir Bartle Frere 1815-84.* London: Able Publications 2002.

Ogawa, Mariko. "Uneasy Bedfellows: Science and Politics in the Refutation of Koch's Bacterial Theory of Cholera." *Bulletin of the History of Medicine* 74,4 (2000):671-707.

Pal, Dharm. *The Administration of Sir John Lawrence in India 1864-1869.* Simla: Minerva Book Shop 1952.

Pati, Biswamoy, and Mark Harrison, eds. *Health, Medicine and Empire: Perspectives on Colonial India.* London: Sangam Books 2001.

Pearson, Karl. *The Life, Letters and Labours of Francis Galton.* Cambridge: Cambridge University Press 1914-30.

Pearson, M.N. "The Thin End of the Wedge: Medical Relativities as a Paradigm of Early Modern Indian-European Relations." *Modern Asian Studies* 29,1 (1995):141-70.

Porter, Roy. *Medicine, a History of Healing: Ancient Traditions to Modern Practices.* London: O'Mara Books 1997.

Quinn, Vincent, and John Prest, eds. *Dear Miss Nightingale: A Selection of Benjamin Jowett's Letters to Florence Nightingale 1860-1893.* Oxford: Clarendon Press 1987.

Roberts, Andrew. *Salisbury: Victorian Titan.* London: Weidenfeld & Nicolson 1999.

Schama, Simon. *A History of Britain: The Fate of Empire 1776-2000.* Toronto: McClelland & Stewart 2002.

Seavoy, Ronald E. *Famine in Peasant Societies.* London: Greenwood Press 1986.

Sen, Amartya. *Poverty and Famines: An Essay on Entitlement and Deprivation.* Oxford: Clarendon Press 1981.

_______. *The Argumentative Indian: Writings on Indian History, Culture and Identity.* London: Penguin 2005.

_______, and Jean Drèze. *Hunger and Public Action.* Oxford: Clarendon Press 1989.

Sen, Priyaranjan, ed. *Florence Nightingale's Indian Letters: A Glimpse into the Agitation for Tenancy Reform, Bengal 1878-82.* Calcutta: Mihir Kumar Sen 1937.

Shrimpton, Charles. *The British Army and Miss Nightingale.* Paris: Galignani 1864.

Singh, S.N. *The Secretary of State for India and His Council 1859-1919.* Delhi: Munshi Ram Manohar Lal 1962.

Skelley, Alan Ramsay. *The Victorian Army at Home: The Recruitment and Terms and Conditions of the British Regular 1859-1899.* Montreal: McGill-Queen's University Press 1977.

Small, Hugh. *Florence Nightingale: Avenging Angel.* London: Constable 1998.

Smith, Reginald Bosworth. *Life of Lord Lawrence.* 2 vols. London: Smith, Elder 1883.

Smith, Robert Angus. *Disinfectants and Disinfection.* Edinburgh: Edmonston & Douglas 1869.

Smith, Vincent A. *The Oxford History of India.* 3rd ed., ed. Percival Spear. Oxford: Clarendon Press 1958.

Stanmore, Lord (Arthur Hamilton-Gordon). *Sidney Herbert: Lord Herbert of Lea, A Memoir.* 2 vols. London: John Murray 1906.

Sterne, Lawrence. *A Sentimental Journey through France and Italy by Mr Yorick.* London: T. Becket and P.A. De Hondt 1768.

Strachey, Sir John. *India: Its Administration and Progress.* London: Macmillan 1911.

Strachey, Richard, and John Strachey. *The Finances and Public Works of India from 1869 to 1881.* London: K. Paul, Trench 1882.

Suleri, Sara. *The Rhetoric of English India.* Chicago: University of Chicago Press 1982.

Sweetman, John. *War and Administration: The Significance of the Crimean War for the British Army.* Edinburgh: Scottish Academic Press 1984.

Talbot, Ian. *India and Pakistan.* Oxford: Oxford University Press 2000.

Verney, Margaret M. *Sir Henry Stewart Cunningham.* London: John Murray 1923.

Waller, John. *The Discovery of the Germ: Twenty Years that Transformed the Way We Think about Disease.* Toronto: Penguin 2002.

Watts, Sheldon J. *Epidemics and History: Disease, Power and Imperialism.* New Haven CT: Yale University Press 1997.

West, Raymond. *A Digest of the Hindu Law of Inheritance, Partition and Adoption.* London: Sweet & Maxwell 1919.

White, Gilbert. *The Natural History and Antiquities of Selborne.* London: T. Bensley 1789.

Williams, Donovan. *The India Office 1858-1869.* Hoshiarpur: Vishveshvaranand Vedia Research Institute 1983.

Wilson, A.N. *The Victorians.* New York: Norton 2003.

Wolpert, Stanley. *A New History of India.* 4th ed. Oxford: Oxford University Press 1993.

Woodruff, Philip. *The Men Who Ruled India.* 2 vols. London: J. Cape 1953-54.

# Index

Space limitations required some compromises in the index. It generally includes proper names, omitting those of acquaintances, employees and persons who appear briefly or are not readily identifiable. Items with identifying information are shown in italics. Persons known by more than one name are indexed under the name most frequently appearing in the text. Biblical references are indexed by book under "Bible." Most Indian place names and Indian words in English are found in an Appendix of *Social Change in India.*